Clinical Cardiac CT
Anatomy and Function

Second Edition

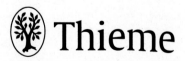

Clinical Cardiac CT
Anatomy and Function

Second Edition

Ethan J. Halpern, MD
Professor and Vice Chairman of Radiology
Director, Cardiac CT
Thomas Jefferson University
Philadelphia, Pennsylvania

Thieme
New York · Stuttgart

Thieme Medical Publishers, Inc.
333 Seventh Ave.
New York, NY 10001

Executive Editor: Timothy Y. Hiscock
Managing Editor: J. Owen Zurhellen IV
Editorial Assistant: Judith Tomat
Editorial Director, Clinical Reference: Michael Wachinger
Production Editor: Kenneth L. Chumbley, Publication Services
International Production Director: Andreas Schabert
Vice President, International Marketing and Sales: Cornelia Schulze
Chief Financial Officer: James W. Mitos
President: Brian D. Scanlan
Compositor: Thomson Digital
Printer: Leo Paper Group

Library of Congress Cataloging-in-Publication Data

Halpern, Ethan J.
  Clinical cardiac CT : anatomy and function / Ethan J. Halpern. –2nd ed.
     p. ; cm.
  Includes bibliographical references and index.
  ISBN 978-1-60406-375-2
  1. Heart–Tomography. I. Title.
  [DNLM: 1. Coronary Disease–radiography. 2. Heart–anatomy & histology.
  3. Tomography, X-Ray Computed–methods. WG 300]
  RC683.5.T66H35 2011
  616.1'20757–dc22
                                          2010036129

Important note: Medical knowledge is ever-changing. As new research and clinical experience broaden our knowledge, changes in treatment and drug therapy may be required. The authors and editors of the material herein have consulted sources believed to be reliable in their efforts to provide information that is complete and in accord with the standards accepted at the time of publication. However, in view of the possibility of human error by the authors, editors, or publisher of the work herein or changes in medical knowledge, neither the authors, editors, nor publisher, nor any other party who has been involved in the preparation of this work, warrants that the information contained herein is in every respect accurate or complete, and they are not responsible for any errors or omissions or for the results obtained from use of such information. Readers are encouraged to confirm the information contained herein with other sources. For example, readers are advised to check the product information sheet included in the package of each drug they plan to administer to be certain that the information contained in this publication is accurate and that changes have not been made in the recommended dose or in the contraindications for administration. This recommendation is of particular importance in connection with new or infrequently used drugs.

Some of the product names, patents, and registered designs referred to in this book are in fact registered trademarks or proprietary names even though specific reference to this fact is not always made in the text. Therefore, the appearance of a name without designation as proprietary is not to be construed as a representation by the publisher that it is in the public domain.

Printed in China

5 4 3 2 1

ISBN 978-1-60406-375-2

Dedicated to my dear wife Sarah. You are my best friend, my partner in all endeavors, and always selflessly devoted to our family. Once again, I could not possibly have completed the second edition of this textbook without your love and support. I love you always.

Ethan J. Halpern

Contents

DVD Contents

xii DVD Contents

Cine 10.17 Calcified aortic valve with moderate stenosis.

Cine 10.18 Calcified aortic valve with moderate stenosis and mild insufficiency.

Cine 10.19 Calcified aortic valve with severe stenosis.

Cine 10.20 Calcified and thickened aortic valve with severe stenosis.

Cine 10.21 Critical aortic stenosis.

Cine 10.22 Porcelain aortic root with aortic stenosis and mild insufficiency.

Bicuspid aortic valve

Cine 10.23 Bicuspid aortic valve; fusion of the commissure between the light and left coronary cusps.

Cine 10.24 Bicuspid aortic valve; fusion of the commissure between the right and left coronary cusps.

Cine 10.25 Bicuspid aortic valve; fusion of the commissure between the right and left coronary cusps.

Cine 10.26 Bicuspid aortic valve; fusion of the commissure between the right and left coronary cusps.

Cine 10.27 Bicuspid aortic valve with one visible commissure–no pseudoraphe.

Cine 10.28 Bicuspid aortic valve with dilated ascending aorta.

Cine 10.29 Functionally bicuspid valve secondary to fusion of the left aortic cusp to the left sinus of Valsalva.

Bicuspid aortic valve with stenosis

Cine 10.30 Bicuspid aortic valve with aneurysm of the ascending aorta.

Cine 10.31 Bicuspid aortic valve with minimal stenosis.

Cine 10.32 Bicuspid aortic valve with mild to moderate aortic stenosis.

Cine 10.33 Bicuspid aortic valve with moderate aortic stenosis.

Cine 10.34 Bicuspid aortic valve with moderate to severe aortic stenosis.

Cine 10.35 Bicuspid aortic valve with moderate to severe aortic stenosis.

Cine 10.36 Bicuspid aortic valve with severe stenosis.

Aortic valve masses/vegetation

Cine 10.37 Fibroelastoma of the aortic valve.

Cine 10.38 Bacterial endocarditis with aortic valve vegetation.

Prosthetic aortic valves

Cine 10.39 Normally functioning bioprosthetic aortic valve.

Cine 10.40 Normally functioning bioprosthetic aortic valve.

Cine 10.41 Normally functioning bioprosthetic aortic valve without metallic struts.

Cine 10.42 Normally functioning Carbomedics prosthetic aortic valve.

Cine 10.43 Normally functioning St. Judes prosthetic aortic valve.

Cine 10.44 Normally functioning St. Judes prosthetic aortic valve.

Cine 10.45 Normally function Medtronic-Hall prosthetic aortic valve.

Normal mitral valve

Cine 10.46 Normally functioning mitral valve.

Cine 10.47 Normally functioning mitral valve with short axis imaging.

Mitral valve prolapse

Cine 10.48 Myxomatous mitral valve with prolapse of the posterior mitral leaflet.

Cine 10.49 Myxomatous mitral valve with prolapse of both leaflets.

Cine 10.50 Prolapse of the posterior mitral leaflet.

Cine 10.51 Prolapse of both mitral leaflets.

Cine 10.52 Redundant posterior mitral leaflet.

Foreword

Introducing a novel imaging technology to clinical practice requires integration by practitioners of both technical and clinical expertise. Cardiac CT applies a new generation of continuously advancing CT technology to an organ that was not previously amenable to CT imaging. Physicians who interpret traditional CT examinations may not have had previous exposure to an evaluation of the beating heart. Echocardiographers seldom have experience in the interpretation of high-resolution CT images of the thorax. However, the functional and anatomic information obtained from CT evaluation of the heart are often complementary. This text–atlas is designed to provide the clinician with adequate tools to perform and interpret high-quality CT imaging of cardiac anatomy and function.

The techniques and images described in this book and DVD are based on a large clinical practice of cardiac CT at Thomas Jefferson University, as well as on contributions from collaborating colleagues at other academic centers. Dr. Ethan Halpern, director of cardiac CT at Thomas Jefferson University, is an experienced cross-sectional CT imager and echocardiographer. He is a prolific researcher who has published a number of outstanding studies pertaining to cardiac CT and has personally performed thousands of these examinations. He currently serves as professor of radiology and vice chair for research in Jefferson's department of radiology. Dr. Halpern is one of a select group of board-certified radiologists who have taken the examination of special competency in adult echocardiography given by the National Board of Echocardiography. This text–atlas represents a joint effort among radiologists, echocardiographers, interventional cardiologists, and cardiac surgeons to highlight the unique capabilities of CT for imaging cardiac anatomy and function in real clinical applications. It is a vital addition to the library of anyone involved in performing or interpreting cardiac CT.

David C. Levin, MD
Professor and Chairman Emeritus
Department of Radiology
Thomas Jefferson University
Philadelphia, Pennsylvania

Preface

Cardiovascular imaging represents about one-third of total noninvasive diagnostic imaging services and continues to grow more rapidly than other types of imaging (Levin DC et al, JACR 2005; 2:736-739). Cost-effective management of cardiac disease requires appropriate application of imaging resources. Multidetector computed tomography provides a unique approach to evaluation of the cardiac patient, allowing the physician to visualize coronary anatomy along with cardiac morphology and function in a single, noninvasive study. *Clinical Cardiac CT: Anatomy and Function* explores the clinically appropriate application of cardiac CT for risk stratification, evaluation of coronary artery disease, pre-operative planning, post-operative assessment, and planning/assessment of percutaneous cardiac procedures.

This new second edition of *Clinical Cardiac CT: Anatomy and Function* has been updated to keep pace with the advances in multidetector CT technology (MDCT) and has been expanded to incorporate additional important topics including the thoracic aorta, congenital heart disease, triple rule-out studies, and perfusion imaging. This text-atlas provides a didactic tutorial to optimize CT technique, as well as CT case material that reflects the full spectrum of normal variations and pathological findings that are seen in an adult cardiology practice. The extensive experience at our own tertiary cardiac care center has been supplemented with contributions from other nationally recognized centers to demonstrate the full gamut of clinical applications possible with state of the art MDCT.

Written by experienced radiologists, cardiologists, and cardiothoracic surgeons, this clinically oriented text-atlas contains hundreds of clearly annotated cases. An accompanying DVD provides cine clips of over 200 cases that are invaluable in demonstrating three-dimensional anatomic relationships, valvular anatomy, and cardiac function. Numerous references are included to classical journal articles describing coronary anatomy, as well as to recent studies evaluating the latest advances in coronary CTA. A comprehensive index provides the reader with quick access to the many different topics included in the text. The combination of didactic text and case material has been selected to systematically teach cardiac CT and to serve as a reference textbook for the accomplished cardiac imager.

This second edition of *Clinical Cardiac CT: Anatomy and Function* is useful/ideal at several levels:

- For residents or fellows preparing for board examinations or spending time on a cardiac imaging rotation
- For practitioners who wish to add cardiac CT to their practice
- For experienced cardiac imagers who will find it to be an excellent text for quick and easy reference in daily practice

◆ Acknowledgments

To my dear friend and mentor, Dr. David C. Levin, who recruited me to my first real job at Thomas Jefferson University and encouraged me to head up the cardiac CT program: thank you for your friendship, dedication, and training.

To my chairperson Dr. Vijay Rao: thank you for your continued support and encouragement of our clinical and research efforts in cardiac CT.

To all the dedicated CT technologists and nursing staff at Thomas Jefferson University: your dedication to our patients on a daily basis is what makes our cardiac CT program a true success.

To Dr. Alex Grieco for his assistance in proofreading the manuscript of this text.

Contributors

Galit Aviram, MD
Lecturer
Sackler Faculty of Medicine
Tel Aviv University
Head of Cardiothoracic Imaging
Department of Radiology
Tel Aviv Sourasky Medical Center
Tel Aviv, Israel

Linda J. Bogar, MD
Assistant Professor of Surgery
Division of Cardiothoracic Surgery
Thomas Jefferson University
Philadelphia, Pennsylvania

C. Douglas Borg, MD
Clinical Fellow
Division of Cardiology
University of Colorado–Denver
Aurora, Colorado

James T. Diehl, MD
Professor and Chief
Division of Cardiothoracic Surgery
Thomas Jefferson University
Philadelphia, Pennsylvania

Panayotis Fasseas, MD
Assistant Professor of Medicine
Department of Cardiovascular Diseases
Medical College of Wisconsin
Milwaukee, Wisconsin

David L. Fischman, MD, FACP, FACC
Associate Professor of Medicine
Co-director, Cardiac Catheterization
    Laboratory
Jefferson Heart Institute
Thomas Jefferson University
Philadelphia, Pennsylvania

Stephanie Fuller, MD
Surgeon, Assistant Professor of Clinical Surgery
Division of Cardiothoracic Surgery
The Children's Hospital of Philadelphia
University of Pennsylvania School of Medicine
Philadelphia, Pennsylvania

Aaron M. Giltner, MD, FACC
Interventional Cardiologist
Summit Cardiovascular Care
Paoli Hospital
Paoli, Pennsylvania

Jonathan Gomberg, MD, FACC
Clinical Assistant Professor of Medicine
Division of Cardiology
University of Pennsylvania
Philadelphia, Pennsylvania

Ethan J. Halpern, MD
Professor and Vice Chairman of Radiology
Director, Cardiac CT
Thomas Jefferson University
Philadelphia, Pennsylvania

Nicholas Hilpipre, MD
Diagnostic Radiology Resident
Department of Radiology
University of Colorado–Denver
Aurora, Colorado

David C. Levin, MD
Professor and Chairman Emeritus
Department of Radiology
Thomas Jefferson University
Philadelphia, Pennsylvania

Daniel J. McCormick, DO, FACC, FSCAI
Director
Cardiac Catheterization Laboratories
Hahnemann University Hospital
Philadelphia, Pennsylvania

Alyson N. Owen, MD
Assistant Professor of Medicine
Director of Quality Assurance,
   Echocardiography Laboratory
Thomas Jefferson University
Philadelphia, Pennsylvania

Behzad B. Pavri, MD, FACC
Associate Professor of Medicine
Department of Medicine
Thomas Jefferson University
Philadelphia, Pennsylvania

Robert A. Quaife, MD
Director
Advanced Cardiac Imaging
Health Sciences Center
Associate Professor of Medicine
   and Radiology
Departments of Medicine (Cardiology)
   and Radiology (Nuclear Medicine)
University of Colorado–Denver
Aurora, Colorado

David M. Shipon, MD, FACC
Instructor of Medicine
Department of Cardiology
Thomas Jefferson University
Philadelphia, Pennsylvania

Scott C. Silvestry, MD
Associate Professor
Department of Surgery
Washington University School of Medicine
Surgical Director
Cardiac Transplantation and Mechanical Circulatory
   Support Program
Barnes Jewish Hospital
St. Louis, Missouri

Jacob Sosna, MD
Section Chief, CT
Director of Research and Imaging Laboratories
Department of Radiology
Hadassah Hebrew University Medical Center
Jerusalem, Israel

David Wang, DO
Clinical Instructor
Department of Radiology
University of Virginia Health System
Charlottesville, Virginia

Donna R. Zwas, MD
Department of Cardiology
Hadassah-Hebrew University Medical Center
Jerusalem, Israel
Adjunct Assistant Professor of Medicine
Thomas Jefferson University
Philadelphia, Pennsylvania

1

Key Issues in Cardiac CT

Ethan J. Halpern

◆ Coronary Heart Disease

Coronary heart disease is the single largest cause of mortality in the United States and is an underlying or contributing cause in one of every five deaths.[1] It is estimated that 785,000 Americans will have a new coronary attack in 2009, and 470,000 will have a recurrent attack. Furthermore, 195,000 silent first myocardial infarctions occur each year. One American will suffer a coronary event every 25 seconds, and one American will die of coronary heart disease every minute. The death rate from coronary heart disease has declined over the past four decades because of secondary preventive therapies used after myocardial infarction, new and improved treatments for angina and heart failure, and reductions in specific risk factors (cholesterol, blood pressure, smoking).[2] However, the favorable improvements in risk factors among Americans have been partially offset by increases in body mass index and diabetes, such that the burden of disease remains high. The prevalence of coronary heart disease is about 6.0% in black Americans and 6.1% among white Americans.[3]

Evaluation of chest pain and related symptoms is the most common reason for an emergency department visit by an adult man and the second most common reason for a visit to the emergency department by an adult woman in the United States.[4] Chest pain accounts for more than six million emergency department visits and almost two million inpatient hospital admissions annually. Acute coronary syndrome (ACS) refers to the patient who presents with an acute myocardial infarction or unstable angina. The number of patients admitted annually to U.S. hospitals with the diagnosis of ACS is close to a million. More than 2% of patients who present to an emergency department with ACS are discharged inappropriately; these missed diagnoses are associated with increased mortality.[5,6] Preventive therapy for coronary disease depends on prospective identification of the patient who is truly at risk for ACS before the appearance of symptoms. Effective treatment of ACS depends on a rapid and accurate diagnosis of this entity in the symptomatic patient. The imprecise predictive value of risk factors, clinical symptoms, and biochemical markers is a major limitation in the treatment of coronary heart disease. Cardiac CT has the potential to improve the accuracy of risk stratification for

preventive therapy[7-9] and efficiently excludes the diagnosis of ACS in the patient with chest pain.[10-13]

◆ Cardiac Computed Tomography Technology

Imaging of the heart and coronary arteries is complicated by the rapid, nonlinear motion of cardiac structures. Coronary CT angiography (CTA) became practical with the introduction of electrocardiographic gating and multislice technology. Among the various modalities capable of cardiac imaging, CT excels in its ability to depict coronary calcification, coronary anatomy, and cardiac-chamber morphology. The information obtained from cardiac CT is often complementary to that provided by other studies, including echocardiography, nuclear scintigraphy, cardiac magnetic resonance (MR) imaging, and conventional catheter angiography. Numerous studies have demonstrated the accuracy and high negative predictive value of CT for evaluation of coronary artery stenosis.[14] Given the lower costs associated with CT compared with conventional angiography, CT provides a cost-effective alternative to diagnostic catheterization for the evaluation of coronary artery disease (CAD) in most patients.[15] Clinical trials continue to establish the utility and cost-effectiveness of cardiac CT coronary angiography for specific clinical indications.[16] Recent improvements in CT technology with faster scans, better temporal resolution, lower radiation exposure, and dual-energy imaging continue to expand the applications of CT to cardiac imaging. Additional clinical trials are needed to demonstrate the utility of CT for newer applications that include stress imaging and evaluation of myocardial perfusion.[17]

Two major categories of advanced CT technology have been applied to cardiac imaging: electron-beam CT (EBCT) and multislice–multidetector computed tomography (MDCT). EBCT is best known for its application to measure coronary artery calcification (**Fig. 1.1**). Calcium scoring provides cardiac risk stratification with a low radiation dose of about 1 mSv. More than one thousand publications have documented the utility of EBCT for coronary calcium scoring. EBCT is distinguished by the absence of moving parts within the scanner and by a short acquisition time, which

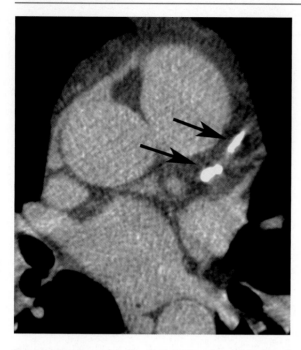

Fig. 1.1 Coronary calcium and calcium scoring. Axial image through the level of the left anterior descending artery demonstrates the presence of calcification in the proximal portion of this vessel (*arrows*). A detailed discussion of calcium scoring is covered in Chapter 5.

reduces motion artifact. The ultrafast scan time of EBCT (33–50 msec) is possible because a rotating electron beam is used to produce thin-section tomographic scans without gantry rotation. However, EBCT is limited in terms of slice thickness (not <1.5 mm) and overall image noise.

MDCT has assumed the dominant role for contrast-enhanced CTA of the coronary arteries (**Fig. 1.2**). The spatial resolution and signal-to-noise characteristics of MDCT are superior to those of EBCT. Overall image quality for coronary CTA is better with MDCT compared with EBCT, especially with heavier patients. MDCT technology is available from competing manufacturers, who are continuously improving their systems to provide the best spatial and temporal resolution and the best techniques to reduce artifact from calcium and metallic stents. "Conventional" 64-slice MDCT technology remains the "workhorse" of cardiac CT imaging, with a temporal resolution in the range of 165 to 210 msec. Several MDCT scanners are now available with 256 or 320 slices to provide greater anatomic coverage. Newer scanners use faster gantry rotation times and dual radiographic sources to achieve a temporal resolution as low as 75 msec with subsecond scan times for the entire heart.[18] Advances in dual-energy and multienergy imaging techniques are poised to provide further improvements in plaque characterization and evaluation of myocardial enhancement. These techniques should provide additional

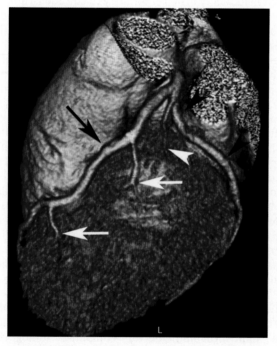

A L

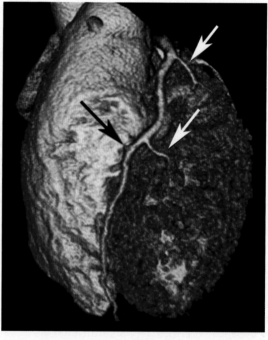

B

Fig. 1.2 Surface-rendered volumetric images of the left coronary circulation provide a three-dimensional prospective and demonstrate positions of the coronary arteries relative to the underlying cardiac structures. **(A)** Left anterior oblique (LAO) projection demonstrates left anterior descending artery (*black arrow*), as well as two diagonal branches (*white arrows*). A normal variant, the ramus medianus, extends from a trifurcation of the left main coronary artery (*white arrowhead*). The third branch from the left main coronary artery is the circumflex (*black arrowheads*), which travels in the left atrioventricular groove. No obtuse marginal branches are identified from the circumflex artery. The territory of left ventricular free wall is supplied entirely by the diagonal branches and the ramus. **(B)** Shallow LAO from a more caudal vantage point demonstrates the left anterior descending (LAD) coronary artery as it courses down the anterior interventricular groove (*black arrow*). The two diagonal branches are again identified (*white arrows*).

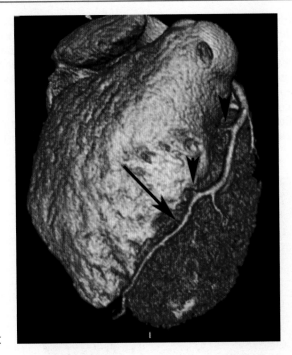

Fig. 1.2 (*Continued*) **(C)** Anteroposterior view again demonstrates the LAD (*arrow*). Two septal perforator branches extend from the LAD into the interventricular septum (*arrowheads*). The septal perforators are identified only in their proximal portions before entering the interventricular septum.

C

prognostic information through assessment of plaque composition and stability[19] and myocardial perfusion studies.[20]

◆ Accuracy of Coronary Computed Tomography Angiography

With respect to the detection of stenosis in native coronary arteries, numerous studies have compared the diagnostic accuracy of coronary CTA with that of invasive catheter angiography, the traditional gold standard. In most of these studies, significant coronary stenosis is defined as diameter reduction of 50% or more. A recent meta-analysis of 64 slice studies demonstrated a sensitivity of 99% (95% confidence interval [CI], 97–99%) and a specificity of 89% (95% CI, 83–94%) for the presence of significant coronary stenosis in a patient-based analysis.[14] In a by-segment analysis, CTA demonstrated a sensitivity of 90% (95% CI, 85–94%) and a specificity of 97% (95% CI, 95–98%). The median negative predictive value of CTA for patient-based detection of coronary disease was 100%.

Although the abundant publications from single-center trials demonstrate very high sensitivity and negative predictive value for significant coronary stenosis, these results have only recently been tested in multicenter trials. Accuracy is often lower in multicenter trials when technology is used in a standardized fashion on a more diverse patient population by multiple investigators. The results of multicenter trials by Budoff and colleagues,[21] Meijboom and coworkers,[22] and Miller and colleagues[23] are summarized in **Table 1.1**, along with meta-analysis results from Mowatt et al,[14] Meijer and associates,[24] and Vanhoenacker et al.[25] All these studies support the high negative predictive value of a normal coronary CTA to exclude the presence of significant coronary stenosis.

◆ Clinical Applications of Cardiac Computed Tomography

Cardiac CT may be performed for a wide range of clinical applications. Technical details related to multislice scanners, scan protocols, and radiation dose are discussed in Chapter 2. The remaining chapters in this text are organized to discuss individual applications of cardiac CT.

Gated CT of the heart without administration of contrast material has proven useful to image coronary calcium as a measure of overall atherosclerotic plaque burden (Chapter 5). Although this technique does not demonstrate the presence or absence of stenosis in a particular patient, it is useful for risk assessment.[26] Clinical trials suggest that coronary calcium scoring can modify the predicted risk based on the Framingham risk score.[27] A consensus has emerged that

Table 1.1 Accuracy of 64-Slice Coronary CT Angiography for Significant Coronary Stenosis

Author	Sensitivity (by Patient)	Specificity (by Patient)
Budoff et al[21]	0.95	0.83
Meijboom et al[22]	0.99	0.64
Miller et al[23]	0.85	0.90
Mowatt et al[14]	0.99	0.89
Meijer et al (40- & 64-slice)[24]	0.98	0.91
Vanhoenacker et al[25]	0.99	0.93

coronary calcium scoring is most appropriate for asymptomatic individuals with an intermediate Framingham risk in whom the calcium score may be used to determine the appropriate levels of lifestyle modification and pharmacologic therapy.[28]

CTA has numerous cardiac applications. It provides a noninvasive assessment of coronary anatomy (Chapter 3) and a clear demonstration of coronary anatomic variations and anomalies (Chapter 4). Because CT demonstrates adjacent anatomic structures as well as coronary arteries, MDCT provides a unique opportunity to assess the origin and course of a coronary artery relative to the aortic root, pulmonary artery, and myocardium (**Fig. 1.3**). Coronary venous anatomy is also visualized (**Fig. 1.4**). With respect to assessment of coronary anatomic variations, CTA is often superior to conventional catheter arteriography.[29]

Coronary CT demonstrates high sensitivity for the detection of coronary artery stenosis (Chapter 6). Although diagnostic

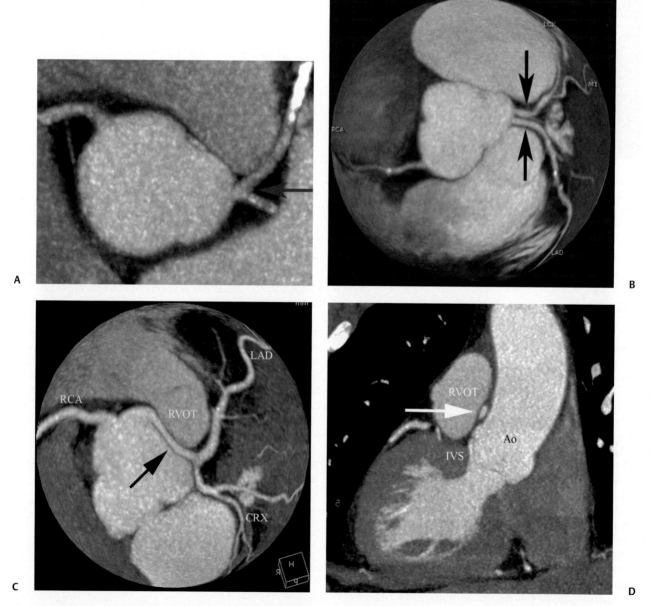

Fig. 1.3 Anatomic variations in the left main coronary artery. **(A)** Slab maximum intensity projection (MIP) demonstrates a cloacal left main coronary artery, which branches immediately into the left anterior descending (LAD) coronary artery and circumflex arteries (*arrow*). **(B)** Globe MIP in a second patient demonstrates independent origins of the LAD and circumflex arteries (*black arrows*). A left main coronary artery is not present. The globe MIP demonstrates three-dimensional relationships of the coronary vessels to the underlying cardiac anatomy. **(C)** Globe MIP in a third patient demonstrates an anomalous left coronary artery (*arrow*) passing between the aorta and right ventricular outflow tract (RVOT). **(D)** Sagittal reconstruction demonstrates the anomalous vessel (*arrow*) passing between the aorta (Ao) and RVOT above the level of the interventricular septum (IVS).

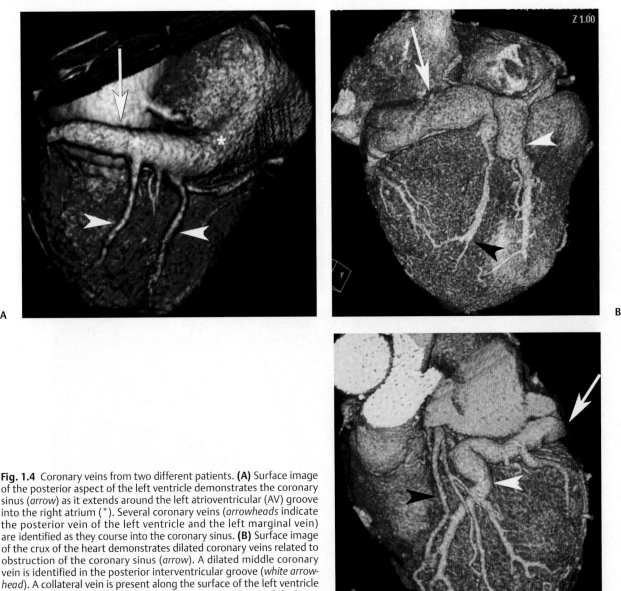

Fig. 1.4 Coronary veins from two different patients. **(A)** Surface image of the posterior aspect of the left ventricle demonstrates the coronary sinus (*arrow*) as it extends around the left atrioventricular (AV) groove into the right atrium (*). Several coronary veins (*arrowheads* indicate the posterior vein of the left ventricle and the left marginal vein) are identified as they course into the coronary sinus. **(B)** Surface image of the crux of the heart demonstrates dilated coronary veins related to obstruction of the coronary sinus (*arrow*). A dilated middle coronary vein is identified in the posterior interventricular groove (*white arrowhead*). A collateral vein is present along the surface of the left ventricle (*black arrowhead*). **(C)** Surface image of the anterior aspect of the heart in the same patient as in part B. The dilated great cardiac vein (*arrow*) represents the continuation of the coronary sinus in the left AV groove. The dilated anterior interventricular vein (*white arrowhead*) courses down the anterior interventricular groove alongside the left anterior descending artery (*black arrowhead*).

accuracy may be limited in patients with heavy coronary calcification, there is a general consensus that "a normal CT coronary angiogram allows the clinician to rule out the presence of hemodynamically relevant coronary artery stenoses with a high degree of reliability."[7] In patients who do not have a high pretest likelihood of coronary stenosis, a normal CT coronary angiogram serves to obviate any further need for a diagnostic coronary workup.[30] Because the radiation dose with state-of-the-art coronary CTA is lower than that of nuclear scintigraphy and the negative predictive value of CT is superior to that of nuclear scintigraphy, CTA provides a reasonable alternative to nuclear scintigraphy for the evaluation of chest pain in a

patient with a low to intermediate risk for CAD. In the setting of an emergency department patient presenting with chest pain, CT can be used for a "triple rule-out" to evaluate the pulmonary arteries for pulmonary embolism, the thoracic aorta for dissection, and the coronary arteries for significant stenosis **(Fig. 1.5)**. With a single examination requiring no more than 100 mL of intravenous contrast, CTA can evaluate all three of these serious vascular causes of chest pain as well as nonvascular extracardiac causes of pain (Chapter 15).[31]

In patients with known coronary disease who have been treated with angioplasty and a stent, the question of in-stent stenosis or stent thrombosis often arises. Current

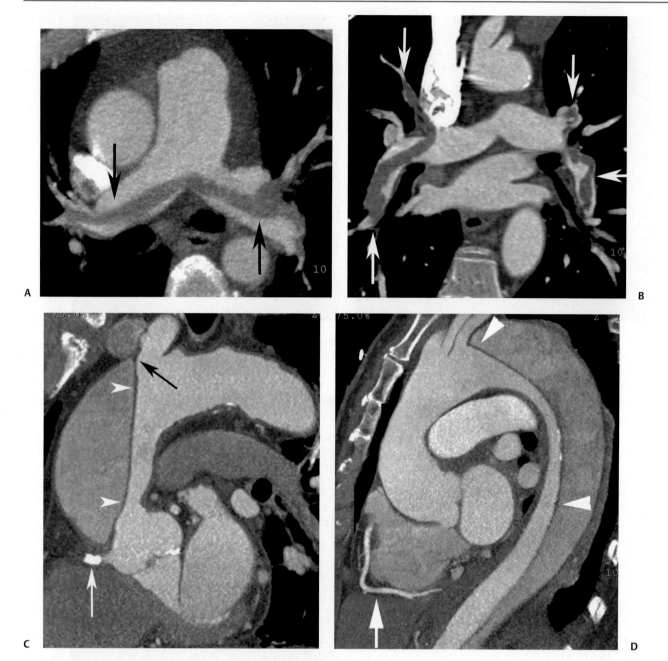

Fig. 1.5 "Triple rule-out" scans in four different patients with evidence of acute pulmonary embolism or aortic dissection. **(A)** Coronal maximum intensity projection (MIP) demonstrates a saddle pulmonary embolism extending across from the right to the left pulmonary artery (*arrows*). **(B)** Coronal MIP demonstrates pulmonary embolism extending into upper and lower lobar branches (*arrows*). **(C)** Oblique MIP demonstrates the ascending aorta and aortic arch with a stent in the proximal right coronary artery (RCA; *white arrow*). A type "A" dissection of the ascending aorta is present with an intimal flap (*arrowheads*) beginning from just above the RCA origin and extending to the origin of the innominate artery (*black arrow*). **(D)** Oblique MIP of the thoracic aorta in a different patient demonstrates a type "B" dissection extending from just beyond the origin of the left subclavian artery down through the thoracic aorta (*arrowheads*). The RCA is identified as it courses around the right atrioventricular groove (*arrow*).

64-slice CT technology is limited in this evaluation because of blooming artifact associated with calcium and metallic stents.[32] Nonetheless, larger stents are often well evaluated, and conventional angiography may be avoided in these patients after demonstration of a normal stent lumen (Chapter 7). Recent studies suggest that the sensitivity and specificity of CT for in-stent stenosis are greater than 90% in adequately visualized stented vessels.[33] Given the current pace of technological advances in CT, it is likely that future improvements will expand further the utility of cardiac CT for imaging of stents.

CTA is useful in both the pre-operative planning of coronary bypass surgery and in the post-operative evaluation of bypass grafts (Chapter 8),[34] especially in the setting of repeat cardiac surgery after previous bypass.[35] CTA clearly demonstrates the location of bypass grafts relative to other cardiac and thoracic anatomic landmarks. Venous bypass grafts are easily evaluated for stenosis or thrombosis. Arterial bypass grafts are more difficult to evaluate because of their smaller size. Native vessels are difficult to evaluate in these patients because of extensive calcification. Future improvements in CT technology are likely to expand this application as well.

Assessment of cardiac morphology and function is usually performed with echocardiography or cardiac MR. The lack of ionizing radiation with these techniques presents a major advantage over CT when detailed imaging of the coronary arteries is not needed. When evaluation of coronary anatomy is required, cardiac CT can provide assessment of coronary anatomy, cardiac morphology, and function (Chapter 9)[36] and cardiac valves (Chapter 10)[37] in a single evaluation (**Fig. 1.6**). A recent review of patients imaged with coronary CTA for suspected CAD identified unsuspected cardiovascular morphologic abnormalities in almost 1% of patients, including aortic aneurysms, hypertrophic cardiomyopathy, valvular heart disease, ventricular septal defects, left ventricular noncompaction, left atrial myxoma, and left ventricular apical aneurysms.[38] Assessment of morphology and function is quite useful in preoperative and postoperative studies for valve surgery and ventricular remodeling as well as in planning for left atrial ablation (Chapter 11) and other percutaneous interventional procedures (Chapter 12). Imaging of the coronary circulation can be combined with imaging of the thoracic aorta for preoperative assessment and post-surgical evaluation of aortic aneurysms and dissections (Chapter 13). Finally, CT imaging of the heart and great vessels may be useful for evaluation of congenital heart disease in the adult (Chapter 14).

Four new category I Current Procedural Terminology (CPT) codes have been introduced for 2010 to replace the former category III codes, which were viewed as "investigational" by many insurance carriers. Calcium scoring is covered by the code for cardiac CT without contrast material (75571). Evaluation of cardiac anatomy and chambers as well as coronary and pulmonary veins is covered by the code for contrast-enhanced cardiac CT (75572). A separate code is used for evaluation of cardiac anatomy in the setting of congenital heart disease (75573). Evaluation of coronary arteries, including evaluation of bypass grafts and stents, is included along with evaluation of cardiac morphology in the code for CTA of the heart (75574). There is no longer an add-on code for cardiac function; evaluation of cardiac function is subsumed into codes 75572–75574.

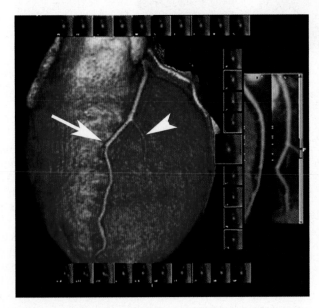

A

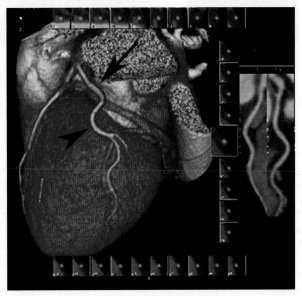

B

Fig. 1.6 Surface-rendered image of the left coronary circulation demonstrating tools for the assessment of coronary stenosis and evaluation of left ventricular (LV) function. In this patient, the circumflex artery supplies the majority of the LV free wall. **(A)** The left anterior oblique surface projection demonstrates the left anterior descending artery (LAD) as it courses into the anterior interventricular groove (*arrow*). A single small diagonal branch is identified (*arrowhead*). Assessment of the vessel lumen is facilitated with orthogonal curved maximum intensity projection (MIP) images of the LAD along the right side of the image and by short-axis images through multiple levels presented as small squares surrounding the surface projection. The LAD appears normal with no stenosis. **(B)** Left lateral projection demonstrates the circumflex artery as it courses in the left atrioventricular groove (*arrow*). The circumflex artery terminates in a large obtuse marginal branch (*arrowhead*), which supplies much of the left ventricular wall. Diagonal branches are not well developed in this patient. Orthogonal curved MIP images along the right side of the image and short-axis images of the circumflex demonstrate a normal vessel. (*Continued on page 8*)

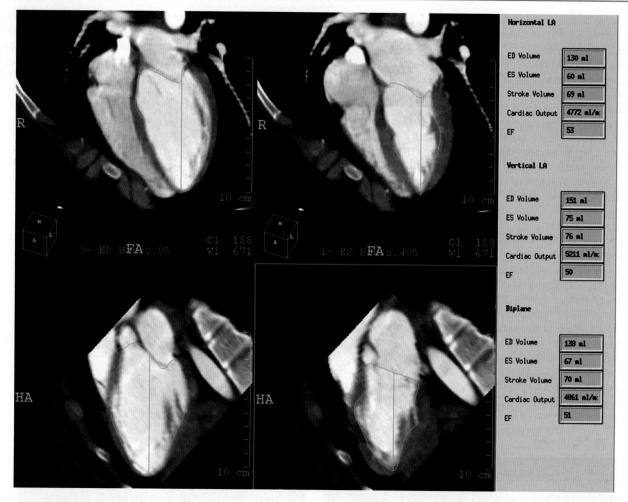

C

Fig. 1.6 (*Continued*) Surface-rendered image of the left coronary circulation demonstrating tools for the assessment of coronary stenosis and evaluation of left ventricular (LV) function. In this patient, the circumflex artery supplies the majority of the LV free wall. **(C)** Calculation of the ejection fraction is performed with a biplane Simpson algorithm using systolic and diastolic images in orthogonal four-chamber and two-chamber views. A low normal ejection fraction of just over 50% is computed.

◆ Appropriate Utilization of Cardiac Computed Tomography

Based on the recent statement of the American Heart Association (AHA), calcium scoring is most appropriate for risk stratification of patients with intermediate risk as suggested by traditional risk factor assessment.[28] Although the AHA criteria for calcium scoring are based on an intermediate Framingham risk score, a logical extension of this position suggests that calcium scoring is appropriate in any asymptomatic population with an intermediate risk of coronary heart disease based either on a Framingham risk calculation or on other risk factors not considered in the Framingham analysis (such as an elevated C-reactive protein, metabolic syndrome, obesity, or a family history of premature coronary disease).[39] An elevated calcium score may alter the expected risk of a coronary event and demonstrate a need for more aggressive lifestyle modifications or medical therapy.

A review of appropriateness criteria for cardiac CT conducted under the auspices of the American College of Cardiology Foundation concluded that cardiac CTA is most appropriate for evaluation of "cardiac structure and function and for diagnosis in symptomatic, intermediate CAD risk patients."[40] CTA evaluation of the patient with chest pain was considered most appropriate in the patient with an uninterpretable electrocardiogram (ECG), in those unable to exercise, or in those who had an uninterpretable or equivocal stress test. Coronary CTA was also rated as appropriate for evaluation of a suspected congenital coronary anomaly and for evaluation of new-onset heart failure to assess the cause. With respect to cardiac morphology, appropriate indications for cardiac CT included CT evaluation of pulmonary vein anatomy before performing ablation for atrial fibrillation, CT evaluation for coronary vein mapping before placement of a biventricular pacemaker, and CT arterial mapping before repeat cardiac surgical revascularization. In patients with technically limited echocardiographic and MR imaging, CT was also considered highly appropriate for evaluation of a cardiac mass or pericardial conditions.

With respect to assessment of the asymptomatic patient with risk factors for CAD, the most recent AHA scientific statement clearly states that "neither coronary CTA nor MRA should be used to screen for CAD in patients who have no signs or symptoms suggestive of CAD."[41] However, multiple studies now suggest that CTA may be useful to identify the presence of vulnerable plaque based on low plaque density, spotty calcifications, the presence of diffuse coronary disease, or arterial remodeling.[42,43] In one recent study of 1059 patients, the presence of CTA risk factors, including low-attenuation plaque or positive remodeling, changed the risk of that patient developing an ACS from 0.5 to 22% during an average follow-up of 27 months.[44] These studies suggest that coronary CTA may have a future role in cardiac risk assessment. Larger clinical trials are necessary to confirm the utility of CTA for this application.

A common indication for coronary CTA is for assessment of the patient with an indeterminate or abnormal stress test. This indication often arises in the patient with atypical chest pain or the asymptomatic high-risk patient who is subjected to a stress test before surgery or before starting a new exercise program. In the Thomas Jefferson university experience, fewer than half of these patients will have significant coronary disease at coronary angiography. Coronary CTA can exclude the presence of significant coronary disease in these patients and preclude the need for coronary angiography. Interestingly, the latest AHA scientific statement maintains that "in the case of equivocal stress-test results, it is conceivable but unproven that MDCT coronary CTA may facilitate a decision for or against invasive coronary angiography."[41] Nonetheless, given the excellent negative predictive value of coronary CTA, it can be demonstrated based on a decision theoretic model that coronary CTA is a cost-effective strategy for such patients and that the use of CTA in these patients will avoid many unnecessary cardiac catheterizations.[45]

Evaluation of the symptomatic patient with a normal stress test is another reasonable clinical indication for coronary CTA. The unstable patient with symptoms suggesting

ACS should be triaged directly to the interventional catheterization laboratory. However, for the clinician who is not satisfied with a negative stress test result on a stable symptomatic patient, the CTA may provide a more definitive answer by demonstrating that there is truly no underlying coronary disease. Alternatively, coronary CTA may detect the significant coronary disease in the setting of a false-negative stress study (**Fig. 1.7**).

In the absence of large randomized outcome trials to compare coronary CTA versus stress testing for the workup of suspected coronary disease, appropriateness criteria are based on the subjective opinions of "experts." Nonetheless, for the hypothetical patient who requires a workup for CAD, it is possible to predict the expected probability of a true- or false-positive result, a true- or false-negative result, the expected imaging cost, and the expected level of radiation exposure based on a theoretical decision analysis model. Such a model was implemented based on published multicenter studies of diagnostic accuracy for coronary CTA and stress testing and based on Medicare fee schedules for coronary CTA, stress testing, and invasive cardiac catheterization. Diagnostic accuracy, imaging costs, and effective dose are related to the expected prevalence of significant coronary disease in a theoretical patient (**Fig. 1.8**).[46] The expected prevalence of significant coronary disease for this model must be estimated based on the clinical presentation.[47]

Several conclusions can be drawn from this decision theoretic model for evaluation of the stable symptomatic patient who is referred for evaluation for CAD with CTA or stress testing:

1. The false-negative rate (or probability that significant coronary disease is missed) is minimized when coronary CTA is used as the primary workup modality.
2. The false-positive rate (or probability that a patient with normal coronary arteries will end up in the catheterization

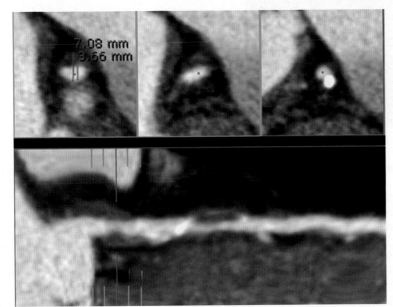

A

Fig. 1.7 Coronary CT angiography performed in a 40-year-old athlete with atypical symptoms and a normal nuclear stress evaluation. Vessel tracking is used to present orthogonal oblique images of each artery along with a straightened lumen view that allows cross-sectional measurements of vessel diameter. **(A)** Tracked imaged of the left main coronary artery and proximal left anterior descending coronary artery (LAD). Noncalcified plaque is present in the left main coronary artery, narrowing the diameter from 7.1 mm to 3.7 mm (see measurements on short-axis image). (Continued on page 10)

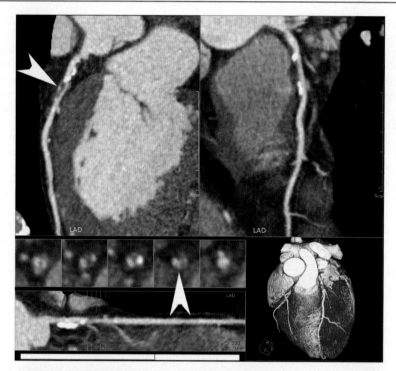

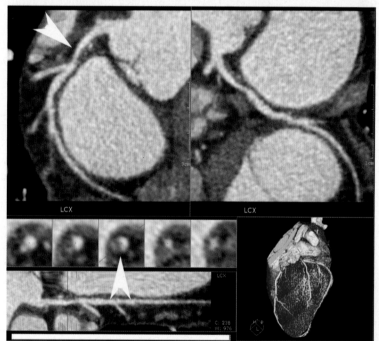

Fig. 1.7 (*Continued*) Coronary CT angiography performed in a 40-year-old athlete with atypical symptoms and a normal nuclear stress evaluation. Vessel tracking is used to present orthogonal oblique images of each artery along with a straightened lumen view that allows cross-sectional measurements of vessel diameter. **(B)** Calcified and noncalcified plaque in the proximal LAD (*arrowheads*). The corresponding diameter reduction is greater than 50%, as demonstrated on the short-axis images. **(C)** Noncalcified plaque in the proximal circumflex artery (*arrowheads*) with approximately 50% narrowing.

laboratory) is minimized when coronary CTA is used in combination with stress echocardiography.

3. Effective radiation dose is minimized when stress ECG or stress echocardiography is performed before coronary CTA (and only patients with a positive stress study are sent for CTA).

4. A strategy that uses stress echocardiography followed by coronary CTA minimizes the false-positive rate and effective radiation exposure. This strategy is associated with relatively low imaging costs and with a false-negative rate only slightly higher than a stress myocardial scintigraphy strategy as long as the pre-test probability of significant coronary disease is low (ie, <20%).

5. A strategy that includes stress echocardiography followed by coronary CTA is appropriate for evaluation of the low-risk CAD patient, whereas cardiac CTA alone may be more appropriate in the intermediate-risk patient. As noted above, the symptomatic, high-risk patient is more likely to benefit from direct triage to cardiac catherization.

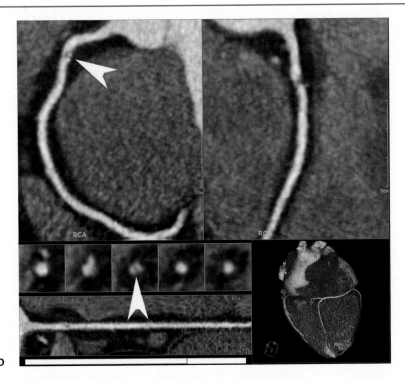

Fig. 1.7 (*Continued*) **(D)** Small focus of noncalcified plaque in the proximal right coronary artery (*arrowheads*) with close to 50% diameter narrowing. The presence of contrast material on both sides of the plaque suggests possible ulceration.

When there is suspicion for pulmonary embolism or aortic dissection as well as coronary disease, a CT angiogram may be more appropriately performed as a "triple rule-out" study. This topic is discussed in greater depth in Chapter 15. Triple rule-out studies are most appropriate in patients with low to intermediate risk of coronary disease who do not have ECG or laboratory evidence of acute myocardial injury. As noted, in patients with acute chest pain and a high suspicion for coronary disease, direct triage to more aggressive interventional therapy may be more appropriate than a diagnostic CTA. However, in patients who would otherwise be observed overnight and evaluated with a stress test, the triple rule-out

study may be used to evaluate quickly for multiple causes of chest symptoms with a single examination.

◆ The Comprehensive Cardiac Examination

A key advantage of cardiac CT is the ability to evaluate simultaneously coronary anatomy, myocardial morphology, and ventricular function with high spatial and temporal resolution.[48] Anatomic and functional information are often

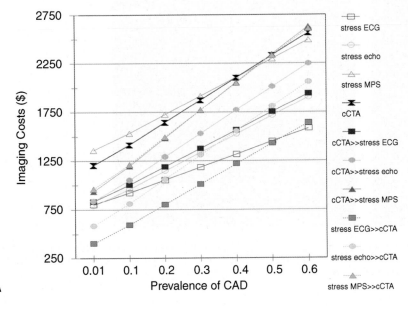

Fig. 1.8 Results of decision analysis model. **(A)** Expected imaging cost for the evaluation of suspected coronary disease as a function of the pre-test probability of significant coronary disease. MPS: myocardial perfusion scintigraphy; cCTA>>stress echo; coronary CTA followed by stress echocardiography. (*Continued on page 12*)

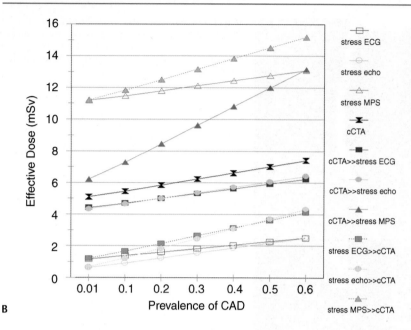

Fig. 1.8 (*Continued*) Results of decision analysis model. **(B)** Expected effective radiation dose for the evaluation of suspected coronary disease as a function of the pre-test probability of significant coronary disease. (From Halpern EJ, Fischman D, Savage MP, Koka AR, DeCaro M, Levin DC. Decision analytic model for evaluation of suspected coronary disease with stress testing and coronary CT angiography. Acad Radiol. 2010;17:577–586. Reprinted with permission.)

complementary. Significant coronary disease is often manifest by changes in ventricular morphology or function. The findings of segmental-wall thinning, fatty change in the endocardium, a focal bulge in the ventricular contour, abnormality in segmental wall motion, or papillary muscle or valvular dysfunction should prompt a search for localized coronary disease to explain the dysfunction. Conversely, a finding of coronary stenosis may be confirmed by demonstrating associated changes in morphology and function

(**Fig. 1.9**). In the absence of coronary disease, morphologic findings such as intracardiac shunts or changes of pulmonary hypertension may provide the explanation for an apparent cardiomyopathy.

A true comprehensive examination of the heart should include evaluation of myocardial perfusion in addition to coronary anatomy, cardiac morphology, and function. Coronary CTA often identifies lesions of uncertain hemodynamic significance. The extent of inducible ischemia associated with

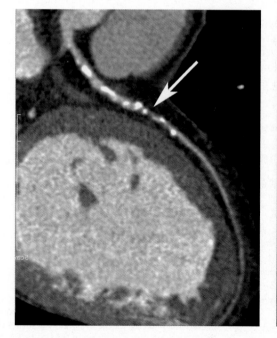

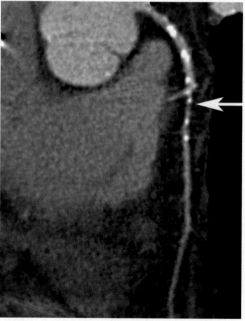

Fig. 1.9 Apical infarct associated with a diseased left anterior descending (LAD) coronary artery and high-grade stenosis in the mid-LAD. **(A,B)** Tracked maximum intensity projection images of the LAD demonstrate diffuse calcified plaque in the proximal LAD, with a focal area of noncalcified plaque associated with high-grade stenosis (*arrow*).

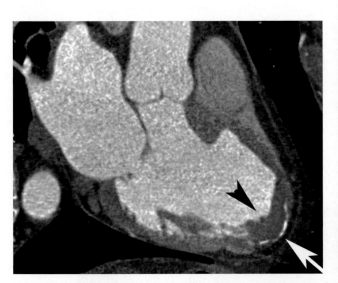
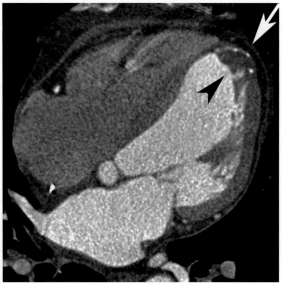

C   D

Fig. 1.9 (*Continued*) **(C)** Three-chamber view of the heart with a calcified apical infarct (*white arrow*) and an apical thrombus (*black arrowhead*). **(D)** Four/five chamber view of the heart with a calcified apical infarct (*white arrow*) and apical thrombus (*black arrowhead*).

coronary disease is predictive of the risk of a coronary event as well as the expected benefit of revascularization compared with medical therapy.[49,50] Studies comparing coronary CTA to gated single-photon emission CT (SPECT) imaging suggest that the perfusion information supplied by SPECT may be complementary to the coronary anatomy defined by CTA.[51,52] Co-registration of coronary CTA and SPECT studies performed independently may improve the diagnostic accuracy of the nuclear perfusion analysis.[53] Recent reports have demonstrated that CT imaging of the myocardium can provide an accurate measure of perfusion[54] and may predict future myocardial function.[55,56] For assessment of myocardial viability, low-dose CT late enhancement scanning is feasible, and

preliminary results look promising.[57] In direct comparison with nuclear scintigraphy, CT perfusion compares favorably for the detection, extent, and severity of myocardial perfusion defects.[58] A recent clinical study of adenosine-induced stress myocardial perfusion with CT demonstrated that the addition of CT perfusion data improved the sensitivity of CTA for coronary stenosis and that CT perfusion imaging had diagnostic accuracy comparable to SPECT.[17]

Assessment of CT perfusion may confirm that a specific coronary lesion results in myocardial ischemia (**Fig. 1.10**). Unfortunately, the findings of decreased myocardial perfusion on conventional CTA studies are often subtle, based on small differences in enhancement that may vary with

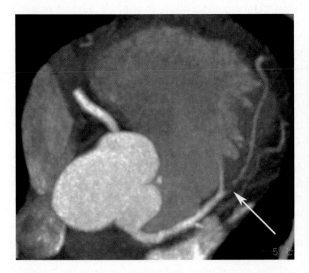
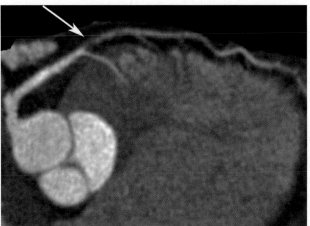

A   B

Fig. 1.10 Acute coronary syndrome with focal high-grade stenosis/occlusion of the left anterior descending (LAD) coronary artery associated with a subendocardial area of decreased perfusion. **(A,B)** Slab maximum intensity projection (MIP) images demonstrates an abrupt cutoff of the

LAD (*arrow*) just beyond the origin of a septal perforator branch. The distal LAD branches beyond this point are smaller and opacified to a lesser degree. (*Continued on page 14*)

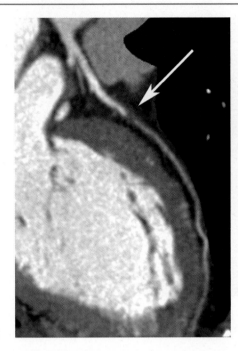

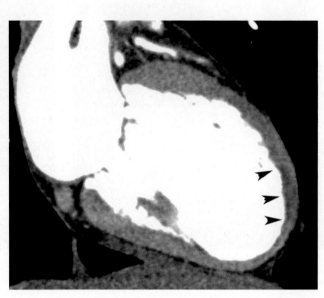

C

D

Fig. 1.10 (*Continued*) Acute coronary syndrome with focal high-grade stenosis/occlusion of the left anterior descending (LAD) coronary artery associated with a subendocardial area of decreased perfusion. **(C)** Tracked MIP image of the LAD demonstrates the same abrupt cutoff (*arrow*). **(D)** Two-chamber view of the left heart demonstrates a subendocardial region of lower density (*arrowheads*) in the distal anterior wall extending to the ventricular apex, corresponding to the territory supplied by the distal LAD.

contrast injection technique and timing of the scan. Recent studies have used various techniques, including dynamic perfusion imaging and dual-energy CT, to improve the quantification of myocardial perfusion during CTA.[59] Further studies are needed to define a standard technique for CT evaluation of myocardial perfusion and to clarify the clinical utility of CT perfusion imaging in clinical practice. The final chapter of this text (Chapter 16) includes a more detailed discussion of CT perfusion imaging along with other new technical innovations that will no doubt expand the applications of cardiac CT in the near future.

◆ Plaque Characterization

In contrast to conventional cardiac catheterization, which images contrast within the coronary vessel lumen, coronary CTA provides detailed images of the lumen as well as the vessel wall surrounding the lumen. Both calcified and non-calcified plaques are visible on coronary CTA (**Fig. 1.11**).[60] Even when plaque is associated with positive remodeling such that there is no detectable narrowing of the lumen, the plaque remains visible on CTA. Atherosclerotic changes within the vessel wall that do not impact the lumen may not be visible with conventional catheter arteriography. However, coronary atherosclerosis can be characterized with CTA on the basis of plaque distribution (proximal–distal), plaque density (calcified, noncalcified, or low density), plaque surface (smooth versus irregular), plaque ulceration, and positive remodeling.

Over the past decade, our understanding of the mechanisms underlying the complications of atherosclerosis, including ACS, have shifted remarkably from an emphasis on flow-limiting lesions to plaque characterization.[61] Acute coronary events most commonly arise from the disruption of a thin-cap fibroatheroma that includes a large lipid pool inside the plaque, now known as vulnerable plaque.[62] Calcified plaque is less likely to be associated with ACS, whereas lipid-laden plaque is more likely to rupture. Several researchers have investigated plaque characterization with MDCT and have suggested that it may be possible to distinguish calcified plaque (>350 HU) from fibrous plaque (70–104 HU) and lipid-laden plaque (14–49 HU).[63–65] Clinical studies have demonstrated a difference in the CT density of coronary plaque and in the presence of positive remodeling between patients with ACS versus stable angina.[66] A recent study demonstrated that the presence of low-density plaque and positive remodeling can be used to predict the risk for subsequent ACS.[44]

Several clinical studies suggest that plaque burden and the distribution of plaque are related to risk of a coronary event. A study of 1127 patients with average follow-up of 15.3 months demonstrated that the presence of left main stenosis, proximal stenosis in a major coronary artery, three vessel disease, the number of involved coronary segments, and severity of stenosis were all independent predictors of mortality.[8] A more recent study demonstrated an increasing frequency of cardiac events when patients are grouped by: normal CTA, presence of coronary disease, obstructive coronary disease, and obstructive coronary disease in the proximal left coronary system.[67]

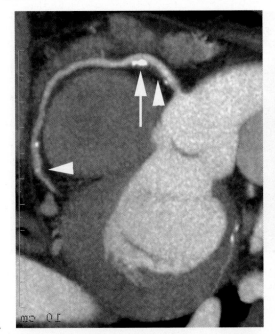

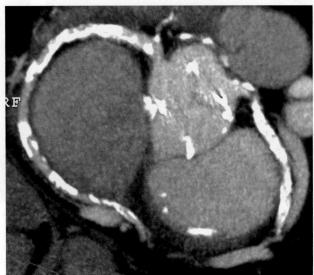

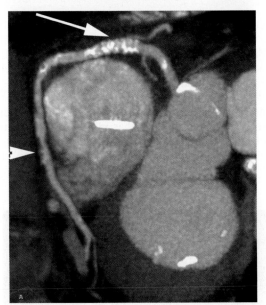

Fig. 1.11 Plaque characterization in three patients with right coronary artery plaque. **(A)** Focal calcified plaque in the proximal right coronary artery (RCA) (*arrow*). Additional areas of noncalcified plaque (*arrowheads*) and small calcified plaques are present without significant narrowing of the vessel lumen. There is positive remodeling in the proximal RCA such that the lumen of the vessel is preserved. The presence of smooth plaque with positive remodeling may be difficult to appreciate on conventional coronary arteriography but is clearly demonstrated on coronary CT angiography. **(B)** Diffusely calcified RCA and circumflex. The vessel lumen is suboptimally visualized on coronary CT in the presence of heavy calcification. Blooming artifact from calcium leads to overcalling of stenosis with loss of specificity. **(C)** Diseased RCA with stent surrounded by calcified plaque in the proximal RCA (*arrow*) and ulcerated, noncalcified plaque in the distal RCA (*arrowhead*).

Although plaque characterization appears promising, there is substantial overlap in the CT density of different types of plaque.[68,69] Technical parameters in the acquisition of a CT image as well as differences between scanners produced by different vendors will impact on the measured CT density of a plaque. Furthermore, it is difficult to quantify objectively plaque volume, plaque distribution, and the surface texture of plaque by CTA. CT plaque characterization is a promising technique that awaits standardization of CT parameters and prospective clinical trials to provide empiric evidence that it can distinguish stable from vulnerable plaque in the management of coronary disease.

◆ Rendering and Display Modes

The basic unit of data acquisition in cardiac CT is the thin axial slice. However, the acquisition of isotropic pixels with equal spatial resolution in all planes allows volumetric reconstruction in any arbitrary plane. Although different display features are provided by various CT three-dimensional (3-D) workstations, several basic features should be available on all systems, including surface-rendered volumetric display, maximum intensity projection (MIP), and vessel tracking.[70,71] Most systems also provide automated software to quantify the degree of stenosis. To evaluate coronary

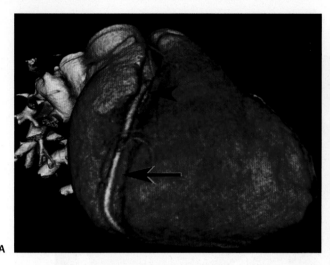

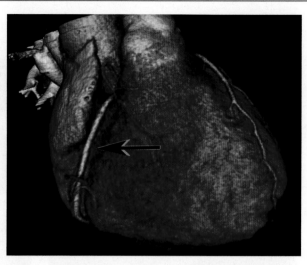

Fig. 1.12 Surface-rendered image of the right coronary artery demonstrates the relationship of the coronary artery to adjacent landmarks and structures. **(A)** The right coronary artery courses through the right atrioventricular groove (*arrow*). The proximal portion of the right coronary artery is partially obscured by the overlying right atrial appendage (*arrowhead*). **(B)** With a slightly different obliquity, the right coronary artery (*arrow*) is visualized as it courses under the atrial appendage.

anatomy properly, a 3-D workstation should provide the ability to rotate any rendered image into any desired imaging plane.

Surface-rendered volumetric images of the coronary vessels provide an excellent overview of the anatomy while also demonstrating the relationship of coronary arteries to the underlying cardiac structures (**Figs. 1.12** and **1.13**). Surface-rendered displays do not demonstrate internal detail within coronary vessels and are not generally useful for the identification of calcified plaque or assessment of coronary stenosis. Surface images may be useful for the

surgeon who wishes to define the course of a vessel relative to adjacent anatomic landmarks.

An MIP image presents a series of contiguous CT images ("the slab") as a single image. The intensity of each pixel in an MIP image is obtained by projecting a ray through the slab and determining the maximum intensity among all the contiguous images at one corresponding location. The number of images included in the slab is adjustable and is determined by the slab thickness. An MIP image provides an angiographic projection of a coronary artery (**Fig. 1.14**) that can be used to assess the degree of stenosis. However,

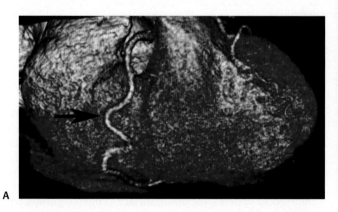

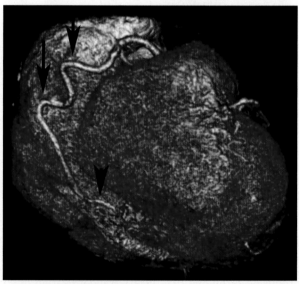

Fig. 1.13 Surface-rendered image demonstrates a tortuous right coronary artery (RCA). **(A)** The RCA courses along the right atrioventricular (AV) groove (*arrow*). **(B)** The more distal portion of the RCA is tortuous and swings out of the AV groove (*arrows*). The proximal posterior descending artery (*arrowhead*) enters the posterior interventricular groove.

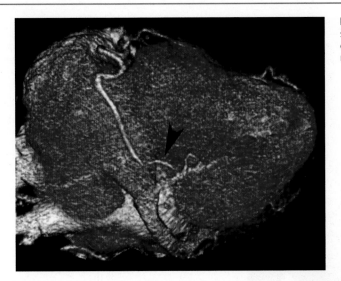

C

Fig. 1.13 (*Continued*) **(C)** View of the crux of the heart demonstrates the posterior descending artery (*arrowhead*). The posterior descending artery often appears more tortuous than do other coronary vessels.

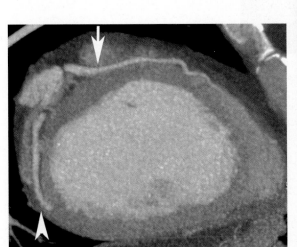

A

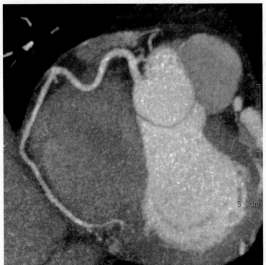

C

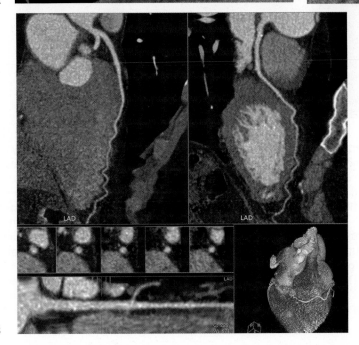

B

Fig. 1.14 Slab maximum intensity projection (MIP), curved MIP, and globe MIP images of the left anterior descending (LAD) coronary artery and right coronary artery (RCA). **(A)** Slab MIP image of the LAD (*arrow*) and circumflex (*arrowhead*) arteries (*arrows*). Neither vessel is visualized in its entirety. **(B)** Tracked images of the LAD with curved MIP demonstrate the entire LAD and provide orthogonal images (*bottom left*) to evaluate the LAD lumen in short axis. **(C)** Slab MIP image of the RCA demonstrates most of this vessel with a characteristic "C" shape. Note the tortuous proximal course of the RCA. (*Continued on page 18*)

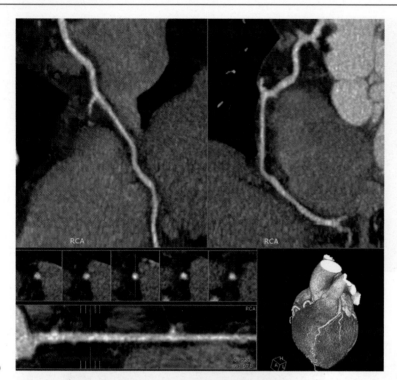

D

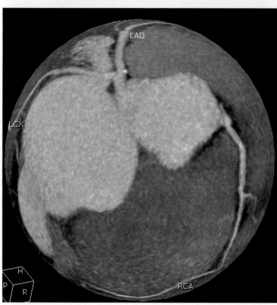

E

Fig. 1.14 (*Continued*) Slab maximum intensity projection (MIP), curved MIP, and globe MIP images of the left anterior descending (LAD) coronary artery and right coronary artery (RCA). **(D)** Tracked RCA images with curved MIP demonstrate the RCA in two orthogonal planes. When compared with the slab MIP, the shape/course of the RCA is distorted to present the entire vessel in a single image. **(E)** Globe MIP of the coronary vessels provides an overview of the relationship of these vessels to the underlying cardiac structures.

because coronary arteries are curved, it is not generally possible to visualize an entire coronary artery on a single-slab MIP image (**Fig. 1.14A**). To evaluate the full length of a coronary artery, a sliding-slab technique may be used for real-time evaluation whereby the location of the slab MIP is controlled with a mouse.

As an alternative to the sliding-slab MIP, automated vessel-tracking algorithms may be combined with curved multi-planar reconstruction to demonstrate the entirety of a vessel on a single curved MIP display (**Figs. 1.14** and **1.15**). Vessel-tracking algorithms and curved MIP projections are very useful for the assessment of stenosis, but the curved

MIP does warp the true contour of the vessel to display the entire vessel in a single image. This distortion of the vessel may impact the interpretation of stenosis. In most cases, the choice of slab MIP versus tracked curved MIP display is a matter of personal preference; either technique will display the required anatomic details. Whichever MIP technique is used, it is imperative that the workstation provide the ability to rotate the vessel in all directions to assess adequately the degree of stenosis.

Many 3-D workstations provide the ability to project a straightened lumen view of the coronary vessels and render orthogonal short-axis images through the artery (**Figs. 1.6**

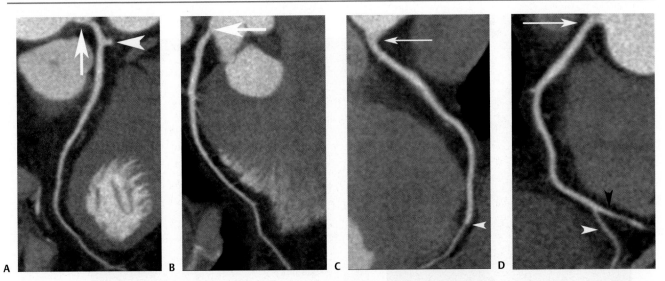

Fig. 1.15 Curved maximum intensity projection (MIP) images of the left anterior descending (LAD) and right coronary arteries (RCAs) in orthogonal projections. **(A)** Curved MIP demonstrates the origin of the left main coronary artery from the aorta (*arrow*). The vessel is tracked beyond the origin of the circumflex artery (*arrowhead*) to demonstrate the entire length of the LAD. The circumflex artery is not visualized as it extends out of the plain of view of this image. **(B)** Orthogonal curved MIP demonstrates the presence of noncalcified plaque in the left main coronary artery with less than 50% narrowing (*arrow*). The remainder of the LAD demonstrates a normal appearance. **(C)** Curved MIP demonstrates the RCA from its origin at the aorta (*arrow*) down to the origin of the posterior descending artery (*arrowhead*). There is no significant plaque or stenosis. **(D)** Orthogonal curved MIP demonstrates the classic "C" shape of this vessel in the left anterior oblique projection. Once again, the origin from the aorta is identified (*arrow*), as is the bifurcation of the distal RCA into a posterior left ventricular branch (*black arrowhead*) and the posterior descending artery (*white arrowhead*). Curved MIP images based on a vessel-tracking algorithm allow visualization of the entire coronary artery to demonstrate the presence of plaque and evaluate the degree of stenosis.

and **1.7**). Short-axis images of a vessel allow one to measure the degree of stenosis at any point within the vessel. Short-axis images are extremely useful when there is circumferential plaque, especially circumferential calcified plaque that may not be amenable to assessment with a slab MIP or curved MIP approach. An important shortcoming of measuring stenosis in the short-axis projection is the lack of a normal adjacent segment for comparison. A slab MIP or curved MIP projection demonstrates the lumen of the adjacent vascular segment that may be compared with the suspected site of stenosis.

A globe MIP display combines the anatomic overview provided by a surface-rendered volumetric display with the angiographic information provided by an MIP image. The globe display demonstrates the underlying cardiac structures but provides an MIP image that can be used to assess vascular patency and calcification (**Figs. 1.14E** and **1.16**).

◆ Limitations and Future Developments

The major limiting factors in cardiac CTA include elevated heart rate, irregularity of cardiac rhythm, patient body habitus, and coronary calcium. Coronary CTA is dependent on accurate gating so that images can be obtained in a relatively quiescent phase of the cardiac cycle. Elevated heart rates, variable heart rates, and irregular heart rates often result in blurring of images.[72] These issues are currently being addressed by improvements in temporal resolution and by single heartbeat scans in the latest generation of scanners.

Large patients are difficult to image because of the high radiation dose necessary to obtain a reasonable signal-to-noise ratio in thin-section images of the coronary arteries. Signal-to-noise issues are being addressed by technical improvements in the delivery of radiographic energy, including better filtration and collimation of the roentgen source, improved pulsing of the roentgen tube during diastole, and tailoring of the roentgen beam profile according to patient thickness, coupled with more efficient detector systems and reconstruction algorithms, such that the overall radiation dose to the patient is decreased while image quality is improved. Imaging of calcified coronary arteries is often limited by blooming artifact that obscures the vessel lumen as well as by the difficulty of distinguishing calcium from the adjacent contrast-enhanced lumen. Artifact from calcium may be reduced in future scanners with improved spatial resolution or by use of radiographic spectral analysis to distinguish calcium from contrast material.[73] Other factors that can limit coronary CTA include patient motion and adequacy of vascular enhancement. Careful attention to patient preparation and technique is critical to overcome these issues.

◆ Ancillary Findings on Cardiac Computed Tomography

Extracardiac findings are identified frequently in patients during coronary CTA (**Fig. 1.17**). A recent study demonstrated incidental noncardiac findings in 41.5% of patients but suggested that only 1.2% of patients had clinically significant

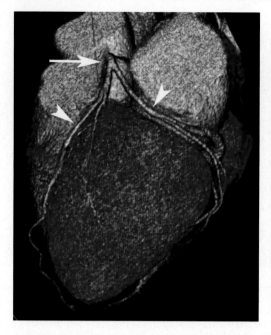
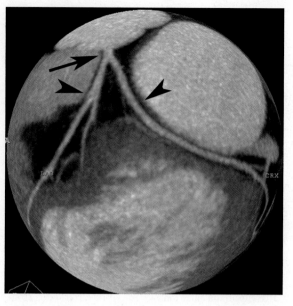

A

B

Fig. 1.16 Surface and globe maximum intensity projection (MIP) images of a short left main coronary artery. **(A)** Surface image demonstrates a short left main coronary artery (*arrow*), which bifurcates into left anterior descending coronary artery and circumflex branches (*arrowheads*). **(B)** Globe MIP view demonstrates the short left main coronary artery (*arrow*) and its two branches (*arrowheads*). Both rendering modes demonstrate the relationship of the vessels to the underlying chambers, but the globe MIP image allows assessment of the internal structure of the vessel for plaque and stenosis.

extracardiac findings.[74] Some extracardiac findings, such as pulmonary embolism, hiatal hernia, or pneumothorax, may explain chest pain. The presence of pulmonary parenchymal disease may explain shortness of breath. Extracardiac findings may also demonstrate the cause of secondary pulmonary hypertension. A judicious evaluation of incidental extracardiac findings should report all clinically significant findings and all findings that might explain the presenting symptoms while attempting to minimize follow-up examinations for nonsignificant findings.

◆ Conclusion

Although cardiac CT is a relative newcomer to the field of cardiac imaging, this technology provides exquisite images for the evaluation of coronary anatomy, cardiac morphology, and valvular function. Large trials have already documented the utility of cardiac CT for calcium scoring and cardiac risk assessment in selected patient populations. Multiple trials have demonstrated high sensitivity and specificity of coronary CTA for the detection of coronary

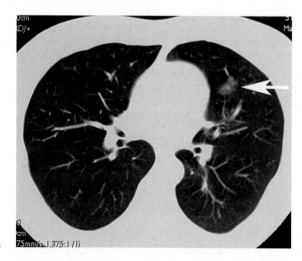
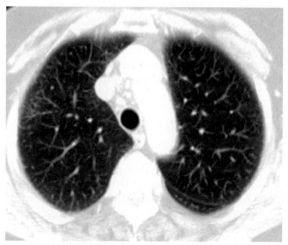

A

B

Fig. 1.17 Incidental findings in patients referred for coronary CT angiography. **(A)** Axial image through the lungs demonstrates the presence of a lung cancer in the left upper lobe (*arrow*). **(B)** A different patient with shortness of breath was found to have peripheral interstitial lung disease.

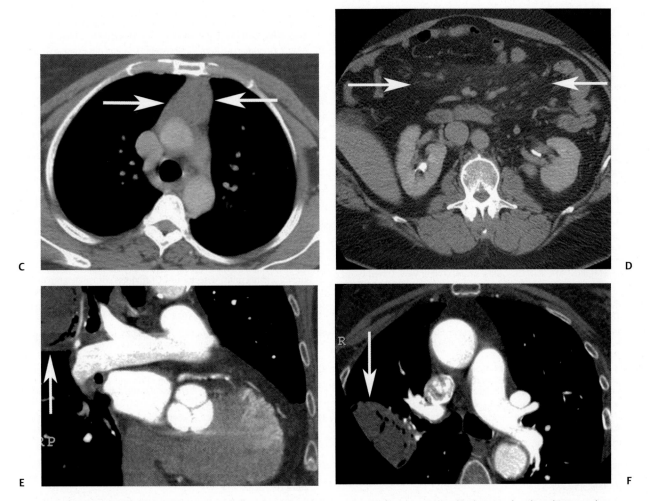

Fig. 1.17 (*Continued*) **(C)** A third patient was diagnosed with lymphoma and an anterior mediastinal mass (*arrows*). **(D)** Substernal chest pain in a fourth patient is related to infiltration at the root of the mesentery in retractile mesenteritis. **(E,F)** Coronal and axial images demonstrate the presence of an air containing a round mass lesion in the right upper lobe. Further evaluation demonstrated a fungal infection.

artery stenosis and, most important, the very high negative predictive value of a normal coronary CTA study. A normal coronary CTA excludes coronary disease from the differential diagnosis. However, visualization of coronary disease on CTA does not necessarily imply myocardial ischemia. The addition of CT perfusion imaging to coronary CTA will define the ischemic burden and help classify coronary lesions as hemodynamically significant to provide a truly comprehensive single modality study for cardiac evaluation. Additional experience and controlled studies are now needed to document the clinical benefit that may be obtained when cardiac CTA is used to guide treatment decisions for CAD. Unfortunately, clinical trial data are quickly outdated as a result of rapidly evolving CT technology. Applications that are technically difficult today are likely to become routine in the future.

References

1. Lloyd-Jones D, Adams R, Carnethon M, et al; American Heart Association Statistics Committee and Stroke Statistics Subcommittee. Heart disease and stroke statistics—2009 update: a report from the American Heart Association Statistics Committee and Stroke Statistics Subcommittee. Circulation. 2009;119(3):480–486

2. Ford ES, Ajani UA, Croft JB, et al. Explaining the decrease in U.S. deaths from coronary disease, 1980–2000. N Engl J Med. 2007;356(23): 2388–2398

3. Pleis JR, Lucas JW. Summary health statistics for U.S. adults: National Health Interview Survey, 2007. Vital Health Stat 10. 2009;(240):1–159

4. Pitts SR, Niska RW, Xu J, Burt CW. National Hospital Ambulatory Medical Care Survey: 2006 emergency department summary. Natl Health Stat Report. 2008;(7):1–38

5. Pope JH, Aufderheide TP, Ruthazer R, et al. Missed diagnoses of acute cardiac ischemia in the emergency department. N Engl J Med. 2000;342(16):1163–1170

6. Lee TH, Rouan GW, Weisberg MC, et al. Clinical characteristics and natural history of patients with acute myocardial infarction sent home from the emergency room. Am J Cardiol. 1987;60(4): 219–224

7. Budoff MJ, Achenbach S, Blumenthal RS, et al; American Heart Association Committee on Cardiovascular Imaging and Intervention; American Heart Association Council on Cardiovascular Radiology and Intervention; American Heart Association Committee on Cardiac Imaging, Council on Clinical Cardiology. Assessment of coronary artery disease by cardiac computed tomography: a scientific statement from the American Heart Association Committee on Cardiovascular Imaging and Intervention, Council on Cardiovascular Radiology and Intervention, and Committee on Cardiac Imaging, Council on Clinical Cardiology. Circulation. 2006;114(16):1761–1791

8. Min JK, Shaw LJ, Devereux RB, et al. Prognostic value of multidetector coronary computed tomographic angiography for prediction of all-cause mortality. J Am Coll Cardiol. 2007;50(12):1161–1170

9. van Werkhoven JM, Gaemperli O, Schuijf JD, et al. Multislice computed tomography coronary angiography for risk stratification in patients with an intermediate pretest likelihood. Heart. 2009;95(19):1607–1611

10. Hoffmann U, Pena AJ, Moselewski F, et al. MDCT in early triage of patients with acute chest pain. AJR Am J Roentgenol. 2006;187(5):1240–1247

11. Hoffmann U, Nagurney JT, Moselewski F, et al. Coronary multidetector computed tomography in the assessment of patients with acute chest pain. Circulation. 2006;114(21):2251–2260

12. Gallagher MJ, Ross MA, Raff GL, Goldstein JA, O'Neill WW, O'Neil B. The diagnostic accuracy of 64-slice computed tomography coronary angiography compared with stress nuclear imaging in emergency department low-risk chest pain patients. Ann Emerg Med. 2007;49(2):125–136

13. Johnson TR, Nikolaou K, Wintersperger BJ, et al. ECG-gated 64-MDCT angiography in the differential diagnosis of acute chest pain. AJR Am J Roentgenol. 2007;188(1):76–82

14. Mowatt G, Cook JA, Hillis GS, et al. 64-Slice computed tomography angiography in the diagnosis and assessment of coronary artery disease: systematic review and meta-analysis. Heart. 2008;94(11):1386–1393

15. Stacul F, Sironi D, Grisi G, Belgrano M, Salvi A, Cova M. 64-Slice CT coronary angiography versus conventional coronary angiography: activity-based cost analysis. Radiol Med (Torino). 2009;114(2):239–252

16. Budoff MJ, Karwasky R, Ahmadi N, et al. Cost-effectiveness of multidetector computed tomography compared with myocardial perfusion imaging as gatekeeper to invasive coronary angiography in asymptomatic firefighters with positive treadmill tests. J Cardiovasc Comput Tomogr. 2009;3(5):323–330

17. Blankstein R, Shturman LD, Rogers IS, et al. Adenosine-induced stress myocardial perfusion imaging using dual-source cardiac computed tomography. J Am Coll Cardiol. 2009;54(12):1072–1084

18. Lell M, Marwan M, Schepis T, et al. Prospectively ECG-triggered high-pitch spiral acquisition for coronary CT angiography using dual source CT: technique and initial experience. Eur Radiol. 2009;19(11):2576–2583

19. Das M, Braunschweig T, Mühlenbruch G, et al. Carotid plaque analysis: comparison of dual-source computed tomography (CT) findings and histopathological correlation. Eur J Vasc Endovasc Surg. 2009;38(1):14–19

20. Ruzsics B, Schwarz F, Schoepf UJ, et al. Comparison of dual-energy computed tomography of the heart with single photon emission computed tomography for assessment of coronary artery stenosis and of the myocardial blood supply. Am J Cardiol. 2009;104(3):318–326

21. Budoff MJ, Dowe D, Jollis JG, et al. Diagnostic performance of 64-multidetector row coronary computed tomographic angiography for evaluation of coronary artery stenosis in individuals without known coronary artery disease: results from the prospective multicenter ACCURACY (Assessment by Coronary Computed Tomographic Angiography of Individuals Undergoing Invasive Coronary Angiography) trial. J Am Coll Cardiol. 2008;52(21):1724–1732

22. Meijboom WB, Meijs MF, Schuijf JD, et al. Diagnostic accuracy of 64-slice computed tomography coronary angiography: a prospective, multicenter, multivendor study. J Am Coll Cardiol. 2008;52(25):2135–2144

23. Miller JM, Rochitte CE, Dewey M, et al. Diagnostic performance of coronary angiography by 64-row CT. N Engl J Med. 2008;359(22):2324–2336

24. Meijer AB, O YL, Geleijns J, Kroft LJ. Meta-analysis of 40- and 64-MDCT angiography for assessing coronary artery stenosis. AJR Am J Roentgenol. 2008;191(6):1667–1675

25. Vanhoenacker PK, Heijenbrok-Kal MH, Van Heste R, et al. Diagnostic performance of multidetector CT angiography for assessment of coronary artery disease: meta-analysis. Radiology. 2007;244(2):419–428

26. Arad Y, Goodman KJ, Roth M, Newstein D, Guerci AD. Coronary calcification, coronary disease risk factors, C-reactive protein, and atherosclerotic cardiovascular disease events: the St. Francis Heart Study. J Am Coll Cardiol. 2005;46(1):158–165

27. Greenland P, LaBree L, Azen SP, Doherty TM, Detrano RC. Coronary artery calcium score combined with Framingham score for risk prediction in asymptomatic individuals. JAMA. 2004;291(2):210–215

28. Greenland P, Bonow RO, Brundage BH, et al; American College of Cardiology Foundation Clinical Expert Consensus Task Force (ACCF/AHA Writing Committee to Update the 2000 Expert Consensus Document on Electron Beam Computed Tomography); Society of Atherosclerosis Imaging and Prevention; Society of Cardiovascular Computed Tomography. ACCF/AHA 2007 clinical expert consensus document on coronary artery calcium scoring by computed tomography in global cardiovascular risk assessment and in evaluation of patients with chest pain: a report of the American College of Cardiology Foundation Clinical Expert Consensus Task Force (ACCF/AHA Writing Committee to Update the 2000 Expert Consensus Document on Electron Beam Computed Tomography). Circulation. 2007;115(3):402–426

29. Kim SY, Seo JB, Do KH, et al. Coronary artery anomalies: classification and ECG-gated multi-detector row CT findings with angiographic correlation. Radiographics. 2006;26(2):317–333, discussion 333–334

30. Achenbach S. Computed tomography coronary angiography. J Am Coll Cardiol. 2006;48(10):1919–1928

31. Halpern EJ. Triple-rule-out CT angiography for evaluation of acute chest pain and possible acute coronary syndrome. Radiology. 2009;252(2):332–345

32. Beohar N, Robbins JD, Cavanaugh BJ, et al. Quantitative assessment of in-stent dimensions: a comparison of 64 and 16 detector multislice computed tomography to intravascular ultrasound. Catheter Cardiovasc Interv. 2006;68(1):8–10

33. Kumbhani DJ, Ingelmo CP, Schoenhagen P, Curtin RJ, Flamm SD, Desai MY. Meta-analysis of diagnostic efficacy of 64-slice computed tomography in the evaluation of coronary in-stent restenosis. Am J Cardiol. 2009;103(12):1675–1681

34. Herzog C, Wimmer-Greinecker G, Schwarz W, et al. Progress in CT imaging for the cardiac surgeon. Semin Thorac Cardiovasc Surg. 2004;16(3):242–248

35. Gasparovic H, Rybicki FJ, Millstine J, et al. Three dimensional computed tomographic imaging in planning the surgical approach for redo cardiac surgery after coronary revascularization. Eur J Cardiothorac Surg. 2005;28(2):244–249

36. Orakzai SH, Orakzai RH, Nasir K, Budoff MJ. Assessment of cardiac function using multidetector row computed tomography. J Comput Assist Tomogr. 2006;30(4):555–563

37. Alkadhi H, Wildermuth S, Plass A, et al. Aortic stenosis: comparative evaluation of 16-detector row CT and echocardiography. Radiology. 2006;240(1):47–55

38. Knickelbine T, Lesser JR, Haas TS, et al. Identification of unexpected nonatherosclerotic cardiovascular disease with coronary CT angiography. JACC Cardiovasc Imaging. 2009;2(9):1085–1092

39. Hecht HS, Budoff MJ, Berman DS, Ehrlich J, Rumberger JA. Coronary artery calcium scanning: clinical paradigms for cardiac risk assessment and treatment. Am Heart J. 2006;151(6):1139–1146

40. Hendel RC, Patel MR, Kramer CM, et al; American College of Cardiology Foundation Quality Strategic Directions Committee Appropriateness Criteria Working Group; American College of Radiology; Society of Cardiovascular Computed Tomography; Society for Cardiovascular Magnetic Resonance; American Society of Nuclear Cardiology; North American Society for Cardiac Imaging; Society for Cardiovascular Angiography and Interventions; Society of Interventional Radiology. ACCF/ACR/SCCT/SCMR/ASNC/NASCI/SCAI/SIR 2006 appropriateness criteria for cardiac computed tomography and cardiac magnetic resonance imaging: a report of the American College of Cardiology Foundation Quality Strategic Directions Committee Appropriateness Criteria Working Group, American College of Radiology, Society of Cardiovascular Computed Tomography, Society for Cardiovascular Magnetic Resonance, American Society of Nuclear Cardiology, North American Society for Cardiac Imaging, Society for Cardiovascular Angiography and Interventions, and Society of Interventional Radiology. J Am Coll Cardiol. 2006;48(7):1475–1497

41. Bluemke DA, Achenbach S, Budoff M, et al. Noninvasive coronary artery imaging: magnetic resonance angiography and multidetector computed tomography angiography: a scientific statement from the American Heart Association Committee on Cardiovascular Imaging and Intervention of the Council on Cardiovascular Radiology and Intervention, and the Councils on Clinical Cardiology and Cardiovascular Disease in the Young. Circulation. 2008;118(5):586–606

42. Rumberger JA. The promise of quantitative computed tomography coronary angiography and noninvasive segmental coronary plaque quantification: pushing the "edge." J Am Coll Cardiol. 2006;47(3):678–680

43. Schmermund A, Magedanz A, Voigtländer T. The role of CT angiography in risk stratification for atherosclerosis. Curr Atheroscler Rep. 2009;11(2):111–117

44. Motoyama S, Sarai M, Harigaya H, et al. Computed tomographic angiography characteristics of atherosclerotic plaques subsequently resulting in acute coronary syndrome. J Am Coll Cardiol. 2009;54(1):49–57

45. Halpern EJ, Savage MP, Fischman DL, Levin DC. Cost-effectiveness of coronary CT angiography in evaluation of patients without symptoms who have positive stress test results. AJR Am J Roentgenol. 2010;194(5):1257–1262

46. Halpern EJ, Fischman DL, Savage MP, Koka AR, DeCaro M, Levin DC. Decision analytic model for evaluation of suspected coronary disease with stress testing and coronary CT angiography. Acad Radiol. 2010;17(5):577–586

47. Diamond GA, Forrester JS. Analysis of probability as an aid in the clinical diagnosis of coronary-artery disease. N Engl J Med. 1979;300(24):1350–1358

48. Mahnken AH, Mühlenbruch G, Günther RW, Wildberger JE. Cardiac CT: coronary arteries and beyond. Eur Radiol. 2007;17(4):994–1008

49. Hachamovitch R, Hayes SW, Friedman JD, Cohen I, Berman DS. Comparison of the short-term survival benefit associated with revascularization compared with medical therapy in patients with no prior coronary artery disease undergoing stress myocardial perfusion single photon emission computed tomography. Circulation. 2003;107(23):2900–2907

50. Hachamovitch R, Kang X, Amanullah AM, et al. Prognostic implications of myocardial perfusion single-photon emission computed tomography in the elderly. Circulation. 2009;120(22):2197–2206

51. Schuijf JD, Wijns W, Jukema JW, et al. A comparative regional analysis of coronary atherosclerosis and calcium score on multislice CT versus myocardial perfusion on SPECT. J Nucl Med. 2006;47(11):1749–1755

52. Schuijf JD, Bax JJ. CT angiography: an alternative to nuclear perfusion imaging? Heart. 2008;94(3):255–257

53. Slomka PJ, Cheng VY, Dey D, et al. Quantitative analysis of myocardial perfusion SPECT anatomically guided by coregistered 64-slice coronary CT angiography. J Nucl Med. 2009;50(10):1621–1630

54. Ko SM, Seo JB, Hong MK, et al. Myocardial enhancement pattern in patients with acute myocardial infarction on two-phase contrast-enhanced ECG-gated multidetector-row computed tomography. Clin Radiol. 2006;61(5):417–422

55. Kato M, Dote K, Sasaki S, et al. Plain computed tomography for assessment of early coronary microcirculatory damage after revascularization therapy in acute myocardial infarction. Circ J. 2006;70(11):1475–1480

56. Wada H, Kobayashi Y, Yasu T, et al. Multi-detector computed tomography for imaging of subendocardial infarction: prediction of wall motion recovery after reperfused anterior myocardial infarction. Circ J. 2004;68(5):512–514

57. Kopp AF, Heuschmid M, Reimann A, et al. Evaluation of cardiac function and myocardial viability with 16- and 64-slice multidetector computed tomography. Eur Radiol. 2005;15(Suppl 4):D15–D20

58. Okada DR, Ghoshhajra BB, Blankstein R, et al. Direct comparison of rest and adenosine stress myocardial perfusion CT with rest and stress SPECT. J Nucl Cardiol. 2010;17(1):27–37

59. Ruzsics B, Schwarz F, Schoepf UJ, et al. Comparison of dual-energy computed tomography of the heart with single photon emission computed tomography for assessment of coronary artery stenosis and of the myocardial blood supply. Am J Cardiol. 2009;104(3):318–326

60. Achenbach S, Moselewski F, Ropers D, et al. Detection of calcified and noncalcified coronary atherosclerotic plaque by contrast-enhanced, submillimeter multidetector spiral computed tomography: a segment-based comparison with intravascular ultrasound. Circulation. 2004;109(1):14–17

61. Libby P. Current concepts of the pathogenesis of the acute coronary syndromes. Circulation. 2001;104(3):365–372

62. Virmani R, Kolodgie FD, Burke AP, Farb A, Schwartz SM. Lessons from sudden coronary death: a comprehensive morphological classification scheme for atherosclerotic lesions. Arterioscler Thromb Vasc Biol. 2000;20(5):1262–1275

63. Nikolaou K, Sagmeister S, Knez A, et al. Multidetector-row computed tomography of the coronary arteries: predictive value and quantitative assessment of non-calcified vessel-wall changes. Eur Radiol. 2003;13(11):2505–2512

64. Schroeder S, Kopp AF, Baumbach A, et al. Noninvasive detection and evaluation of atherosclerotic coronary plaques with multislice computed tomography. J Am Coll Cardiol. 2001;37(5):1430–1435

65. Schroeder S, Kuettner A, Leitritz M, et al. Reliability of differentiating human coronary plaque morphology using contrast-enhanced multislice spiral computed tomography: a comparison with histology. J Comput Assist Tomogr. 2004;28(4):449–454

66. Hoffmann U, Moselewski F, Nieman K, et al. Noninvasive assessment of plaque morphology and composition in culprit and stable lesions in acute coronary syndrome and stable lesions in stable angina by multidetector computed tomography. J Am Coll Cardiol. 2006;47(8):1655–1662

67. Pundziute G, Schuijf JD, Jukema JW, et al. Prognostic value of multislice computed tomography coronary angiography in patients with known or suspected coronary artery disease. J Am Coll Cardiol. 2007;49(1):62–70

68. Ferencik M, Chan RC, Achenbach S, et al. Arterial wall imaging: evaluation with 16-section multidetector CT in blood vessel phantoms and ex vivo coronary arteries. Radiology. 2006;240(3):708–716

69. Pohle K, Achenbach S, Macneill B, et al. Characterization of non-calcified coronary atherosclerotic plaque by multi-detector row CT: comparison to IVUS. Atherosclerosis. 2007;190(1):174–180

70. Lell MM, Anders K, Uder M, et al. New techniques in CT angiography. Radiographics. 2006;26(Suppl 1):S45–S62

71. Fishman EK, Ney DR, Heath DG, Corl FM, Horton KM, Johnson PT. Volume rendering versus maximum intensity projection in CT angiography: what works best, when, and why. Radiographics. 2006;26(3):905–922

72. Leschka S, Wildermuth S, Boehm T, et al. Noninvasive coronary angiography with 64-section CT: effect of average heart rate and heart rate variability on image quality. Radiology. 2006;241(2):378–385

73. Boll DT, Hoffmann MH, Huber N, Bossert AS, Aschoff AJ, Fleiter TR. Spectral coronary multidetector computed tomography angiography: dual benefit by facilitating plaque characterization and enhancing lumen depiction. J Comput Assist Tomogr. 2006;30(5):804–811

74. Machaalany J, Yam Y, Ruddy TD, et al. Potential clinical and economic consequences of noncardiac incidental findings on cardiac computed tomography. J Am Coll Cardiol. 2009;54(16):1533–1541

2

Technique, Protocols, Instrumentation, and Radiation Dose

Ethan J. Halpern

Technique is the major determinant of image quality for cardiac CT. Patient preparation before the examination, coaching of the patient during the examination, and appropriate CT technique are critical to image quality. Post-processing techniques may enhance the diagnostic information present in a suboptimal examination, but they cannot compensate for information that is lacking in an improperly performed examination. This chapter addresses technical aspects of the cardiac CT evaluation, including those aspects of imaging physics relevant to optimization of image quality and reduction of radiation dose—the practical "how-to" guide for cardiac CT.

◆ Patient Related Issues

Patient Preparation

A high-quality cardiac CT begins with proper patient preparation. To minimize ectopy in the cardiac rhythm, patients are asked to refrain from stimulants such as caffeine on the day of the examination. Solid foods should not be ingested for 4 hours before the study to reduce the risk of emesis. Liquid intake (water, milk, or juice) is encouraged up to 1 hour preceding the examination to maintain a well-hydrated patient before the administration of contrast.

A patient interview before the CT examination should include questions about prior treatment and/or interventions for coronary disease. The presence of bypass grafts or stents will impact the protocol used for the study. If the patient has a paced heart rhythm, temporary reprogramming of the pacemaker to a slower rate may be helpful to obtain high-quality images of the coronary arteries.

Each patient is questioned for a history of asthma, allergy to iodinated contrast material, or any history of a severe allergic reaction. β-blockers should be used with extreme caution in any patient with a history of asthma requiring treatment. Patients with a history of allergy to iodinated contrast should be pretreated with steroids to reduce the risk of an allergic reaction. A history of an anaphylactic reaction to iodinated contrast or other medication should serve as a red flag; contrast-enhanced studies should be performed in these patients only as an option of last resort. The protocol for steroid pre-medication at Thomas Jefferson University includes pretreatment with oral Medrol (methylprednisolone), 32 mg given 12 hours before the procedure and repeated again 2 hours before the procedure.

Intravenous Access

Adequate intravenous (IV) access is necessary to ensure delivery of a rapid, tight contrast bolus. An 18-gauge IV line in the antecubital fossa is preferred, although a 20-gauge line may suffice. Once the IV access is placed, the line should be tested with a rapid hand injection of saline to ascertain that there is no extravasation and that the patient does not experience pain with injection. The test injection of saline should simulate the rate of 5.0 to 5.5 mL/sec that will be required for the subsequent injection during CT angiography (CTA). Injections performed at this rate are often pressure limited when the IV line is smaller than 18 gauge.

To optimize the IV flow rate, the arm with the IV line should be positioned anterior to the patient rather than above the head. When an arm is extended above the head, the subclavian vein may be compressed under the clavicle with resultant obstruction of flow. Experience with evaluation of thoracic outlet compression shows that compression of venous structures is increased as the arm is extended further above the head.[1] Because the arm cannot be left down at the patient's side within the bore of the gantry, it should be positioned anterior to the patient in a vertical orientation where it can rest.

Patient Monitoring

To avoid artifact from electrocardiographic (ECG) leads, the two arm leads should be placed cephalad to the level of the heart; the left lower lead is placed in the region of the left midabdomen. Leads should be positioned in an area that is clean and free of hair to obtain good contact. An adequate

ECG tracing with clearly defined R-waves must be observed before proceeding. When necessary, the position of the ECG leads should be adjusted to optimize the ECG tracing.

A regular sinus rhythm is optimal for a gated cardiac examination. If the rhythm is irregular, the risks and benefits of the examination should be considered because an irregular rhythm is often associated with a suboptimal examination. When a coronary CTA examination is performed in a patient with an irregular rhythm, prospective ECG gating should not be used (see below).

A baseline blood pressure should be obtained before the administration of β-blockers. Monitoring of blood pressure and heart rate should continue during and after administration of β-blockers to document stable vital signs before discharge.

◆ Planning the Scan

Calcium Scoring Preceding Coronary CT Angiography

A low-dose, noncontrast calcium examination may be useful before coronary CTA is performed. The radiation exposure of a typical calcium study (about 1 mSv) is 10% of the dose associated with conventional helical coronary CTA.[2,3] The presence of heavy coronary calcification, specifically an Agatston-130 calcium score above 1000, is associated with reduced image quality and diagnostic accuracy on coronary CTA **(Figs. 2.1** and **2.2)**.[4] When an elevated calcium score above 1000 is identified before coronary CTA, the option of proceeding directly to cardiac catheterization should be considered because CTA is unlikely to exclude the presence of stenosis. In patients who do proceed to coronary CTA,

the calcium examination can be used to determine the proper superior and inferior endpoints for the coronary CTA study. The heart rate pattern during calcium scoring should also be evaluated because it may be predictive of the changes in rhythm that will be observed during coronary CTA. Calcium scoring is discussed in more detail in Chapter 5.

Scan Position

In-plane spatial resolution varies within the axial plane and is highest near the center of the CT gantry. For this reason, it is important to center the scan on the heart. Most cardiac scans are performed with a field of view of 22 to 25 cm. The heart should be centered within this field of view in both the left–right and anterior–posterior axes. In our protocol, centering of the heart is performed when the bolus-tracking region of interest is defined **(Fig. 2.3)**.

A basic coronary CTA scan should begin at about 2 cm above the most superior point in the left anterior descending artery and extend 1 to 2 cm below the cardiac apex **(Fig. 2.4)**. If a calcium scoring study is performed before coronary CTA, table positions for the CTA may be determined from the noncontrast calcium scoring images. If a calcium scoring study is not performed, coronary CTA should begin at the carina and extend 2 cm below the estimated lower margin of the heart on the topogram. When the ascending aorta is tortuous or the left heart border bulges superiorly, imaging should begin 1 to 2 cm above the carina to allow for a cranial angulation of the proximal left coronary artery (LCA).

In a patient with venous bypass grafts or radial artery grafts from the ascending aorta, CTA begins at the top of the aortic arch. When evaluating a patient with internal

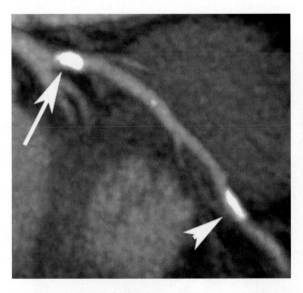

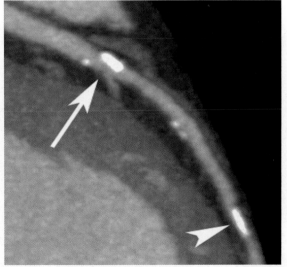

A **B**

Fig. 2.1 Mild coronary calcification with diagnostic-quality coronary CT angiography of the left anterior descending artery (LAD). **(A)** Maximum intensity projection (MIP) through the LAD demonstrates two areas of calcification, one at the origin of the vessel (*arrow*) and a second area more distally (*arrowhead*). The calcified plaque at the origin of the vessel obscures the entire lumen, and the more distal plaque results in approximately a 50% diameter narrowing. **(B)** Orthogonal MIP image through the LAD demonstrates that the proximal calcified plaque results in no more than 50% narrowing (*arrow*). In this projection, however, the more distal plaque appears to cover a larger portion of the vessel lumen. By combining the information from both images, one can conclude that there is no more than a 50% narrowing of the LAD. The absence of significant narrowing was confirmed at cardiac catheterization.

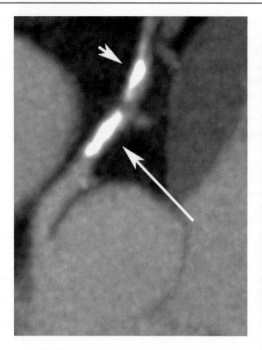
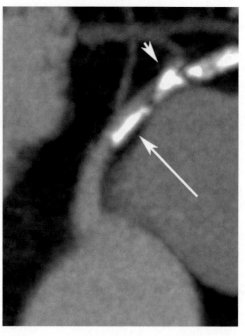

A

B

Fig. 2.2 Extensive coronary calcification limits the value of coronary CT angiography. **(A)** Maximum intensity projection (MIP) image of the left anterior descending artery demonstrates diffuse calcification in the proximal portion of the vessel (*large and small arrows*). The calcified plaques appear to obstruct much of the lumen of the vessel. **(B)** Orthogonal MIP image demonstrates that the more proximal calcified plaque (*large arrow*) results in less than 50% narrowing; the more distal calcification (*small arrow*) overlies the entire width of the vessel. Coronary angiography demonstrated less than 50% narrowing. Dense calcification is often associated with blooming artifact that causes plaque to appear larger than its true size and results in overestimation of stenosis.

mammary artery bypass grafts, the scan starts just above the level of the clavicles to include the origins of the internal mammary arteries. A "triple rule-out" scan usually begins just below the level of the clavicles to image the upper lobe pulmonary artery branches and the origins of the great vessels. The lower extent of the scan should extend just below the expected lower margin of the heart. In a patient with a gastroepiploic bypass graft, the scan should be extended further down into the abdomen to visualize the origin of this graft.

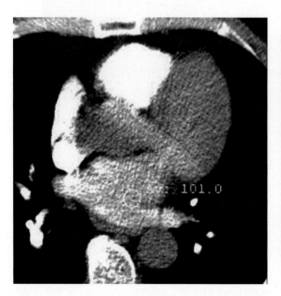
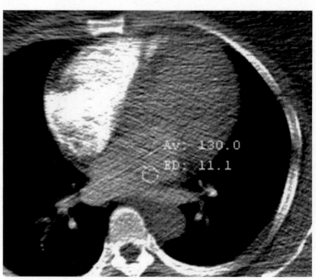

A

B

Fig. 2.3 Locator image for tracking of the injection bolus during coronary angiography. **(A)** Axial locator through the level of the left atrium demonstrates a region of interest along the left side of the left atrium. The region of interest is placed posteriorly and to the left so that the examination is not inadvertently triggered by contrast in the right side of the heart. **(B)** Axial locator with region of interest in the left atrium. The coronary angiogram is triggered when the contrast bolus arrives in the left atrium. After the scan is triggered, this system requires 5 seconds to begin the actual CT angiogram series. This additional short delay provides adequate time for full arterial enhancement of the aorta and coronary circulation.

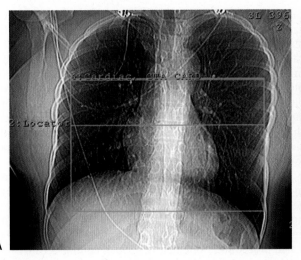
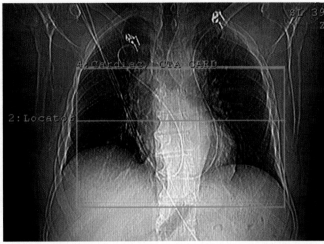

A   B

Fig. 2.4 Topogram for planning of coronary CT angiography. **(A)** Anteroposterior scout demonstrates the cardiac silhouette with the planned levels for coronary angiography. The superior extent of the scan is just above the carina. The inferior extent of the scan is 2 cm below the cardiac apex. The inferior extent is positioned to provide adequate coverage of the coronary circulation in the event that the patient takes a deeper breath during the angiographic phase of the study. The locator image that is used to monitor enhancement during the injection is positioned below the carina at the level of the left atrium. **(B)** Planned levels for coronary angiography in a patient with a tortuous ascending aorta. The superior extent of the scan is positioned slightly higher because the left anterior descending artery may course superiorly from its origin. The left-right centering places the heart in the center of the image.

It is important to realize that patient dose is proportional to the length of the scan. Patient dose is minimized by limiting the scan to the levels necessary to visualize the coronary arteries. The rationale for imaging above the coronaries and below the heart is to ensure that the coronary arteries are visualized in their entirety in the event that the inspiratory effort during the coronary CTA is different from the effort during the acquisition of the scout topogram or the calcium scoring study. Based on the Jefferson experience, the optimal starting and ending positions for coronary CTA include a 1–2 cm margin of error for respiratory variation.

◆ Optimizing Patient-Related Factors

Heart Rate

The ideal heart rate for this examination is regular sinus bradycardia in the range of 50 to 60 beats per minute. Regular sinus bradycardia is critical for single-source scanners with temporal resolution greater than 150 msec. Although this requirement may be relaxed for dual-source scanners with a temporal resolution of 75 to 83 msec and single-source scanners that acquire the entire coronary circulation in one or two cardiac cycles, a regular sinus bradycardia results in better image quality with all scanners. Even scans obtained with the most advanced equipment may be adversely impacted by a premature beat at an inopportune time during image acquisition.

Coronary CTA may be performed without pre-medication in a minority of patients who present with a stable sinus bradycardia. However, it is important to determine whether the observed sinus bradycardia actually represents a stable rhythm. Anxiety may result in elevation of an initially

favorable heart rate. Many patients will experience a sudden change in heart rate or rhythm while holding their breath or immediately after administration of IV contrast material. For the patient who presents in sinus bradycardia, stability of the heart rate should be confirmed on a continuous ECG tracing while speaking with the patient and practicing a breath-hold on the CT table before the study. Pre-medication should be administered to maintain stability of the rhythm for any patient who demonstrates heart rate variability before the study.

Various techniques have been advocated for controlling patient heart rate during cardiac CT. The generally preferred method is to administer a β-blocker to the patient before performing the study. The most commonly used β-blocker for cardiac CT, metoprolol, may be administered orally or intravenously. Metoprolol has a half-life of about 4 hours after IV administration and is relatively cardioselective at low doses.[5] The maximum effect of an orally administered dose might not be observed for an hour, whereas the maximum effect of an intravenously administered dose is apparent in 3 to 5 minutes.

For patients who cannot tolerate prolonged β-blockade, a fast-acting β-blocker with a short half-life is an option. Esmolol is an ultrashort-acting cardioselective IV β-blocker with a half-life of approximately 9 minutes.[6] Esmolol is administered as an IV bolus followed by an infusion. The effect of esmolol begins to wane almost immediately after the drug is discontinued. Unfortunately, maintaining a steady heart rate for cardiac CT with an esmolol infusion can be technically challenging because changes in the rate of infusion are associated with rapid changes in heart rate.

For the typical patient, metoprolol is administered either orally or intravenously. Oral administration requires pretreatment of the patient at least 1 hour before the examination. A 50-mg oral dose is well tolerated by most adults. If the reduction in heart rate is not sufficient with one dose, a second or third dose may be required. Because of variable absorption and sensitivity to this drug, it is difficult to predict *a priori* how long it will take to regulate the heart rate with oral metoprolol. To maintain a fixed patient schedule and to avoid long waiting times for our patients, IV administration of metoprolol is the preferred technique for control of heart rate at our institution. IV administration provides rapid regulation of heart rate that can be carefully monitored while the patient is placed on the CT table before the examination.

Regulation of the heart rate with IV metoprolol is usually accomplished within 5 to 10 minutes while the patient is on the CT table. To save time, administration of the IV β-blocker is performed during acquisition of the topogram, calcium scoring images, and tracker images that are obtained before coronary CTA. Patients who arrive with a heart rate in the range of 60 to 65 beats per minute are given an initial IV dose of 2.5 mg of metoprolol. Patients who arrive with a heart rate above 65 beats per minute are given an initial IV dose of 5 mg. After allowing several minutes to observe the effect of the first dose, additional doses of 5 mg are administered every 3 to 5 minutes until the target heart rate is achieved. Blood pressure is monitored after every dose to maintain a systolic blood pressure greater than 100 mm Hg. The maximum dose of IV metoprolol in my practice is 30 mg, although it is rare to administer more than 20 mg. If the heart rate has not decreased substantially with the first 15 to 20 mg, it is unlikely that further dosing will be beneficial.

When an oral β-blocker is given before coronary CTA, some centers prescribe 100 mg of metoprolol 1 hour before the examination. It is important to question the patient about any history of asthma, bradycardia, hypotension, or cocaine use before the β-blocker is prescribed. Ideally, a blood pressure should be obtained before metoprolol is prescribed. Although this dose is usually well tolerated, there is variation in patient sensitivity to the drug. Any patient who does not routinely take a β-blocker should be monitored after taking the oral dose because this medication can result in bradycardia, hypotension, and dizziness.

Asthma represents a relative contraindication to β-blockade. In a patient with mild asthma, the referring physician should be consulted to decide whether the patient may tolerate 5 or 10 mg of IV metoprolol before the examination. A higher dose should not be administered because the cardioselective action of metoprolol may be lost at higher doses, with the potential to cause an acute asthmatic reaction. Administration of a β-blocker in a patient who has recently used cocaine may predispose to coronary vasospasm and should therefore be avoided.

Calcium channel blockers may be considered as an alternative to β-blockers in an asthmatic patient or in the patient with atrial fibrillation. Diltiazem and verapamil suppress atrioventricular nodal function and, to a lesser extent, sinoatrial nodal function.[7] Unlike β-blockers, calcium channel blockers do not induce bronchospasm; however, they are not as effective in slowing down sinus rhythm. Calcium channel blockers are more effective than β-blockers in slowing the ventricular rate of a patient in atrial fibrillation. If a

calcium channel blocker is to be used for cardiac CT, diltiazem may be preferred because this drug demonstrates the least negative inotropic effect among the commonly used calcium channel blockers. Diltiazem may be given as an initial bolus of up to 0.25 mg/kg. Careful monitoring of blood pressure is advised when giving IV calcium channel blockers because these medications are potent vasodilators and tend to lower the blood pressure even more quickly than β-blockers. The combination of β-blockers with calcium channel blockers tends to cause an even more precipitous drop in blood pressure.

The protocol for IV administration of β-blockers presented in this chapter is somewhat more aggressive than that suggested by the prevailing literature.[8] Judicious IV administration of metoprolol and diltiazem with the patient in a supine position and with careful monitoring of the blood pressure is a safe procedure. Nonetheless, anyone administering IV β-blockers or calcium channel blockers should have training in cardiac resuscitation. A full discussion of the pharmacology of these drugs is beyond the scope of this chapter. Treatment of hypotension or bradycardia that results from administration of a β-blocker or calcium channel blocker should be titrated to the patient's blood pressure and mental status. Basic treatment for hypotension includes elevating the patient's legs and administering fluid to maintain blood pressure. Glucagon should be available for treatment of β-blocker overdose.[9] Calcium gluconate or calcium chloride should be available for treatment of overdose with a calcium channel blocker.[10] If these methods fail, more aggressive resuscitation with atropine and catecholamines may be required.[11]

Coronary Vasodilatation

Nitroglycerin is routinely administered to promote coronary vasodilatation during cardiac catheterization. Nitroglycerin spray is simple to administer and provides a metered dose of nitroglycerin that is rapidly absorbed. Sublingual nitroglycerin is also simple to administer. The vasodilatory effect on heart rate and blood pressure is usually evident within 2 minutes, with a maximum effect at 5 to 10 minutes. Administration of sublingual nitroglycerin before cardiac CT results in an average increase of 12 to 21% in the diameters of the proximal coronary arteries.[12] In addition to increasing the diameter of coronary arteries, pre-treatment with sublingual nitroglycerin increases the number of visualized coronary side branches.[13] Vasodilatation of the normal coronary artery will make the presence of nondistensible atherosclerotic plaque more obvious and can help to distinguish fixed lesions from arterial spasm.[14] Finally, the use of nigroglycerin may improve the diagnostic accuracy of coronary CTA.[15]

It is important to realize that the combination of nitroglycerin with a β-blocker may precipitate hypotension on the CT table. Furthermore, administration of nitroglycerin is associated with a reflex tachycardia and transiently increased variability of the heart rate, which may actually degrade image quality.[16] Using a conventional 64-slice CT scanner with a temporal resolution of 165 to 210 msec, the mild variation in heart rate caused by nitroglycerin can impact negatively on image quality. However, this variability of heart rate related to nitroglycerin is less of an issue in newer scanners with better temporal resolution.

Although there is a paucity of controlled trials to demonstrate the benefit of sublingual nitroglycerin prior to coronary CTA, our experience suggests that nitroglycerin is beneficial to coronary image quality. For this reason, our protocol includes sublingual nitroglycerin (800 mcg), administered on the CT table 2 to 3 minutes before the scan, provided the heart rate is well controlled, blood pressure is adequate, and the patient is not currently taking a phosphodiesterase inhibitor for erectile dysfunction.

◆ Optimizing Study Parameters

Contrast Injection

The goal of contrast injection for coronary CTA is to achieve a steady, high level of arterial enhancement (ie, >300 HU) during the examination. For a dedicated cardiac study, the goal is to achieve a high level of enhancement in the left heart and coronary arteries. A biphasic injection technique is used to clear dense contrast out of the superior vena cava during imaging of the coronary vessels to reduce streak artifact **(Fig. 2.5)**. For a triple rule-out study, the goal is to achieve sufficient contrast enhancement on both sides of the heart to allow simultaneous evaluation of the coronary

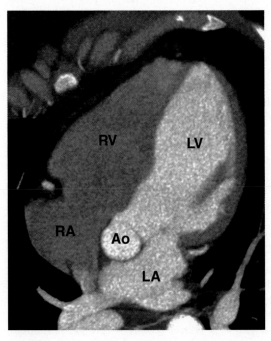

Fig. 2.5 Five-chamber view during coronary CT angiography demonstrates intense contrast opacification of the left atrium (LA) and left ventricle (LV) as well as the aortic root (Ao). The right atrium (RA) and right ventricle (RV) have been cleared of contrast by a saline flush, providing clear visualization of the right coronary artery as it courses in the right atrioventricular groove. The saline flush is useful for coronary angiography, but it should not be used for a "triple rule-out" scan during which the pulmonary artery must also be opacified.

and pulmonary arteries. Although some clinicians have described three-phase injection protocols, the two-phase techniques are simpler and generally adequate.

The volume and rate to be used for contrast injection depend on the scan time. As a general rule, the contrast injection time should be approximately 3 seconds longer than the scan time. Using a 16-detector system with a scan time of about 20 to 25 seconds, the duration of the contrast injection should be at least 25 seconds (100 mL at 4 mL/sec), followed by a saline flush (40 mL at 4 mL/sec). Using a 40-detector system with a scan time of about 15 seconds, the duration of the contrast injection should be at least 18 seconds (100 mL at 5.5 mL/sec), followed by a saline flush (40 mL at 4 mL/sec). Using a 64-detector system with a scan time of about 10 seconds, the duration of the contrast injection should be 13 seconds (70 mL at 5.5 mL/sec), followed by a saline flush (40 mL at 4 mL/sec). Using a 256-detector system with a scan time of 5 to 6 seconds, the duration of the contrast injection should be 8 to 9 seconds (50 mL at 5.5 mL/sec), followed by a saline flush (40 mL at 4 mL/sec). When evaluating a post-bypass patient with a 64-detector system, the contrast injection rate is reduced to 5 mL/sec to compensate for an increased scan time of 12 to 13 seconds that is required to include the origins of the bypass grafts.

When performing a triple rule-out study for coronary disease, dissection, and pulmonary embolism, a saline flush cannot be used because it would wash the contrast out of the pulmonary arteries. For these studies, the saline flush is replaced by a 1:1 dilution of contrast material with saline. Using a 64-detector system with a scan time of ~15 seconds, the duration of the contrast injection should be 14 seconds (70 mL at 5 mL/sec), followed by a second phase with dilute contrast (60 mL at 4 mL/sec). These injection protocols for helical coronary CTA are summarized in **Table 2.1**. A more detailed discussion of technique for triple rule-out studies is presented in Chapter 15. When imaging is performed with prospective ECG gating with a "step-and-shoot" technique, contrast volume may need to be adjusted to accommodate a slightly shorter or longer scan time, depending on the number of acquisition cycles ("steps") required in the step and shoot protocol.

The plateau level of enhancement obtained within the heart is related both to the rate of injection and to the iodine concentration used.[17] To increase the level of arterial enhancement, one may increase either the rate of contrast injection or the iodine concentration in the contrast material. Based on pressure limitations, an injection rate above 5 to 6 mL/sec is often not possible. The maximum iodine concentration currently available for contrast material in the United States is 350 mg/mL. European studies have demonstrated better arterial enhancement with a concentration of 400 mg/mL.[18,19]

Scan Timing

To obtain diagnostic quality coronary CTA, it is important that the CTA scan be performed during the peak of contrast enhancement in the coronary arteries. Several different

Table 2.1 Contrast Injection Protocols: Biphasic Injection

	First phase	Second phase (mL at 4 mL/sec)	Second phase
Basic coronary CTA (16-slice system)	100cc @ 4cc/sec	40	Saline
Basic coronary CTA (40-slice system)	100cc @ 5.5cc/sec	40	Saline
Basic coronary CTA (64-slice system)	75cc @ 5.5cc/sec	40	Saline
Post-bypass CTA (64-slice system)	80cc @ 5 cc/sec	40	Saline
Triple rule-out study (64-slice system)	70cc @ 5cc/sec	60	50:50 mixture of contrast and saline
Basic coronary CTA (256-slice system)	50cc @ 5.5cc/sec	40 mL	Saline
Modification for prospective electrocardiographic gating	Alter contrast volume as needed to accommodate increased or decreased scan time based on heart rate and the number of "steps" in the acquisition		

Abbreviations: CTA, computed tomographic angiography.

algorithms are available for determining when to start the scan. The time required for the contrast to travel from the arm to the right side of the heart varies substantially from one individual to another (usually 5–10 seconds) and from the right side of the heart to the left side of the heart (usually 4–6 seconds). The time delay from the right side to the left side of the heart may be considerably longer in patients with pulmonary hypertension or left-sided heart failure. Thus, it is not possible simply to initiate the scan at a set time delay after injection. However, in almost all patients, enhancement of the aorta and coronary vessels occurs within 2 to 3 seconds after contrast reaches the left atrium. Timing of coronary CTA may be based on a test injection that determines the delay between injection in the arm and peak opacification of the left heart, or by the use of a dynamic bolus tracking algorithm to initiate image acquisition immediately after contrast has opacified the left side of the heart and aorta.

Our protocol utilizes the bolus tracking technique, which requires only one injection (no test injection), minimizes the contrast load to the patient, and is quicker to perform. Low-dose bolus tracking scans are performed over the left atrium every other second, beginning 5 seconds after the start of the contrast injection (**Fig. 2.3**). The coronary CTA study is triggered to begin about 5 seconds after the contrast material has begun to opacify the left atrium. This delay of 5 seconds after the time of triggering allows the scanner to be repositioned from the left atrium to a position just above the coronary arteries, where the CT angiogram will begin. Furthermore, the 5 second delay allows the level of contrast enhancement in the coronary arteries to increase to a peak plateau level.

For the protocols summarized in **Table 2.1**, the injection time is typically 3 seconds longer than the CTA scan time. However, the coronary CTA scan begins 5 seconds after the contrast reaches the left heart. Although one might expect to run out of contrast before the end of the scan, the contrast bolus spreads out temporally by the time it reaches the left side of the heart so that left-sided opacification is maintained for the entire length of the coronary CTA. The degree of temporal spreading of the contrast bolus is related to

cardiac function, but even in patients with normal function the bolus usually spreads out to provide left-sided enhancement that lasts several seconds longer than the injection time.

Breath-hold

The cardiac examination must be performed during suspended respiration to eliminate motion. However, the patient should be instructed not to take a large breath because the negative intrathoracic pressure resulting from a sudden, large inspiratory effort will draw unopacified blood from the inferior vena cava into the heart. The optimum inspiratory effort is a small to medium-size breath taken slowly over 2 to 3 seconds. It is important to practice the breath-hold technique with the patient before performing the actual scan. The practice run provides the patient with a general idea of how large an inspiratory effort is required and how long inspiration will be suspended. The patient should be warned about a warm sensation and a possible feeling of nausea during the administration of contrast material. The patient should be instructed to remain still without moving or breathing during the scan.

Scan Parameters

The output capability of multidetector roentgen tubes has increased dramatically over the past few years as a result of technical improvements in tube design and cooling. Several years ago most scanners came with a peak tube capacity of 500 mA at 120 kVp. Newer scanners have tubes that can provide a sustained tube current of 1000 mA at 120kVp, allowing for thin-slice imaging of large patients. The effective milliamperes for the scan are computed as the tube current measured in milliamperes multiplied by the rotation time for 360 degrees, divided by the pitch. A typical-size patient scanned at a tube kilovoltage setting of 120 kVp will require 600 mA to image the coronary arteries with

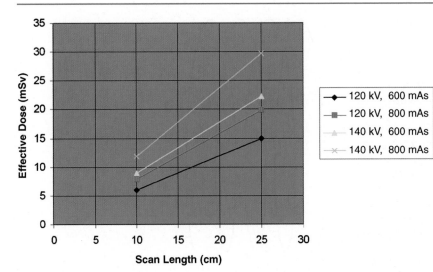

Fig. 2.6 Using CT angiography, the relationship of an effective patient dose as measured in milliSieverts (mSv) to tube current (mA), voltage (kVp), and scan length for the Brilliance CT 64-channel unit (Philips Medical Systems, Cleveland, OH) using a conventional retrospectively gated helical acquisition is shown. A linear relationship exists between effective dose and both scan length and milliamperes. The relationship of dose to peak kilovoltage is exponential. The effective patient dose is cut by almost 50% with electrocardiographically (ECG)-pulsed tube-current modulation and may be reduced by 75 to 80% with a prospective ECG-triggered acquisition (not shown in this graph). (Calculations and figure courtesy of Eric Gingold, PhD, Thomas Jefferson University.)

0.5- to 0.6-mm slice thickness. For heavier patients, the milliamperes or peak kilovoltage will need to be increased to prevent a noise-limited scan. Noise is proportional to the reciprocal of the square root of the milliamperes. Patient dose is proportional to milliamperes.

Whereas the tube current (mA) controls the number of roentgen photons created, the voltage applied across the tube (kVp) determines the peak energy of the roentgen photons. Traditionally, most coronary scans are performed at 120 kVp. The effective energy is generally about half of this value. For very heavy patients or patients with heavily calcified or stented vessels, peak kilovoltage may be increased to 140. The higher peak kilovoltage is associated with better radiographic penetration and decreased blooming artifact from calcium and stents. Thus, a higher peak kilovoltage (at constant milliamperes) will allow more roentgens to reach the detectors and will reduce image noise. However, it is important to remember that patient dose is exponentially related to peak kilovoltage. Theoretically, a higher peak kilovoltage may decrease image contrast. The lower contrast obtained at a higher peak kilovoltage is not usually detrimental for coronary angiography so long as there is ample contrast material within the coronary arteries, although a higher peak kilovoltage may reduce sensitivity for detection of subtle findings on myocardial perfusion imaging (Chapter 16).

There is a clear trade-off between image noise and patient dose. Image noise can be decreased by using higher values of milliamperes and kilovoltage. These higher values may be useful in obese patients. However, this improvement in image quality comes at the expense of radiation dose **(Fig. 2.6)**. A typical cardiac scan performed in helical mode with retrospective ECG gating using 600 mA at120 kVp will result in an exposure of approximately 10 mSv.[20,21] However, the exposure can be twice as high if these parameters are increased to 800 mA at 140 kVp. In thin patients, both the mA and kVp can be reduced to minimize dose. Several studies suggest that cardiac CT imaging may be obtained routinely with a kVp of 80 to 100 when using adaptive iterative techniques for image reconstruction (see section

on dose-reduction techniques). As a general rule, coronary CTA should be performed with the lowest dose (kVp and mA) that will provide diagnostic images.

The pitch of a multidetector scanner is the table travel distance per gantry rotation divided by the total beam collimation **(Fig. 2.7)**. Conversely, the z-axis coverage = pitch × beam collimation × number of gantry rotations. Thus, z-axis coverage and pitch will determine the scan time for a coronary CTA examination. For conventional cardiac scanning with a helical approach, the pitch is generally set in the range of 0.2 to 0.3. Scanners with faster gantry rotations times (<300 msec) typically use a slightly lower pitch of 0.14 to 0.2. Although some systems allow the operator to modify the pitch to adjust the scan time, this parameter is usually adjusted automatically for heart rate. A complex relationship exists between pitch and temporal resolution, depending on the heart rate and speed of gantry rotation.[22] Automated algorithms adjust the pitch to optimize temporal resolution for the heart rate detected during ECG gating.

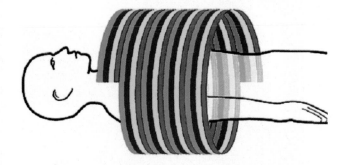

Fig. 2.7 Multidetector CT data acquisition and pitch. Image acquisition is demonstrated for a four-detector scanner at a pitch of 1.0. The four detectors are symbolized by the green, blue, yellow, and red rings that surround the patient. At a pitch of 1.0, the patient advances through the scanner such that the adjacent rings of the helix are immediately contiguous without an overlap. Cardiac CT is typically performed with many more detectors and with a pitch of 0.2 that provides substantial overlap between the adjacent rings of acquisition.

◆ Temporal Resolution

Single-Cycle Reconstruction

Temporal resolution refers to the time required to acquire the data for a single CT image. The temporal resolution of a CT scanner with a single radiographic source is approximately half the gantry rotation time, typically 165 to 210 msec for most 64-slice scanners (**Fig. 2.8**). Unfortunately, the coronary arteries will move several millimeters during this time, resulting in a blurred image. To compensate for this cardiac motion, ECG gating is used in combination with β-blockers to image the coronary arteries during quiescent phases of the cardiac cycle. ECG gating is based on detection of sequential R-waves that are used to mark the beginning of systole in each cardiac cycle.

With a heart rate below 65 beats per minute, the most quiescent portion of the cycle is generally mid-diastole. Thus, data acquired in mid-diastole will present the best image quality. However, as the heart rate accelerates, there is selective shortening of diastole such that the most quiescent phase may occur at end systole or early diastole.[23] Empirically, the optimal time for imaging of the LCA and its branches is at about 70 to 80% of the R-R interval. The optimal time for imaging the right coronary artery (RCA) is frequently at the 70 to 80% phase, but RCA anatomy is more clearly demonstrated in end systole in about 50% of patients (**Fig. 2.9**).[24] Although research has focused on automatic determination of the optimal image phase for reconstruction,[25,26] images from multiple phases of the cardiac cycle are required in up to 25% of clinical

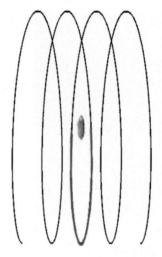

Fig. 2.8 Reconstruction of an image requires data acquisition through 180 degrees of detector rotation (indicated in color). Temporal resolution is limited by the time required for 180 degrees of gantry rotation.

cases imaged with a single-source multislice scanner for optimal assessment of both the LCA and RCA.

Multicycle Reconstruction

For a CT scanner with a gantry rotation time of 330 msec, temporal resolution will be 165 msec. When the heart rate is in the range of 50 to 60 beats per minutes, the quiescent

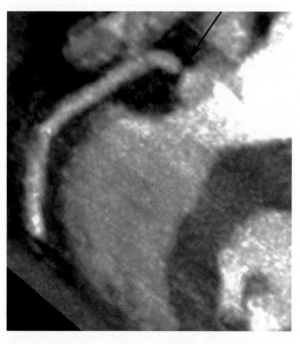

A

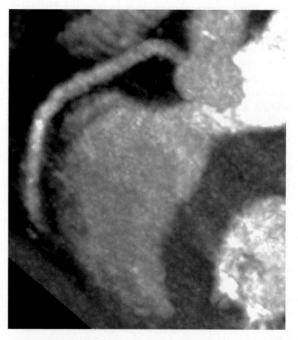

B

Fig. 2.9 Phase artifact mimicking high-grade stenosis in the right coronary artery. **(A)** Maximum intensity projection of the right coronary artery (RCA) obtained at 70% of the R-R interval suggests the presence of a band-like high-grade stenosis at the RCA origin (*arrow*).

(B) Reconstruction of the same vessel during the late systolic phase at 40% of the R-R interval demonstrates a patent RCA with no significant stenosis. The apparent stricture demonstrated in the diastolic image is related to cardiac motion during this phase of reconstruction.

phase in mid-diastole is sufficiently long to allow acquisition of a complete image during a single cardiac cycle. However, as the heart rate rises, the length of diastole is shortened and the quiescent period may be shorter than the temporal resolution of the scanner. To accommodate for this, helical scan data may be pooled from multiple adjacent cardiac cycles rather than from a single cardiac cycle. Conventional helical cardiac CTA with a pitch of 0.2 to 0.3 acquires overlapping data such that individual axial images may be reconstructed from multiple adjacent cardiac cycles. Temporal resolution may be improved by a factor of 2 when half the data for image reconstruction are obtained from each of two adjacent cycles. If the data are obtained from four adjacent cycles, the temporal resolution may be improved by up to a factor of 4 (**Fig. 2.10**). This process, referred to as *multicycle reconstruction*, can result in a significant improvement in image quality.[27]

Multicycle reconstruction provides an advantage of improved temporal resolution. However, because the images are obtained from multiple cycles, this technique must assume that the heart is in exactly the same position in each subsequent heartbeat. If there is a slight variation in heart rate, the position of the coronary arteries may change during a particular part of the cycle, resulting in blurring of the image. Thus, multicycle reconstruction will provide improved images as long as the heart rate is stable. Multicycle reconstruction in a patient with a variable heart rate will provide blurred images. Most CT scanners will automatically

choose multicycle reconstruction and will automatically determine the number of cycles to combine for a single CT slice based on patient heart rate. However, the operator may choose to override the option for multicycle reconstruction in a patient with a variable heart rate.

Improving Temporal Resolution: Gantry Rotation Speed versus Dual-Source CT

Temporal resolution is clearly a major limiting factor in cardiac CT. Although temporal resolution is improved with multicycle reconstruction, variability in heart rate may limit the usefulness of this technique. Furthermore, since CT image reconstruction requires 180° of x-ray attenuation data, multicycle reconstruction becomes inefficient when the heart rate and gantry rotation speed are in phase such that overlapping arcs of data are acquired in consecutive cycles. When using multicycle reconstruction, a lower pitch increases the number of cycles per voxel, thereby improving temporal resolution. To obtain maximal temporal resolution with multicycle reconstruction for a given heart rate, gantry rotation speed and pitch can be optimized to ensure that the gantry rotation is out of phase with respect to the heart rate. The optimal gantry rotation speed for multicycle reconstruction should minimize the time required to acquire 180° of data during consecutive cardiac cycles.

One obvious method to improve temporal resolution without multicycle reconstruction is to increase the gantry rotation speed. Conventional 64-slice scanners provide a gantry rotation time in the range of 330 to 420 msec. Newer commercial scanners are now available with gantry rotation times as fast as 270 msec. Gantry rotation speed is limited by technical issues, including the high centripetal force generated by rapid gantry rotation, the need to minimize wobble of the roentgen tube in the z-axis, the need to deliver a sufficient radiographic radiation dose in a short interval to achieve adequate image quality, and the speed with which detector data can be acquired and downloaded.

Dual-source CT represents another approach to improve temporal resolution while acquiring each CT slice during a single cardiac cycle. The first commercial dual-source CT uses two roentgen tubes oriented at 90 degrees to each other, reducing temporal resolution to 82.5 msec at a gantry rotation time of 330 msec based on conventional single-cycle reconstruction.[28] The combination of multicycle dual-segment reconstruction with this dual-source scanner provides a mean temporal resolution of 60 msec (minimum temporal resolution of 42 msec), yielding excellent image quality even with elevated heart rates and potentially eliminating the need for administration of a β-blocker.[29] A second-generation dual-source scanner now provides temporal resolution of 75 msec based on conventional single-cycle reconstruction. As temporal resolution is improved, the impact of premature or ectopic beats on image quality is less of an issue. Functional evaluation of heart valves and myocardium is also facilitated by improved image quality throughout the cardiac cycle with better temporal resolution. Finally, faster temporal resolution may provide a reduction

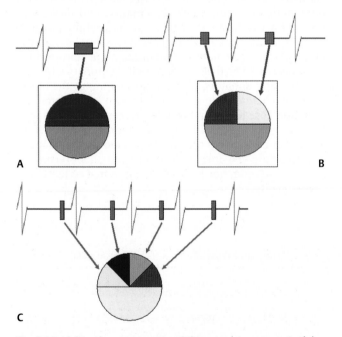

Fig. 2.10 Multicycle reconstruction. **(A)** Image data are acquired during a single heartbeat for single-cycle reconstruction. Temporal resolution equals the time required to acquire data from 180 degrees of gantry rotation. **(B)** Double-cycle reconstruction acquires 180 degrees of data from two consecutive heartbeats. Only 90 degrees of data are acquired in each cycle, resulting in up to a twofold improvement in temporal resolution. **(C)** Four-cycle reconstruction requires 45 degrees of data acquisition during each cardiac cycle, resulting in up to a fourfold improvement in temporal resolution.

in radiation dose by allowing a smaller pulsing window with prospective ECG gating. Limitations of this technique may be related to the additional weight of two roentgen tubes in the gantry that may limit maximum gantry rotation speeds and the additional cost of using two sets of roentgen tubes and detectors. Finally, special techniques must be used to reduce the impact of cross-scatter radiation between the two tubes to maintain the stability of CT density measurements and image quality across the image.

◆ Dose-Reduction Techniques (Table 2.2)

Tube-Current Modulation

ECG-pulsed tube-current modulation was the first widely available dose-reduction technique for retrospectively gated helical coronary CTA. In the patient with a regular sinus bradycardia, the optimal phase for reconstruction of coronary CTA images is nearly always in mid-diastole. With ECG-pulsed tube-current modulation, roentgen generation is modulated such that the peak milliamperes are delivered only during a predetermined phase of the cardiac cycle, usually corresponding to mid-diastole. The typical dose reduction if peak milliamperes is delivered only during mid-diastole is dependent on heart rate, but it approaches 50%.[30] One study described dose reduction of as much as 88% for thin patients without loss of image quality by lowering the kilovoltage setting to 80 kVp in combination with ECG-pulsed tube-current modulation.[31] A more recent study measured a 47% dose reduction with ECG-pulsed tube-current modulation and achieved a mean effective dose of 5.3 mSv by combining ECG-pulsed tube-current modulation with a reduced tube voltage of 100 kVp.[32] A major advantage of ECG-pulsed tube-current modulation over newer dose savings techniques described below is the ability to image cardiac function throughout the cycle. Although the tube current in systole is reduced below a level that would allow adequate signal-to-noise for coronary imaging, the tube current remains sufficient throughout the cardiac cycle to provide imaging of myocardial motion. Furthermore, if the heart rate changes during the scan, tube-current modulation often allows sufficient leeway to alter the phase of reconstruction to a slightly earlier or later phase in diastole. Finally, if there is an arrhythmia during the scan, the scan can continue with automatic cancellation of tube-current modulation for the remainder of the acquisition. When tube-current modulation is applied during the incorrect phase of the cardiac cycle as the result of a premature or ectopic beat, the error can often be corrected by ECG editing (see next section).

Prospective Electrocardiographic Gating "Step-and-Shoot"

Newer scanning techniques have been developed that provide greater dose savings compared with ECG-pulsed tube-current modulation. These techniques reduce the imaging redundancy that is typical in a conventional low-pitch single-source helical CTA scan. The nonhelical "step-and-shoot" technique uses axial imaging during diastole, with prospective ECG gating to turn the roentgen tube on only during a short interval in mid-diastole when optimal coronary imaging is performed. The prospective gating technique analyzes the ECG to predict the duration of diastole and the time of the next R-wave. The roentgen tube is activated, and imaging is performed only during the short interval that is predicted to correspond to mid-diastole. In patients with a relatively regular cardiac rhythm, prospective ECG gating can provide image quality and diagnostic performance equivalent to that of the more conventional retrospectively gated helical approach.[33] Coronary CTA with the step-and-shoot axial technique can image the entire coronary circulation in a 12-cm scan with a mean effective radiation dose just over 4 mSv.[34,35] A recent comparison of helical coronary CTA with tube-current modulation versus axial step-and-shoot coronary CTA demonstrated a mean effective dose of 4.3 mSv for the step-and-shoot technique (a 79% dose reduction) with only a minimal reduction in image quality.[36]

Table 2.2 Dose-Reduction Techniques

Technique	Helical/Axial	Functional data	Arrhythmia correction	Typical dose
Tube current modulation	Helical	Yes	Flexible window during diastole	7–8 mSv
Prospective electrocardiographic gating (triggering)	Axial	No	Real time; must repeat slice	4–4.5 mSv
High-pitch helical scanning	Helical	No	Not possible	1–2 mSv
Statistical iterative reconstruction	Both	In helical mode	Yes	32–65% dose reduction
Pre-patient Z-collimation	Both	In helical mode	Yes	
Anatomic-based tube current modulation	Axial	No	Yes	

A major limitation of prospective ECG gating is the lack of image data in phases of the cardiac cycle, other than the small interval used for coronary imaging. High-resolution imaging of cardiac function and valve motion requires data from the entire cardiac cycle and cannot be obtained when prospective ECG gating is used to limit radiation exposure to mid-diastole. At least one vendor allows a hybrid acquisition that combines prospective tube-current modulation with step-and-shoot axial imaging to allow functional imaging with a step-and-shoot technique. With this hybrid technique, each axial acquisition is extended to include a complete cardiac cycle, but the full tube current is applied only during a short period in mid-diastole. Although the radiation dose with the hybrid technique is greater than

pure prospective ECG triggering in mid-diastole, the hybrid technique allows reconstruction of functional images throughout the cardiac cycle.

A second limitation of prospective ECG gating is loss of image quality as a result of changes in heart rate or arrhythmia. Because each cycle of the study is an independent axial acquisition, demarcation lines are often visible between the individual steps of a step-and-shoot acquisition and may be associated with step-off artifacts in the coronary arteries. When an R-wave arrives earlier than expected, the scan at that particular level may be obtained during systole and demonstrate blurring caused by systolic cardiac motion (**Fig. 2.11**). It is possible to allow for a certain degree of "phase tolerance" in prospective ECG triggering by irradiating a

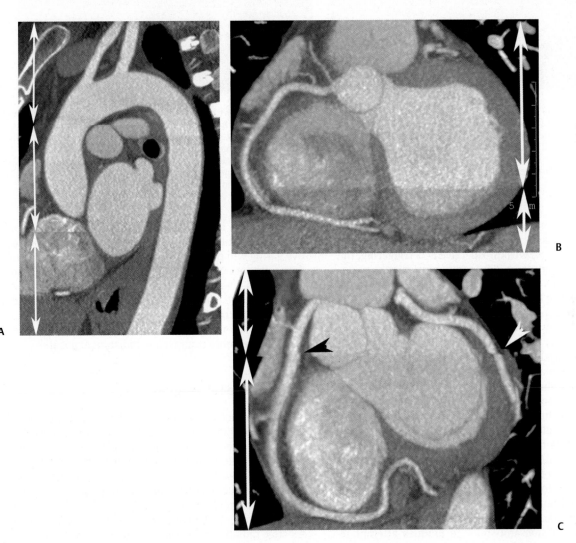

Fig. 2.11 Artifacts related to prospective electrocardiographic (ECG) gating. **(A)** Slab maximum intensity projection (MIP) of the thoracic aorta from a scan obtained on a 256-slice scanner. This MIP was reconstructed from a three-cycle acquisition using prospective ECG gating with "step-and-shoot" axial technique. The upper, middle, and lower thirds of the image are imaged as three independent axial acquisitions (*arrows*), and subtle lines are visible at the junctions of these acquisitions. **(B)** Left anterior oblique (LAO) MIP projection of the right

coronary artery (RCA) from a scan obtained on a 256-slice scanner. Two cycles are demonstrated (*arrows*) in this image, with a clear line of demarcation between the cycles. The level of contrast opacification is decreased in the second cycle, which was acquired two heartbeats after the first cycle. **(C)** LAO MIP projection from a scan obtained on a 256-slice scanner. Two cycles are demonstrated (*arrows*). A step-off is visible in the RCA (*black arrowhead*) and the circumflex artery (*white arrowhead*) at the junction of the two cycles.   (*Continued on page 36*)

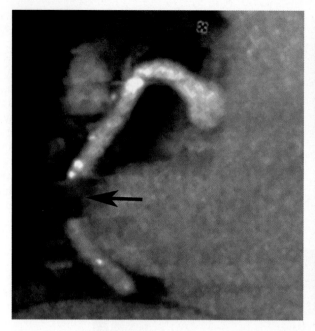

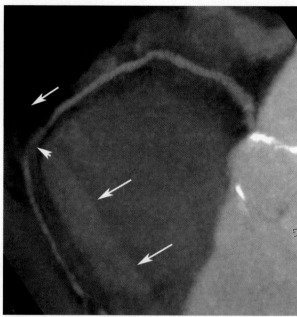

D

E

Fig. 2.11 (*Continued*) Artifacts related to prospective electrocardio-graphic (ECG) gating. **(D)** MIP projection of the RCA obtained on a 16-slice scanner. A segment in the mid- to distal portion of the RCA appears absent (*arrow*). This segment is sharply defined and corresponds to a single premature ventricular contraction during data acquisition with a 16-detector scanner. The individual cycles in this acquisition have a much shorter z-axis coverage compared with the 256-slice scanner. Many more cycles are required for imaging, thus increasing the likelihood of artifact related to a change in rhythm between cycles. **(E)** Image of the RCA in a different patient with a 16-detector scanner demonstrates a sharply demarcated blurred segment of the mid- to distal RCA associated with a linear artifact traversing the soft tissues (*arrows*). A single premature atrial contraction shortened the cardiac cycle and resulted in blurring of a segment of the RCA (*arrowhead*).

wider phase of the cardiac cycle, but phase tolerance results in a marked increase in radiation exposure. To achieve a phase tolerance of 5% with prospective ECG triggering, the wider window results in a 70% increase in radiation exposure, although this exposure is still lower than the traditional retrospective ECG gating.

Compared with retrospectively gated scans, prospective ECG triggering may result in a higher rate of nondiagnostic imaging, especially at higher heart rates or in the presence of an irregular rhythm. The likelihood of artifact related to arrhythmia within a prospective ECG-gated scan is proportional to the number of individual cycles required for the study acquisition and is therefore inversely related to detector length (or the number of slices). With helical scans, the anatomy of a single level may be retrospectively reconstructed from different phases of the cardiac cycle, or even from different cardiac cycles, to compensate for changes in cardiac rhythm or for errors in ECG gating (see next section). The options for ECG editing and to reconstruct images from additional phases are limited with prospective ECG gating. Newer intelligent algorithms incorporated into prospective axial step-and-shoot techniques attempt to overcome this limitation by recognizing ectopic beats in real time and rescanning the same level during the next normal beat before moving to the next level. In the setting of a sustained arrhythmia, however, these techniques remain inferior to retrospective ECG gating.

The decision about whether to use prospective ECG gating with axial aquisition or retrospectively gated helical coronary CTA in a particular patient is not to be taken lightly. In a patient with regular sinus bradycardia, prospective gating will provide a substantial reduction in radiation dose without loss of image quality. However, when there is a substantial variation in cardiac rate or rhythm immediately before the coronary CTA, prospective gating should be avoided. An error in prospective gating can render the entire examination nondiagnostic and can force a repeat study requiring yet more contrast and radiation exposure.

High-Pitch Spiral Imaging

A recent method introduced to speed up coronary CTA and reduce dose is high-pitch spiral acquisition. The relatively low pitch used in conventional coronary CTA entails substantial redundancy in data acquisition, providing functional data over the entire cardiac cycle, allowing for multi-cycle reconstruction of coronary anatomy and providing the ability to correct retrospectively any ECG gating errors. Unfortunately, the low pitch also results in a relatively high effective radiation dose. Even when scans are acquired with prospective ECG triggering using step-and-shoot mode, there is an overlap between sequential axial acquisitions, which is needed to accommodate the cone beam reconstruction algorithms used in multidetector CT. In a high-pitch helical mode, this redundancy is eliminated such that the entire acquisition is performed in a "flash spiral" during the diastolic phase of a single heartbeat. To date, this technique has been implemented for commercial purposes only with dual-source CT for patients with a relatively stable bradycardia (<60 beats/min).[37] Early clinical studies have demonstrated promising image quality with this technique, with effective radiation doses in the range of 1 to 2 mSv.[38,39] Because this technique employs a single, continuous helical acquisition, there are no step artifacts between individual axial scans as might be seen with a prospectively triggered step-and-shoot technique. Furthermore, because the acquisition takes place with a rapid temporal resolution of 75 msec during a single heartbeat, the technique requires only a single adequate diastolic phase for acquisition and is less likely to be impacted by an arrhythmia. It is likely that future variations of this technique will be applied to other commercial scanners.

Iterative Reconstruction Algorithms

The most basic method for reducing radiation dose is to reduce the output of the roentgen tube.[40] However, scans obtained at lower milliampers and peak kilovoltage will have a lower signal-to-noise ratio and will appear noisy. Iterative reconstruction algorithms provide one option for reducing image noise with low milliampere/peak kilovolt settings (**Figs. 2.12** and **2.13**). These algorithms use initial estimates of voxel attenuation to predict projection data; estimates of voxel attenuation are iteratively adjusted to minimize the difference between the predicted projection data and the measured projection data. Iterative techniques have traditionally been used for image reconstruction from

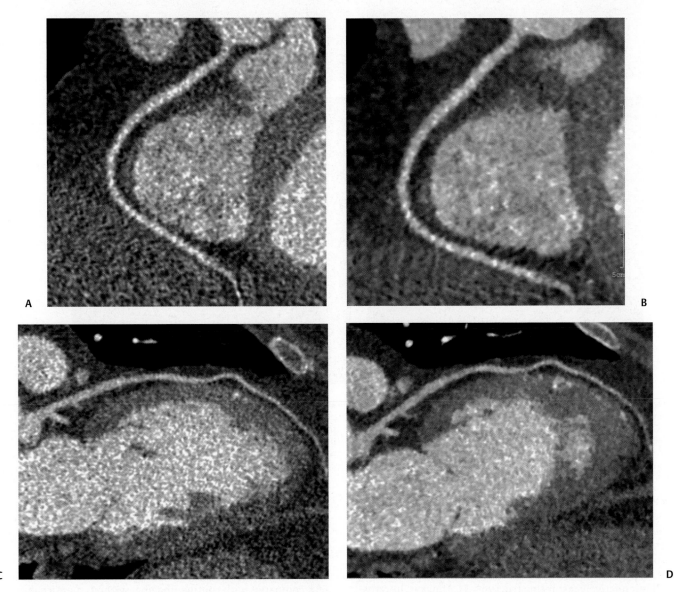

Fig. 2.12 Iterative reconstruction of the right coronary artery (RCA) and left anterior descending artery (LAD) in an obese patient. **(A)** Curved thin-slab maximum intensity projection (MIP) of the RCA with reconstruction using standard filtered back projection. **(B)** Similar curved thin-slab MIP of the RCA using an iterative reconstruction technique demonstrates a reduction in image noise. **(C)** Curved thin-slab MIP of the LAD with reconstruction using standard filtered back projection. **(D)** Similar curved thin-slab MIP of the LAD using an iterative reconstruction technique demonstrates a reduction in image noise.

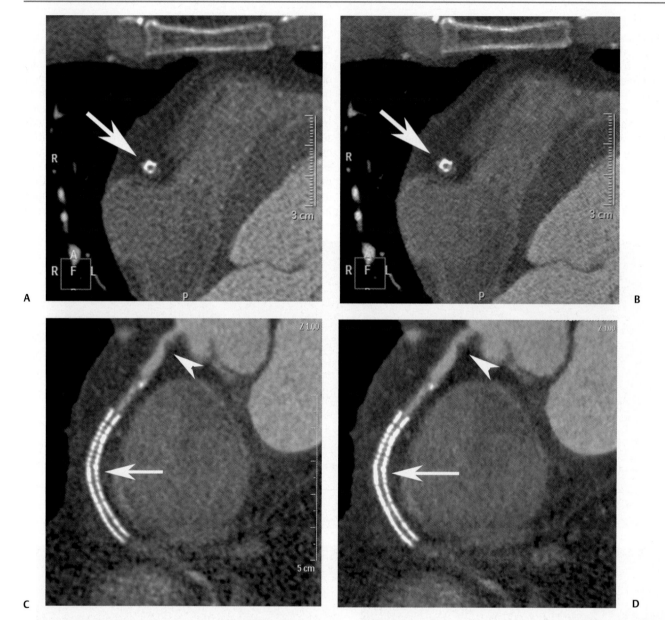

Fig. 2.13 Iterative reconstruction of an occluded stent within the mid-right coronary artery (RCA) of an obese patient. **(A)** Axial image of the RCA stent (*arrow*) with reconstruction using standard filtered back projection. **(B)** Axial image from the same examination processed with an iterative reconstruction technique demonstrates a reduction in image noise and slightly sharper definition of the stent. **(C)** Curved thin-slab MIP of the RCA using standard filtered back projection demonstrates proximal plaque (*arrowhead*) and occlusion of the stent in the mid-RCA (*arrow*). **(D)** Curved thin-slab MIP from the same examination processed with an iterative reconstruction technique demonstrates a reduction in image noise with improved delineation of the noncalcified plaque in the proximal RCA.

raw data in the data projection space, but techniques have been developed to use iterative methods in the image space domain as well. Statistical modeling or maximum likelihood estimates have recently been used to guide the iterative reconstruction process. Most current CT scanners use a reconstruction method known as *filtered-back projection*, which allows relatively fast reconstruction of CT images. Iterative reconstruction algorithms for creating CT images were used with early CT scanners but are more computationally intensive compared with filtered-back projection. Recent advances in computer hardware and software design have resulted in a resurgence of interest in iterative reconstruction algorithms for CT images.[41] Iterative reconstruction techniques provide signal-to-noise ratios that are superior to filtered-back projection without loss of spatial resolution.[42] A recent phantom and in vivo study of one iterative reconstruction technique demonstrated dose reductions of 32 to 65% compared with routine imaging, without a noticeable increase in image noise.[43] Clinical trials are needed to determine whether iterative reconstruction techniques can provide equivalent diagnostic image quality with reduced radiation exposure.

Additional Dose-Reduction Measures

Additional techniques that have been applied to reduce radiation dose include improved filtration of the roentgen beam, pre-patient Z-collimation, and anatomic-based tube-current modulation. Overscanning in the z-axis occurs when radiographic exposure includes portions of the patient that lie outside the planned scan length. Dynamic Z-collimation may be introduced at the beginning and at the end of an acquisition to limit exposure to the region of interest. Anatomic-based tube-current modulation can be used in cardiovascular imaging to optimize tube current based on the thickness of tissue that must be traversed by the roentgen as the tube rotates around the patient.[44] This technique can also be used to minimize exposure to specific areas such as the breast tissue of a woman.[45] Unfortunately, this technique interferes with ECG-based tube-current modulation in helical acquisitions. However, anatomic-based tube-current modulation may be applicable in combination with prospective ECG-triggered step-and-shoot acquisition.

◆ Electrocardiographic Editing

As described, ECG gating techniques identify the R-wave and use this information to determine the beginning of the cardiac cycle. For image acquisition with prospective ECG gating, the R-R interval is used to trigger the roentgen generator during a limited interval in mid-diastole. With retrospective gating, data are obtained continuously throughout the cardiac cycle; data are then selected from specific phases of the cardiac cycle for image reconstruction. An ectopic beat or an error in the identification of an R-wave will result in improper triggering of the roentgen tube in a prospectively gated scan and may result in reconstruction from a suboptimal phase of the cardiac cycle. It is not possible to correct for an error in prospective ECG gating because the necessary data have not been acquired at the appropriate part of the cardiac cycle. However, ECG editing may be used in conjunction with retrospective gating to provide superior images from the most optimal portion of the cardiac cycle (**Fig. 2.14**).[46]

When a premature contraction results in a shortened diastolic phase, the quiescent period during this heartbeat might not be sufficient to acquire diagnostic images of the coronary arteries. ECG editing may be used to remove this single beat from the reconstruction algorithm, thereby providing sharper detail of the coronary arteries (**Fig. 2.15**). Rarely the amplitude of a t-wave is observed to change after contrast injection. When a "peaked" t-wave is inappropriately gated, ECG editing can be used to correct the reconstruction (**Fig. 2.16**). Gating errors may cause an apparent blurring of an artery but may also simulate a stenosis (**Fig. 2.17**). It is important to be aware of this technical issue and of its potentially profound effect on the imaging of coronary disease with CTA.

◆ Image Reconstruction

Coronary CTA scan data are usually acquired with the best z-axis resolution provided by the scanner, but images can be reconstructed at different slice thicknesses by combining

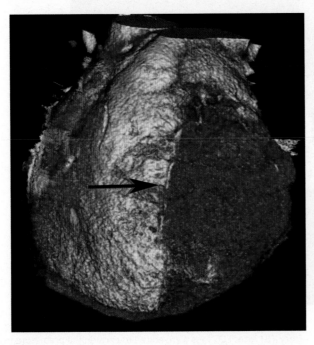
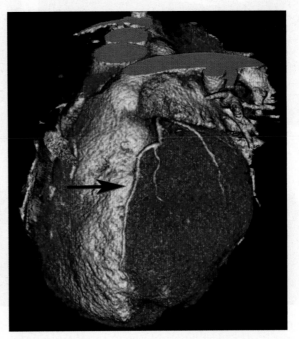

A   B

Fig. 2.14 Impact of electrocardiographic (ECG) editing on image quality. **(A)** Surface-rendered image in the left anterior oblique projection demonstrates a poorly visualized left anterior descending artery (LAD) (*arrow*), with multiple nonvisualized segments. **(B)** After editing of the ECG tags, the reconstructed surface-rendered image clearly demonstrates a normal LAD as well as additional diagonal branches over the left ventricular anterior wall.   (*Continued on page 40*)

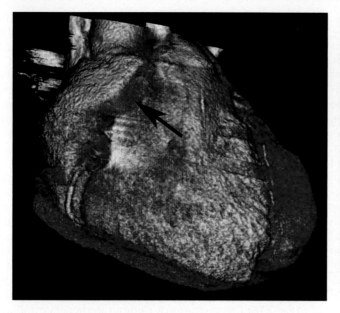

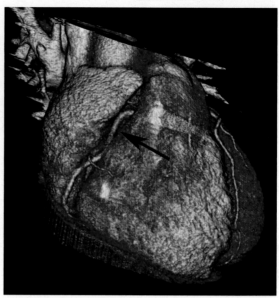

Fig. 2.14 (*Continued*) Impact of electrocardiographic (ECG) editing on image quality. **(C)** Surface views of the right coronary artery (RCA) in the same patient before ECG editing demonstrates nonvisualization of the RCA (*arrow*). **(D)** After editing of ECG tags, the RCA is visualized in its entirety (*arrow*).

data from adjacent detector rows. Although modern scanners provide isotropic voxels with a z-axis resolution of down to 0.5 mm, thin-section images obtained at a resolution of 0.5 to 0.6 mm often appear grainy because of a reduced signal-to-noise ratio. It is therefore common to evaluate the coronary arteries with a slice thickness of 0.7 to 1.0 mm. In heavier patients, the scans are often evaluated with a slice thickness of 1.0 to 1.2 mm. These images are

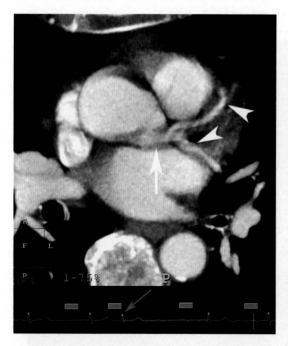

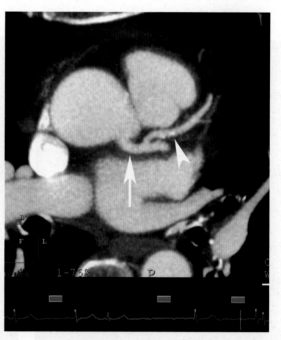

Fig. 2.15 Electrocardiographic (ECG) editing to correct a nondiagnostic image related to a premature atrial contraction. **(A)** Axial image at the level of the bifurcation of the left main coronary artery demonstrates marked blurring of the left main coronary artery (*arrow*) as well as the left anterior descending artery (LAD) and circumflex branches (*arrowheads*).The ECG demonstrates a premature atrial contraction (*arrow*) corresponding to the acquisition of the left main coronary artery. **(B)** After ECG tags were edited to exclude the premature beat, the resulting image reconstruction demonstrates a normal left main coronary artery (*arrow*) as well as minimal calcification in the proximal LAD without significant narrowing (*arrowhead*).

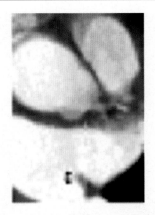
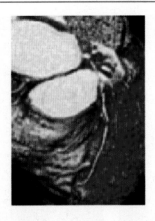

Fig. 2.16 Gating error related to increased amplitude of the t-wave. **(A)** Automated electrocardiographic (ECG) gating misidentified a large t-wave (*blue arrow*) as an R-wave. As a result of this error, a single cardiac cycle was misinterpreted as two cycles. Axial and surface-rendered images through the left main coronary artery were not of diagnostic quality. **(B)** After removing the ECG tag from the t-wave, repeat surface-rendered views of the left main coronary artery demonstrate a normal vessel.

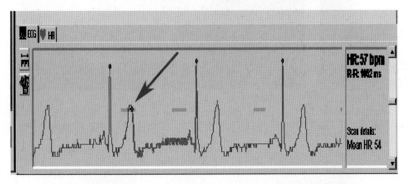

A

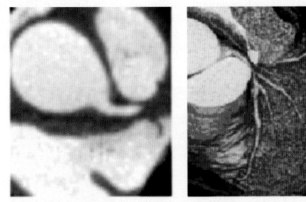

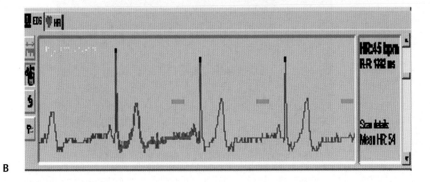

B

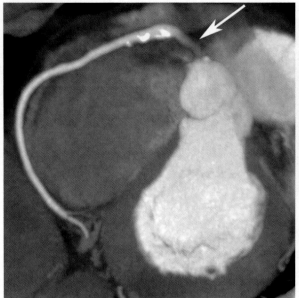

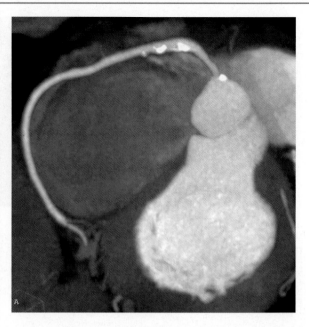

A   B

Fig. 2.17 Gating error resulting in apparent stenosis of the proximal right coronary artery (RCA). **(A)** Maximum intensity projection of the right coronary artery suggests the presence of narrowing in the proximal RCA (*arrow*). **(B)** After editing of the electrocardiographic tags and repeat reconstruction, the proximal RCA was demonstrated to be normal.

reconstructed with a 50% overlap between adjacent slices. Images that are obtained for functional analysis are reconstructed at 1.5- to 3-mm thickness.

Various reconstruction kernels are available to reconstruct images of the coronary arteries. The standard cardiac

reconstruction kernels provide a balance between edge enhancement and image noise. Unfortunately, there is a substantial blooming artifact and dropout artifact related to vascular calcifications **(Fig. 2.18)** and stents **(Fig. 2.19)**. A sharper reconstruction kernel will reduce blooming

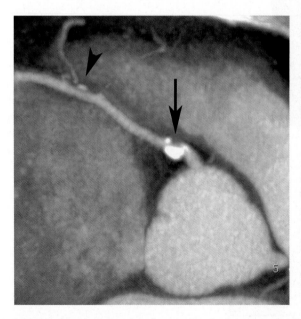

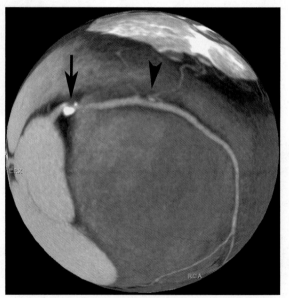

A   B

Fig. 2.18 Beam hardening and dropout artifact in the proximal right coronary artery (RCA). **(A)** Maximum intensity projection (MIP) image demonstrates focally calcified plaque just beyond the origin of the RCA. Just above the calcified plaque, a hypodense area suggests high-grade stenosis (*arrow*). Minimal disease was found at this level on coronary angiography. The extent of the calcified plaque is exaggerated by blooming artifact, while the adjacent dropout in the contrast-enhanced lumen creates the artifactual appearance of stenosis. A noncalcified plaque with ulceration is identified more distally within the vessel (*arrowhead*), which is adjacent to the origin of an acute marginal branch. **(B)** Globe MIP image again demonstrates calcified proximal RCA plaque with associated beam hardening and dropout artifact (*arrow*), suggesting the presence of high-grade stenosis. The ulcerated plaque is also identified (*arrowhead*).

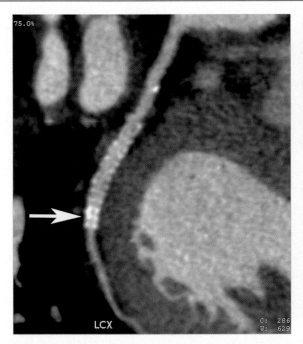

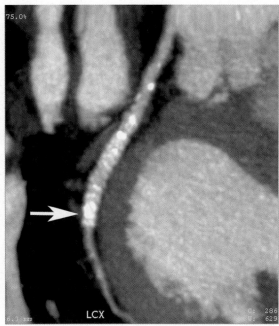

Fig. 2.19 Metallic stent artifact. **(A)** Maximum intensity projection (MIP) image through the left circumflex artery demonstrates a patent stent. At the distal aspect of the stent, there is increased density (*arrow*) that obscures the underlying vessel. The distal stent is underexpanded, resulting in increased density of the metal within the stent. Blooming artifact from the stent results in an apparent narrowing of the lumen. **(B)** Orthogonal MIP image through the stent fails to demonstrate the underlying lumen, which is obscured by stent artifact as well as vascular calcification (*arrow*).

associated with high-density materials **(Fig. 2.20)**. For the evaluation of calcified vessels and stents, a sharper kernel combined with a thinner slice will improve evaluation of the underlying lumen **(Fig. 2.21)**. However, sharper kernels and thinner slices are also associated with increased image noise. In some situations, a sharp kernel reconstruction may be followed by a smoothing filter used to reduce the noise. Before scanning a patient with pacemaker wires, it is important to realize that moving metallic structures often cause severe artifact that cannot be corrected with a sharper reconstruction kernel **(Fig. 2.22)**. Further discussion of reconstruction kernels is included with the discussion of stents in Chapter 7.

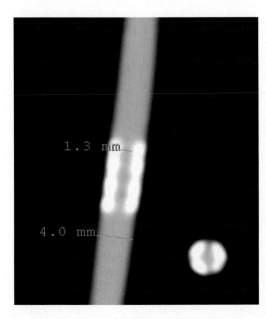

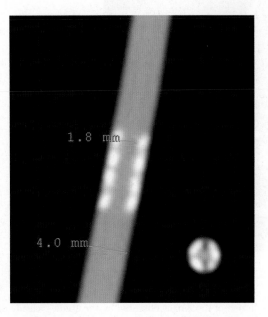

Fig. 2.20 Impact of reconstruction kernel on metallic stent artifact. **(A)** Standard reconstruction kernel demonstrates blooming of the stent with narrowing of the internal lumen. **(B)** Sharp kernel (stent detail kernel) demonstrates reduced blooming with a larger apparent internal lumen.

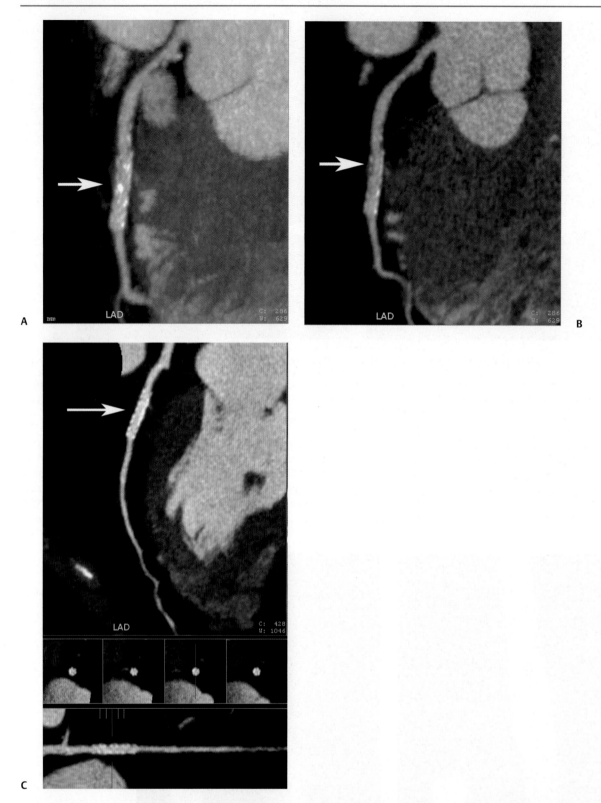

Fig. 2.21 Patent stent in the left anterior descending artery (LAD) evaluated with a stent detail kernel. **(A)** Maximum intensity projection (MIP) of the LAD with 5-mm slice thickness demonstrates a stent (*arrow*). The underlying lumen of the LAD is obscured by the stent struts and vascular calcification. **(B)** MIP with 1-mm slice thickness demonstrates the internal lumen with minimal noncalcified plaque along the proximal aspect of the stent without significant narrowing. **(C)** Curved MIP with 0.6-mm slice thickness through the stent more clearly demonstrates patency of the LAD. Short-axis images through the stent demonstrate the struts and the inner patent lumen.

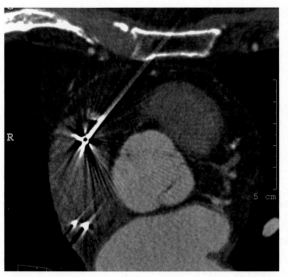

A

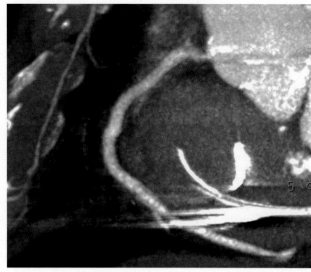

B

Fig. 2.22 Pacemaker wire artifact. **(A)** Axial image through the aortic root demonstrates multiple pacer wires in the right atrium. Both bright and dark streak artifacts extend in a star configuration from the wires.

(B) Maximum intensity projection of the right coronary artery demonstrates that the mid- to distal portion of the vessel is obscured by streak artifact from the pacer wires.

Images obtained for coronary CTA are typically reconstructed with a 22- to 25-cm field of view. However, the x-ray beam traverses the entire patient, and thus the scan usually contains raw data from a much larger field of view. Additional images may be reconstructed with a larger field of view without any additional imaging time or radiation exposure to the patient. For triple rule-out studies, additional 3-mm slice thickness images may be reconstructed with a 30- to 3-cm field of view to evaluate the pulmonary arteries. Following every coronary CTA study, an additional set of 3- to 5-mm slice thickness images should be reconstructed with a large field of view to evaluate the lung fields and surrounding structures in each patient.

◆ Conclusion

Advances in CT technology over the past decade continue to provide scanners with more slices, improved temporal resolution, and lower radiation exposure. Nonetheless, the diagnostic quality of coronary CTA is highly dependent on technical factors. Imaging must be performed during the appropriate phase of contrast distribution with careful attention to patient preparation and scanning technique. A basic understanding of scan parameters—including injection rate, temporal resolution, milliamperes, peak kilovoltage, pitch, and prospective or retrospective ECG gating is necessary to tailor the examination for optimal image quality with a minimum radiation dose.

References

1. Novak CB, Mackinnon SE. Thoracic outlet syndrome. Orthop Clin North Am. 1996;27(4):747–762

2. Morin RL, Gerber TC, McCollough CH. Radiation dose in computed tomography of the heart. Circulation. 2003;107(6):917–922

3. Hunold P, Vogt FM, Schmermund A, et al. Radiation exposure during cardiac CT: effective doses at multi-detector row CT and electron-beam CT. Radiology. 2003;226(1):145–152

4. Kuettner A, Trabold T, Schroeder S, et al. Noninvasive detection of coronary lesions using 16-detector multislice spiral computed tomography technology: initial clinical results. J Am Coll Cardiol. 2004;44(6):1230–1237

5. Everts B, Karlson BW, Herlitz J, Abdon NJ, Hedner T. Effects and pharmacokinetics of high dose metoprolol on chest pain in patients with suspected or definite acute myocardial infarction. Eur J Clin Pharmacol. 1997;53(1):23–31

6. Covinsky JO. Esmolol: a novel cardioselective, titratable, intravenous beta-blocker with ultrashort half-life. Drug Intell Clin Pharm. 1987;21(4):316–321

7. Kawai C, Konishi T, Matsuyama E, Okazaki H. Comparative effects of three calcium antagonists, diltiazem, verapamil and nifedipine, on the sinoatrial and atrioventricular nodes. Experimental and clinical studies. Circulation. 1981;63(5):1035–1042

8. Pannu HK, Alvarez W Jr, Fishman EK. Beta-blockers for cardiac CT: a primer for the radiologist. AJR Am J Roentgenol. 2006;186(6, Suppl 2)S341–S345

9. Bailey B. Glucagon in beta-blocker and calcium channel blocker overdoses: a systematic review. J Toxicol Clin Toxicol. 2003;41(5):595–602

10. Kenny J. Treating overdose with calcium channel blockers. BMJ. 1994;308(6935):992–993

11. Shepherd G. Treatment of poisoning caused by beta-adrenergic and calcium-channel blockers. Am J Health Syst Pharm. 2006;63(19): 1828–1835

12. Dewey M, Hoffmann H, Hamm B. Multislice CT coronary angiography: effect of sublingual nitroglycerine on the diameter of coronary arteries. Rofo. 2006;178(6):600–604

13. Decramer I, Vanhoenacker PK, Sarno G, et al. Effects of sublingual nitroglycerin on coronary lumen diameter and number of visualized septal branches on 64-MDCT angiography. AJR Am J Roentgenol. 2008;190(1):219–225

14. Hamon M, Hamon M. Images in clinical medicine. Asymptomatic coronary-artery spasm. N Engl J Med. 2006;355(21):2236

15. Chun EJ, Lee W, Choi YH, et al. Effects of nitroglycerin on the diagnostic accuracy of electrocardiogram-gated coronary computed tomography angiography. J Comput Assist Tomogr. 2008;32(1):86–92

16. Leschka S, Wildermuth S, Boehm T, et al. Noninvasive coronary angiography with 64-section CT: effect of average heart rate and heart rate variability on image quality. Radiology. 2006;241(2):378–385

17. Cademartiri F, Mollet NR, van der Lugt A, et al. Intravenous contrast material administration at helical 16-detector row CT coronary angiography: effect of iodine concentration on vascular attenuation. Radiology. 2005;236(2):661–665

18. Cademartiri F, de Monye C, Pugliese F, et al. High iodine concentration contrast material for noninvasive multislice computed tomography coronary angiography: iopromide 370 versus iomeprol 400. Invest Radiol. 2006;41(3):349–353

19. Rist C, Nikolaou K, Kirchin MA, et al. Contrast bolus optimization for cardiac 16-slice computed tomography: comparison of contrast medium formulations containing 300 and 400 milligrams of iodine per milliliter. Invest Radiol. 2006;41(5):460–467

20. Morin RL, Gerber TC, McCollough CH. Radiation dose in computed tomography of the heart. Circulation. 2003;107(6):917–922

21. Hunold P, Vogt FM, Schmermund A, et al. Radiation exposure during cardiac CT: effective doses at multi-detector row CT and electron-beam CT. Radiology. 2003;226(1):145–152

22. Hoffmann MH, Shi H, Manzke R, et al. Noninvasive coronary angiography with 16-detector row CT: effect of heart rate. Radiology. 2005;234(1):86–97

23. Herzog C, Arning-Erb M, Zangos S, et al. Multi-detector row CT coronary angiography: influence of reconstruction technique and heart rate on image quality. Radiology. 2006;238(1):75–86

24. Zhang S, Halpern EJ. Optimal ECG phases for coronary assessment with cardiac CTA angiography. Proceedings of the Radiological Society of North America. Abstract #LL-CA4098–H04. December 2006:668

25. Vembar M, Garcia MJ, Heuscher DJ, et al. A dynamic approach to identifying desired physiological phases for cardiac imaging using multislice spiral CT. Med Phys. 2003;30(7):1683–1693

26. Manzke R, Köhler T, Nielsen T, Hawkes D, Grass M. Automatic phase determination for retrospectively gated cardiac CT. Med Phys. 2004;31(12):3345–3362

27. Dewey M, Müller M, Teige F, et al. Multisegment and halfscan reconstruction of 16-slice computed tomography for assessment of regional and global left ventricular myocardial function. Invest Radiol. 2006;41(4):400–409

28. Johnson TR, Nikolaou K, Wintersperger BJ, et al. Dual-source CT cardiac imaging: initial experience. Eur Radiol. 2006;16(7):1409–1415

29. Flohr TG, McCollough CH, Bruder H, et al. First performance evaluation of a dual-source CT (DSCT) system. Eur Radiol. 2006;16(2):256–268

30. Gerber TC, Stratmann BP, Kuzo RS, Kantor B, Morin RL. Effect of acquisition technique on radiation dose and image quality in multidetector row computed tomography coronary angiography with submillimeter collimation. Invest Radiol 2005;40(8):556–563

31. Abada HT, Larchez C, Daoud B, Sigal-Cinqualbre A, Paul JF. MDCT of the coronary arteries: feasibility of low-dose CT with ECG-pulsed tube current modulation to reduce radiation dose. AJR Am J Roentgenol. 2006;186(6, Suppl 2):S387–S390

32. Feuchtner GM, Jodocy D, Klauser A, Haberfellner B, Aglan I, Spoeck A, Hiehs S, Soegner P, Jaschke W. Radiation dose reduction by using 100-kV tube voltage in cardiac 64-slice computed tomography: a comparative study. Eur J Radiol. 2009;Aug 9 (Epub ahead of print)

33. Pontone G, Andreini D, Bartorelli AL, et al. Diagnostic accuracy of coronary computed tomography angiography: a comparison between prospective and retrospective electrocardiogram triggering. J Am Coll Cardiol. 2009;54(4):346–355

34. Hirai N, Horiguchi J, Fujioka C, et al. Prospective versus retrospective ECG-gated 64-detector coronary CT angiography: assessment of image quality, stenosis, and radiation dose. Radiology. 2008;248(2):424–430

35. Shuman WP, Branch KR, May JM, et al. Prospective versus retrospective ECG gating for 64-detector CT of the coronary arteries: comparison of image quality and patient radiation dose. Radiology. 2008; 248(2):431–437

36. Maruyama T, Takada M, Hasuike T, Yoshikawa A, Namimatsu E, Yoshizumi T. Radiation dose reduction and coronary assessability of prospective electrocardiogram-gated computed tomography coronary angiography: comparison with retrospective electrocardiogram-gated helical scan. J Am Coll Cardiol. 2008;52(18):1450–1455

37. Achenbach S, Marwan M, Schepis T, et al. High-pitch spiral acquisition: a new scan mode for coronary CT angiography. J Cardiovasc Comput Tomogr. 2009;3(2):117–121

38. Hausleiter J, Bischoff B, Hein F, et al. Feasibility of dual-source cardiac CT angiography with high-pitch scan protocols. J Cardiovasc Comput Tomogr. 2009;3(4):236–242

39. Lell M, Marwan M, Schepis T, et al. Prospectively ECG-triggered high-pitch spiral acquisition for coronary CT angiography using dual source CT: technique and initial experience. Eur Radiol. 2009;19(11): 2576–2583

40. Bischoff B, Hein F, Meyer T, et al. Impact of a reduced tube voltage on CT angiography and radiation dose: results of the PROTECTION I study. JACC Cardiovasc Imaging. 2009;2(8):940–946

41. Wang G, Yu H, De Man B. An outlook on x-ray CT research and development. Med Phys. 2008;35(3):1051–1064

42. Thibault JB, Sauer KD, Bouman CA, Hsieh J. A three-dimensional statistical approach to improved image quality for multislice helical CT. Med Phys. 2007;34(11):4526–4544

43. Hara AK, Paden RG, Silva AC, Kujak JL, Lawder HJ, Pavlicek W. Iterative reconstruction technique for reducing body radiation dose at CT: feasibility study. AJR Am J Roentgenol. 2009;193(3):764–771

44. Herzog C, Mulvihill DM, Nguyen SA, et al. Pediatric cardiovascular CT angiography: radiation dose reduction using automatic anatomic tube current modulation. AJR Am J Roentgenol. 2008;190(5):1232–1240

45. Angel E, Yaghmai N, Jude CM, et al. Monte Carlo simulations to assess the effects of tube current modulation on breast dose for multidetector CT. Phys Med Biol 2009;54(3):497–512

46. Cademartiri F, Mollet NR, Runza G, et al. Improving diagnostic accuracy of MDCT coronary angiography in patients with mild heart rhythm irregularities using ECG editing. AJR Am J Roentgenol. 2006; 186(3):634–638

3

Normal Coronary Anatomy

Ethan J. Halpern and David C. Levin

Coronary artery blood flow is critical for the normal development and function of the heart. Although some variations in coronary anatomy may result in cardiac dysfunction, many variations provide adequate blood flow to the myocardium. For the purposes of this chapter, however, the definition of normal coronary anatomy is based on the commonly observed anatomy rather than on an assessment of healthy versus pathologic state. In accordance with the definition of "normal" coronary anatomy by Angelini, the spectrum of normal coronary anatomy includes observed variations in coronary anatomy present in 1% or more of the population.[1] Based on this criterion, less frequent variations are classified as anomalies, whether or not they result in a pathologic state. Selected coronary anomalies are discussed along with related common variants in this chapter, but most clinically significant coronary anomalies are discussed in Chapter 4.

◆ Aortic Root

Our discussion of coronary anatomy begins with the aortic root, which extends from the aortic annulus to the sinotubular junction and consists of the aortic valve, the three sinuses of Valsalva, and the sinotubular junction. Although the tubular portion of the aorta is circular in shape beyond the sinotubular junction, the aortic root has a cloverleaf shape in short axis. Three equally spaced sites of minimal tethering within the aortic root mark the junctions of the sinuses of Valsalva (**Fig. 3.1**). Each sinus is associated with a leaflet of the aortic valve; the junctions between adjacent sinuses are aligned with the commissures between the aortic valve leaflets. The sinuses of Valsalva represent a normal dilation at the root of the aorta, with a diameter that is greater than that in the tubular portion of the ascending aorta.

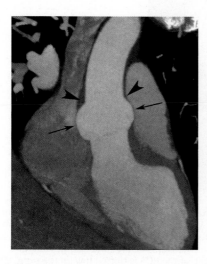

A

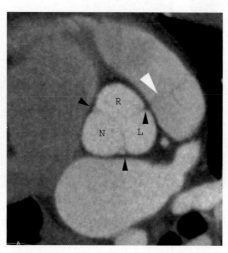

B

Fig. 3.1 Aortic root, including aortic valve, sinuses of Valsalva, and sinotubular junction. **(A)** Sagittal maximum intensity projection (MIP). There is a normal dilatation of the aortic root related to the sinuses of Valsava (*arrows*). The sinotubular junction is marked by a caliber change just above the aortic root (*arrowheads*). **(B)** Axial MIP at the level of the aortic valve. The root demonstrates a cloverleaf shape with three sinuses of Valsalva named for their coronary arteries: R, right, L, left, and N, noncoronary. The commissures of the aortic valve are visible (*black arrowheads*) as is the pulmonary valve (*white arrowhead*). The commissure between the right and left aortic leaflets is aligned with an adjacent commissure in the pulmonic valve. (*Continued on page 48*)

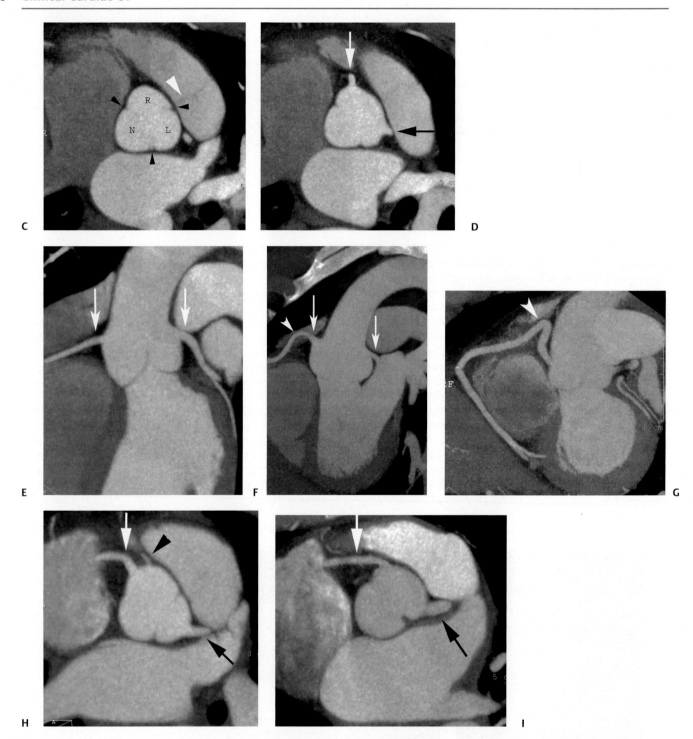

Fig. 3.1 (*Continued*) Aortic root, including aortic valve, sinuses of Valsalva, and sinotubular junction. **(C)** Axial MIP at a slightly higher level again demonstrates the cloverleaf shape of the aortic root. **(D)** Axial MIP just below the sinotubular junction demonstrates normal origins of the coronary arteries from the center of the right (*white arrow*) and left (*black arrow*) coronary sinuses. **(E)** Slab MIP in the left anterior oblique projection. The right (RCA) and left (LCA) coronary arteries originate from the sinuses of Valsava, just below the level of the sinotubular junction (*arrows*). **(F)** The coronary origins in a different patient demonstrate a shepherd's crook curvature of the proximal RCA (*arrowhead*). A shepherd's crook proximal RCA is a common variation (approximately 5%) that may present as a technical challenge during angioplasty. **(G)** Slab MIP of the RCA in another patient with a more obvious shepherd's crook (*arrowhead*). **(H)** Axial MIP in a patient with independent origins of the conus artery (*black arrowhead*) and RCA (*white arrow*). The origin of the RCA is shifted toward the right, while the conus artery and the LCA (*black arrow*) originate from the center of their respective sinuses. **(I)** Axial MIP in a patient with bicuspid aortic valve. Only two sinuses of Valsalva are present. Both coronary arteries arise from the anterior-left sinus. The RCA (*white arrow*) originates at an acute angle from the aortic root.

The proper anatomic names for the three sinuses of Valsalva are the posterior, right, and left sinuses. The common names for the sinuses—noncoronary sinus, right coronary sinus, and left coronary sinus—refer to the coronary arteries, which normally originate from the center of two of the sinuses. The right coronary artery (RCA) originates from the more anterior right sinus of Valsalva, and the left coronary artery (LCA) originates from the left sinus of Valsalva. The coronary arteries originate from the superior portions of the sinuses of Valsalva, just below the sinotubular junction. The ostia of the arteries are located just above the free margins of the aortic leaflets during systole. A normal coronary artery origin is situated at a right angle to the wall of the aortic root. Coronary ostia that arise at an acute angle are typical of anomalous vessels, described in more detail in Chapter 4.

The right ventricular outflow tract is normally located anteriorly and to the left of the aortic root. During embryologic development, the pulmonary artery separates from the aortopulmonary truncus. The commissure between the right and left cusps of the aortic valve is aligned with the posterior commissure of the pulmonic valve. The alignment of these two commissures is related to the origin of both valves from the aortopulmonary truncus. The commissure between the right and left coronary sinuses within the aortic root remains adjacent to the embryologic aortopulmonary septum. During embryologic development, the infundibulum is resorbed below the aortic valve but is preserved within the right ventricular outflow tract. This resorption results in caudal displacement of the aortic annulus relative to the pulmonic valve. To maintain its relationship with the pulmonary artery, the aortic annulus becomes angled off the axial plane such that the aortopulmonary contact point remains the most superior point within the aortic root. The coronary arteries arise on both sides of this contact point (the embryologic aortopulmonary septum) from the right and left coronary sinuses. As a result of this angulation of the aortic root out of the axial plane, the proximal coronary arteries are often directed superiorly. Anomalies of septation of the aorta and pulmonary artery—tetralogy of Fallot, truncus arteriosus, pulmonary atresia, and transposition—are often associated with anatomic variations in coronary anatomy.[2–5]

◆ Main Coronary Arteries

The left main coronary artery typically originates as a single vessel from the left sinus of Valsalva. This artery courses between the right ventricular outflow tract and the left atrium and under the left atrial appendage (**Fig. 3.2**). To visualize the left main coronary artery on surface-rendered images of the heart, the left atrial appendage must be removed. As the left main coronary artery emerges from under the left atrial appendage, it typically divides into two major branches: the left anterior descending (LAD) artery and the circumflex (LCX) artery.

The LAD courses in the epicardial space along the anterior interventricular groove between the right and left ventricles

down to the apex of the heart. The LAD supplies blood flow to the interventricular septum through the anterior septal perforators and to the anterior and anterolateral walls of the left ventricle through diagonal branches. Septal branches are often difficult to visualize with coronary CT angiography (CTA) because of their small size as well as the enhancement of the surrounding septal myocardium. Diagonal branches course in the epicardial space over the left ventricular free wall and are more readily visible on coronary CTA. The LAD may end slightly before the apex, or it may wrap around the apex into the posterior interventricular groove.

The LCX courses in the left atrioventricular groove between the left atium and left ventricle. The LCX provides flow to the lateral and posterior lateral walls of the left ventricle through obtuse marginal branches. The LCX and obtuse marginal arteries are epicardial in location and generally well visualized on coronary CTA. The extent of myocardial territory supplied by the LCX is highly variable. The LCX may end as an obtuse marginal branch. In a minority of people, the circumflex artery courses around the left atrioventricular groove to the crux of the heart and supplies the posterior descending artery (PDA). The *crux* is defined as the point on the diaphragmatic surface of the heart where the right atrioventricular groove, the left atrioventricular groove, and the posterior interventricular groove converge. The PDA courses along the posterior interventricular groove from the crux to the cardiac apex.

The RCA courses within the right atrioventricular groove, between the right atrium and right ventricle, where it supplies

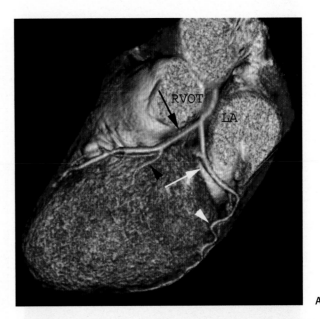

Fig. 3.2 Left coronary artery anatomy. **(A)** Volumetric surface rendering demonstrates the course of the left main coronary artery between the right ventricular outflow tract (RVOT) and left atrium (LA). The left main coronary artery bifurcates into the left anterior descending (LAD) (*black arrow*) and circumflex (LCX) (*white arrow*) arteries. A diagonal branch (*black arrowhead*) arises from the LAD. The circumflex terminates as an obtuse marginal branch (*white arrowhead*). (*Continued on page 50*)

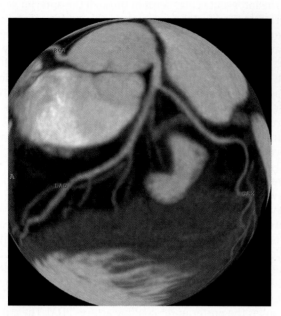

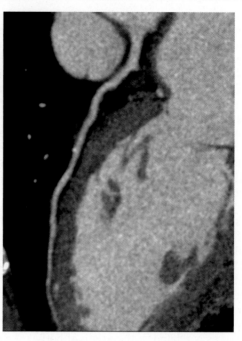

B

C

Fig. 3.2 (*Continued*) Left coronary artery anatomy. **(B)** Globe MIP of the same patient demonstrates the LAD in the anterior interventricular groove and the circumflex in the left atrioventricular groove.

(C) Curved MIP demonstrates the entire length of the LAD as it courses along the anterior interventricular groove to the apex of the left ventricle.

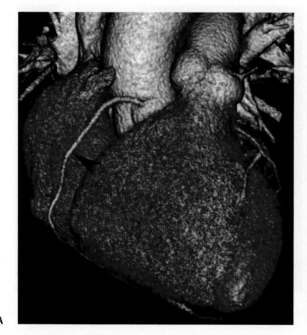

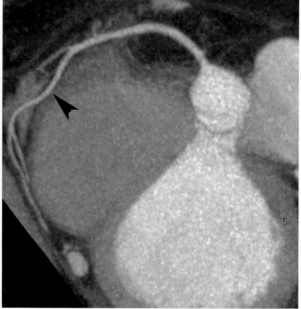

A

B

Fig. 3.3 Right coronary anatomy in surface and maximum intensity projections (MIPs). **(A)** Surface image in a shallow left anterior oblique (LAO) projection demonstrates the right coronary artery (RCA) (*black arrowhead*) coursing along the right atrioventricular (AV) groove.

(B) MIP image in the LAO projection again demonstrates the RCA (*black arrowhead*), coursing in a classic "C" shape toward the crux of the heart. In this patient, the RCA bifurcates into the posterior descending artery and a posterior left ventricular branch proximal to the crux.

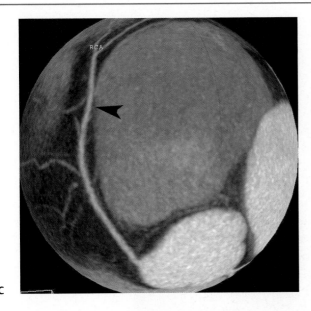

C

Fig. 3.3 (*Continued*) **(C)** Globe MIP demonstrates the RCA (*black arrowhead*) within the AV groove adjacent to the right atrium.

small acute marginal branches to the free wall of the right ventricle (**Fig. 3.3**). The proximal portion of the RCA is often covered by the right atrial appendage. The RCA is often embedded within a deep right atrioventricular groove but is generally well visualized because of its epicardial location. In most people, the RCA continues around the right atrioventricular groove to the crux of the heart, where it supplies a PDA that descends in the posterior interventricular groove

(**Fig. 3.4**). The PDA supplies numerous small branches into the septum, the posterior septal perforating arteries. The RCA generally continues beyond the crux of the heart to supply additional posterior left ventricular branches. In the setting of coronary disease, the posterior septal perforating arteries may collateralize with the LAD via the anterior septal perforators, and the posterior left ventricular branches may collateralize with the LCX via distal obtuse marginal branches.

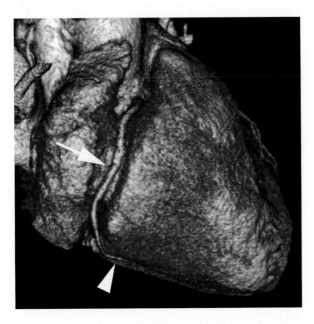

A

Fig. 3.4 Right coronary artery (RCA) and posterior descending artery (PDA) in surface and maximum intensity projections (MIPs). **(A)** The RCA courses in the right atrioventricular groove (*arrow*) to the crux of the heart. The PDA arises from the RCA at the crux and courses down the posterior interventricular groove (*arrowhead*). (*Continued on page 52*)

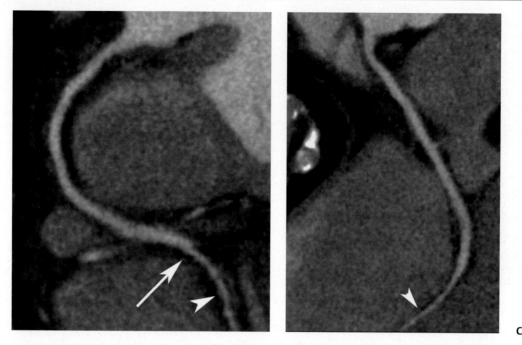

B

C

Fig. 3.4 (*Continued*) Right coronary artery (RCA) and posterior descending artery (PDA) in surface and maximum intensity projections (MIPs). **(B)** The classic "C" shape of the RCA is demonstrated in a curved MIP LAO projection. The vessel narrows in caliber at the crux of the heart (*arrow*), where it bifurcates into the PDA (*arrowhead*) and posterior left ventricular branches (not shown). **(C)** Orthogonal MIP image again demonstrates the RCA throughout its course to the PDA.

◆ Coronary Dominance

A commonly described variation in coronary anatomy is the degree to which the left ventricular myocardium is supplied by the LCA and RCA. *Coronary dominance* refers to the supply of the PDA and the posterior left ventricular branches. In a right-dominant system, the RCA supplies the PDA as well as additional posterior left ventricular branches (**Fig. 3.5**). In a superdominant right circulation, the LCX is very small and the RCA continues to supply the posterior and lateral wall of the left ventricle (**Fig. 3.6**). In a left-dominant system, the LCX supplies the posterior left ventricular branches as well as the PDA (**Fig. 3.7**). In the setting of a wraparound LAD, the LAD may actually supply the PDA in a left-dominant

circulation (**Fig. 3.7**). In a balanced circulation, the RCA supplies the PDA, and the circumflex supplies the posterior left ventricular branches (**Fig. 3.8**).

A right-dominant circulation is present in the vast majority of the population. In one study of 1950 people, right dominance was observed in 89.1%, left dominance in 8.4%, and codominance in 2.5%.[6,7] Right-dominant, left-dominant, and codominant circulations all represent normal variations of the coronary arterial tree. Of note, the term *right-dominant system* is somewhat of a misnomer because the left main coronary artery and its branches almost always supply most of the blood flow to the left ventricle, even in the presence of a right-dominant system.

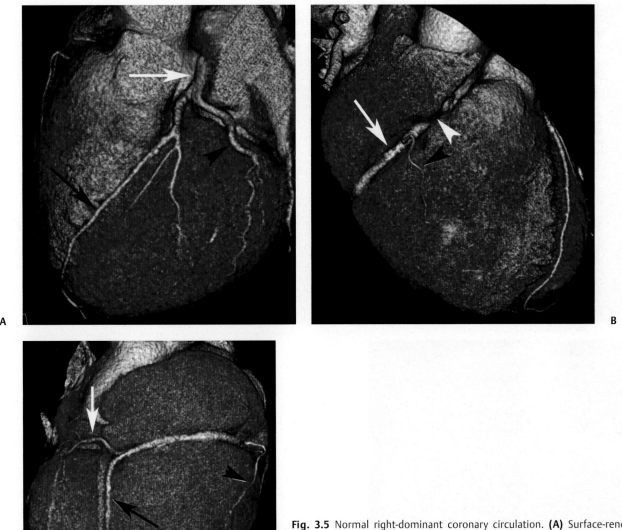

Fig. 3.5 Normal right-dominant coronary circulation. **(A)** Surface-rendered image in a steep left anterior oblique (LAO) projection demonstrates the bifurcation of the left main coronary artery (*white arrow*) into the left anterior descending (*black arrow*) and circumflex (*black arrowhead*) arteries. **(B)** Right anterior oblique projection demonstrates the right coronary artery (RCA) (*arrow*) as it courses in the right atrioventricular groove. The proximal portion of the RCA is obscured by the overlying right atrial appendage (*white arrowhead*). A small acute marginal branch of the RCA is demonstrated (*black arrowhead*). **(C)** The heart is rotated further so that the crux is visible. The distal RCA bifurcates into the posterior descending artery (*black arrow*), which courses in the posterior interventricular groove and a posterior left ventricular branch (*white arrow*). An acute marginal branch is again identified (*black arrowhead*).

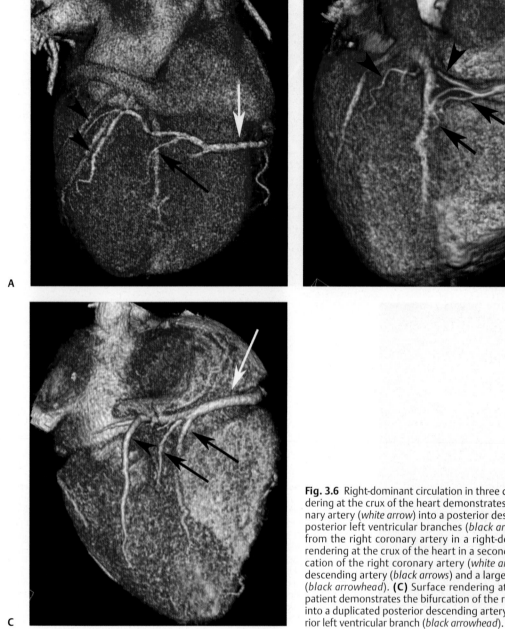

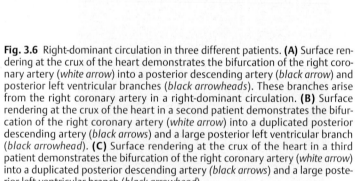

Fig. 3.6 Right-dominant circulation in three different patients. **(A)** Surface rendering at the crux of the heart demonstrates the bifurcation of the right coronary artery (*white arrow*) into a posterior descending artery (*black arrow*) and posterior left ventricular branches (*black arrowheads*). These branches arise from the right coronary artery in a right-dominant circulation. **(B)** Surface rendering at the crux of the heart in a second patient demonstrates the bifurcation of the right coronary artery (*white arrow*) into a duplicated posterior descending artery (*black arrows*) and a large posterior left ventricular branch (*black arrowhead*). **(C)** Surface rendering at the crux of the heart in a third patient demonstrates the bifurcation of the right coronary artery (*white arrow*) into a duplicated posterior descending artery *(black arrows)* and a large posterior left ventricular branch (*black arrowhead*).

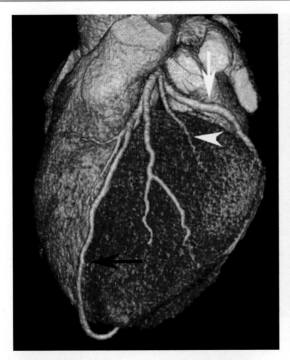

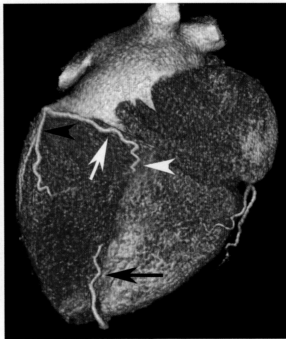

A

B

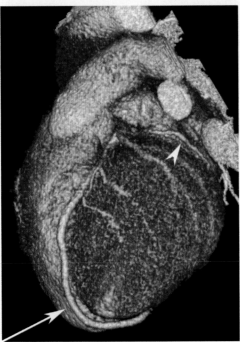

C

Fig. 3.7 Left-dominant coronary circulation in two different patients. Patient 1: **(A)** Surface-rendered image in the left anterior oblique projection demonstrates the circumflex artery as it courses through the left atrioventricular (AV) groove (*white arrow*). A ramus medianus (*white arrowhead*) supplies the lateral wall of the left ventricle. The left anterior descending artery (*black arrow*) courses around the apex of the heart. **(B)** The heart is rotated further so that the crux is visible. The distal circumflex artery (*white arrow*) continues around the AV groove. The posterior wall of the left ventricle is supplied by a posterolateral branch of the circumflex (*black arrowhead*). The circumflex artery (*white arrow*) terminates as a short posterior descending artery (*white arrowhead*), which supplies the basal inferoseptum. Termination of the circumflex artery as the posterior descending artery is the most common form of left-dominant circulation. In this patient, a wraparound left anterior descending artery (*black arrow*) continues in the posterior interventricular groove to supply the distal posterior descending artery. Patient 2: **(C)** Surface-rendered image in the left anterior oblique projection demonstrates a large left anterior descending artery (*white arrow*) that courses around the apex of the heart. A small circumflex artery is visible (*white arrowhead*). (Continued on page 56)

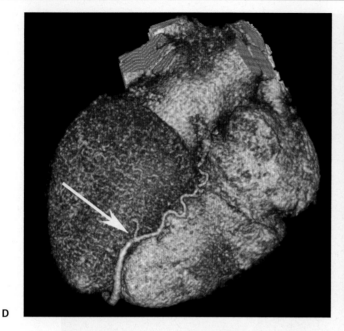

D

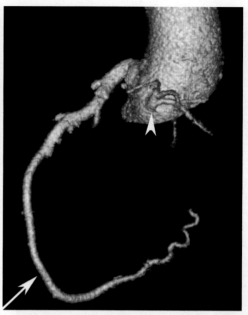

E

Fig. 3.7 *(Continued)* Left-dominant coronary circulation in two different patients. **(D)** Surface-rendered image of the undersurface of the heart demonstrates that the left anterior descending artery (*white arrow*) wraps around the apex and continues in the posterior interventricular groove as the posterior descending artery. Neither the circumflex nor the right coronary artery is visible near the crux of the heart. **(E)** Extracted tree view of the coronary circulation in a steep left anterior oblique projection demonstrates the large left anterior descending artery (*white arrow*), which wraps around the apex of the heart. The right coronary artery origin is visible (*white arrowhead*) with several small branches. In this uncommon variation of a left dominant circulation, the left anterior descending artery supplies the entire posterior descending artery territory.

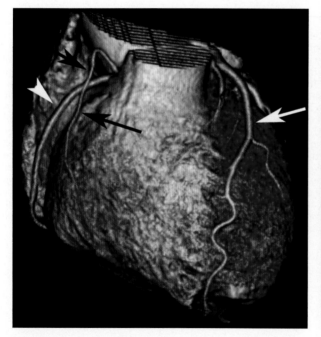

A

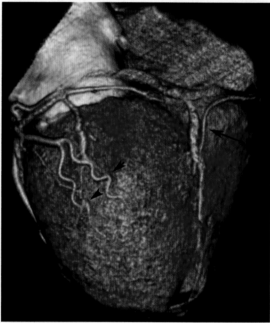

B

Fig. 3.8 Balanced (co-dominant) coronary circulation. **(A)** Surface-rendered view in the anteroposterior projection demonstrates the left anterior descending artery (*white arrow*) as it courses in the anterior interventricular groove. The right coronary artery (*arrowhead*) has a large conus branch that supplies the free wall of the right ventricle. **(B,C)** Posterior views of the left ventricle and the crux of the heart demonstrate terminal branches of the circumflex artery, which supply the inferolateral left ventricular wall (*black arrowheads*) as well as the inferior wall (*white arrowhead*). The posterior descending artery (*arrow*) arises from the right coronary artery.

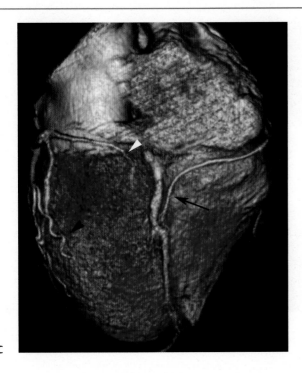

C

Fig. 3.8 *(Continued)* **(B,C)** Posterior views of the left ventricle and the crux of the heart demonstrate terminal branches of the circumflex artery, which supply the inferolateral left ventricular wall (*black arrowheads*) as well as the inferior wall (*white arrowhead*). The posterior descending artery (*arrow*) arises from the right coronary artery.

◆ Variations in Left Coronary Circulation

In most patients, the LCA bifurcates into LAD and circumflex branches. However, a trifurcation of the LCA into the LAD, ramus medianus, and circumflex is present in about 37% of people (**Fig. 3.9**).[8] The ramus medianus courses between the diagonal and obtuse marginal branches and supplies a territory of the left ventricle that might otherwise be supplied by a first diagonal or a first obtuse marginal branch. In the presence of a large ramus branch, diagonal or obtuse marginal branches may be smaller or absent.

The distribution of diagonal branches, the ramus branch, and obtuse marginal branches demonstrates considerable variability. When large diagonal branches or a large ramus medianus is present, the obtuse marginal branches are often underdeveloped. Conversely, in the presence of large obtuse marginal branches, the diagonal branches are often smaller. These variations in anatomic supply are of considerable importance when there is disease in the LAD or LCX. The extent of myocardium in jeopardy depends on the region supplied by the diseased vessel.

Although the LAD is always an important artery, the extent of myocardium supplied by the LAD is quite variable (**Fig. 3.10**). When the LAD artery ends proximal to the apex, there may be a large diagonal branch that extends down to the apex and supplies this territory. Conversely, when the LAD artery is large and wraps around the apex, the PDA is often smaller. In such situations, the LAD artery may supply the cardiac apex as well as the posterior septal branches. The presence of a dual LAD is a rare variation, more appropriately classified as a coronary anomaly.[9] In rare individuals there may be a congenital intercoronary communication between the distal LAD and the distal PDA. Congenital anatomic variations of the LAD must be distinguished from variations that arise based on collateral supply resulting from vascular disease (**Fig. 3.11**).

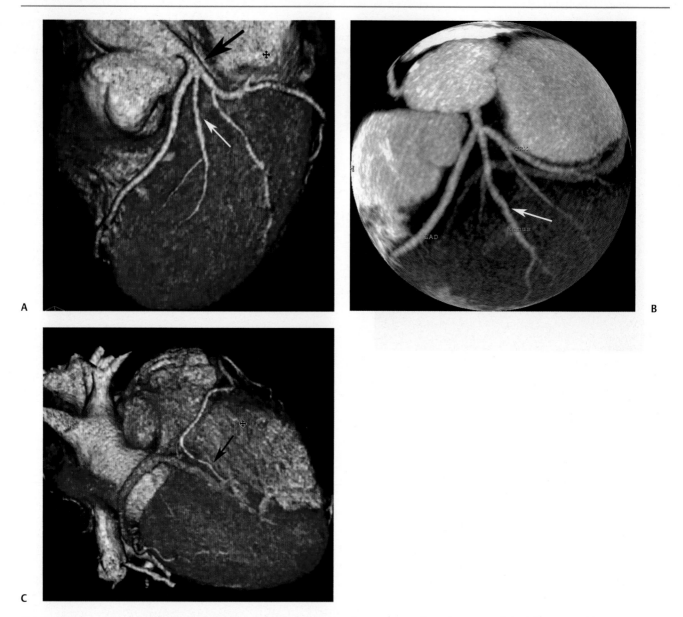

Fig. 3.9 Ramus medianus. **(A)** Surface-rendered view of the left coronary circulation demonstrates a trifurcation of the left main coronary artery (*black arrow*). The additional branch that rises between the left anterior descending artery and the circumflex artery is the ramus medianus (*white arrow*). **(B)** Globe maximum intensity projection demonstrates the trifurcation of the left main coronary artery into the left anterior descending artery, circumflex, and ramus (*arrow*). **(C)** Surface- rendered image at the crux demonstrates that the right coronary artery supplies the posterior descending artery (*black arrow*).

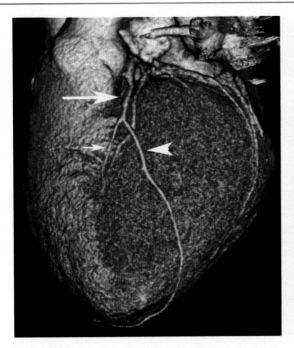

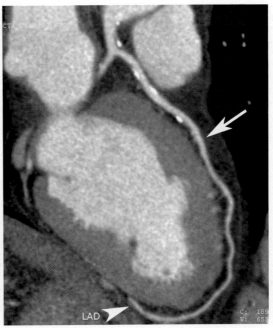

Fig. 3.10 Variations of left anterior descending (LAD) anatomy. **(A)** Absent distal LAD. Surface-rendered view in the left anterior oblique (LAO) projection demonstrates the LAD (*large arrow*) in the proximal anterior interventricular groove. A large first diagonal branch (*arrowhead*) arises from the LAD and extends around the cardiac apex. The LAD persists as a small vessel (*small arrow*) in the anterior interventricular groove, but it terminates proximal to the cardiac apex. In this variation of normal anatomy, the apex of the left ventricle is supplied by a large diagonal branch rather than the LAD. **(B)** Wraparound LAD in a different patient. Tracked maximum intensity projection view of the LAD demonstrates a normal course of the LAD in the anterior interventricular groove (*arrow*). This vessel continues around the apex to supply the distal posterior descending artery (*arrowhead*).

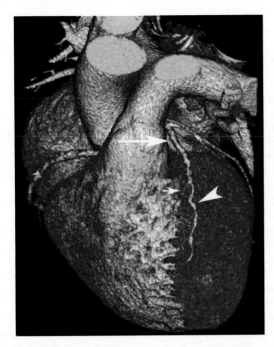

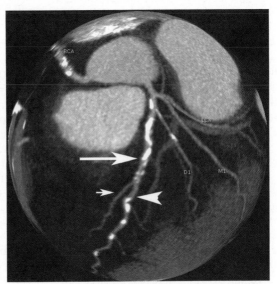

Fig. 3.11 Proximal termination of the left anterior descending artery (LAD) related to extensive atherosclerotic disease. **(A)** The LAD (*arrow*) terminates proximal to the cardiac apex secondary to extensive atherosclerotic disease in the midportion of this vessel (*arrowhead*). There is an associated infarct of the left ventricular apex. A septal perforator branch is identified (*small arrow*). **(B)** Globe maximum intensity potential confirms extensive calcification along the LAD (*large arrow*) and again demonstrates a large septal branch (*small arrow*).

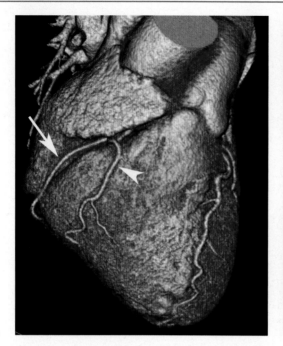
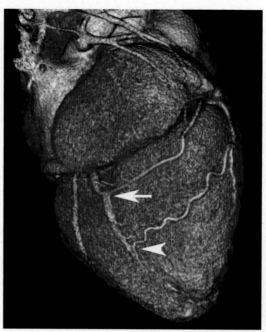

A

B

Fig. 3.12 Variant anatomy of the posterior descending artery. **(A)** Surface-rendered image in an anteroposterior projection demonstrates the right coronary artery (RCA) in the right atrioventricular groove (*arrow*). A large proximal acute marginal artery originates from the RCA and courses over the free wall of the right ventricle (*arrowhead*). **(B)** Surface view of the distal right coronary circulation demonstrates the origin of the posterior descending artery (PDA) from the distal RCA at the crux of the heart (*arrow*). A second PDA is present in the more distal posterior interventricular groove, originating from the acute marginal branch of the RCA (*arrowhead*).

◆ Variations in Right Coronary Circulation

As it courses in the right atrioventricular groove, the RCA supplies a variable number of acute marginal branches to the right ventricular free wall. In about 25% of people with a right-dominant circulation, there are variations of PDA anatomy, including partial supply of the PDA territory by acute marginal branches, a duplicated PDA, or a PDA origin from the RCA proximal to the crux **(Fig. 3.12)**.[10] As the RCA courses beyond the crux, the number and size of posterior left ventricular branches are highly variable.

◆ Conus Artery

The conus artery is a small vessel, typically arising as the first branch of the proximal RCA. The conus branch courses around the right ventricular outflow tract and terminates on the anterior aspect of the heart **(Fig. 3.13A)**. In up to 50% of Americans, the conus artery demonstrates an independent origin from the right sinus of Valsalva adjacent to the RCA origin **(Figs. 3.1G** and **3.13)**.[11] There may be large geographic differences in the frequency of an independent origin of the conus artery; this variation is found in only 10% of Japanese,[12] 27% of Pakistanis, and 38% of Britons.[13] In rare cases, a conus artery may originate from the LAD. An intracoronary communication between the conus branches arising from the RCA and LAD may represent a rare congenital anomaly **(Fig. 3.14)**. More frequently, communicating arteries develop anterior to the conus as collateral pathways in the setting of a diseased RCA or LAD.

◆ SA Nodal Artery

In 50% of patients, the sinoatrial (SA) nodal artery arises from the proximal RCA, usually beyond the origin of the conus artery. In the remaining cases, the SA nodal artery branches from the midportion of the RCA or the proximal LCX.[14] When the SA nodal artery originates from the RCA, it is observed to course posteriorly between the aortic root and the right atrium, toward the cavoatrial junction. When the artery originates from the LCX, it courses posteriorly and to the right, between the aortic root and the left atrium, toward the cavoatrial junction **(Fig. 3.15)**. The distal SA nodal artery may course anterior or posterior to the superior vena cava to enter the SA node in the sulcus terminalis. In about 3% of people, SA nodal arteries arise from both the RCA and the LCX.[15] Rare patients may demonstrate a congenital intracoronary communication between SA nodal arteries from the RCA and LCX, resulting in bidirectional blood flow. In the setting of a diseased proximal RCA or LCX, this intracoronary communication may serve as the source of collateral flow between these two vessels.

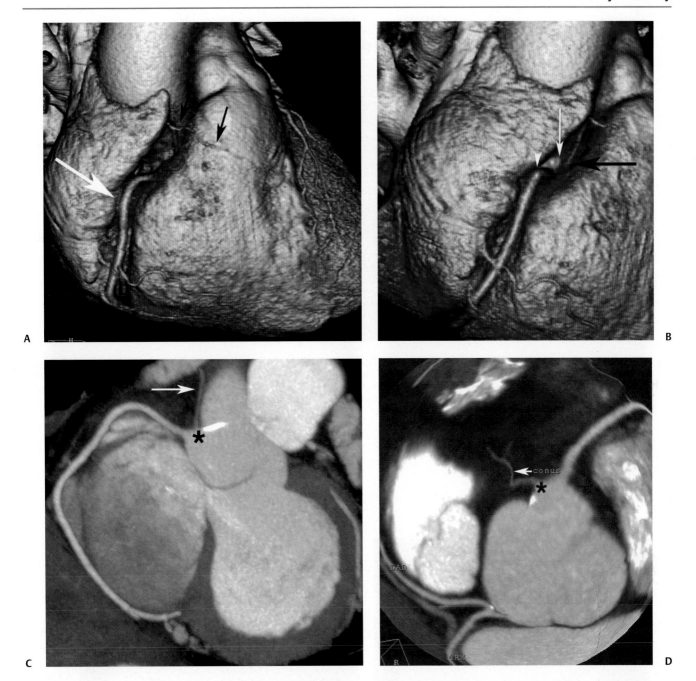

Fig. 3.13 Conus artery. **(A)** Surface-rendered image in an right anterior oblique projection demonstrates the right coronary artery (RCA) in the right atrioventricular (AV) groove (*white arrow*). A small conus branch (*black arrows*) arises from the proximal portion of the RCA and courses across the right ventricular outflow tract. **(B)** An independent origin of the conus artery (*black arrow*) is immediately adjacent to the RCA origin (*white arrow*). The RCA courses into the right AV groove below an overlying venous structure (*arrowhead*). **(C)** Maximum intensity projection (MIP) view of the RCA in the left anterior oblique projection. An independent origin of the conus branch is adjacent to the RCA origin (*black asterisk*). The conus branch courses superiorly from its origin (*arrow*). **(D)** Globe MIP again demonstrates the independent origin of the conus branch (*black asterisk*) as well as the short course of this vessel over the right ventricular outflow tract (*arrow*).

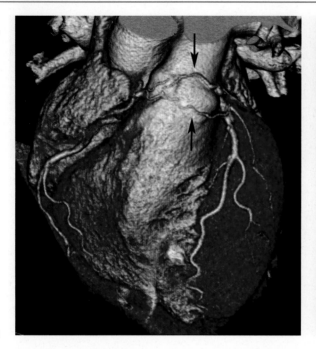

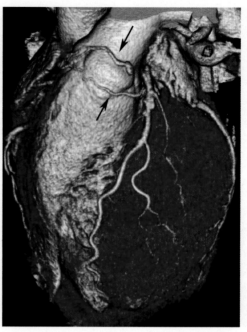

A

B

Fig. 3.14 Conus branch intercoronary communication. **(A,B)** Surface-rendered images in the anteroposterior and left anterior oblique projection demonstrate two small branches crossing anterior to the right ventricular outflow tract (*arrows*). This intercoronary communication connects the proximal right coronary artery and the proximal left anterior descending artery. Although this type of communication is often associated with collateral flow in the setting of coronary artery disease, this patient had no significant coronary disease.

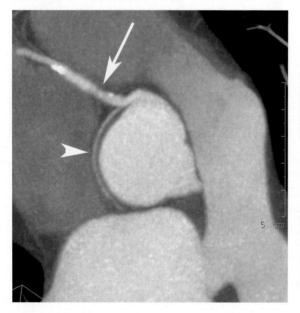

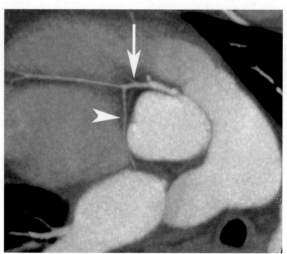

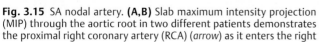

A

B

Fig. 3.15 SA nodal artery. **(A,B)** Slab maximum intensity projection (MIP) through the aortic root in two different patients demonstrates the proximal right coronary artery (RCA) (*arrow*) as it enters the right atrioventricular groove. The artery to the SA node arises from the RCA just before it enters the groove (*arrowhead*) but beyond the origin of the conus artery.

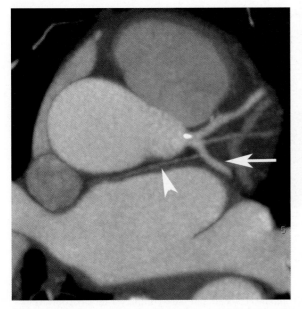

C

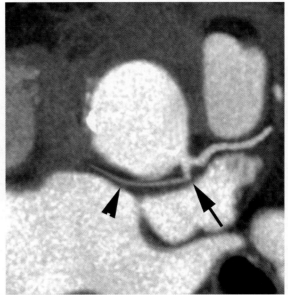

D

Fig. 3.15 (*Continued*) **(C,D)** Slab MIP in two additional patients demonstrates the SA nodal artery (*arrowhead*) arising from the circumflex artery (*arrow*). This artery courses between the aortic root and the left atrium to the interatrial septum. The short left main coronary arteries in C and D bifurcate just beyond their origins.

◆ Variations in the Left Main Coronary Artery

Anatomic variations in the origin and course of the left coronary system are rare (<1%) and are covered in Chapter 4 with coronary anomalies. However, there is considerable variation in the normal length of the left main coronary artery. Note the difference in the length of the left main coronary artery in **Figs. 2.2A,B** and **2.15C,D**. Absence of the left main coronary artery with independent origins of the LAD and LCX from the left sinus of Valsalva may be classified as a variation of coronary anatomy; in one series, it was reported in up to 1% of the population.[16] In patients with an absent left main coronary artery, special techniques may be used for selective catheterization and angioplasty. In this case, ostia of the LAD and LCX are generally adjacent to each other **(Fig. 3.16)** but may be slightly separated **(Fig. 3.17)**. The ostia are slightly smaller than might be expected for a single left main coronary

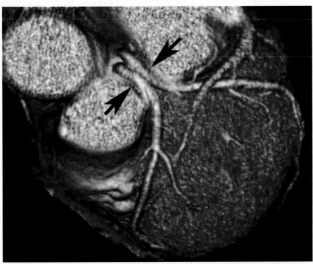

A

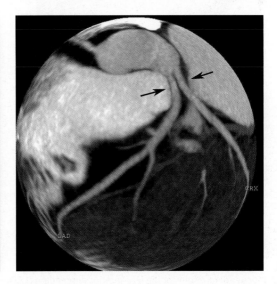

B

Fig. 3.16 Absent left main coronary artery. **(A)** Surface rendering demonstrates two arteries, the left anterior descending (LAD) and the circumflex, originating independently from the left sinus of Valsalva (*arrows*). **(B)** Globe maximum intensity projection (MIP) confirms independent origins of the LAD and circumflex arteries from the aorta (*arrows*). (*Continued on page 64*)

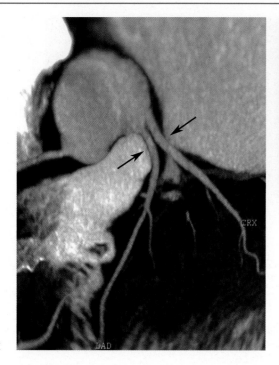

C

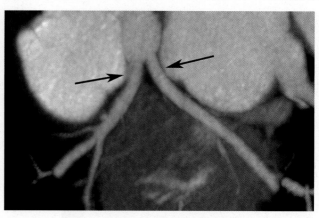

D

Fig. 3.16 (*Continued*) Absent left main coronary artery. **(C)** Surface-map MIP flattens out the globe display and again demonstrates independent origins of the LAD and circumflex arteries (*arrows*). **(D)** Slab MIP image demonstrates independent origins of the circumflex and LAD vessels (*arrows*).

artery. This is a benign variation with no other clinical significance. Nonetheless, the absence of the left main coronary artery is classified in most studies as a coronary anomaly because the incidence is reported as less than 1%. In the largest North American trial, absence of the left main coronary artery was identified in 0.4% of patients.[17]

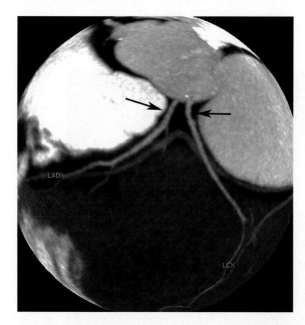

Fig. 3.17 Independent origins of the left anterior descending (LAD) and circumflex arteries. Globe maximum intensity projection image demonstrates independent origins of the LAD and circumflex vessels (*arrows*).

◆ Myocardial Bridging

Myocardial bridging is a congenital coronary variation in which a segment of a coronary artery that is normally epicardial in location is tunneled intramurally through the myocardium. Estimated frequency in angiographic series varies from 1.5 to 16%,[18] but it may be as high as 80% in autopsy series.[19,20] Myocardial bridges are most common in the LAD (**Figs. 3.18** and **3.19**).[21] Bridges may be classified by their length, depth within the myocardium, and degree of reduction in diameter during ventricular contraction. The large number of bridges found on autopsy series are likely related to short, shallow bridges that are not detected by angiography. These bridges may be more easily recognized with coronary CTA (**Figs. 3.20** and **3.21**). The bridged segment appears slightly narrowed, with slight angulation of the vessel as it enters and leaves the myocardium.

The vast majority of myocardial bridges are benign and of no clinical significance. However, complications, including arrhythmias, ischemia, and even sudden death, have been reported.[22] Unfortunately, it is difficult to establish a causal relationship between the myocardial bridge and clinical complications in many of the case reports. Doppler studies have demonstrated hemodynamic effects of bridging throughout the cardiac cycle and suggest that bridges may be associated with decreased coronary reserve. It has been hypothesized that the clinical significance of myocardial bridges may be suggested on the basis of the degree of arterial narrowing during systole on intracoronary Doppler studies, but there are no generally accepted criteria to assess which patients should have percutaneous or surgical intervention.[23]

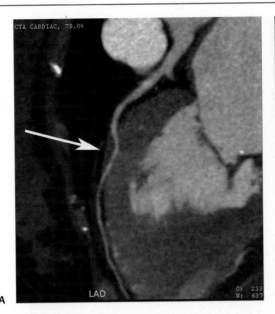

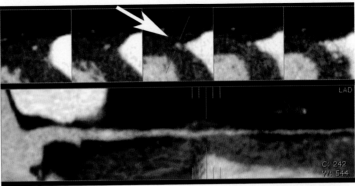

Fig. 3.18 Myocardial bridge of the left anterior descending artery (LAD). **(A)** Curved maximum intensity projection of the LAD demonstrates a short bridged segment that courses below the surface of the myocardium (*arrow*). **(B)** Short-axis images demonstrates the bridged segment of the LAD (*arrow*) surrounded by myocardium.

There appears to be a protective effect of myocardial bridges on the tunneled artery. The intima of the tunneled artery is significantly thinner than that of the more proximal vessel, and it is hypothesized that high shear stress within the bridged segment may be protective.[23] In our experience, a diffusely diseased artery may demonstrate a spared intramural segment that does not appear to be involved by atherosclerosis **(Fig. 3.22)**. Paradoxically, others have suggested that systolic kinking of the bridged segment may damage the endothelium and result in thrombosis with acute coronary syndrome. Additional studies are needed to establish the clinical significance of myocardial bridging and to determine the criteria for therapy of this condition.

◆ Capillary Level Arterial Communications

Normal coronary arteries subdivide into smaller branches that terminate in a capillary network. Although coronary arteries are generally of the terminal type, diminutive connections (20-250 μm in size) can be found between adjacent myocardial territories. These communications can enlarge to form collaterals in the setting of coronary disease and occlusion. Histopathological examination also demonstrates coronary-cameral communications between a minority of small terminal coronary branches and the intracardiac cavity. In addition, there are normal coronary venous communications to the

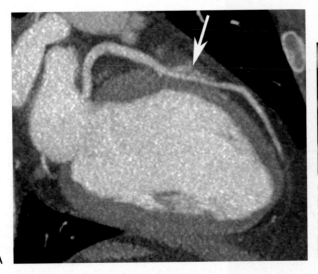

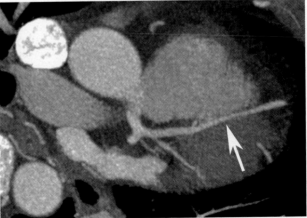

Fig. 3.19 Myocardial bridge of the mid-left anterior descending artery (LAD) with physiologic narrowing. **(A)** Long-axis slab maximum intensity projection (MIP) of the LAD demonstrates a bridged segment of the mid-LAD (*arrow*) that appears narrowed relative to the more proximal and distal segments of the LAD. **(B)** Orthogonal slab MIP again demonstrates narrowing of the bridged segment of the LAD (*arrow*) with no evidence of atherosclerotic disease.

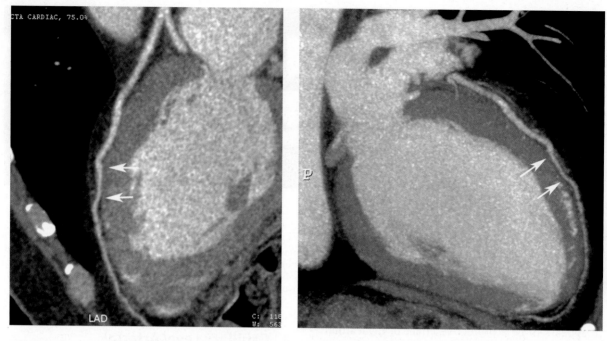

Fig. 3.20 Shallow myocardial bridge of the left anterior descending artery (LAD). **(A)** Curved maximum intensity projection (MIP) of the LAD demonstrates a short bridged segment that courses below a thin layer of myocardium (*arrows*). **(B)** Slab MIP image again demonstrates the bridged segment of the LAD (*arrows*). The diameter of the LAD is slightly decreased by the bridge.

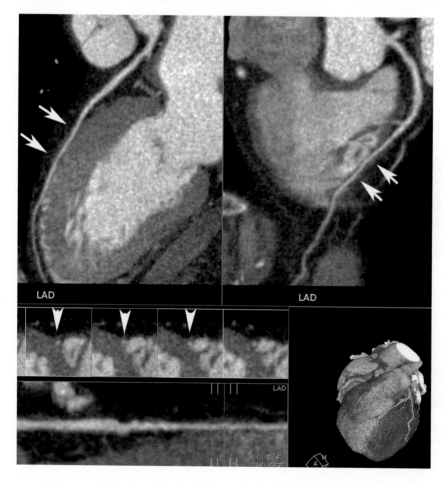

Fig. 3.21 Shallow myocardial bridge of the left anterior descending artery (LAD) on orthogonal curved maximum intensity projection (MIP) images. The myocardial bridge presents as a straightened segment along the surface of the left ventricle (*arrows*). Short-axis images of the LAD in this segment demonstrate a thin layer of myocardium anterior to the vessel (*arrowheads*), confirming the diagnosis of a myocardial bridge.

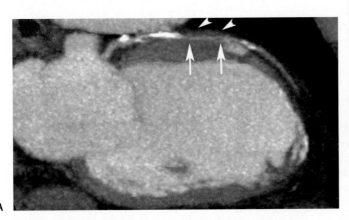

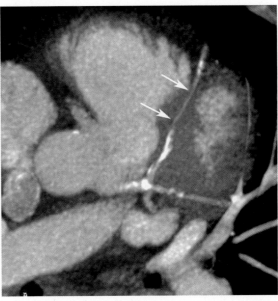

A   B

Fig. 3.22 Diseased left anterior descending artery (LAD) with a myocardial bridge. **(A)** Slab maximum intensity projection (MIP) of the LAD in the long axis of the left ventricle demonstrates a myocardial bridge (*arrows*). The LAD is calcified both proximal and distal to the bridge, but there is no atherosclerotic disease within the bridged segment. A small amount of myocardium is appreciated overlying this portion of the LAD (*arrowheads*). **(B)** Slab MIP in a slightly oblique axial projection again demonstrates the bridged segment (*arrows*), which appears smaller in diameter but free of atherosclerotic disease. Bridged segments of the coronary arteries may be protected from atherosclerotic disease.

cardiac cavities, known as *thebesian* veins. These communications are generally under 250 μm in size and are not visible on cardiac CT.[14] Larger communications with the cardiac chambers can occur and are included in the discussion of coronary anomalies in Chapter 4.

◆ Conclusion

The most common variation of the coronary circulation includes a dominant RCA that supplies the inferior septum (via the PDA) and the inferior wall of the left ventricle (via posterior left ventricular branches). The LCA branches into the LAD and LCX. The LAD typically supplies the anterior septum (via septal perforators) as well as the anterior and lateral walls (via diagonal branches). The LCX typically supplies the lateral and inferolateral walls (via obtuse marginal branches). The supply of the inferior and inferolateral walls is quite variable and defines the dominance of the coronary circulation. Variations in coronary anatomy are common, most frequently involving the distribution of diagonal, ramus medianus, and obtuse marginal branches. Other common variations include an increased number of coronary ostia in the aortic root related to independent origins of the conus artery, LAD, and LCX. With the advent of coronary CTA, a larger number of myocardial bridge segments are appreciated, most commonly in the LAD.

Cine 3.1 Normal right-dominant coronary circulation (see **Fig. 3.5**). Cine begins in a left anterior oblique (LAO) projection, demonstrating the origin of the left coronary artery with the left atrial appendage cut away. The heart rotates into a standard LAO projection to demonstrate the left anterior descending artery and then turns right anterior oblique to demonstrate the right coronary artery (RCA) in the right atrioventricular groove. Further rotation follows the RCA to the origins of the posterior descending artery and posterior left ventricular branches at the crux of the heart, demonstrating a right-dominant circulation. The cine loop is completed with further rotation to demonstrate the circumflex branches and finally back to the initial LAO projection.

Cine 3.2 Normal right-dominant coronary circulation (see **Fig. 3.6B**). Cine begins in a left lateral projection, demonstrating a small circumflex artery ending as an obtuse marginal branch. The heart is then rotated into an left anterior oblique projection to demonstrate the left anterior descending and diagonal branches. Further rotation follows the right coronary artery (RCA) around the right atrioventricular groove to the crux of the heart. The posterior descending artery and posterior left ventricular branches arise from the distal RCA.

(Continued on page 68)

Cine 3.3 (A,B) Normal right-dominant coronary circulation. **(A)** Cine begins in the left anterior oblique projection, demonstrating the left anterior descending artery. The heart is then rotated into a right anterior oblique projection to follow the right coronary artery (RCA) around the right atrioventricular groove. Further rotation demonstrates bifurcation of the RCA into a large posterior descending artery and small left ventricular branch at the crux of the heart. **(B)** Cine illustrates the same patient with the left atrial appendage removed to demonstrate the circumflex artery.

Cine 3.4 (A,B) Normal left-dominant coronary circulation. **(A)** Cine begins in the left anterior oblique (LAO) projection with the left atrial appendage removed to reveal the bifurcation of the left main coronary artery into the left anterior descending artery (LAD) and circumflex. Caudal rotation demonstrates the LAD, followed by rotation into the right anterior oblique (RAO) projection to demonstrate the right coronary artery (RCA) in the right atrioventricular (AV) groove. The RCA ends as a small acute marginal branch. The heart then rotates back to follow the circumflex artery in the left AV groove around to the crux. Multiple left ventricular branches arise from the large circumflex artery that ends as the posterior descending artery. **(B)** The same patient anatomy as **(A)** but beginning in the RAO projection with a view of the RCA. The heart then rotates into the LAO, rotates further

to demonstrate the crux, and completes a full 360 rotation to end back at the RCA.

Cine 3.5 Weakly left-dominant coronary circulation. Cine begins in the left anterior oblique projection, demonstrating a duplicated left anterior descending artery in the anterior interventricular groove. The heart then rotates to demonstrate a large circumflex artery and its branches: several obtuse marginal branches, a posterior left ventricular branch, and a small posterior descending artery (PDA) ending in the proximal portion of the posterior interventricular groove. The distal portion of the posterior interventricular groove is supplied by a large terminal branch of the right coronary artery. The PDA territory in this patient is therefore supplied by both the left circumflex artery (proximally) and the right coronary artery (distally).

Cine 3.6 Codominant (balanced) coronary circulation. Cine begins in the left anterior oblique projection demonstrating a mildly diseased left anterior descending artery. The heart then rotates to demonstrate a large circumflex artery with obtuse marginal and posterior left ventricular branches. The posterior descending artery (PDA) is visualized at the crux of the heart as a small branch of the diseased distal right coronary artery (RCA) entering the posterior interventricular groove. This is a balanced circulation with a left circumflex artery supplying the posterior left ventricular branches and a RCA supplying the PDA.

References

1. Angelini P. Normal and anomalous coronary arteries: definitions and classification. Am Heart J. 1989;117(2):418–434
2. Neufeld HN, Schneeweiss A. Coronary artery disease in infants and children. Philadelphia: Lea & Febiger, 1983
3. Dabizzi RP, Teodori G, Barletta GA, Caprioli G, Baldrighi G, Baldrighi V. Associated coronary and cardiac anomalies in the tetralogy of Fallot: an angiographic study. Eur Heart J. 1990;11(8):692–704
4. Dabizzi RP, Barletta GA, Caprioli G, Baldrighi G, Baldrighi V. Coronary artery anatomy in corrected transposition of the great arteries. J Am Coll Cardiol. 1988;12(2):486–491
5. Mainwaring RD, Lamberti JJ. Pulmonary atresia with intact ventricular septum. Surgical approach based on ventricular size and coronary anatomy. J Thorac Cardiovasc Surg. 1993;106(4):733–738
6. Angelini P, Velasco JA, Flamm S. Coronary anomalies: incidence, pathophysiology, and clinical relevance. Circulation. 2002;105(20):2449–2454
7. Angelini P. Coronary Artery Anomalies. Philadelphia: Lippincott Williams & Wilkins, 1999
8. Levin DC, Harrington DP, Bettmann MA, Garnic JD, Davidoff A, Lois J. Anatomic variations of the coronary arteries supplying the anterolateral aspect of the left ventricle: possible explanation for the "unexplained" anterior aneurysm. Invest Radiol. 1982;17(5):458–462
9. Spindola-Franco H, Grose R, Solomon N. Dual left anterior descending coronary artery: angiographic description of important variants and surgical implications. Am Heart J. 1983;105(3):445–455
10. Levin DC, Baltaxe HA. Angiographic demonstration of important anatomic variations of the posterior descending coronary artery. Am J Roentgenol Radium Ther Nucl Med. 1972;116(1):41–49
11. Schlesinger MJ, Zoll PM, Wessler S. The conus artery; a third coronary artery. Am Heart J. 1949;38(6):823–836

12. Cheng TO. Anomalous coronary arteries. Int J Cardiol. 1993;40(2):183
13. Topaz O, DeMarchena EJ, Perin E, Sommer LS, Mallon SM, Chahine RA. Anomalous coronary arteries: angiographic findings in 80 patients. Int J Cardiol. 1992;34(2):129–138
14. Baroldi G, Scomazzoni G. Coronary circulation in the normal heart, and the pathologic heart. Washington, DC: Department of the Army: US Government Printing Office, 5-90, 1967
15. Kyriakidis MK, Kourouklis CB, Papaioannou JT, Christakos SG, Spanos GP, Avgoustakis DG. Sinus node coronary arteries studied with angiography. Am J Cardiol. 1983;51(5):749–750
16. Vlodaver Z, Neufeld HN, Edwards JE. Pathology of coronary disease. Semin Roentgenol. 1972;7(4):376–394
17. Yamanaka O, Hobbs RE. Coronary artery anomalies in 126,595 patients undergoing coronary arteriography. Cathet Cardiovasc Diagn. 1990;21(1):28–40
18. Soran O, Pamir G, Erol C, Kocakavak C, Sabah I. The incidence and significance of myocardial bridge in a prospectively defined population of patients undergoing coronary angiography for chest pain. Tokai J Exp Clin Med. 2000;25(2):57–60
19. Rossi L, Dander B, Nidasio GP, et al. Myocardial bridges and ischemic heart disease. Eur Heart J 1980;1(4):239–245
20. Geiringer E. The mural coronary. Am Heart J 1951;41(3):359–368
21. Irvin RG. The angiographic prevalence of myocardial bridging in man. Chest. 1982;81(2):198–202
22. Cutler D, Wallace JM. Myocardial bridging in a young patient with sudden death. Clin Cardiol 1997;20(6):581–583
23. Alegria JR, Herrmann J, Holmes DR Jr, Lerman A, Rihal CS. Myocardial bridging. Eur Heart J. 2005;26(12):1159–1168

4

Coronary Anomalies

Ethan J. Halpern and David C. Levin

Coronary anomalies have been implicated as the cause of sudden death in up to 19% of athletes.[1] A study of deaths in U.S. high school and college athletes reported that coronary anomalies were responsible for 11.8% of deaths.[2] Among 14- to 40-year-old individuals, coronary anomalies are involved in 12% of sports-related sudden cardiac deaths.[3] Hemodynamically significant coronary anomalies may manifest with angina, arrhythmia, myocardial infarction, or sudden death and may promote the onset and progression of coronary atherosclerosis.[4] Unfortunately, it is often difficult to establish a definite causal relationship between coronary anomalies and clinical events. The discussion of normal coronary anatomy in the previous chapter included common coronary variations. The present chapter expands the discussion to include coronary anomalies, defined as anatomic features that are present in less than 1% of the population. Although it might be useful to classify coronary anomalies based on clinical significance, physiologic correlation is often lacking.[5] Nonetheless, coronary anomalies are classified as benign or potentially serious based on anatomic considerations and anecdotal clinical observation.

◆ Anatomic Considerations in the Diagnosis of Coronary Anomalies

Coronary CT angiography (CTA) is particularly well suited to demonstrate anatomic detail for clinical evaluation and research study of coronary anomalies. Features of coronary anatomy that should be evaluated include the coronary artery ostium, course of the artery, arterial termination, and arterial size. The number of coronary ostia should be noted, and each ostium should be evaluated for location, size, and angle of origin.[6]

The presence of two coronary ostia, one in the right coronary sinus and one in the left coronary sinus, is a minimum requirement for normalcy.[7] As discussed in the previous chapter, up to four coronary ostia may be present, including independent origins of the right coronary artery (RCA), conus artery, left anterior descending artery (LAD), and left circumflex artery (LCX). The presence of a solitary coronary ostium in the aortic root or the presence of a right and a left coronary ostia originating from a single coronary sinus is

anomalous. Ectopic origin of a coronary artery above the sinotubular junction, or from a vessel other than the aorta, is anomalous.

Anomalous coronary artery origins may be associated with anomalies of the aortic root (**Fig. 3.1**) or anomalous course of a coronary artery. In these situations, coronary flow may be compromised by narrowing of the ostium or by compression of the anomalous coronary artery between the aorta and right ventricular outflow tract.

The spectrum of coronary anomalies also includes less common anatomic variations, such as distal connections to other coronary arteries (intercoronary communication) and fistulae to the cardiac chambers, to cardiac veins, or to extracardiac arteries or veins. Anomalies of coronary artery size are not defined by specific size criteria, but the diagnosis can be made in the setting of a focally atretic, hypoplastic, or ectatic coronary segment. The criteria for this diagnosis are less well defined when an entire artery is involved.

◆ Frequency of Coronary Anomalies

In the large series reported from the Cleveland Clinic Foundation, coronary anomalies were identified in 1.3% of 126,595 patients undergoing coronary arteriography.[8] Among 1686 patients with anomalies, 87% had anomalies of origin and distribution of the coronary arteries, whereas 13% had coronary artery fistulae. A frequently cited smaller study documented coronary anomalies in 5.6% of 1950 consecutive cineangiograms.[9] The higher incidence in this study may be related to the author's strict definition of coronary anomalies, to meticulous technique, or to referral bias. Some studies demonstrate a higher prevalence of coronary anomalies in men,[10] whereas other studies demonstrate a higher prevalence in women.[11] Most studies report the overall prevalence of coronary anomalies at about 1%, although a review of the literature suggests that the true incidence of coronary anomalies "in the general population is variable and depends on genetic and geographic factors."[12]

Based on the data from the Cleveland Clinic study, clinically benign coronary anomalies are present in 1.07% of the population. The most common anomalies are absent left main coronary artery with independent origins of the LAD and LCX in 0.41% and anomalous LCX from the right coronary sinus or the RCA in 0.37%. Less common benign anomalies include anomalous origin of a coronary artery from the posterior sinus of Valsalva or from above the sinotubular junction, absent LCX ("superdominant RCA"), intercoronary communications, and small coronary artery fistulae.

In the Cleveland Clinic series, potentially serious anomalies were identified in 0.26% of the population. The most common serious anomalies include origin of the RCA from the left sinus of Valsalva in 0.11%, origin of the left coronary artery (LCA) or LAD from the right sinus of Valsalva in 0.05%, and multiple or large fistulae in 0.05%. Less common serious anomalies include origin of a coronary artery from the pulmonary artery and single coronary artery. Anomalous origin of a coronary artery from the pulmonary artery involves the left main coronary in approximately 75% of cases, with the remaining cases involving the RCA or LAD. Most of these patients present in early childhood, with 75% of these patients developing symptoms in the first 4 months of life and a minority surviving into adulthood.[13] The overall frequency of an anomalous coronary artery arising from a pulmonary artery was 0.01% in the Cleveland Clinic study.

◆ Anomalies of Origin and Course

Left Coronary Artery

An anomalous origin of the LCA is most frequently from the right anterior sinus of Valsalva in a common origin with the RCA or adjacent to the ostium of the RCA. The LCA may then course anterior to the aorta in the space between the aorta and right ventricular outflow tract (**Fig. 4.1**), anterior to right ventricular outflow tract (**Fig. 4.2**), or posterior to the aorta (**Fig. 4.3**). When the LCA courses anterior to the aorta, a sagittal image should be obtained to distinguish an interarterial course from a septal course. An interarterial course is diagnosed when the anomalous vessel passes between the aorta and the right ventricular outflow tract. The interarterial course is considered a serious congenital anomaly[14] and can present with angina, myocardial infarction, syncope, ventricular tachycardia, or sudden death.[15] Various hypotheses explain these consequences based on a slit-like origin, kinking of the anomalous vessel, or compression between the right and left ventricular outflow tracts.

When an anomalous LCA passes anterior to the pulmonary artery or posterior to the aorta, the variant is considered benign. Likewise, a "septal" course that passes between the great vessels below the level of the pulmonary valve is generally considered a benign variation (**Fig. 4.4**).[16] However, coronary CTA clearly demonstrates that even when the anomalous LCA drops directly into the intraventricular septum, a short segment of the proximal LCA will usually course between the aorta and the right ventricular outflow tract at the level of the aortic root (**Fig. 4.5**). A recent report suggests that the distinction between the malignant interarterial variant and the benign septal variant is too simplistic.[17] The course of an anomalous LCA behind the pulmonary artery is often a combination of interarterial and septal segments.

An uncommon anomaly involving the main LCA is a posteriorly displaced origin of the LCA from the posterior,

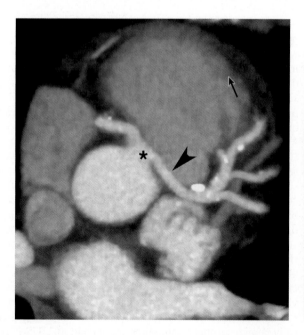
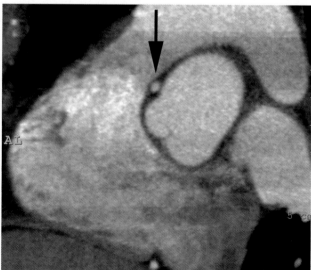

A

B

Fig. 4.1 Anomalous left coronary artery passing between the aorta of the right ventricular pulmonary outflow tract. **(A)** Axial image demonstrates a common origin of the right coronary artery and left coronary artery (*arrowhead*) from a common trunk at the right coronary sinus of Valsalva (***). The left coronary artery passes posterior to the right ventricular outflow tract (*arrowhead*). **(B)** Sagittal reconstruction demonstrates the left coronary artery as it passes anterior to the aortic root and posterior to the pulmonic outflow tract (*arrow*).

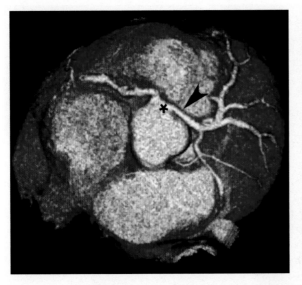

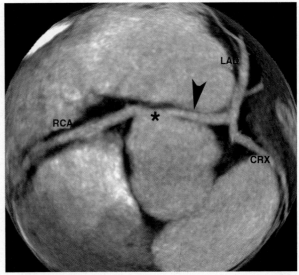

C

D

Fig. 4.1 *(Continued)* **(C, D)** Surface rendering and globe maximum intensity projection demonstrate the common origin of both coronary arteries (*). The left coronary artery (*arrowhead*) passes between the aortic root and the right ventricular outflow tract. LAD, left anterior descending; RCA, right coronary artery; CRX, circumflex artery.

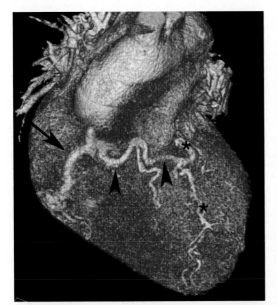

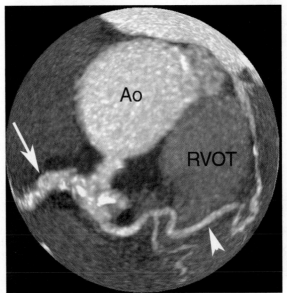

A

B

C

Fig. 4.2 Anomalous left coronary artery passing anterior to the right ventricular outflow tract (RVOT). **(A)** Volumetric surface image demonstrates a large right coronary artery (*arrow*), with a left coronary artery that originates from a common ostium with the right coronary artery and courses anterior to the RVOT (*arrowheads*). Left anterior descending (LAD) and circumflex branches are seen to arise from the left coronary artery (*asterisks*). **(B)** Globe MIP demonstrates a single coronary artery arising from the anterior sinus of the aorta (Ao). The left coronary artery (*arrowhead*) originates from the right coronary artery (*arrow*) and courses anterior to the RVOT. **(C)** Slab maximum intensity projection image demonstrates that the left coronary artery (*arrowhead*) passes anterior to the RVOT.

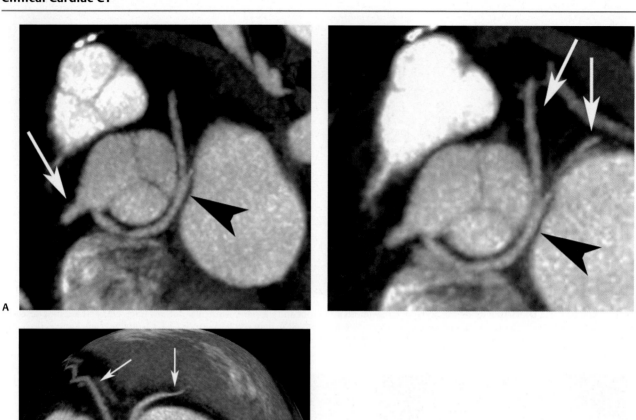

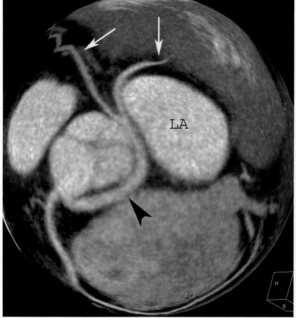

Fig. 4.3 Anomalous left coronary artery (LCA) passing behind the aortic root. **(A)** Axial image demonstrates the right coronary artery (*arrow*) and LCA (*arrowhead*), both originating from the right coronary sinus of Valsava. The LCA courses posterior to the aortic root, between the aortic root and left atrium (*arrowhead*). **(B)** Slab maximum intensity projection (MIP) demonstrates the LCA as it courses posterior to the aortic root (*arrowhead*) and bifurcates into the left anterior descending artery (LAD) and circumflex arteries (*arrows*). **(C)** Globe MIP image again demonstrates the LCA as it courses around the aortic root posteriorly (*arrowhead*). There is a long left main coronary artery, which then bifurcates into the LAD and circumflex arteries (*arrows*). These vessels assume their normal positions in the anterior interventricular groove and the left atrioventricular groove, respectively. LA, left atrium.

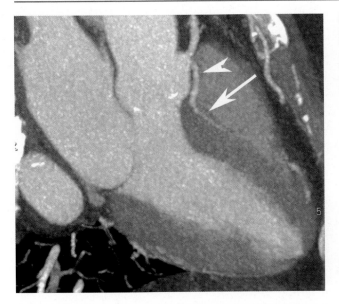

Fig. 4.4 Intramyocardial "septal" course of an anomalous left coronary artery (*arrowhead*), which arises from the right sinus of Valsalva just below the right coronary origin but courses directly down into the myocardium of the interventricular septum (*arrow*). Although an anomalous course of a coronary artery anterior to the aorta is generally considered a dangerous variation, it is often stated that the intramyocardial course of the anomalous vessel is protective.

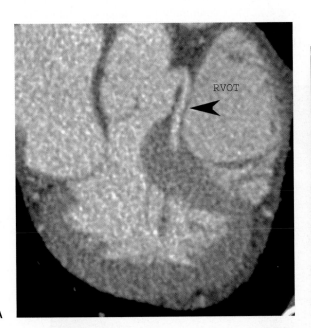

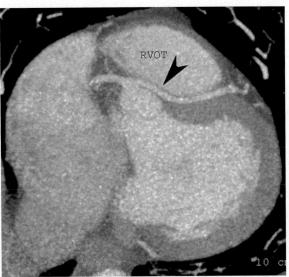

A   B

Fig. 4.5 Anomalous left coronary artery with an intramyocardial course. The anomalous vessel demonstrates a short proximal segment that courses between the aortic root and right ventricular outflow tract (RVOT). **(A)** Slab maximum intensity projection (MIP) demonstrates an anomalous anterior origin of the left coronary artery (*arrowhead*) coursing directly down into the myocardium of the interventricular septum. **(B)** Slab MIP in a different obliquity demonstrates the proximal course of this anomalous vessel (*arrowhead*) between the aorta and right ventricular outflow tract.   (Continued on page 74)

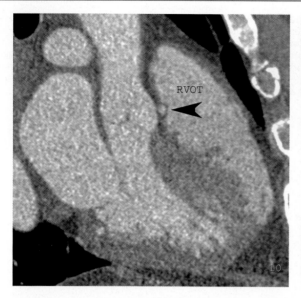

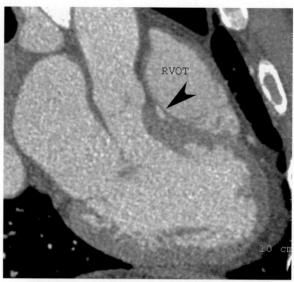

C

D

Fig. 4.5 (*Continued*) Anomalous left coronary artery with an intramyocardial course. The anomalous vessel demonstrates a short proximal segment that courses between the aortic root and right ventricular outflow tract (RVOT). **(C)** Sagittal MIP near the origin of the anomalous vessel demonstrates its course between the outflow tracts (*arrowhead*). **(D)** Sagittal MIP slightly to the left of the image in (C) demonstrates the intramyocardial course of the left anterior descending artery (*arrowhead*).

right-sided cusp of the aorta, which is generally designated as the noncoronary cusp **(Fig. 4.6)**. In this benign anomaly, the left main coronary artery courses posterior to the aorta.

In some patients, the anomalous course may involve the LAD or LCX rather than the left main coronary. In the rare patient with no left main coronary artery, both the LAD and LCX arteries may demonstrate an anomalous course **(Fig. 4.7)**. More commonly, an isolated anomalous LAD may be associated with a normal position of the circumflex artery **(Fig. 4.8)**. When an anomalous LAD passes between the aorta and the right ventricular outflow tract, the imaging

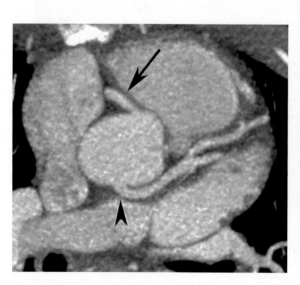

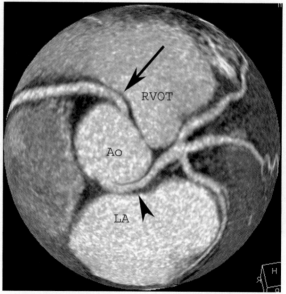

A

B

Fig. 4.6 Posterior origin of the left coronary artery (LCA). **(A)** Axial maximum intensity projection (MIP) demonstrates the origin of the right coronary artery (RCA) (*arrow*) from the anterior sinus of Valsalva. The LCA (*arrowhead*) originates more posteriorly than normal, from the margin of the posterior or right sinus of Valsalva, which is normally the noncoronary sinus. The left main coronary artery courses between the aorta and left atrium (LA) before branching into the left anterior descending and circumflex arteries. **(B)** Globe MIP again demonstrates a posterior origin of the LCA (*arrowhead*) and also suggests that the RCA (*arrow*) may originate slightly more to the left than usual. The RCA courses to the right for a short distance before entering the right atrioventricular groove. RVOT, right ventricular outflow tract.

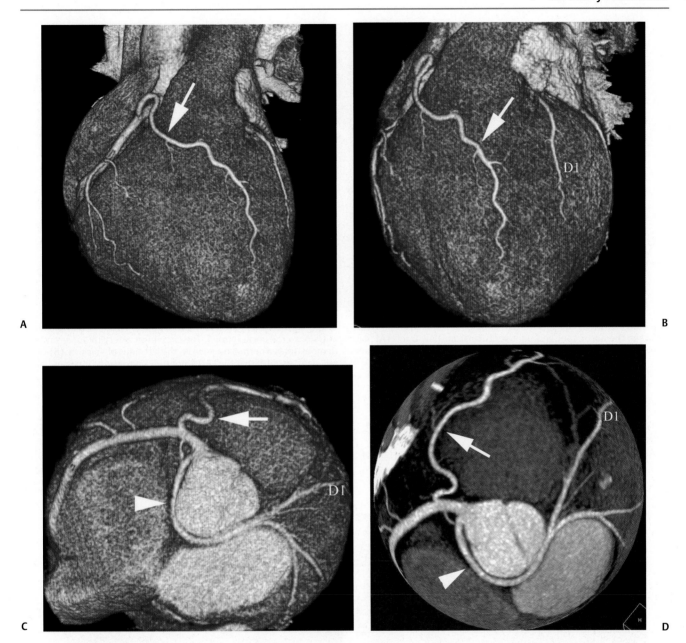

Fig. 4.7 Single coronary artery originating from the anterior sinus of Valsalva. Anomalous left anterior descending artery (LAD) courses anterior to the right ventricular outflow tract (RVOT) while the anomalous circumflex passes behind the aorta (Ao). **(A)** Volumetric surface rendering in the anteroposterior projection demonstrates a large right coronary artery (RCA). The LAD (*arrow*) originates from the RCA and courses anterior to the RVOT. **(B)** LAO projection demonstrates the anomalous LAD with an adjacent diagonal artery (D1) that arises from an anomalous circumflex artery. **(C)** View from above demonstrates the LAD (*arrow*) as well as the anomalous circumflex (*arrowhead*) as they originate from the RCA. The circumflex artery courses behind the aorta and supplies a large first diagonal branch (D1). **(D)** Globe maximum intensity projection image demonstrates similar anatomy.

and clinical considerations are similar to those posed by a left main coronary artery that passes between them. An anomalous circumflex from the right sinus of Valsalva almost always passes posterior to the aorta (**Fig. 4.9** and **4.10**), and is not in danger of compression by the outflow

tracts. However, when a patient with this anomaly undergoes cardiac surgery, the surgeon should be informed of the anomalous course to avoid accidental compression of the circumflex during valve replacement.[18] Furthermore, at least one study suggests that an anomalous retroaortic

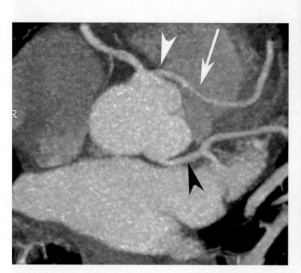

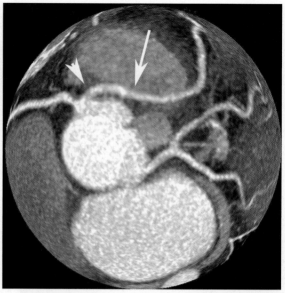

A

B

Fig. 4.8 Anomalous course of the left anterior descending artery (LAD) between the aortic root and right ventricular outflow tract. **(A)** Slab maximum intensity projection (MIP) image just off the axial plane demonstrates the origin of the left anterior descending artery (LAD) (*white arrowhead*) from the right sinus of Valsalva, adjacent to the origin of the right coronary artery. The LAD appears narrowed as it courses anterior to the aorta (*arrow*). The circumflex artery (*black arrowhead*) demonstrates a normal origin from the left sinus of Valsalva. **(B)** Globe MIP demonstrates that the LAD is not truly narrowed as it passes behind the right ventricular outflow tract.

circumflex artery is more likely to be affected by atherosclerotic disease **(Fig. 4.11)**.[19]

An uncommon, serious anomaly is the anomalous origin of the LCA from the pulmonary artery, also know as ALCAPA **(Fig. 4.12)**. Most of these patients are identified as infants or during early childhood because of myocardial ischemia or infarction or congestive heart failure, and about 90% die within the first year.[20] Those patients who do survive into adulthood

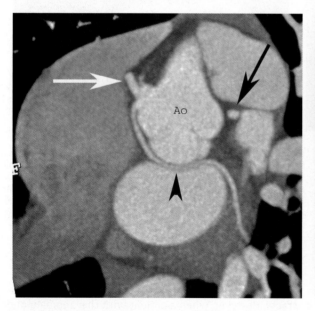

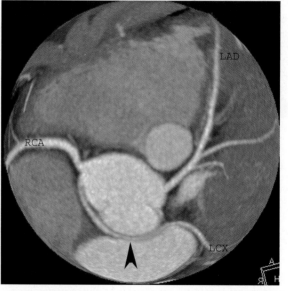

A

B

Fig. 4.9 Anomalous course of the circumflex artery between the aortic root and left atrium. **(A)** Slab maximum intensity projection (MIP) demonstrates the right coronary artery (RCA) originating from the right sinus of Valsava in a normal anterior location (*white arrow*). A segment of the left anterior descending artery (LAD) is identified as it enters the anterior interventricular groove (*black arrow*). The circumflex artery originates from the base of the RCA and courses posteriorly behind the aorta (Ao) to pass between the aortic root and left atrium (*black arrowhead*). **(B)** Globe MIP demonstrates similar anatomy but demonstrates the LAD more clearly. The circumflex artery passes between the aortic root and left atrium (*arrowhead*) into the left atrioventricular groove.

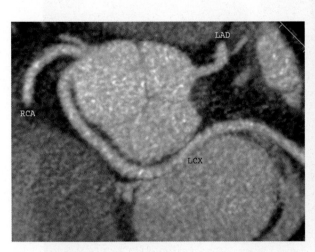

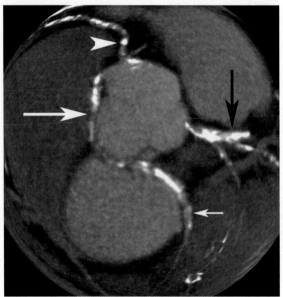

Fig. 4.10 Anomalous course of the circumflex artery (LCX) between the aortic root and left atrium. **(A)** Axial image demonstrates the origins of three coronary arteries. The circumflex originates from the right sinus of Valsalva, adjacent to the right coronary artery (RCA). **(B)** Globe maximum intensity projection (MIP) demonstrates similar anatomy. LAD, left anterior descending artery.

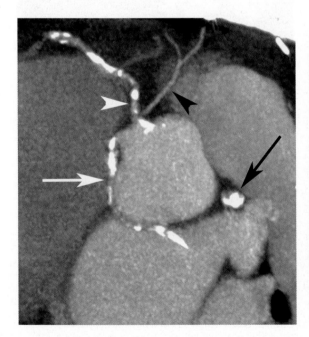

Fig. 4.11 Anomalous circumflex artery in a patient with severe triple vessel coronary disease. **(A)** The right coronary artery (RCA) is in standard location, originating from the right sinus of Valsava (*white arrowhead*). The conus branch originates with a common trunk from the RCA (*black arrowhead*). The circumflex artery originates from the right sinus of Valsava, adjacent to the RCA origin, and courses around the aortic root (*white arrow*) posteriorly. The proximal left coronary artery is seen adjacent to the left coronary sinus (*black arrow*). Diffuse vascular calcifications are identified in all three major coronary arteries. **(B)** Globe maximum intensity oprojection (MIP) image again demonstrates the RCA originating from the right sinus of Valsalva (*arrowhead*). The circumflex artery originates adjacent to the RCA (*arrow*) and courses around the aorta posteriorly. On the globe MIP, the circumflex artery can be traced as it enters the left atrioventricular groove (*small arrow*).

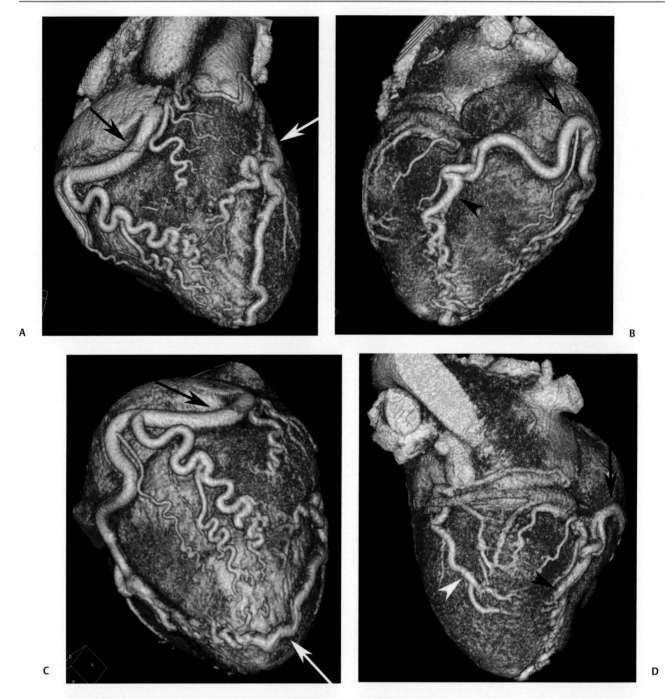

Fig. 4.12 Anomalous left coronary artery from the pulmonary artery (ALCAPA) presenting in adulthood. **(A)** Surface volumetric image in a slight left anterior oblique (LAO) projection demonstrates marked enlargement of the right coronary artery (RCA) (*black arrow*) and left coronary artery (LCA) (*white arrow*) as well as numerous enlarged, tortuous collateral vessels over the free wall of the right ventricle. **(B)** Volumetric projection of the crux of the heart again demonstrates an enlarged RCA (*black arrow*) feeding an enlarged posterior descending artery (PDA) (*black arrowhead*). **(C)** Volumetric projection at the apex of the heart demonstrates enlarged collateral vessels extending from the PDA to the distal left anterior descending artery (LAD) (*white arrow*). **(D)** Volumetric projection in a steep LAO projection demonstrates large obtuse marginal branches of the circumflex artery (*white arrowhead*) that appear to be extending toward other posterior left ventricular branches arising from the PDA (*black arrowhead*).

will have numerous collateral vessels between the left and right coronary circulations. In these cases, the RCA supplies the left coronary circulation, but it also supplies a left-to-right shunt into the pulmonary artery. Increased flow through the coronary arteries results in marked dilatation and tortuosity of numerous vessels over the surface of the myocardium. Shunt physiology may result in pulmonary hypertension. ALCAPA can present as a cause of sudden cardiac death in the adult.

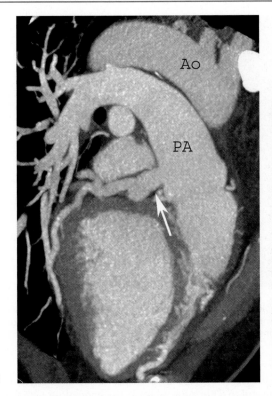

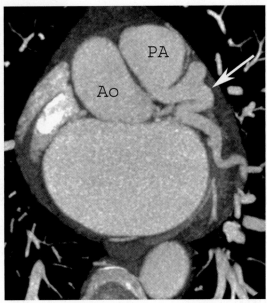

E

F

Fig. 4.12 (*Continued*) **(E)** Slab MIP in a sagittal projection demonstrates the anomalous origin of the left coronary artery (*arrow*) from the posterior surface of the pulmonary artery (PA). **(F)** Slab MIP in the axial plane again demonstrates the anomalous origin of the LCA (*arrow*) from the posterior surface of the pulmonary artery (PA). The normal origin of this left coronary artery should have been from the adjacent left side of the aorta (Ao).

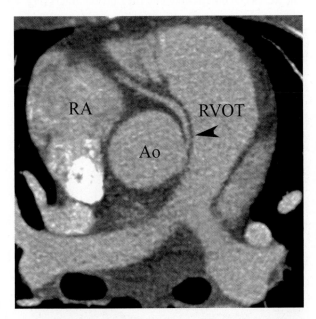

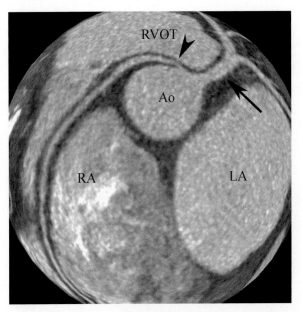

A

B

Fig. 4.13 Anomalous right coronary artery (RCA) passing between the aorta (Ao) and right ventricular outflow tract (RVOT). **(A)** Axial maximum intensity projection (MIP) demonstrates the RCA origin (*arrowhead*) from the left sinus of Valsalva. The RCA passes between the Ao root and RVOT. **(B)** Globe MIP demonstrates the RCA origin (*arrowhead*) immediately anterior to the origin of the left coronary artery (LCA) (*arrow*) from the left sinus of Valsalva. The RCA courses between the RVOT and the Ao root into the right atrioventricular groove, adjacent to the right atrium (RA). Note that the RCA appears narrowed at its angulated origin (*arrowhead*) compared with the remainder of its course. LA, left atrium. (Continued on page 80)

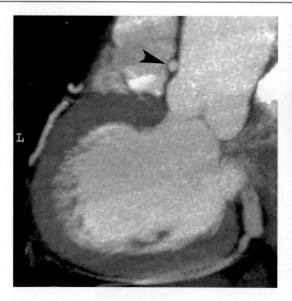

C

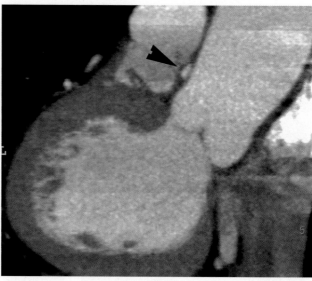

D

Fig. 4.13 (*Continued*) Anomalous right coronary artery (RCA) passing between the aorta (Ao) and right ventricular outflow tract (RVOT). **(C)** Sagittal image again demonstrates the RCA (*arrowhead*) as it passes anterior to the Ao root root at the level of the sinotubular junction. The artery passes immediately posterior to the RVOT above the level of the interventricular septum. **(D)** Sagittal image to the left of the image in (B) demonstrates compression of the RCA (*arrowhead*) just beyond its origin.

Right Coronary Artery

Anomalous origin of the RCA is most frequently from the left sinus of Valsalva or from the ascending aorta. The RCA may originate from the left sinus of Valsalva in a common ostium with the LCA or adjacent to the ostium of the LCA. In either case, treatment decisions will be based on the course of the RCA relative to the aorta and right ventricular outflow tract.

When the RCA traverses anterior to the aorta, a sagittal image is useful to determine whether the anomalous vessel has an interarterial or septal course **(Fig. 4.13)**. When the RCA crosses between the aorta and the pulmonary artery above the level of the interventricular septum, there is risk for occlusion during systolic aortic expansion.[21,22] In some patients, it may be possible to demonstrate compression of the RCA as it courses between the outflow tracts **(Fig. 4.14)**.

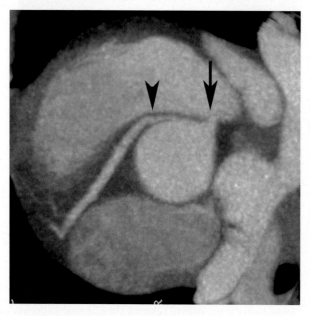

A

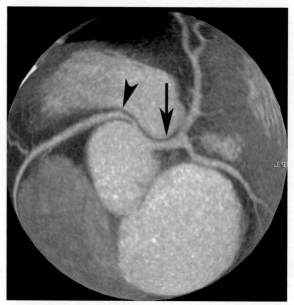

B

Fig. 4.14 Anomalous right coronary artery (RCA) passing between the aorta (Ao) and right ventricular outflow tract (RVOT). **(A)** Axial maximum intensity projection (MIP) demonstrates the origin of the left main coronary artery (*arrow*) from the left coronary sinus of Valsava. The RCA (*arrowhead*) originates from the left sinus of Valsava, although not quite as close to the origin of the left coronary artery as in Fig. 4.13. The RCA passes between the aortic root and RVOT (*arrowhead*). **(B)** Globe MIP demonstrates the course of the RCA (*arrowhead*) and LCA (*arrow*). The RCA is narrowed to 1.3 mm as it passes behind the RVOT but measures 4 mm as it emerges into the right atrioventricular groove.

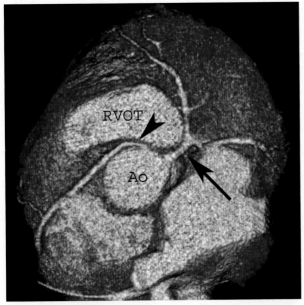

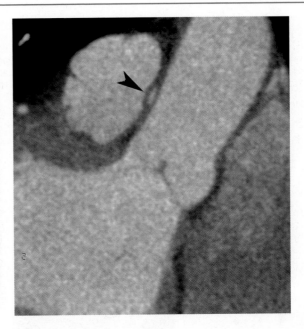

Fig. 4.14 (*Continued*) **(C)** Surface-rendered image demonstrates compression of the RCA as it passes between the Ao and RVOT. **(D)** Sagittal

MIP demonstrates compression of the RCA between the Ao and RVOT into a slit-like contour (*arrowhead*).

Anomalous origin of the RCA above the sinotubular junction is actually more common than anomalous origin from the left sinus of Valsalva (**Fig. 4.15**). This anomaly is generally considered benign, although it may be associated with a relatively long length of vessel that crosses between the aorta and pulmonary artery (**Fig. 4.16**).

When assessing a coronary artery with an anomalous course, the origin of the artery should be carefully evaluated. Ectopic origin of a coronary artery may be associated with an angulated ostium (**Figs. 4.13** and **4.14**). Acute angulation of the coronary origin may result in a stenotic orifice or accelerated development of atherosclerosis. One question

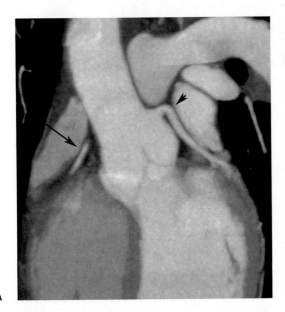

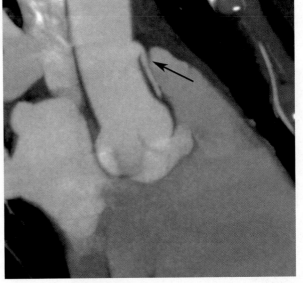

Fig. 4.15 Origin of the right coronary artery (RCA) from the tubular portion of the aorta. **(A)** Slab maximum intensity projection (MIP) of the aortic root in a left anterior oblique projection demonstrates the origin of the left coronary artery (*arrowhead*) just below the sinotubular

junction. The RCA is visualized at this level (*arrow*), but its origin from the aorta is not identified. **(B)** Slab MIP in a steep right anterior oblique projection demonstrates the origin of the RCA (*arrow*) well above the sinuotubular junction. (*Continued on page 82*)

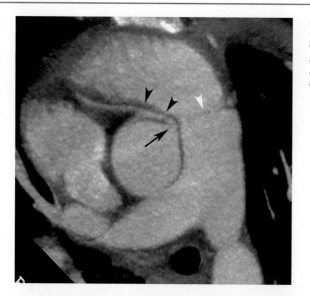

Fig. 4.15 (*Continued*) Origin of the right coronary artery (RCA) from the tubular portion of the aorta. (C) Olique axial MIP at the level of the right ventricular outflow tract. The pulmonic valve (*white arrowhead*) is anterior and to the left of the aorta. The origin of the RCA is visualized along the anterior wall of the aorta (*arrow*). The RCA courses between the ascending aorta and right ventricular outflow tract (*black arrowheads*).

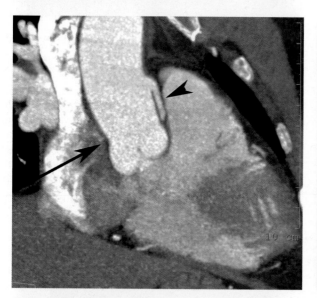

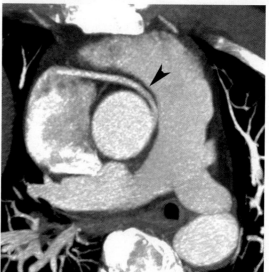

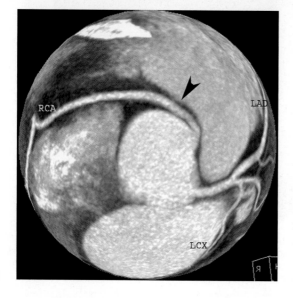

Fig. 4.16 Origin of the right coronary artery (RCA) from the tubular portion of the aorta with long interarterial course. (A) Slab maximum intensity projection (MIP) of the aortic root demonstrates a superior displaced origin of the RCA (*arrowhead*) well above the sinotubular junction (*arrow*). (B) Slab MIP in an angled axial projection demonstrates a relatively long interarterial course of the RCA (*arrowhead*) between the aorta and the pulmonary artery. (C) Globe MIP demonstrates similar anatomy. LAD, left anterior descending artery; LCX, left circumflex artery.

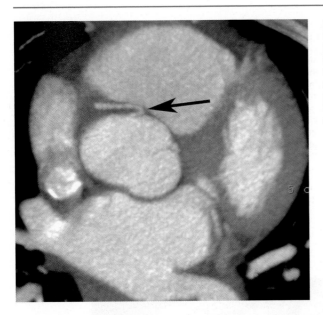

Fig. 4.17 Kink in the proximal right coronary artery (RCA). A knuckle of the RCA is situated between the aorta and right ventricular outflow tract. Axial image demonstrates a nondominant RCA that courses first to the left, into the space between the aorta and right ventricular outflow tract (*arrow*), and then courses back into the right atrioventricular groove. In a right-dominant situation, this is a potentially serious anomaly because the RCA may be compressed between the aorta and right ventricular outflow tract. No intervention was offered to this patient because she was left dominant with no significant left ventricular myocardium at risk from RCA compression.

that has not been addressed in the literature is whether a kinked proximal coronary artery may present a similar potential for compression and stenosis in the absence of an ectopic origin (**Fig. 4.17**).

As discussed in the previous chapter on normal anatomy, the ostia of the coronary arteries develop on both sides of the embryologic aorticopulmonary septum. Anomalies in the development of the aortic root are associated with an increasing frequency of coronary anomalies.

Bicuspid aortic valve may be associated with anomalies in the location and angulation of the coronary ostia (**Fig. 4.18**). Anomalies of septation of the aortopulmonary truncus—tetralogy of Fallot, truncus arteriosus, pulmonary atresia and transposition—are often associated with anatomic variations in coronary anatomy.[23–26] Tetralogy of Fallot is characterized by hypoplasia of the pulmonary infundibulum and can be associated with anomalous origin of the LAD from the RCA (**Fig. 4.19**).[27]

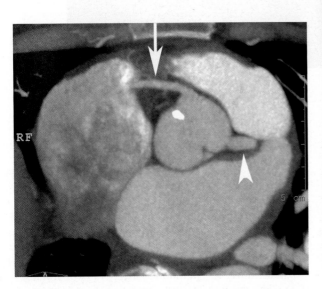

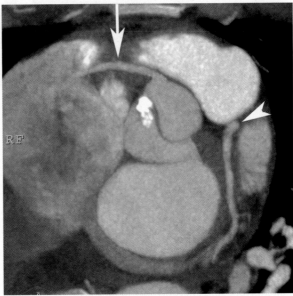

A   B

Fig. 4.18 Anomalous position and angle of origin of the right coronary artery (RCA) in the setting of a bicuspid aortic valve. **(A)** Axial maximum intensity projection (MIP) demonstrates origins of the RCA (*arrow*) and left coronary artery (*arrowhead*). The RCA originates just behind the right ventricular outflow tract (RVOT), slightly to the left of its normal position of origin. The RCA angles to the right side immediately at is origin but does not course between the aorta and RVOT. **(B)** Angled MIP demonstrates the calcified bicuspid aortic valve.

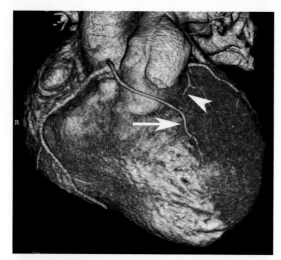

A

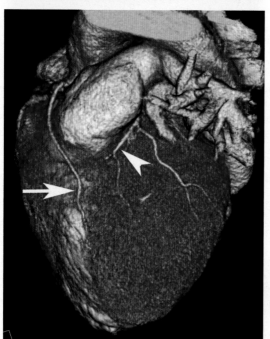

B

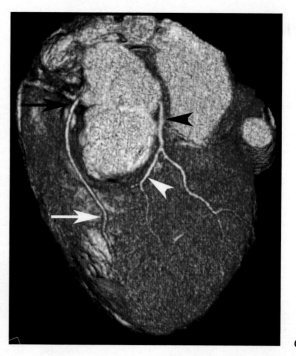

C

Fig. 4.19 Origin of the left anterior descending artery (LAD) from the conus artery. **(A,B)** Surface-rendered images in the anteroposterior and left anterior oblique (LAO) projections. The proximal LAD (*white arrowhead*) arises from the left coronary artery, but this short vessel ends in the upper portion of the anterior interventricular groove. The remainder of the LAD (*white arrow*) arises from the conus artery. **(C)** Surface-rendered LAO view from above. The great vessels and left atrial appendage have been removed to demonstrate that the proximal LAD (*white arrowhead*) is a branch of the left main coronary artery (*black arrowhead*) and the remainder of the LAD (*white arrow*) arises from the conus artery (*black arrow*). The conus artery arises from the aorta immediately adjacent to the right coronary artery. Abnormal origin of the LAD from the conus artery is often associated with tetrology of Fallot.

◆ Anomalies of Termination

Intercoronary communication that is visible on coronary CT is a rare anatomic situation in which there is congenital communication between coronary arteries. Intercoronary communication may be present between right-and-left sided sinoatrial nodal arteries, between the RCA and distal LCX, or between the distal LAD and posterior descending artery. Rarely, such a communication may be visible between the conus artery and the LAD in the absence of coronary disease (**Fig. 3.14**). Compared with acquired collateral circulation, intercoronary arterial connections are generally larger in diameter, extramural in location, have histologic structure of a normal arterial wall, and have a straight course.[28,29] In the

setting of coronary stenosis, intercoronary communications may enlarge and supply collateral flow (**Fig. 4.20**) but will appear less tortuous than acquired collateral vessels (**Figs. 4.12** and **6.28**), which are often intramyocardial in location and poorly visualized by coronary CTA (see **Fig. 6.27**).

Coronary fistulae represent a more common form of abnormal termination. Most coronary fistulae are congenital, arising from either the RCA (50–60%) or the LCA (30–40%).[30] Coronary fistulae may drain into the right ventricle (41%), right atrium (26%), pulmonary artery (17%), coronary sinus (7%), left atrium (5%), left ventricle (3%), or superior vena cava (1%).[31] Rare cases of iatrogenic coronary artery fistulae have been reported secondary to interventional procedures such as angioplasty.[32] As noted in the previous chapter, very

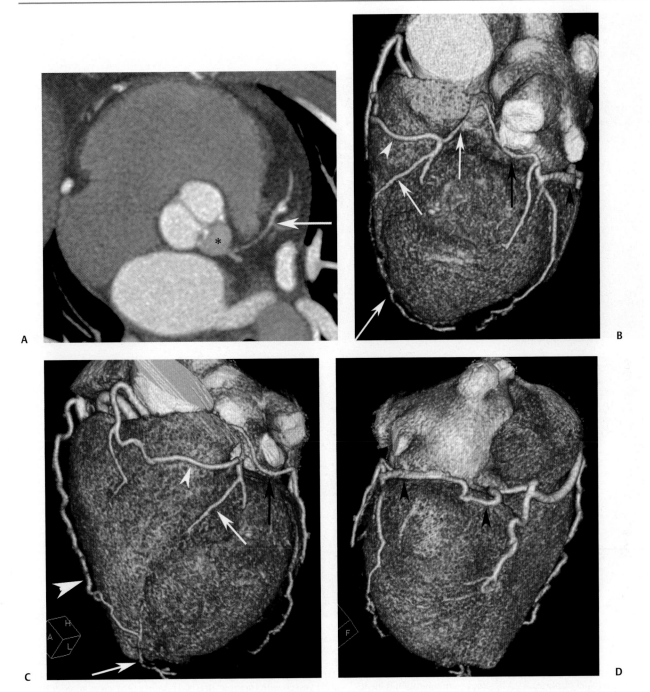

Fig. 4.20 Congenital occlusion of the left coronary artery with reconstitution of the left anterior descending artery (LAD) and circumflex via intercoronary communications from conus, marginal, and posterolateral branches of the right coronary artery (RCA). **(A)** Short axis MIP through the aortic root demonstrates that occlusion of the left coronary artery is related to lack of flow into the left sinus of Valsalva (*). Reconstitution of the LAD (*arrow*) results in retrograde filling of the left sinus of Valsalva on delayed images. **(B)** Surface-rendered image in the left lateral projection demonstrates very small proximal LAD (*white arrows*) and circumflex (*black arrow*) arteries. A conus branch (*white arrowhead*) reconstitutes the proximal LAD. A large posterolateral branch of the RCA (*black arrowhead*) reconstitutes the circumflex. Both the conus and posterolateral branches demonstrate a straight course characteristic of an intercoronary communication. **(C)** Surface-rendered image in the left anterior oblique projection. The LAD (*white arrows*) is segmentally patent. The proximal LAD is reconstituted from the conus artery (*small white arrowhead*); the distal LAD is reconstituted from a large acute marginal branch of the RCA (*large white arrowhead*). These intercoronary communications are large and demonstrate a relatively straight extramural course. **(D)** Surface-rendered view looking at the undersurface of the left heart. A large posterolateral branch from the RCA serves as a collateral which travels in the posterior left atrioventricular groove (*arrowheads*) and reconstitutes the circumflex artery. (See also Fig. 10.12.)

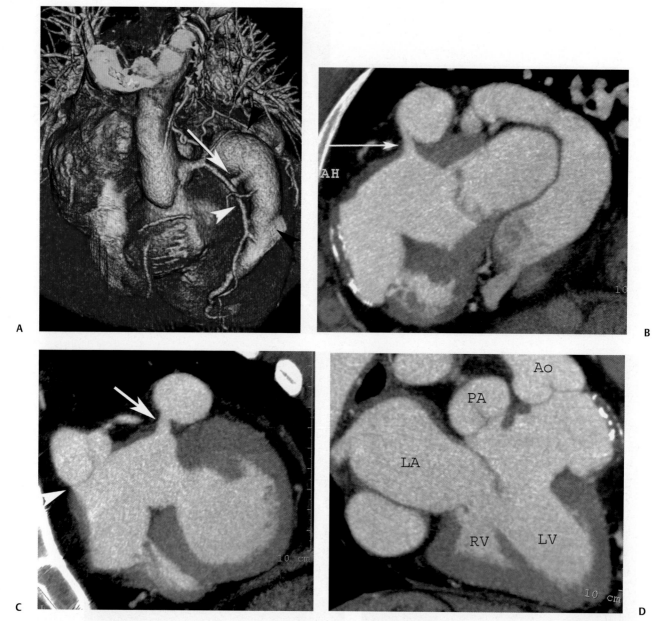

Fig. 4.21 Congenital fistula between the left ventricle (LV) and an anterior coronary vein. **(A)** Surface rendering in the anterior projection demonstrates a normal-sized left anterior descending artery (LAD) (*white arrowhead*). Alongside this artery, there is a markedly dilated venous structure (*black arrowheads*). A fistulous communication is identified between this dilated venous structure and the underlying ventricle (*white arrow*) immediately behind the LAD. **(B)** Oblique maximum intensity projection (MIP) view through the fistula (*arrow*) demonstrates the communication between the dilated venous structure and the ventricular chamber. **(C)** Sagittal MIP image again demonstrates the fistula (*arrow*) between the dilated venous structure and the ventricular outflow tract. The root of the aorta (Ao) arises from this outflow tract (*arrowhead*). **(D)** This patient has surgically corrected congenital transposition of the great vessels with tricuspid atresia. The aorta (Ao) arises anterior to the pulmonary artery (PA) from the left ventricle (LV). A hypoplastic right ventricle (RV) is present posteriorly, with a ventroseptal defect (VSD) connecting it to the left ventricle (LV). LA, left atrium.

small arterial cameral communications under 250 μm in size may represent a normal anatomic finding. Visible arterial fistulae are found in less than 1% of patients and may occur in association with other forms of congenital heart disease in 5 to 30% **(Fig. 4.21)**.[33] Many coronary fistulae are small, and at least half of patients with coronary fistulae remain asymptomatic.[34] Larger coronary fistulae may cause enlargement of the affected coronary artery **(Fig. 4.22)** and may present with episodic myocardial ischemia or arrhythmia secondary to arterial steal **(Fig. 4.23)** or heart failure secondary to left-to-right shunting with right-sided volume overload **(Fig. 4.24)**. Rare complications include endocarditis or rupture of an aneurysmal fistula.

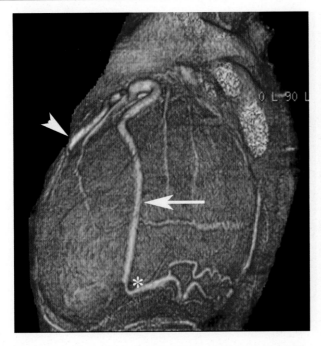

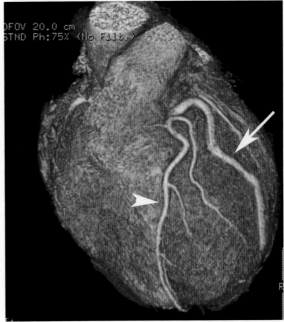

A   B

Fig. 4.22 Arteriovenous fistula between a diagonal branch of the left anterior descending artery (LAD) and a coronary vein. **(A,B)** Volumetric images demonstrate a normal LAD (*arrowhead*) with a dilated first diagonal branch (*arrow*). This diagonal branch communicates with an enlarged coronary vein along the lateral wall of the left ventricle (*). As confirmed by cardiac catheterization, this vessel drained into a venous structure along the posterior aspect of the base of the left ventricle. (The images in this figure were obtained at the Medical College of Wisconsin, courtesy of Drs. W. Dennis Foley and Panayotis Fasseas.)

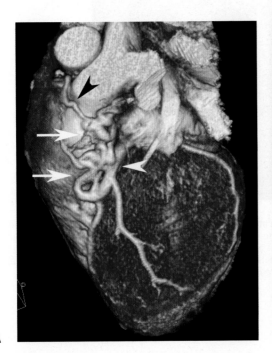

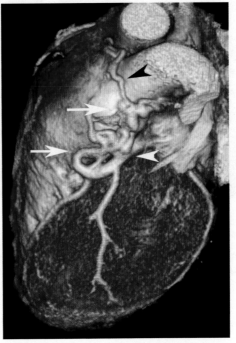

A   B

Fig. 4.23 Coronary arterial fistula from the left anterior descending artery (LAD) to the main pulmonary artery (PA). Fistulas from the LAD to the pulmonary artery (PA) are typically multiple and serpiginous. **(A,B)** Volumetric renderings demonstrate a large proximal LAD (*white arrowhead*) associated with a plexus of vessels (*arrows*) that communicate with the conus branch of the right coronary artery (*black arrowhead*) as well as the PA. The communication between the arterial malformation and PA was along the posterior margin of the PA and is not demonstrated. The patient experienced intermittent arrhythmias and syncope, likely related to a vascular steal physiology.

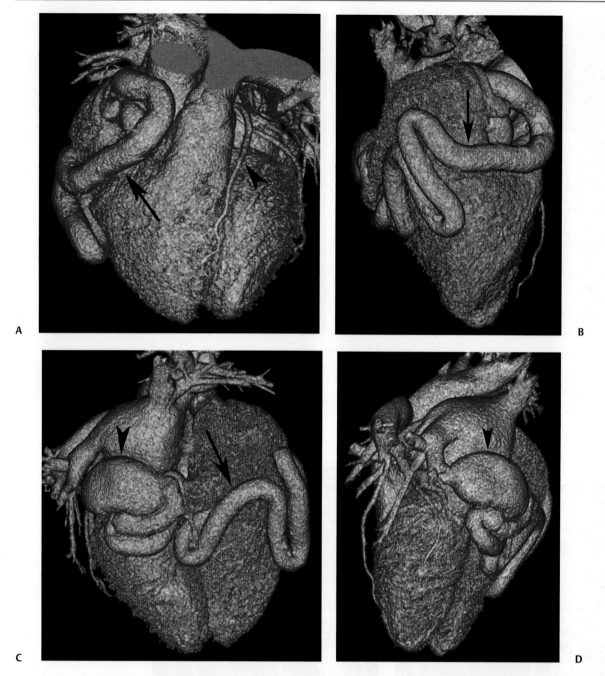

Fig. 4.24 Arterial venous fistula of the right coronary artery (RCA) to the coronary sinus. **(A)** Surface-rendered image in the left anterior oblique (LAO) projection demonstrates a normal-caliber left anterior descending artery (*arrowhead*). A markedly dilated and tortuous RCA is identified (*arrow*). **(B)** Surface-rendered image in the right anterior oblique projection demonstrates the dilated RCA as it courses around the right atrioventricular (AV) groove (*arrow*). **(C)** Surface-rendered image at the crux of the heart demonstrates a dilated distal RCA (*arrow*) as well as a dilated coronary sinus (*arrowhead*). **(D)** Surface-rendered left posterior oblique view demonstrates the dilated coronary sinus (*arrowhead*) posterior to the left atrium.

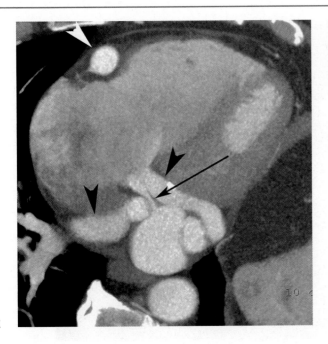

E

Fig. 4.24 *(Continued)* **(E)** Arterial venous fistula of the right coronary artery (RCA) to the coronary sinus. Curved maximum intensity projection through the crux of the heart demonstrates the dilated RCA as it courses along the anterior AV groove (*white arrowhead*). A dilated and tortuous distal RCA is also identified (*black arrowheads*). The site of fistulous communication between the distal RCA and the coronary sinus was identified (*black arrow*).

◆ Coronary Atresia, Hypoplasia, or Ectasia

Congenital coronary stenosis or atresia rarely occurs as an isolated anomaly but may be present in association with calcific coronary sclerosis, supravalvular aortic stenosis, homocystinurea, Friedreich ataxia, Hurler syndrome, progeria, and rubella syndrome.[31] These patients may present with evidence of myocardial infarction.

Although coronary aneurysms are typically acquired secondary to a primary disease process of the coronary arteries, discussion of this entity is included in this chapter on anomalies because ectasia or aneurysms can occur as a congenital anomaly. Focal coronary ectasia or aneurysm is defined by dilatation of a coronary segment to greater than 1.5 to 2.0 times the diameter of the normal adjacent segments.[35] Coronary aneurysms involve less than 50% of the length of a coronary vessel, whereas ectasia involves greater than 50% of the vessel length.[36] The incidence of coronary aneurysms in angiographic studies varies from 0.3 to 4.9%.[37] With the advent of coronary multidetector CTA, coronary aneurysms are more frequently seen as incidental findings.[38] Most coronary aneurysms are true aneurysms containing all three layers of arterial wall: intima, media, and adventitia.[39]

The most common cause of coronary aneurysms is atherosclerotic. Atherosclerotic aneurysms may present as a focal saccular aneurysm (**Figs. 4.25** and **4.26**), as a tubular

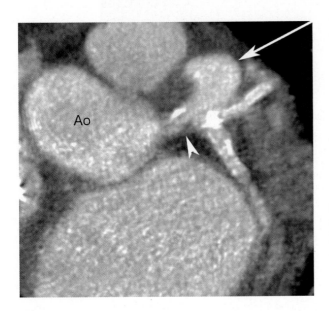

Ao

Fig. 4.25 Aneurysm of the left main coronary artery. Axial maximum intensity projection (MIP) demonstrates the left main coronary artery (*arrowhead*) as it originates from the aorta (Ao). There is a large saccular aneurysm or pseudoaneurysm of the left main coronary artery (*arrow*). Extensive atherosclerotic disease is visible in the left coronary system. Stents are present in the proximal LAD and circumflex arteries. The aneurysm could represent either an atherosclerotic aneurysm or a pseudoaneurysm related to prior instrumentation for stent placement.

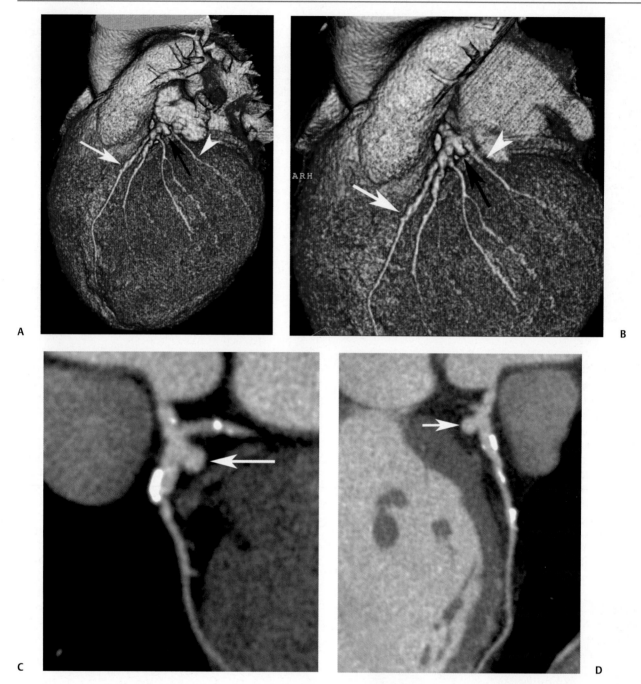

Fig. 4.26 Aneurysm at the origin of the left anterior descending artery (LAD). **(A)** Surface-rendered image demonstrates the LAD (*white arrow*) and a large first obtuse marginal branch of the circumflex artery (*arrowhead*). Just beyond the origin of this circumflex branch, there is a focal aneurysm of the proximal LAD (*black arrow*). **(B)** Surface-rendered image with the left atrial appendage shaved away demonstrates the obtuse marginal branch (*white arrowhead*) and adjacent aneurysm (*black arrow*) with better detail. **(C)** Curved maximum intensity projection (MIP) image along the LAD demonstrates a focal aneurysm (*white arrow*) just beyond the origin of the circumflex artery. Calcified plaque is present in both the circumflex and LAD. **(D)** Orthogonal curved MIP image again demonstrates the aneurysm in the proximal LAD (*arrow*), as well as calcific plaque within the more distal LAD.

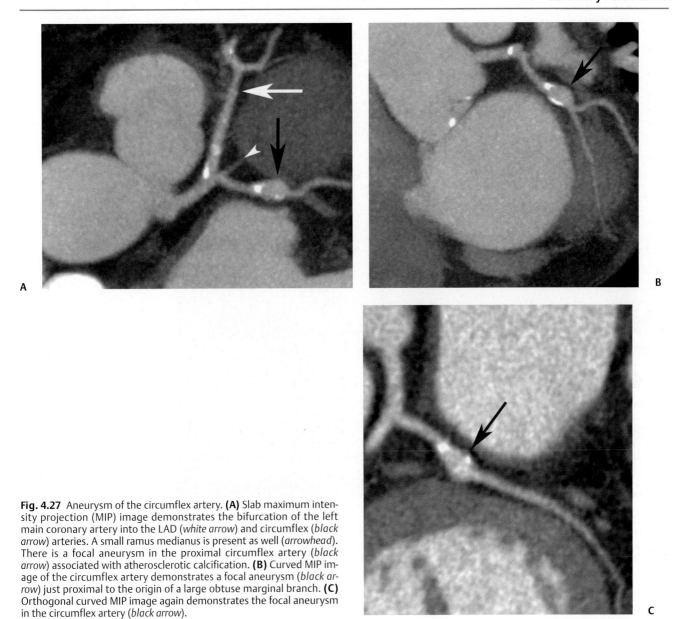

Fig. 4.27 Aneurysm of the circumflex artery. **(A)** Slab maximum intensity projection (MIP) image demonstrates the bifurcation of the left main coronary artery into the LAD (*white arrow*) and circumflex (*black arrow*) arteries. A small ramus medianus is present as well (*arrowhead*). There is a focal aneurysm in the proximal circumflex artery (*black arrow*) associated with atherosclerotic calcification. **(B)** Curved MIP image of the circumflex artery demonstrates a focal aneurysm (*black arrow*) just proximal to the origin of a large obtuse marginal branch. **(C)** Orthogonal curved MIP image again demonstrates the focal aneurysm in the circumflex artery (*black arrow*).

aneurysm (**Fig. 4.27**), or as fusiform dilatation of the coronary artery (**Fig. 4.28**). Arteriomegaly involving the coronary arteries may represent an expression of atherosclerotic disease (**Fig. 4.29**) and may be associated with

aneurysms in other arteries, including the aorta, iliac arteries, and popliteal arteries. Approximately half of coronary aneurysms result from nonatherosclerotic causes.[37] Congenital aneurysms account for 20 to 30%.[40] Inflammatory and

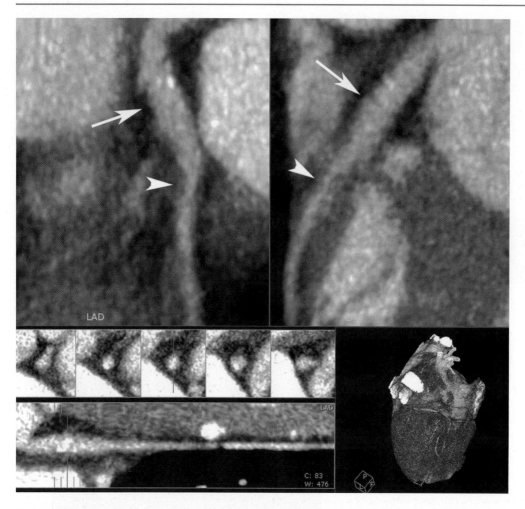

Fig. 4.28 Diffuse mild dilatation of the proximal left anterior descending artery (LAD). Orthogonal maximum intensity projection (MIP) images demonstrate a dilated proximal LAD (*arrow*) that measures 7 mm in maximum diameter. The left main coronary artery measures 5 mm in diameter; the more distal LAD measured just under 3 mm in diameter. Immediately beyond the area of dilatation, there is noncalcified plaque with moderate stenosis in the LAD (*arrowhead*).

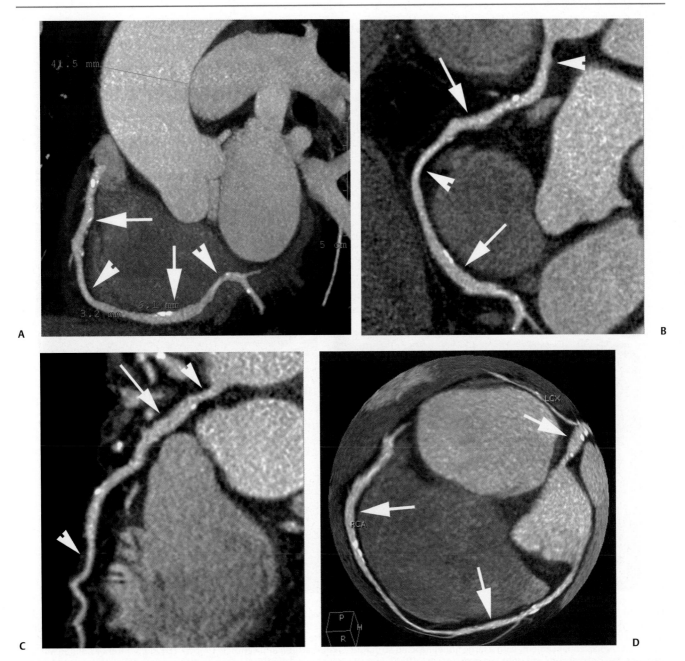

Fig. 4.29 Coronary arteriomegaly. Multiple areas of coronary ectasia associated with atherosclerotic calcifications are shown but no significant stenosis. **(A)** Areas of mild dilatation (*arrows*) interspersed among areas of normal diameter (*arrowheads*) in the right coronary artery (RCA) associated with mild dilatation of the ascending aorta (4.15 cm). **(B)** Curved maximum intensity projection (MIP) again demonstrates areas of dilatation (*arrows*) and normal caliber (*arrowheads*) in the RCA. **(C)** Curved MIP demonstrates a similar, but less marked, pathology in the left anterior descending artery. **(D)** Globe MIP demonstrates areas of arteriomegaly in both the right and left coronary arteries. LCX, left circumflex artery.

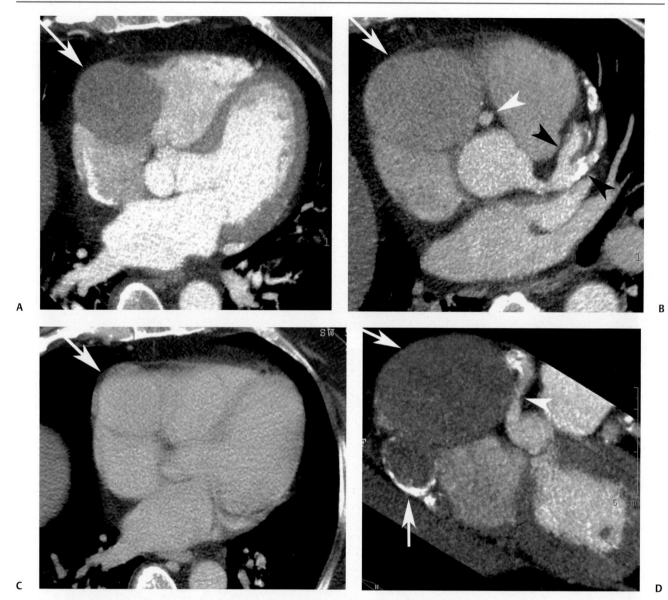

Fig. 4.30 Multiple large aneurysms of the coronary circulation in an asymptomatic patient, likely related to previous Kawaski disease. **(A)** Axial image through the heart in the arterial phase demonstrates left-sided cardiac enhancement, with a large nonenhancing structure between the right atrium and right ventricle (*arrow*). **(B)** Slab maximum intensity projection (MIP) image demonstrates enhancement of the left main coronary artery as well as a dilated proximal left anterior descending artery (LAD) and circumflex branches (*black arrowheads*). The proximal right coronary artery (RCA) is also demonstrated to be enhancing (*white arrowhead*). Again demonstrated is a large nonenhancing structure immediately adjacent to the RCA (*arrow*). **(C)** Delayed phase demonstrates clear enhancement of this structure between the right atrium and ventricle (*arrow*). **(D)** Right anterior oblique MIP projection of the RCA (*arrowhead*) demonstrates enhancement of the RCA, which appears to terminate in a large nonenhancing structure (*white arrows*). This structure represents a large aneurysm of the RCA with peripheral calcification and delayed enhancement.

connective tissue diseases account for 10 to 20%, including Kawasaki disease,[41] Takayasu disease,[42] adult polycystic kidney disease,[43] lupus erythematosus,[44] and Ehlers-Danlos syndrome.[45] A minority of aneurysms may develop secondary to a fistula or as a consequence of infectious diseases. Pseudoaneurysms of coronary arteries are less common than true aneurysms but are reported as a complication after 2 to 10% of percutaneous interventional coronary procedures.[46,47] Coronary CTA provides an excellent tool to evaluate coronary fistulae and aneurysms.[48]

Coronary aneurysms may be detected in asymptomatic individuals (**Fig. 4.30**) or in patients with angina. Potential complications related to coronary aneurysms include thrombosis or distal embolization with myocardial infarction and sudden death. Aneurysm rupture and fistula formation are rare complications. Analysis of findings in the National Institutes of Health–sponsored Coronary Artery Surgery Study, including 978 patients with coronary ectasia or aneurysm, demonstrated no difference in the 5-year survival of patients with coronary aneurysms and coronary artery disease versus

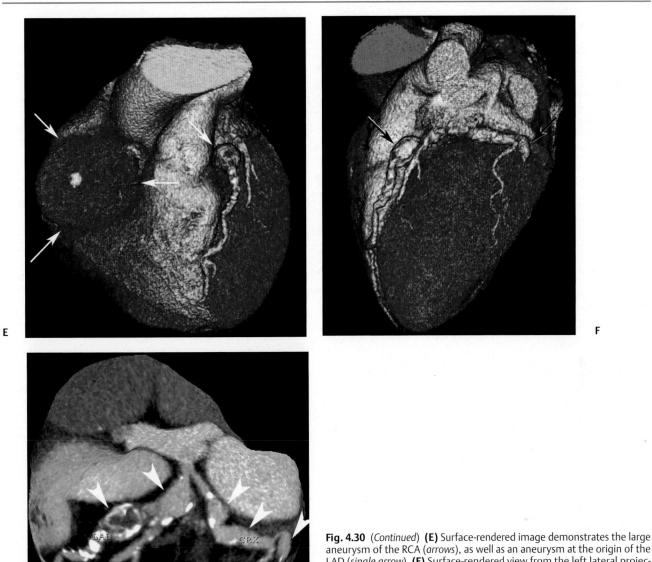

Fig. 4.30 (*Continued*) **(E)** Surface-rendered image demonstrates the large aneurysm of the RCA (*arrows*), as well as an aneurysm at the origin of the LAD (*single arrow*). **(F)** Surface-rendered view from the left lateral projection demonstrates the aneurysm at the origin of the LAD, as well as an additional aneurysm in the distal circumflex artery (*arrows*). **(G)** Globe MIP image demonstrates diffuse aneurysmal dilatation involving LAD and circumflex arteries (*arrowheads*). At least one of the aneurysms in the LAD demonstrates the presence of nonenhancing material compatible with thrombus.

those with only coronary artery disease after controlling for the overall extent of coronary artery disease.[49] Others have reported increased rates of myocardial infarction with coronary aneurysms.[50,51] Optimal therapy of coronary aneurysms is controversial, but anticoagulation and antiplatelet therapy are generally recommended.

◆ Conclusion

Coronary anomalies include numerous rare variations of coronary artery anatomy. Coronary anomalies may be associated with other forms of congenital heart disease. Most

anomalies are compatible with a normal coronary circulation. Although anecdotal reports link coronary anomalies to cardiac complications, there are no population-based prospective imaging trials with documented clinical follow-up to substantiate which anomalies are truly associated with clinically significant complications. In the absence of such evidence, patients with coronary anomalies are treated based on the perceived risk of compromise to coronary blood flow. Coronary CTA provides an excellent noninvasive anatomic demonstration of the coronary anatomy along with adjacent structures and is therefore an appropriate first-line modality for research studies and clinical evaluation of coronary anomalies.

References

1. Maron BJ, Thompson PD, Puffer JC, et al. Cardiovascular preparticipation screening of competitive athletes. A statement for health professionals from the Sudden Death Committee (clinical cardiology) and Congenital Cardiac Defects Committee (cardiovascular disease in the young), American Heart Association. Circulation. 1996;94(4):850–856

2. Van Camp SP, Bloor CM, Mueller FO, Cantu RC, Olson HG. Nontraumatic sports death in high school and college athletes. Med Sci Sports Exerc. 1995;27(5):641–647

3. Burke AP, Farb A, Virmani R, Goodin J, Smialek JE. Sports-related and non-sports-related sudden cardiac death in young adults. Am Heart J. 1991;121(2 Pt 1):568–575

4. Rigatelli G, Gemelli M, Zamboni A, et al. Are coronary artery anomalies an accelerating factor for coronary atherosclerosis development? Angiology. 2004;55(1):29–35

5. Angelini P. Functionally significant versus intriguingly different coronary artery anatomy: anatomo-clinical correlations in coronary anomalies. G Ital Cardiol. 1999;29(6):607–615

6. Angelini P. Coronary artery anomalies—current clinical issues: definitions, classification, incidence, clinical relevance, and treatment guidelines. Tex Heart Inst J. 2002;29(4):271–278

7. Angelini P. Normal and anomalous coronary arteries: definitions and classification. Am Heart J. 1989;117(2):418–434

8. Yamanaka O, Hobbs RE. Coronary artery anomalies in 126,595 patients undergoing coronary arteriography. Cathet Cardiovasc Diagn. 1990;21(1):28–40

9. Angelini P, Velasco JA, Flamm S. Coronary anomalies: incidence, pathophysiology, and clinical relevance. Circulation. 2002;105(20):2449–2454

10. Barriales Villa R, Morís C, López Muñiz A, et al. [Adult congenital anomalies of the coronary arteries described over 31 years of angiographic studies in the Asturias Principality: main angiographic and clinical characteristics]. Rev Esp Cardiol. 2001;54(3):269–281

11. Diez JD, Angelini P, Lee VV. Does the anomalous congenital origin of a coronary artery predispose to the development of stnotic atherosclerotic lesions in its proximal segment? Circulation. 1997;96(Suppl): I-154

12. Cademartiri F, Runza G, Luccichenti G, et al. Coronary artery anomalies: incidence, pathophysiology, clinical relevance and role of diagnostic imaging. Radiol Med (Torino). 2006;111(3):376–391

13. Wesselhoeft H, Fawcett JS, Johnson AL. Anomalous origin of the left coronary artery from the pulmonary trunk. Its clinical spectrum, pathology, and pathophysiology, based on a review of 140 cases with seven further cases. Circulation. 1968;38(2):403–425

14. Cheitlin MD, De Castro CM, McAllister HA. Sudden death as a complication of anomalous left coronary origin from the anterior sinus of Valsalva, a not-so-minor congenital anomaly. Circulation. 1974; 50(4):780–787

15. Leberthson RR, Dinsmore RE, Bharati S, et al. Aberrant coronary artery origin from the aorta. Diagnosis and clinical significance. Circulation. 1974;50(4):774–779

16. Schmitt R, Froehner S, Brunn J, et al. Congenital anomalies of the coronary arteries: imaging with contrast-enhanced, multidetector computed tomography. Eur Radiol 2005;15(6):1110–1121

17. Barry MO, Seeck BA, Virgilio C, Woodard PK. Left main coronary anomaly arising from the right sinus of Valsalva-interarterial, septal, or a continuum? J Thorac Imaging. 2008;23(1):31–34

18. Roberts WC, Morrow AG. Compression of anomalous left circumflex coronary arteries by prosthetic valve fixation rings. J Thorac Cardiovasc Surg. 1969;57(6):834–838

19. Samarendra P, Kumari S, Hafeez M, Vasavada BC, Sacchi TJ. Anomalous circumflex coronary artery: benign or predisposed to selective atherosclerosis. Angiology. 2001;52(8):521–526

20. Peña E, Nguyen ET, Merchant N, Dennie G. ALCAPA syndrome: not just a pediatric disease. Radiographics. 2009;29(2):553–565

21. Benge W, Martins JB, Funk DC. Morbidity associated with anomalous origin of the right coronary artery from the left sinus of Valsalva. Am Heart J. 1980;99:96–100

22. Bekedam MA, Vliegen HW, Doornbos J, Jukema JW, de Roos A, van der Wall EE. Diagnosis and management of anomalous origin of the right coronary artery from the left coronary sinus. Int J Card Imaging. 1999;15(3):253–258, discussion 259

23. Neufeld HN, Schneeweiss A. Coronary artery disease in infants and children. Philadelphia: Lea & Febiger, 1983

24. Dabizzi RP, Teodori G, Barletta GA, Caprioli G, Baldrighi G, Baldrighi V. Associated coronary and cardiac anomalies in the tetralogy of Fallot. An angiographic study. Eur Heart J. 1990;11(8):692–704

25. Dabizzi RP, Barletta GA, Caprioli G, Baldrighi G, Baldrighi V. Coronary artery anatomy in corrected transposition of the great arteries. J Am Coll Cardiol. 1988;12(2):486–491

26. Mainwaring RD, Lamberti JJ. Pulmonary atresia with intact ventricular septum. Surgical approach based on ventricular size and coronary anatomy. J Thorac Cardiovasc Surg. 1993;106(4):733–738

27. Dabizzi RP, Caprioli G, Aiazzi L, et al. Distribution and anomalies of coronary arteries in tetralogy of fallot. Circulation. 1980;61(1): 95–102

28. Atak R, Güray U, Akin Y. Images in cardiology: intercoronary communication between the circumflex and right coronary arteries: distinct from coronary collaterals. Heart. 2002;88(1):29

29. Sokmen A, Tuncer C, Sokmen G, Akcay A, Koroglu S. Intercoronary communication between the circumflex and right coronary arteries: a very rare coronary anomaly. Hellenic J Cardiol. 2009;50(1):66–67

30. Angelini P. Coronary artery anomalies: a comprehensive approach. Philadelphia: Lippincott Williams & Wilkins, 1999

31. Levin DC, Fellows KE, Abrams HL. Hemodynamically significant primary anomalies of the coronary arteries: angiographic aspects. Circulation. 1978;58(1):25–34

32. Lipiec P, Peruga JZ, Krzemiska-Pakula M, Flory J, Drozdz J, Kasprzak JD. Right coronary artery-to-right ventricle fistula complicating percutaneous transluminal angioplasty: case report and review of the literature. J Am Soc Echocardiogr. 2004;17(3):280–283

33. Sunder KR, Balakrishnan KG, Tharakan JA, et al. Coronary artery fistula in children and adults: a review of 25 cases with long-term observations. Int J Cardiol. 1997;58(1):47–53

34. Ata Y, Turk T, Bicer M, Yalcin M, Ata F, Yavuz S. Coronary arteriovenous fistulas in the adults: natural history and management strategies. J Cardiothorac Surg. 2009;4:62

35. Robinson FC. Aneurysms of the coronary arteries. Am Heart J. 1985;109(1):129–135

36. Pahlavan PS, Niroomand F. Coronary artery aneurysm: a review. Clin Cardiol. 2006;29:439–443

37. Villines TC, Avedissian LS, Elgin EE. Diffuse nonatherosclerotic coronary aneurysms: an unusual cause of sudden death in a young male and a literature review. Cardiol Rev. 2005;13(6):309–311

38. Díaz-Zamudio M, Bacilio-Pérez U, Herrera-Zarza MC, et al. Coronary artery aneurysms and ectasia: role of coronary CT angiography. Radiographics. 2009;29(7):1939–1954

39. Aqel RA, Zoghbi GJ, Iskandrian A. Spontaneous coronary artery dissection, aneurysms, and pseudoaneurysms: a review. Echocardiography. 2004;21(2):175–182

40. Sayin T, Döven O, Berkalp B, Akyürek O, Güleç S, Oral D. Exercise-induced myocardial ischemia in patients with coronary artery ectasia without obstructive coronary artery disease. Int J Cardiol. 2001; 78(2):143–149

41. Beiser AS, Takahashi M, Baker AL, Sundel RP, Newburger JW; US Multicenter Kawasaki Disease Study Group. A predictive instrument for coronary artery aneurysms in Kawasaki disease. Am J Cardiol. 1998;81(9):1116–1120

42. Endo M, Tomizawa Y, Nishida H, et al. Angiographic findings and surgical treatments of coronary artery involvement in Takayasu arteritis. J Thorac Cardiovasc Surg. 2003;125(3):570–577

43. Hadimeri H, Lamm C, Nyberg G. Coronary aneurysms in patients with autosomal dominant polycystic kidney disease. J Am Soc Nephrol. 1998;9(5):837–841

44. Uchida T, Inoue T, Kamishirado H, et al. Unusual coronary artery aneurysm and acute myocardial infarction in a middle-aged man with systemic lupus erythematosus. Am J Med Sci. 2001;322(3):163–165

45. Eriksen UH, Aunsholt NA, Nielsen TT. Enormous right coronary arterial aneurysm in a patient with type IV Ehlers-Danlos syndrome. Int J Cardiol. 1992;35(2):259–261

46. Slota PA, Fischman DL, Savage MP, Rake R, Goldberg S; STRESS Trial Investigators. Frequency and outcome of development of coronary artery aneurysm after intracoronary stent placement and angioplasty. Am J Cardiol. 1997;79(8):1104–1106

47. Oyama N, Urasawa K, Kitabatake A. Detection and treatment of coronary artery pseudoaneurysms following coronary stent deployment. J Invasive Cardiol. 2004;16(9):521–523

48. Hara H, Moroi M, Araki T, et al. Coronary artery fistula with an associated aneurysm detected by 16-slice multidetector row computed tomographic angiography. Heart Vessels. 2005;20(4):184–185

49. Swaye PS, Fisher LD, Litwin P, et al. Aneurysmal coronary artery disease. Circulation. 1983;67(1):134–138

50. al-Harthi SS, Nouh MS, Arafa M, al-Nozha M. Aneurysmal dilatation of the coronary arteries: diagnostic patterns and clinical significance. Int J Cardiol. 1991;30(2):191–194

51. Rath S, Har-Zahav Y, Battler A, et al. Fate of nonobstructive aneurysmatic coronary artery disease: angiographic and clinical follow-up report. Am Heart J. 1985;109(4):785–791

5

Calcium Scoring

Ethan J. Halpern and David M. Shipon

◆ Cardiac Risk Stratification

Based on 2009 estimates, the annual incidence of heart disease in the United States will include 785,000 new coronary attacks, 470,000 recurrent attacks, and 195,000 silent first attacks.[1] The prevalence of coronary heart disease among persons over 20 years of age in the United States is estimated at 16,800,000, or 7.6% of the population. Coronary heart disease is the single largest cause of mortality among Americans and is implicated in 1 of every 5 deaths. Conventional risk factors fail to identify one third of deaths caused by coronary heart disease.[2] Conventional screening tools for coronary artery disease include Framingham risk assessment, clinical examination, and stress testing.

In 1948, the Framingham heart study was initiated under the auspices of the National Heart Institute (now known as the National Heart, Lung and Blood Institute, or NHLBI). This project was designed to identify risk factors for cardiovascular disease by following a cohort who had not yet developed overt symptoms. The initial study began in the town of Framingham, Massachusetts, with 5209 men and women. In 1971 the study enrolled a second-generation group consisting of 5124 children and spouses of the original group. A third generation is currently being recruited to investigate further the relationship of genetic factors to cardiovascular disease.

The Framingham study identified major cardiovascular risk factors, including high blood pressure, high blood cholesterol, smoking, obesity, diabetes, and physical activity.[3] A risk assessment formula has been extrapolated from the Framingham data to compute the 10-year risk of hard coronary heart events (myocardial infarction and coronary death) based on age, gender, total cholesterol, high-density lipoprotein (HDL), smoking status, systolic blood pressure, and use of medication to treat high blood pressure. A calculator for estimating this risk is available online under the auspicious of the National Cholesterol Education Program and NHLBI *(http://hp2010. nhlbihin.net/atpiii/calculator.asp)*. It is important to note that that several important risk factors for coronary disease, including metabolic syndromes, obesity, and family history are not included in the Framingham risk calculation.

Based on the results of the Framingham study data, evaluations of cardiovascular risk factors have become an important part of prevention and treatment strategies for cardiovascular disease. Patients are assigned a 10-year risk, and treatment goals are modified based on patient risk (see National Cholesterol Program Adult Education Treatment Plan guidelines).[4] With respect to patient therapy, risk categories are divided into high risk (10-year risk >20%), moderate high risk (10-year risk 10–20%), moderate risk (10-year risk <10%), and low risk (patients with 0–1 cardiac risk factors). The distinction between the moderate- and low-risk categories is based on additional risk factors not included in the Framingham 10-year risk calculation. The risk category into which a patient is placed will impact recommendations for therapeutic lifestyle changes as well as target goals for lowering of low-density lipoprotein (LDL) levels.

Coronary Calcium and Cardiac Risk

It is of interest that most coronary events occur in the territory of coronary arteries that do not demonstrate prior high-grade stenosis.[5] Although atherosclerotic plaque is invariably present as a substrate for an acute coronary event, significant stenosis is not necessary. However, complications of atherosclerotic plaque, such as rupture or erosion with subsequent thrombus formation, are important events leading to acute coronary syndrome. Many different factors, including plaque composition, hemodynamics, endothelial function, and blood thrombogenicity may influence which plaques lead to hemodynamically significant events.[6] Nonetheless, there is a strong relation between the extent of coronary plaque burden and the risk of a coronary event.[7] Because atherosclerosis is the only disease process associated with calcification of the coronary arteries, the degree of coronary calcification as demonstrated by CT is predictive of the overall burden of atherosclerotic plaque.[8]

The role of coronary calcium scoring in assessing the risk for future coronary events has been a subject of considerable controversy.[9] Updated guidelines for coronary calcium scoring were scheduled for publication by the American Heart Association (AHA) in 2004. However, the publication was canceled after an article in the *Wall Street Journal* on September 21, 2004, suggested that the guidelines would endorse calcium scoring for risk stratification. A subsequent statement from the AHA concluded that "EBCT has undergone a 20-year period of testing for reliability and validity and is now established as a useful technique in identifying individuals with or at risk for CHD. . . . The most promising use of these technologies is calcium scoring for risk assessment of the asymptomatic individual."[10] Interestingly, the AHA/American College of Cardiology (AHA/ACC) consensus statement published in 2007 provides a lukewarm endorsement of coronary calcium scoring, suggesting only that asymptomatic individuals with an intermediate Framingham risk score may be reasonable candidates for coronary calcium scoring as a potential means of modifying risk prediction and altering therapy.[11] European guidelines on cardiovascular disease prevention in clinical practice more clearly state that "coronary calcium scanning is especially suited for patients at medium risk" and advocate the use of coronary calcium scores to qualify conventional risk analysis.[12] More recently, a large observational outcomes study of more than 25,000 people demonstrated conclusively that coronary calcium provides independent and incremental predictive value to traditional cardiovascular risk factors for all cause mortality.[13] Another large study demonstrated that these results hold true across racial and ethnic groups including blacks, Hispanics, and Chinese.[14] An elevated coronary calcium burden may not indicate the direct presence of significant coronary stenosis, but it is associated with a higher risk for a coronary events.

CT Technique for Calcium Scoring

Calcium scoring is based on the identification of high-density material within the coronary circulation on a noncontrast CT scan. Both electron-beam CT (EBCT) and multislice–multidetector CT (MDCT) have been used for evaluation of coronary calcium. The largest databases are available for EBCT. However, a strong linear association is present between calcium score as provided by EBCT and MDCT, with an r-value in the range of 0.96 to 0.99.[15] Current literature suggests that MDCT is comparable to EBCT for coronary calcium screening.[16,17]

The effective radiation dose from a calcium scoring examination with EBCT is in the range of 0.7 to 1.0 mSv for men and 0.9 to 1.3 mSv for women. The effective radiation dose from a calcium scoring examination with MDCT is in the range of 1.0 to 1.5 mSv for men and 1.3 to 1.8 mSv for women.[18,19] This compares favorably to the expected dose of MDCT cardiac angiography. The effective radiation dose from a nuclear stress test is in the same range as that of a diagnostic cardiac CT angiogram performed with retrospective electrocardiographic (ECG) gating (10–12 mSv).

Calcium scoring is a simple test that should take no more than 5 minutes. ECG leads are placed on the patient. A CT scout image is obtained to determine the location of the heart. A prospective ECG-gated scan with 3-mm slice thickness is then obtained from the level of the carina through the bottom of the heart. To obtain an accurate calcium score, calcium within the coronary arteries must be distinguished from calcification involving other parts of the heart, especially the annulus of the aortic or mitral valve (**Fig. 5.1**). Aortic annular calcification may be present adjacent to the left anterior descending artery, whereas mitral annular calcification may be present adjacent to the circumflex artery.

Once the location of coronary calcium is identified on a CT examination, an automated program is used to compute a calcium score. The Agatston method has been traditionally

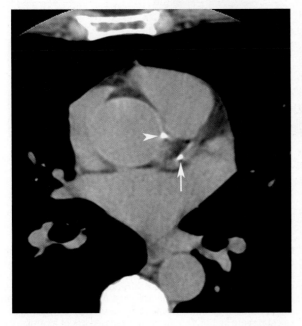
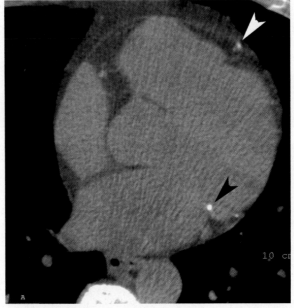

Fig. 5.1 Coronary calcification versus annular calcification. **(A)** Noncontrast axial image at the level of the left main coronary artery demonstrates focal calcification within the left coronary artery (*arrow*), as well as focal calcification of the aortic root (*arrowhead*). **(B)** Axial image at the level of the mitral valve demonstrates focal calcification of the left anterior descending artery (*white arrowhead*), as well as focal calcification of the mitral annulus (*black arrowhead*). The mitral annulus is deep to the circumflex artery, which is found along the left atrioventricular groove.

used to score the amount of coronary calcium with CT.[20] For each focus of calcified coronary plaque, plaque area and maximum attenuation are measured on each CT slice. An attenuation cofactor is assigned to each plaque based on CT attenuation measured in Hounsfield units (HU). The cofactor is assigned as 1 for 131 to 200 HU, 2 for 201 to 300 HU, 3 for 301 to 400 HU, and 4 for greater than 400 HU. The area of each plaque is multiplied by the appropriate attenuation cofactor to achieve a calcium score. Although an Agatston score may be computed for each coronary vessel, the scores of all the individual plaques in all the vessels are generally summed to obtain a single total Agatston calcium score for risk analysis.

The Agatston method does have its shortcomings. Modern CT units are capable of submillimeter resolution, but the Agatston score uses attenuation cofactors determined at a 3-mm slice thickness. Depending on which adjacent tissues are included in this slice thickness, cofactors in the Agatston method may be altered by partial volume averaging. A volumetric method has been proposed that is less dependent on volume averaging and slice thickness.[21] Mass scores have also been defined to combine the volume and density of coronary calcium in a manner that is relatively more independent of slice thickness and spatial resolution. Although volumetric scores of coronary calcium may be more representative of the total plaque burden, volume scores may differ from the Agatston score.[22] More recently, calcium scoring methods have been proposed that combine both the spatial distribution and the amount of calcified plaque to improve risk assessment.[23] Although these newer methods may provide improved risk stratification, most clinicians continue to use the Agatston method for calcium scoring because of the large amount of published data relating the risk of coronary events to the Agatston score.

Calcium Scores, Percentiles, and Cardiac Risk

Coronary calcium scores are generally divided into normal (no calcium), mildly elevated (1–100), moderately elevated (101–400), or severely elevated (>400). Mildly elevated coronary calcium scores are often present without significant stenosis (**Figs. 5.2** and **5.3**). Calcified plaque is frequently associated with positive remodeling, resulting in no significant narrowing of the internal vessel lumen. Positive remodeling is discussed more extensively with atherosclerotic disease in Chapter 6. As the level of coronary calcium increases, the risk of significant stenosis is higher, but there is not a one-to-one correlation. Moderately elevated calcium scores may be associated with normal coronary vessels on

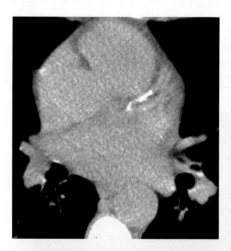

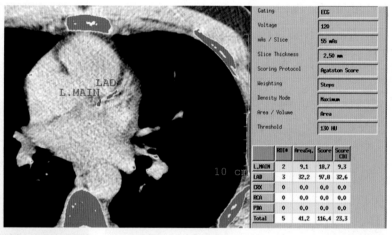

	ROI#	AreaSq.	Score	Score CBI
L.MAIN	2	9.1	18.7	9.3
LAD	3	32.2	97.8	32.6
CRX	0	0.0	0.0	0.0
RCA	0	0.0	0.0	0.0
PDA	0	0.0	0.0	0.0
Total	5	41.2	116.4	23.3

Gating	ECG
Voltage	120
mAs / Slice	55 mAs
Slice Thickness	2.50 mm
Scoring Protocol	Agatston Score
Weighting	Steps
Density Mode	Maximum
Area / Volume	Area
Threshold	130 HU

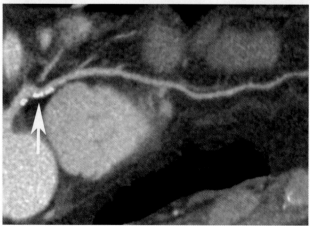

Fig. 5.2 Mild calcification of the left coronary artery without significant stenosis. **(A)** Calcium scoring study demonstrates calcification in the left main coronary artery, as well as the proximal left anterior descending artery (LAD). **(B)** Calcification in the left main and LAD arteries is color-coded by the automated calcium detection algorithm. No other coronary calcification was noted. The total Agatston calcium score of 116.4 suggests an increased risk of a cardiac event relative to an individual with no coronary calcium. **(C)** CT angiogram performed following the calcium scoring study demonstrates calcified plaque in the proximal LAD (*arrow*) without significant stenosis in the LAD.

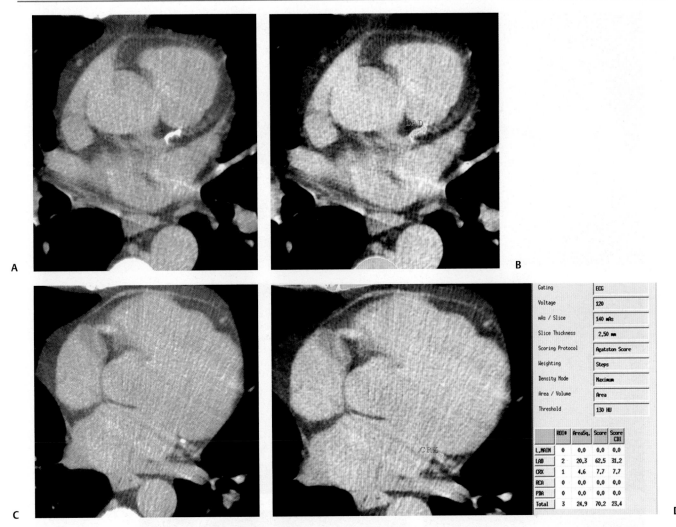

Fig. 5.3 Two-vessel coronary calcium without significant stenosis. **(A)** Axial image through the proximal left coronary artery demonstrates the presence of calcification in the proximal left anterior descending artery (LAD). **(B)** LAD calcium is color-coded by the automated detection algorithm. **(C)** Axial image at a slightly lower level demonstrates calcium within the mid circumflex artery along the left atrioventricular groove. Note the difference in position between this circumflex calcification and the mitral annular calcification demonstrated in Fig. 5.1. **(D)** Calcium in the circumflex artery is color-coded. Although the calcified plaque involves two vessels, the total calculated Agatston calcium score of 70.2 is less than the calcium score calculated for the patient in Fig. 5.2.

angiography (**Fig. 5.4**). Patients with severely elevated calcium scores are more likely to have a significant stenosis; these patients are also the most challenging to study with CT coronary angiography because of artifact from calcification (**Fig. 5.5**). Although very high calcium scores are often associated with coronary stenosis, calcium scoring is generally advocated to assess patient risk for a cardiac event, not to detect the presence of coronary stenosis.

Several large trials have documented a strong correlation between calcium score and the risk of a coronary event. Compared with conventional cardiac risk factors, coronary calcium is an important predictor of future coronary events.[24,25] Furthermore, coronary artery calcification provides incremental information beyond that defined by a single or combined conventional coronary artery disease risk factor assessment.[26] Coronary artery calcium scores can modify the risk assessment based on a traditional Framingham score, especially among patients in the intermediate-risk categories for whom critical decision making is the most uncertain.[27] Among patients who have been evaluated with rest–stress positron emission tomography and found to have either normal myocardial perfusion or ischemia, calcium score provides additional independent data to predict the risk of adverse cardiac events.[28] Based on a meta-analysis of several studies, tables are available to predict the relative increase in risk of a coronary event based on the calcium score and patient's age and sex.[29] As a rough estimate, a calcium score in the range of 1 to 100 provides an increased risk odds ratio of 2, whereas a calcium score in the range of 100 to 400 provides an increased risk odds ratio of 5, and a score above 400 provides an increased risk odds ratio of 10 to 11.

There is a documented change in the distribution of coronary calcium with patient age and sex.[30] Based on the

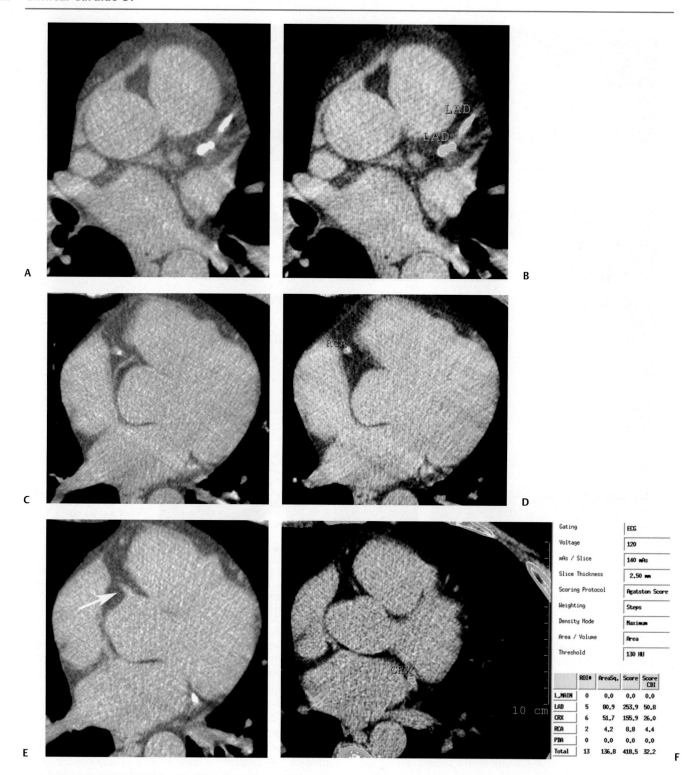

Fig. 5.4 Moderate three-vessel calcification without significant stenosis. **(A)** Axial image demonstrates heavy calcification in the proximal left anterior descending artery (LAD). **(B)** LAD calcium is color-coded by the automated detection algorithm. **(C)** A small calcified plaque is present in the proximal right coronary artery (RCA). **(D)** RCA calcium is color-coded by the automated detection algorithm. **(E)** Axial image at the level of the RCA origin (*arrow*) demonstrates the calcium within the circumflex artery. **(F)** Circumflex calcium is color-coded by the automated detection algorithm. The overall Agatston calcium score of 418.5 suggests that the risk of a coronary event is significantly higher compared with that of a patient without coronary calcium.

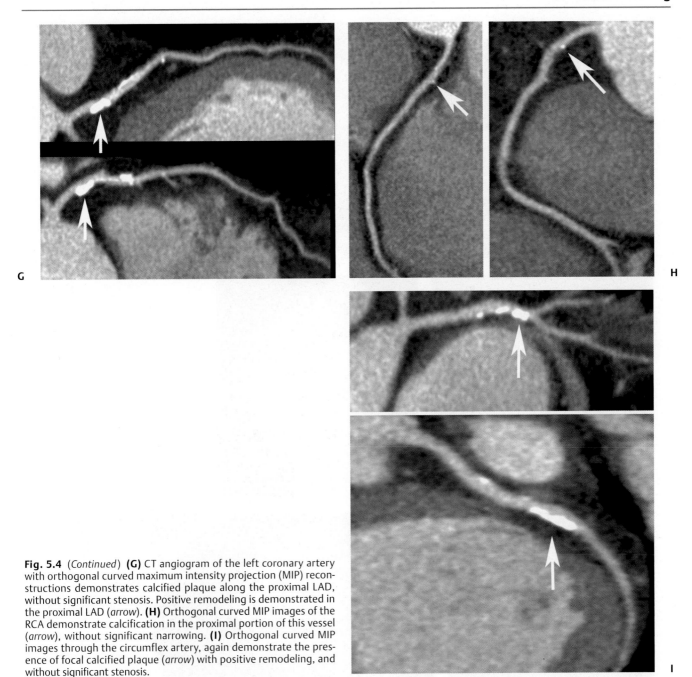

Fig. 5.4 (*Continued*) **(G)** CT angiogram of the left coronary artery with orthogonal curved maximum intensity projection (MIP) reconstructions demonstrates calcified plaque along the proximal LAD, without significant stenosis. Positive remodeling is demonstrated in the proximal LAD (*arrow*). **(H)** Orthogonal curved MIP images of the RCA demonstrate calcification in the proximal portion of this vessel (*arrow*), without significant narrowing. **(I)** Orthogonal curved MIP images through the circumflex artery, again demonstrate the presence of focal calcified plaque (*arrow*) with positive remodeling, and without significant stenosis.

known distribution of calcium scores with age and sex, a patient can be given a calcium score percentile rank.[31,32] Nonetheless, a recent study based on the Multi-Ethnic Study of Atherosclerosis cohort demonstrated that absolute calcium scores are better predictors of cardiovascular outcomes compared with age-, sex-, and race- or ethnicity-specific percentiles.[33] From a clinician's standpoint, the most important clinical application of calcium scores is to modify the pre-test probability of risk for a coronary event based on the Framingham score. Absolute calcium scores facilitate a straightforward application of coronary calcium assessment to risk stratification.

Current literature suggests that coronary artery calcium scores may be incorporated into a set of practice guidelines that include the Framingham score to establish a new paradigm for risk assessment of coronary events.[34] Calcium scoring is most useful as a risk assessment tool for adults who are at intermediate risk of coronary disease based on a Framingham risk score that demonstrates a 10 to 20% risk of a coronary event in the next 10 years. However, in patients with a lower Framingham risk score who have other well-established risk factors—an elevated C-reactive protein, metabolic syndrome, obesity, or a family history of premature coronary disease—calcium scoring may elevate the

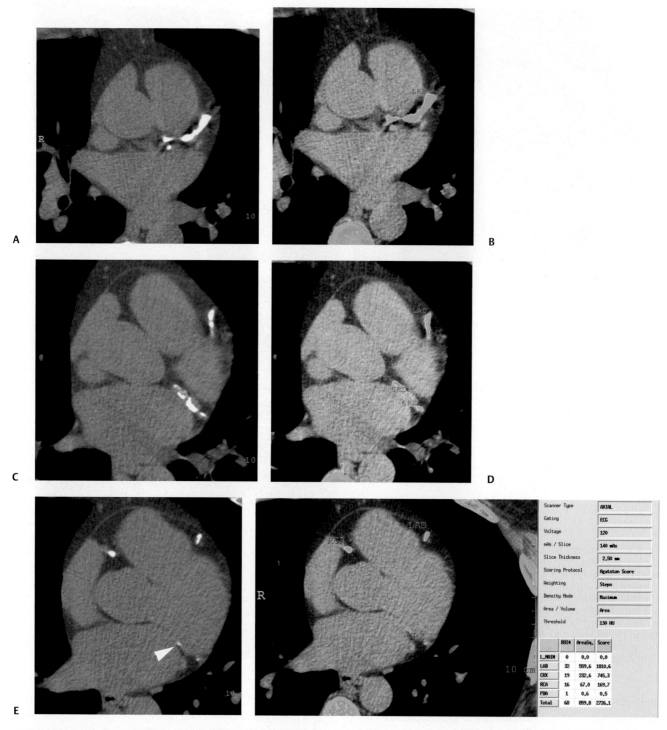

Fig. 5.5 Markedly elevated calcium score with associated stenosis in the right coronary artery (RCA). **(A)** Axial image demonstrates extensive calcification of the proximal left coronary artery and left anterior descending artery (LAD). **(B)** LAD calcium is color-coded. **(C)** Axial image at a slightly lower level demonstrates calcium within both the LAD and circumflex arteries. **(D)** Calcium within the LAD and circumflex arteries is color-coded. **(E)** Axial image at a slightly lower level demonstrates calcification in the LAD, circumflex, and RCA. Mild calcification is also identified in the posterior mitral annulus (*arrowhead*). **(F)** Calcium in the three major coronary arteries is color-coded. The mitral annular calcification is labeled in pink and is not included in the calcium score. The total Agatston calcium of 2726.1 is markedly elevated, suggesting increased risk for a coronary event.

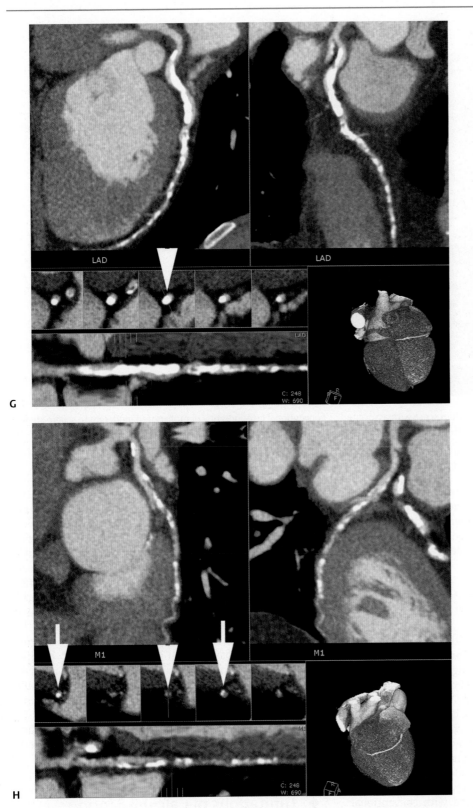

Fig. 5.5 (*Continued*) **(G)** Orthogonal curved maximum intensity projection (MIP) images of the LAD obtained with CT angiography demonstrate diffuse calcification. Calcified plaque appears to fill most of the LAD lumen on short axis-images (*arrowhead*). Conventional coronary angiography demonstrated only mild disease in the LAD. **(H)** Orthogonal curved MIP images through the circumflex artery demonstrate diffuse calcified plaque. Short-axis images demonstrate extensive calcified plaque (*arrows*), as well as noncalcified plaque with ulceration (*arrowhead*). Conventional arteriography demonstrated only mild disease in the circumflex artery. (*Continued on page 106*)

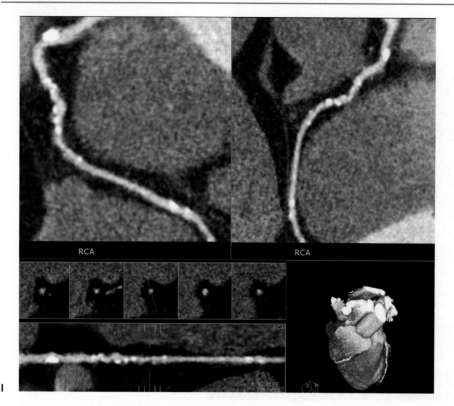

Fig. 5.5 *(Continued)* Markedly elevated calcium score with associated stenosis in the right coronary artery (RCA). **(I)** Orthogonal curved MIP images of the RCA demonstrate diffuse calcified and noncalcified plaque. Of the three major coronary arteries, the RCA was the least suspicious for significant stenosis on CT angiography. Nonetheless, conventional arteriography demonstrated moderate to severe stenosis in the midportion of the RCA. This area was treated by angioplasty. The accuracy of coronary CT angiography is degraded in patients with markedly elevated calcium scores.

patient into a higher risk category and demonstrate a need for aggressive therapy with aspirin and blood pressure or cholesterol-lowering medication. Furthermore, knowledge of the calcium score may motivate patients to comply with a healthier lifestyle and the prescribed medical regimen.

◆ Serial Calcium Scoring to Monitor Medical Therapy

Although most studies have evaluated the utility of calcium scoring as a one-time assessment of cardiac risk, it seems logical that repeated calcium scoring examinations can demonstrate the impact of medical therapy on overall coronary atherosclerotic burden. A study of patients treated with lipid-lowering therapy concluded that "the extent to which atherosclerotic plaque is decreased, stabilized, or increased . . . can be determined noninvasively by EBCT and quantified with use of a calcium-volume score."[35] Furthermore, these researchers claim that evidence of disease progression or regression can be obtained within a shorter time frame with calcium scoring compared with conventional angiography. A more recent study by the same group suggests that progression of coronary artery calcium in patients started on statin therapy may be associated with a 17.2-fold relative risk for myocardial infarction.[36] Given the relatively low radiation dose and noninvasive nature of calcium scoring,

application of calcium scoring to monitor changes in the atherosclerotic plaque burden would appear to represent a practical option for the management of coronary disease.

Nonetheless, recent studies have questioned the utility of serial calcium scores to monitor statin therapy. One study of more than 1000 subjects evaluated treatments that reduced total cholesterol and LDL, but these therapies had no effect on the progression of coronary calcification.[37] In another study involving postmenopausal women, more intensive statin therapy resulted in greater reduction of LDL levels but did not decrease the progression of coronary calcium scores.[38] It is possible that the more "stable" calcified plaque associated with elevated calcium scores is relatively resistant to statin therapy, whereas the more "vulnerable" noncalcified plaque regresses. Given the cost and radiation exposure associated with serial calcium scoring and the lack of conclusive evidence that serial calcium scoring adequately reflects risk reduction with statin therapy, serial calcium scoring is not recommended at this time.

◆ Limitations of Calcium Scoring

Calcium scoring can improve patient risk stratification, above and beyond the stratification provided by the Framingham risk analysis. In the patient who is at intermediate risk based on a Framingham risk stratification, the calcium score may be useful to guide therapy. However, calcium scoring cannot detect uncalcified plaque and cannot distinguish stable from unstable plaque. The magnitude of the calcium score within a coronary artery is significantly related to the mean degree of stenosis, but it does not define the severity of stenosis in a particular patient.[39] A calcium score of 0 is associated with a low probability of obstructive coronary disease (<5%) and a remarkably benign prognosis (event rate of about 0.17%/year),[40] but it cannot entirely exclude a stenosis.[41] Furthermore, among patients presenting with acute coronary syndrome, noncalcified plaques are highly prevalent and may be more likely to represent the culprit lesions.[42] Thus, calcium scoring should not be used to exclude coronary disease in a symptomatic patient. Given the presence of symptoms that are likely to be related to coronary heart disease, diagnostic assessment should focus on determining the location and severity of coronary disease. Calcium scoring may be useful in a patient with atypical chest pain if noninvasive tests are not feasible or inconclusive. At least one study suggests that a calcium score less than 100 is associated with a very low risk of myocardial ischemia. Conversely, in symptomatic patients calcium scores greater 400 are associated with significant myocardial ischemia.[43] This study suggests that calcium scoring may be used to "obviate the need for subsequent noninvasive testing." Nonetheless, given the inability of calcium scoring to detect stenosis related to noncalcified plaque and given the recent technical improvements in coronary CT angiography, low-risk symptomatic patients may be more appropriately evaluated with CT angiography compared with coronary calcium scoring.[44]

◆ Conclusion

Coronary artery calcium scoring provides a quick, noninvasive method for risk assessment of coronary heart events. Calcium scoring is most appropriate in the asymptomatic population with a coronary heart disease risk of 10 to 20% based on the Framingham risk calculation or in patients with other risk factors not considered in the Framingham analysis. In these patients, a coronary calcium score greater than 100 suggests that the patient should be moved to a higher-risk status. A calcium score in the range of 0 to 10 may suggest that the risk is lower than that projected by the Framingham risk score alone. Serial calcium scoring tests to follow up on therapies have not been validated at this time. The executive statement from a working group of the NHLBI issued in December 2005 suggests a modified Framingham risk score with additional risk indicators, including calcium scoring. Incorporation of the coronary calcium score and other tests for subclinical atherosclerosis, together with traditional risk assessment, should improve preventive therapy for future coronary events.

References

1. Lloyd-Jones D, Adams R, Carnethon M, et al; American Heart Association Statistics Committee and Stroke Statistics Subcommittee. Heart disease and stroke statistics—2009 update: a report from the American Heart Association Statistics Committee and Stroke Statistics Subcommittee. Circulation 2009;119(3):e21–e181

2. Grover SA, Coupal L, Hu XP. Identifying adults at increased risk of coronary disease. How well do the current cholesterol guidelines work? JAMA 1995;274(10):801–806

3. Wilson PW, D'Agostino RB, Levy D, Belanger AM, Silbershatz H, Kannel WB. Prediction of coronary heart disease using risk factor categories. Circulation 1998;97(18):1837–1847

4. Grundy SM, Cleeman JI, Merz CN, et al; National Heart, Lung, and Blood Institute; American College of Cardiology Foundation; American Heart Association. Implications of recent clinical trials for the National Cholesterol Education Program Adult Treatment Panel III guidelines. Circulation 2004;110(2):227–239

5. Falk E, Shah PK, Fuster V. Coronary plaque disruption. Circulation 1995;92(3):657–671

6. Maseri A, Fuster V. Is there a vulnerable plaque? Circulation 2003; 107(16):2068–2071

7. Schmermund A, Möhlenkamp S, Erbel R. Coronary artery calcium and its relationship to coronary artery disease. Cardiol Clin 2003;21(4): 521–534

8. Rumberger JA. Clinical use of coronary calcium scanning with computed tomography. Cardiol Clin 2003;21(4):535–547

9. Hecht HS. The deadly double standard (the saga of screening for subclinical atherosclerosis). Am J Cardiol 2008;101(12):1805–1807

10. Budoff MJ, Achenbach S, Blumenthal RS, et al; American Heart Association Committee on Cardiovascular Imaging and Intervention; American Heart Association Council on Cardiovascular Radiology and Intervention; American Heart Association Committee on Cardiac Imaging, Council on Clinical Cardiology. Assessment of coronary artery disease by cardiac computed tomography: a scientific statement from the American Heart Association Committee on Cardiovascular Imaging and Intervention, Council on Cardiovascular Radiology and Intervention, and Committee on Cardiac Imaging, Council on Clinical Cardiology. Circulation 2006;114(16):1761–1791

11. Greenland P, Bonow RO, Brundage BH, et al; American College of Cardiology Foundation Clinical Expert Consensus Task Force (ACCF/AHA Writing Committee to Update the 2000 Expert Consensus Document on Electron Beam Computed Tomography); Society of Atherosclerosis Imaging and Prevention; Society of Cardiovascular Computed Tomography. ACCF/AHA 2007 clinical expert consensus document on coronary artery calcium scoring by computed tomography in global cardiovascular risk assessment and in evaluation of patients with chest pain: a report of the American College of Cardiology Foundation Clinical Expert Consensus Task Force (ACCF/AHA Writing Committee to Update the 2000 Expert Consensus Document on Electron Beam Computed Tomography). Circulation 2007;115(3):402–426

12. De Backer G, Ambrosioni E, Borch-Johnsen K, et al; Third Joint Task Force of European and Other Societies on Cardiovascular Disease Prevention in Clinical Practice. European guidelines on cardiovascular disease prevention in clinical practice. Eur Heart J 2003;24(17): 1601–1610

13. Budoff MJ, Shaw LJ, Liu ST, et al. Long-term prognosis associated with coronary calcification: observations from a registry of 25,253 patients. J Am Coll Cardiol 2007;49(18):1860–1870

14. Detrano R, Guerci AD, Carr JJ, et al. Coronary calcium as a predictor of coronary events in four racial or ethnic groups. N Engl J Med 2008; 358(13):1336–1345

15. Stanford W, Thompson BH, Burns TL, Heery SD, Burr MC. Coronary artery calcium quantification at multi-detector row helical CT versus electron-beam CT. Radiology 2004;230(2):397–402

16. Becker CR, Kleffel T, Crispin A, et al. Coronary artery calcium measurement: agreement of multirow detector and electron beam CT. AJR Am J Roentgenol 2001;176(5):1295–1298

17. Knez A, Becker CR, Becker A, et al. Determination of coronary calcium with multi-slice spiral computed tomography: a comparative study with electron-beam CT. Int J Cardiovasc Imaging 2002;18(4):295–303

18. Morin RL, Gerber TC, McCollough CH. Radiation dose in computed tomography of the heart. Circulation 2003;107(6):917–922

19. Hunold P, Vogt FM, Schmermund A, et al. Radiation exposure during cardiac CT: effective doses at multi-detector row CT and electron-beam CT. Radiology 2003;226(1):145–152

20. Agatston AS, Janowitz WR, Hildner FJ, Zusmer NR, Viamonte M Jr, Detrano R. Quantification of coronary artery calcium using ultrafast computed tomography. J Am Coll Cardiol 1990;15(4):827–832

21. Callister TQ, Cooil B, Raya SP, Lippolis NJ, Russo DJ, Raggi P. Coronary artery disease: improved reproducibility of calcium scoring with an electron-beam CT volumetric method. Radiology 1998;208(3): 807–814

22. Nasir K, Raggi P, Rumberger JA, et al. Coronary artery calcium volume scores on electron beam tomography in 12,936 asymptomatic adults. Am J Cardiol 2004;93(9):1146–1149

23. Brown ER, Kronmal RA, Bluemke DA, et al. Coronary calcium coverage score: determination, correlates, and predictive accuracy in the Multi-Ethnic Study of Atherosclerosis. Radiology 2008;247(3):669–675

24. Raggi P, Callister TQ, Cooil B, et al. Identification of patients at increased risk of first unheralded acute myocardial infarction by electron-beam computed tomography. Circulation 2000;101(8):850–855

25. Keelan PC, Bielak LF, Ashai K, et al. Long-term prognostic value of coronary calcification detected by electron-beam computed tomography in patients undergoing coronary angiography. Circulation 2001; 104(4):412–417

26. Kondos GT, Hoff JA, Sevrukov A, et al. Electron-beam tomography coronary artery calcium and cardiac events: a 37-month follow-up of 5635 initially asymptomatic low- to intermediate-risk adults. Circulation 2003;107(20):2571–2576

27. Greenland P, LaBree L, Azen SP, Doherty TM, Detrano RC. Coronary artery calcium score combined with Framingham score for risk prediction in asymptomatic individuals. JAMA 2004;291(2):210–215

28. Schenker MP, Dorbala S, Hong EC, et al. Interrelation of coronary calcification, myocardial ischemia, and outcomes in patients with intermediate likelihood of coronary artery disease: a combined positron emission tomography/computed tomography study. Circulation 2008; 117(13):1693–1700

29. Pletcher MJ, Tice JA, Pignone M, Browner WS. Using the coronary artery calcium score to predict coronary heart disease events: a systematic review and meta-analysis. Arch Intern Med 2004;164(12): 1285–1292

30. Pletcher MJ, Tice JA, Pignone M, McCulloch C, Callister TQ, Browner WS. What does my patient's coronary artery calcium score mean? Combining information from the coronary artery calcium score with information from conventional risk factors to estimate coronary heart disease risk. BMC Med 2004;2:31

31. Schmermund A, Erbel R, Silber S; MUNICH Registry Study Group. Multislice Normal Incidence of Coronary Health. Age and gender

32. Knez A, Becker A, Leber A, et al. Relation of coronary calcium scores by electron beam tomography to obstructive disease in 2,115 symptomatic patients. Am J Cardiol 2004;93(9):1150–1152

33. Budoff MJ, Nasir K, McClelland RL, et al. Coronary calcium predicts events better with absolute calcium scores than age-sex-race/ethnicity percentiles: MESA (Multi-Ethnic Study of Atherosclerosis). J Am Coll Cardiol 2009;53(4):345–352

34. Hecht HS, Budoff MJ, Berman DS, Ehrlich J, Rumberger JA. Coronary artery calcium scanning: clinical paradigms for cardiac risk assessment and treatment. Am Heart J 2006;151(6):1139–1146

35. Callister TQ, Raggi P, Cooil B, Lippolis NJ, Russo DJ. Effect of HMG-CoA reductase inhibitors on coronary artery disease as assessed by electron-beam computed tomography. N Engl J Med 1998;339(27): 1972–1978

36. Raggi P, Callister TQ, Shaw LJ. Progression of coronary artery calcium and risk of first myocardial infarction in patients receiving cholesterol-lowering therapy. Arterioscler Thromb Vasc Biol 2004;24(7): 1272–1277

37. Arad Y, Spadaro LA, Roth M, Newstein D, Guerci AD. Treatment of asymptomatic adults with elevated coronary calcium scores with atorvastatin, vitamin C, and vitamin E: the St. Francis Heart Study randomized clinical trial. J Am Coll Cardiol 2005;46(1):166–172

38. Raggi P, Davidson M, Callister TQ, et al. Aggressive versus moderate lipid-lowering therapy in hypercholesterolemic postmenopausal women: Beyond Endorsed Lipid Lowering with EBT Scanning (BELLES). Circulation 2005;112(4):563–571

39. Rosen BD, Fernandes V, McClelland RL, et al. Relationship between baseline coronary calcium score and demonstration of coronary artery stenoses during follow-up MESA (Multi-Ethnic Study of Atherosclerosis). JACC Cardiovasc Imaging 2009;2(10):1175–1183

40. Hecht HS. Coronary artery calcium: the cup is 96% full. JACC Cardiovasc Imaging 2009;2(10):1184–1186

41. Haberl R, Becker A, Leber A, et al. Correlation of coronary calcification and angiographically documented stenoses in patients with suspected coronary artery disease: results of 1,764 patients. J Am Coll Cardiol 2001;37(2):451–457

42. Henneman MM, Schuijf JD, Pundziute G, et al. Noninvasive evaluation with multislice computed tomography in suspected acute coronary syndrome: plaque morphology on multislice computed tomography versus coronary calcium score. J Am Coll Cardiol 2008;52(3):216–222

43. Berman DS, Wong ND, Gransar H, et al. Relationship between stress-induced myocardial ischemia and atherosclerosis measured by coronary calcium tomography. J Am Coll Cardiol 2004;44(4):923–930

44. Hausleiter J, Meyer T, Hadamitzky M, Kastrati A, Martinoff S, Schömig A. Prevalence of noncalcified coronary plaques by 64-slice computed tomography in patients with an intermediate risk for significant coronary artery disease. J Am Coll Cardiol 2006;48(2):312–318

6

Coronary Artery Disease

Jonathan Gomberg and Ethan J. Halpern

Following the introduction of coronary angiography in the 1960s, the diagnosis and treatment of coronary artery disease (CAD) focused on the arterial lumen. Treatments such as bypass surgery and angioplasty relieve ischemia by reducing the severity or impact of coronary artery stenoses while leaving the underlying disease process unchanged. In more recent years therapies for CAD have expanded to include the earlier stages of atherosclerosis, before the development of flow-limiting stenoses. These treatments are directed toward preventing or retarding plaque formation or stabilizing existing plaques. Early medical intervention can lessen the likelihood of plaque rupture and the resulting acute coronary syndromes (ACS), which may manifest as unstable angina or myocardial infarction.

Coronary CT angiography (CTA) can demonstrate several important aspects of CAD. Quantification of coronary calcium allows a global assessment of risk, as discussed in detail in Chapter 5. The ability to define the arterial lumen and the arterial wall provides an important noninvasive means of assessing the symptomatic patient with suspected CAD. Combining pharmacologic "stress testing" with coronary CTA expands on this utility.

The determination of which patients should receive lifelong preventative treatment can be difficult. The ability of coronary CTA noninvasively to define plaque morphology may lead to more focused strategies. Identification of the so-called vulnerable plaques that are prone to rupture would be an invaluable aid in the prevention of ACS. If these plaques could be accurately identified, targeted interventions could be performed to prevent myocardial infarctions.

◆ Risk Factors for Coronary Artery Disease

Atherosclerosis is a chronic, systemic, and multifactorial disease. Risk factors contribute to the initial arterial injury and subsequent response, which leads to atherosclerosis. Hyperlipidemia, especially in the form of an elevated serum low-density lipoprotein (LDL), plays an important role in the development of coronary atherosclerosis and is the most powerful risk factor for the development of CAD.

Inflammation also plays a critical role. It has been well demonstrated that C-reactive protein, a marker of systemic inflammation, offers additional independent prognostic information with a predictive value similar to that of LDL.[1]

The most common risk factors for CAD are summarized in **Table 6.1**. Many of these factors have been used in scoring systems, such as the Framingham risk score, the Interheart study, and the Reynolds risk score. Risk factor data are combined in these risk scores to calculate a patient's risk of developing clinically significant CAD. Several additional biomarkers may be relevant in the pathogenesis of CAD but have not been shown to add clinically useful prognostic information beyond the traditional risk factors.[2]

◆ Pathogenesis of Atherosclerosis

The progression of atherosclerosis from a clinically insignificant "fatty streak" to a stenotic lesion is not a linear process of plaque deposition over time. Rather, atherosclerosis is a complex systemic arterial disease that can evolve at varying rates and manifest as different stages at different locations within the arterial tree of a single patient. Atherosclerotic plaques differ in their behavior and their clinical manifestations at different points in their life cycle (**Fig. 6.1**).[3] The American Heart Association (AHA) classification of atherosclerotic lesions[4] and a subsequent modification[5] are summarized in **Tables 6.2** and **6.3**. Whereas a detailed description of the pathophysiology of atherosclerosis is beyond the scope of this book, familiarity with the stages of atherosclerosis should help clarify the clinical implications of the radiographic features of this disease.

Atherosclerosis begins when normal endothelium is damaged. Sources of endothelial injury include hypercholesterolemia, irritants in cigarette smoke, vasoactive substances, metabolic end products in diabetics, and circulating immunocomplexes. Mechanical stresses such as abnormal flow and increased shear forces may be related to hypertension. The resultant endothelial dysfunction leads to a "response to injury" that evolves into an atherosclerotic plaque. This process can begin as early as the second decade of life.[3,6]

Table 6.1 Common Factors Used for Determining the Risk of Coronary Artery Disease

	Framingham Risk Score	Interheart	SCORE	ASSIGN-SCORE	QRISK1&2	PROCAM	Reynolds Risk Score
Gender (male)	+		+	+	+		
Age	+		+	+	+	+	+
Family history of CVD	+			+		+	+
Weight/BMI		+			+		
Cigarette smoking	+	+	+	+	+		
Blood pressure	+	+	+	+	+		+
Diabetes	+	+			+		
Hypercholesterolemia	+	ApoB/ApoA1	+	+	+	+	+
Hypertriglyceridemia						+	
LDL						+	
HDL	+			+	+	+	+
Lipoprotein (a)							
LVH on ECG	+						
C-Reactive Protein							+
Sedentary lifestyle		+					
Psychosocial stress		+					
Lack of dietary fruit, vegetables		+					
Lack of moderate alcohol use		+					
Chronic kidney disease					+		
Homocysteine level							
BNP/pro-N-terminal BNP							
Troponin I							
Carotid plaque							
Ankle–brachial index							
Metabolic syndrome *							
Coronary calcification							

*Abdominal obesity, hypertension, dyslipidemia with hypercholesterolemia, hypertriglyceridemia, low HDL, insulin resistance with hyperglycemia or type 2 diabetes mellitus.

Abbreviations: BMI, body mass index; BNP, brain natriuretic peptide; CVD, cardiovascular disease; HDL, high-density lipoprotein; LDL, low-density lipoprotein; LVH, left ventricular hypertrophy.

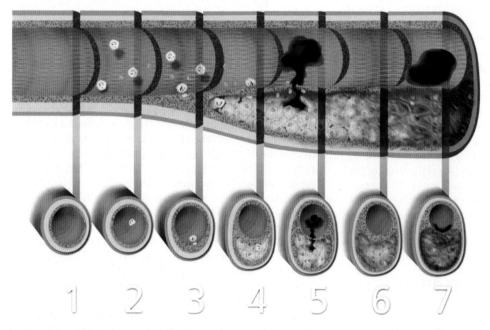

Fig. 6.1 Stages of development of atherosclerotic plaque. Longitudinal schematic of an artery depicts a timeline beginning with (1) a normal artery. Smooth muscle cells migrate into the intima early in life. (2) Lesion initiation is associated with inflammatory leukocytes and extracellular lipid. (3) The fibrofatty stage is characterized by monocytes that transform into macrophages and become lipid-laden foam cells. (4) The inflammatory process continues with matrix degrading proteinases that weaken the fibrous cap. (5) Rupture of the fibrous cap may result in vascular thrombosis. (6) The healing process may result in a fibrous and often calcified plaque. (7) In some cases vascular thrombosis may be related to superficial endothelial erosions rather than to plaque rupture. In this figure the erosion is superimposed on a complex plaque. However, endothelial erosion may occur in the absence of an underlying complex plaque. (Reprinted with permission from Libby P. Current concepts of the pathogenesis of the acute coronary syndromes. Circulation. 2001;104(3):365–72.)

Table 6.2 American Heart Association Classification of Atherosclerotic Lesions (1995)

Early lesions; young patients without clinical disease		
Type I lesion	**Initial lesion**	Fatty streak
	Intimal macrophage-derived foam cells containing lipid droplets	
Type II lesion	*Macrophages and smooth muscle cells, mild extracellular lipid deposits*	
IIa	**Progression-prone type II lesion**	
IIb	**Progression-resistant type II lesion**	
Type III lesion	**Intermediate lesion (preatheroma)**	
	Smooth muscle cells w/extracellular connective tissue, fibrils, lipid deposits, early microcalcification can occur	
Atheromas with high lipid content, increased inflammation, some with thin fibrous cap, positive remodeling		
Type IV lesion	**Atheroma**	
	Confluent cellular lesions, extracellular lipids, and normal intima microcalcifications can occur	
Va	**Fibroatheroma (type V lesion)** *extracellular lipid core covered by a fibrous cap*	Advanced, raised lesions
Vb	**Calcific lesion (type VII lesion)** *may be stenotic, may cause angina*	
Vc	**Fibrotic lesion (type VIII)** *may be stenotic, may cause angina*	
Acute, complicated lesions		
Type VI lesion	**Complex lesion with surface defect or hematoma/hemorrhage or thrombotic deposit**	
	complicated plaque	

Modified from Stary HC, Chandler AB, Dinsmore RE, et al. Committee on Vascular Lesions of the Council on Arteriosclerosis, American Heart Association. Arterioscler Thromb Vasc Biol. 1995;15:1512–1531.

Injured endothelium results in production of proteins that attract circulating monocytes, which become incorporated into the arterial wall as tissue macrophages. Oxidized LDLs become incorporated into the intima, binding with proteins and inducing an inflammatory response. More monocytes migrate into the arterial wall, and smooth muscle cells migrate from the media into the intima. These cells transform into lipid-laden foam cells, collections of which create the "fatty streak" of early atherosclerosis. These early atherosclerotic lesions are seen in young people and can regress. Later stages of atherosclerosis cannot regress.

Cytokines activate smooth muscle cells and cause extracellular protein and matrix deposition and fibrosis. Neovascularization of the intimal plaques arises from the media via the vasa vasorum. Proteins that regulate calcification are expressed by macrophages, smooth muscle cells, and adventitial cells. Microcalcifications can occur in AHA III and IV transitional lesions. Coronary calcification becomes denser with continued fibrosis.[4]

As atherosclerosis progresses, the involved vessel may enlarge, allowing eccentric plaque growth within the vessel wall without impinging upon the arterial lumen. This process

Table 6.3 Modified American Heart Association Classification Based on Morphologic Description (2000)

Lesion	Description	Thrombosis
Nonatherosclerotic intimal lesions		
Intimal thickening	The normal accumulation of SMCs in the intima in the absence of lipid or macrophage foam cells	Absent
Initial xanthoma or fatty streak	Luminal accumulation of foam cells without a necrotic core or fibrous cap. These lesions may regress.	Absent
Progressive atherosclerotic lesions		
Pathologic intimal thickening	SMCs in a proteoglycan-rich matrix with areas of extracellular lipid accumulation without necrosis	Absent
With erosion	Plaque the same as above, with luminal thrombosis	Mostly mural
Fibrous cap atheroma	Well-formed necrotic core with an overlying fibrous cap	Absent
With erosion	Plaque the same as above, with luminal thrombosis No communication of thrombus with necrotic core	Mostly mural infrequently occlusive
Thin fibrous cap atheroma	A thin fibrous cap infiltrated by macrophages and lymphocytes with rare SMCs and an underlying necrotic core	Absent, may have intraplaque hemorrhage
With plaque rupture	Fibroatheroma with cap disruption; luminal thrombus communicates with the bunderlying necrotic core.	Usually occlusive
Calcified nodule	Eruptive nodular calcification with underlying fibrocalcific plaque	Usually nonocclusive
Fibrocalcific plaque	Collagen-rich plaque with significant stenosis, usually contains large areas of calcification with few inflammatory cells; a necrotic core may be present.	Absent

Modified from Virmani R, Kolodgie FD, Burke AP, Farb A, Schwartz SM. Lessons from sudden coronary death: a comprehensive morphological classification scheme for atherosclerotic lesions. Arterioscler Thromb Vasc Biol. 2000;20:1262–1275.

Abbreviation: SMC, smooth muscle cells.

of positive remodeling allows atherosclerosis to evolve without causing a stenosis or any clinical evidence of ischemic disease.[7] Such plaques can grow to a significant size, developing a large lipid core with extensive macrophage infiltration and few smooth muscle cells. Eccentric plaque growth and vascular remodeling can result in disruption of the internal elastic lamina and neovascularization. Intraplaque hemorrhage, inflammation, and apoptosis result in softening of the lipid-rich core and weakening of the overlying fibrous cap. Metabolic processes, including enzymatic degradation of the extracellular matrix, apoptosis and inflammation, and physical factors such as wall stress and blood flow both contribute to thinning of the fibrous cap. Macrophages and mast cells present at the shoulder of an eccentric plaque or between the plaque and the adjacent vessel wall participate in the inflammatory process. These are the two sites where plaque rupture most frequently occurs.

Different mechanisms of ACS may be associated with different types of plaque (**Table 6.3**). The most common mechanism for ACS is related to infiltration by inflammatory cells and plaque rupture at a site of fibrous cap thinning as described above. Several characteristics make a plaque more likely to rupture. In most cases the fibrous cap overlying the lipid core has thinned to less than 65 μm; these plaques are characterized as a thin-cap fibroatheroma (TCFA).

A less common mechanism of ACS is related to a small, nonulcerated erosion of the endothelium that generates a platelet-rich mural thrombus. The thrombus that covers the denuded endothelium is most commonly nonocclusive and often asymptomatic. The aggregate of many of these events throughout the coronary tree results in asymptomatic progression of CAD. However, approximately one third of occlusive thrombi within the coronary arteries occur at a site of endothelial erosion without rupture into a lipid core.[8] The least common mechanism for coronary thrombosis is related to eruptive nodular calcification with underlying fibrocalcific plaque. In this scenario, the unstable plaque responsible for ACS may be calcified.

◆ "Vulnerable" Plaque

The precursor of a ruptured plaque is known as a *vulnerable plaque*. If these vulnerable plaques could be reliably identified before rupture, targeted therapy could be applied to prevent acute coronary events. This simple construct is attractive, but unfortunately it is not currently possible to classify a plaque accurately as stable or vulnerable.

Most plaque ruptures occur in TCFAs. Plaque rupture often occurs in large plaques that are not associated with obstructive coronary disease. These lesions often demonstrate positive remodeling and serve as the nidus for occlusive thrombus. There is a systemic component to CAD; patients with an ACS often have two or more TCFA lesions scattered throughout the coronary artery tree. Therefore, although the presence of TCFAs increases the risk of a clinical event, it is not possible to predict whether an individual TCFA will, within a specified time frame, rupture and become the cause of an acute coronary event.

The heterogeneity of plaque morphologies that presage clinical events complicates the radiographic identification of the vulnerable plaque. TCFA is not the only morphology that leads to acute coronary artery occlusion. Occlusive, platelet-rich intracoronary thrombosis can form on the eroded surface of a plaque without frank rupture. Identification of plaque characteristics that are associated with an increased risk of a clinically relevant coronary event may warrant more aggressive risk factor modification. However, there is no clearly defined morphology or characteristic that can distinguish a stable plaque from a vulnerable plaque with enough accuracy to be immediately predictive of an acute coronary event.

◆ Consequences of Coronary Atherosclerosis

The progression of CAD can manifest in many ways. Atherosclerosis can develop slowly over years as a series of nonclinically significant steps, or it may present suddenly in a young patient as an acute coronary occlusion of a previously nonstenotic plaque. Furthermore, there is a wide range of how people feel angina; some patients experience typical angina when a coronary stenosis limits the blood flow, whereas others have atypical or no symptoms despite myocardial ischemia. These factors, among others, are responsible for the wide range of clinical presentations of CAD.

The clinical consequences of endothelial disruption depend largely on the extent of thrombus that develops. A small disruption of the intima may be covered by a platelet-rich thrombus, which may not cause any limitation of blood flow. Such an intimal disruption can be a clinically silent event that contributes incrementally to the existing coronary stenosis. Factors that affect thrombus formation include the degree of pre-existing stenosis and the thrombogenicity of the plaque. The lipid-rich core of large eccentric plaques is the most thrombogenic substrate in the coronary circulation, and the rupture of this type of plaque is the most frequent cause of ACS. Hypercoagulable states caused by cigarette smoke, elevated LDL levels, catecholamines, or metabolic syndrome also promote thrombus formation.[3,5,6,9] The stenosis caused by the plaque itself (without the overlying thrombus) is often not hemodynamically significant, but the abrupt thrombotic occlusion can cause acute ST elevation or non-ST elevation myocardial infarction or unstable angina.

The factors that determine the clinical course of a plaque rupture include the acuity of the occlusion, the size and distribution of the affected artery, the presence or absence of collaterals, the status of the other coronary arteries, and the underlying ventricular function. Secondary events such as arrhythmias or mechanical complications of an infarction (eg, ventricular septal defect, acute mitral regurgitation secondary to papillary muscle dysfunction or free wall rupture) can also affect the clinical course.

The process of acute plaque rupture with secondary thrombosis explains how a patient can suffer a myocardial infarction shortly after a negative stress test, and more broadly explains why screening tests for CAD based on luminal stenoses has been a disappointing strategy overall. However, the long preclinical phase of atherosclerotic CAD does provide opportunity for early diagnosis and treatment with aggressive risk factor modification. Statins and angiotensin-converting enzyme inhibitors have been demonstrated to decrease cardiac events in prevention trials. The mechanism of action appears to be plaque stabilization and suppression of inflammation rather than regression of stenosis.[10]

◆ CT Angiographic Assessment of Coronary Artery Disease: Stenosis

CTA is an excellent tool for visualization of both calcified and noncalcified plaque and for the assessment of coronary stenosis. Because CTA obtains a volumetric data set, vessels can be visualized in any desired orientation. Each coronary segment can be rotated into an optimal orientation to visualize the vessel lumen and plaque (**Figs. 6.2** and **6.3**).

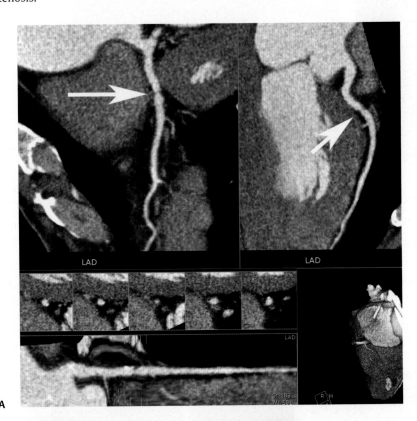

A

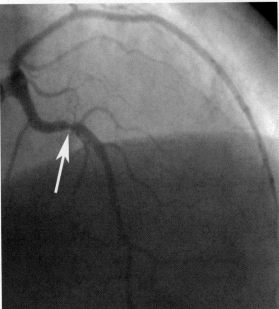

B

Fig. 6.2 Multiple projections demonstrate a focal stenosis in the left anterior descending artery (LAD) with coronary CT angiography. **(A)** Orthogonal curved maximum intensity projections demonstrate a bandlike stenosis in the proximal LAD (*arrows*). The straightened lumen view also demonstrates focal stenosis related to noncalcified plaque at this level. Cross-sectional images of the LAD at the level of the stenosis confirm a 70 to 80% narrowing. **(B)** Conventional coronary arteriography confirms a 70 to 80% narrowing of the LAD (*arrow*).

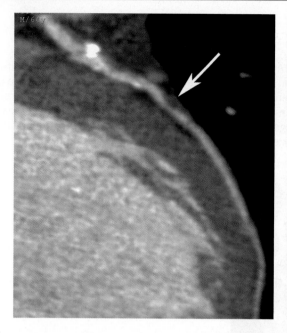

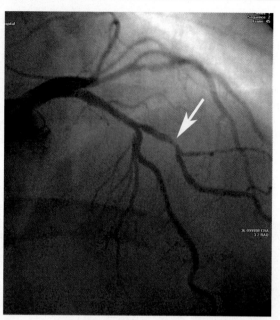

A   **B**

Fig. 6.3 Maximum intensity projection (MIP) image rotated to demonstrate optimally moderate stenosis in a first diagonal branch. **(A)** Slab MIP image through the proximal left anterior descending artery (LAD) and extending into the first diagonal branch demonstrates calcified atherosclerotic disease in the proximal portion of the vessel with positive remodeling. Focal noncalcified plaque in the proximal first diagonal branch results in moderate stenosis of 50 to 70% (*arrow*). **(B)** Conventional arteriography confirms the CT angiographic findings, again demonstrating focal stenosis in the diagonal branch. Because the plaque can be rotated so that it is clearly defined adjacent to the luminal narrowing on CT, the severity of the disease is more easily appreciated by CT angiography compared with conventional arteriography.

Maximum intensity projection (MIP) images provide the most useful technique to assess for vascular stenosis. In the setting of positive remodeling, vessels with calcified plaque can be rotated so that the calcified plaque projects beyond the expected lumen of the vessel (**Figs. 6.4, 6.5, 6.6, 6.7, 6.8,** **6.9,** and **6.10**). Small calcified plaques are generally easy to assess with simple MIP rendering. Vessel tracking tools may be useful in the assessment of more diseased vessels (**Figs. 6.7, 6.8, 6.9,** and **6.10**). Vessel tracking provides straightened lumen and cross-sectional views through the

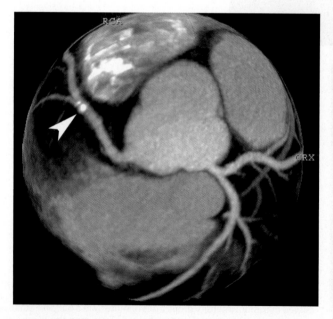

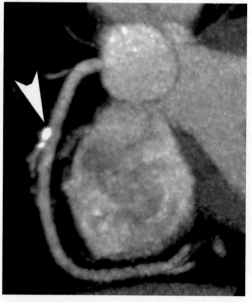

A   **B**

Fig. 6.4 Calcified atherosclerotic plaque in the right coronary artery (RCA) with positive remodeling. **(A)** Globe maximum intensity projection (MIP) demonstrates a focal calcified plaque overlying the proximal RCA (*arrowhead*). The plaque appears to involve the vessel lumen in this view. **(B)** Slab MIP projection of the RCA in a left anterior oblique projection demonstrates that the calcified plaque is mostly outside the lumen of the RCA (*arrowhead*) and is diagnostic of positive remodeling with no significant stenosis.

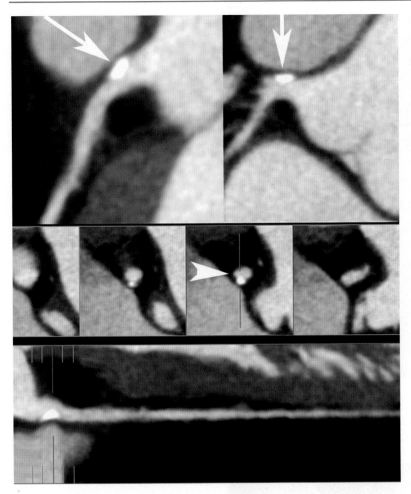

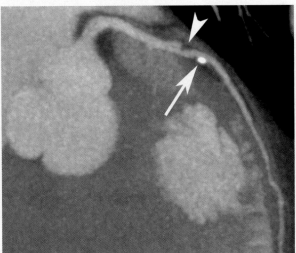

Fig. 6.5 Calcified plaque in the left main coronary artery with positive remodeling. Slab maximum intensity projections (MIPs) of the left main coronary artery (two top images) demonstrate eccentrically located calcified plaque without narrowing of the lumen (*arrows*). A straightened lumen MIP projection at the bottom of the image confirms the eccentric location of the plaque. Cross-sectional images through the left main coronary artery demonstrate that the calcified plaque is extruded from the vessel lumen (*arrowhead*), diagnostic of positive remodeling. There is no associated stenosis of the lumen.

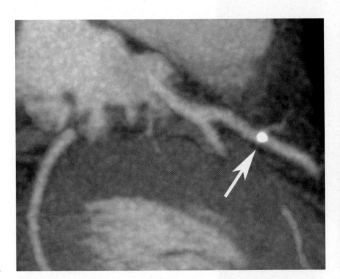

A

B

Fig. 6.6 Noncalcified and calcified plaque in the proximal left anterior descending artery (LAD) without significant narrowing. **(A)** Slab maximum intensity projection (MIP) demonstrates calcified plaque in the proximal LAD overlying the vessel lumen (*arrow*). **(B)** Slab MIP in a different projection demonstrates that the calcified plaque is eccentric with positive remodeling (*arrow*). Just proximal to this calcified plaque, there is noncalcified plaque (*arrowhead*) that was not visible in (A). (*Continued on page 116*)

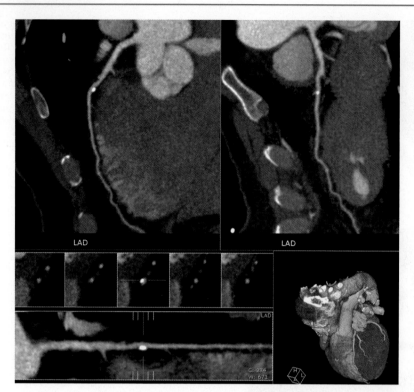

C

Fig. 6.6 (*Continued*) Noncalcified and calcified plaque in the proximal left anterior descending artery (LAD) without significant narrowing. **(C)** Orthogonal curved MIP images demonstrate both noncalcified and calcified plaques with less than 50% luminal narrowing. At the bottom of the figure, the straightened lumen view and associated cross-sectional images through the LAD demonstrate positive remodeling of the calcified LAD plaque.

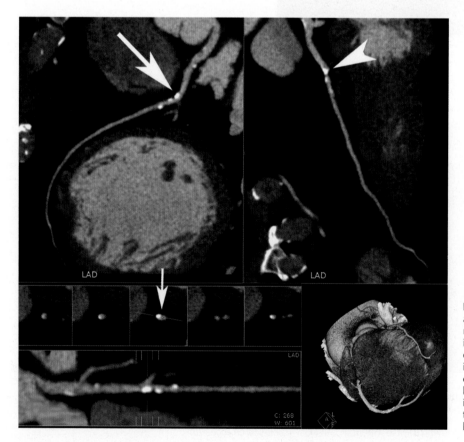

Fig. 6.7 Calcified plaque in the proximal left anterior descending artery (LAD) with positive remodeling. Orthogonal curved maximum intensity projections of the LAD. Although the calcified plaque appears to overlie the vessel in one view (*arrowhead*), it is clearly eccentric on the second view (*arrow*). The straightened lumen view and associated cross-sectional images through the vessel demonstrate positive remodeling with extrusion of the calcium beyond the vessel lumen (*small arrow*).

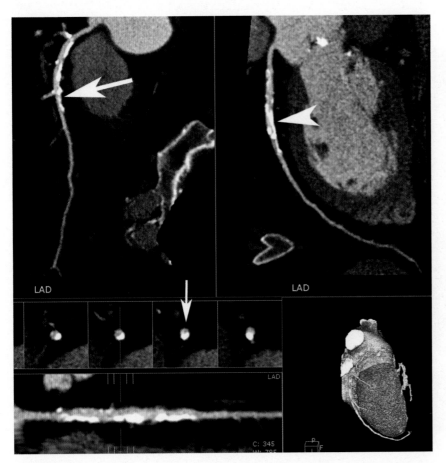

Fig. 6.8 Calcified atherosclerotic plaque in the proximal to the mid-left anterior descending artery (LAD) with less than 50% diameter reduction. Orthogonal curved MIP projections of the LAD demonstrate moderate calcification in the proximal to midportion of the vessel. Although the calcified plaque appears to cause greater than 50% luminal narrowing on one projection (*arrowhead*), only mild narrowing is observed on the second projection (*arrow*). The straightened lumen view and cross-sectional images of the LAD suggest an approximate 50% diameter narrowing with positive remodeling (*small arrow*). The degree of narrowing associated with densely calcified plaque is often overestimated because the extent of the calcium is exaggerated by blooming artifact.

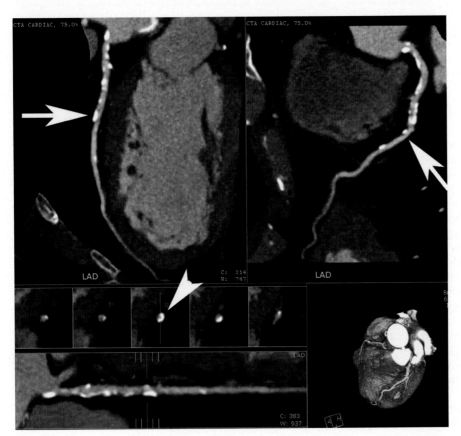

Fig. 6.9 Calcified left main and proximal left anterior descending (LAD) arteries with less than 50% narrowing. Orthogonal curved maximum intensity projection (MIP) images of the LAD demonstrate mild diffuse calcified plaque in the proximal to midportion of the LAD (*arrows*). Cross-sectional images through the LAD at the level of the arrows demonstrate that some of the calcium is circumferential, but the degree of vessel narrowing is less than 50% (*arrowhead*). The circumferential nature of the calcified plaque is not appreciated on the orthogonal MIP views because each thin orthogonal MIP image includes the calcification along only one side of the vessel wall.

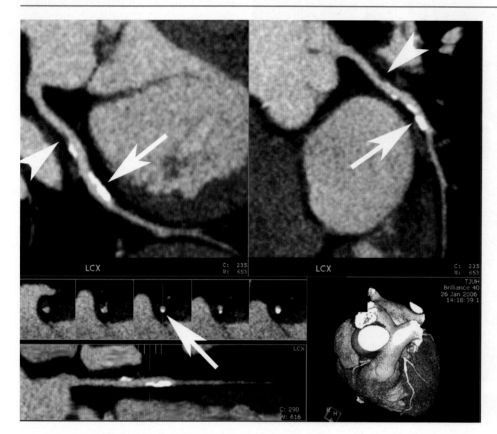

Fig. 6.10 Noncalcified and calcified plaque in the proximal to mid-circumflex artery with mild stenosis. Orthogonal curved maximum intensity projection (MIP) images at the top of the figure demonstrate noncalcified (*arrowheads*) and calcified (*arrows*) plaque in the proximal to mid-circumflex artery with less than 50% luminal narrowing. There is no remodeling associated with the noncalcified plaque, but there is positive remodeling associated with the calcified plaque. The straightened lumen and cross-sectional views at the bottom of the figure confirm that the degree of narrowing is less than 50%. LCX, left circumflex artery.

artery that may be useful for assessment of circumferential plaque. A complete discussion of different rendering and display techniques is included in Chapter 2.

In the setting of extensive coronary calcification, the underlying lumen is often obscured. Calcium in the arterial wall creates blooming artifact, which limits assessment of the adjacent lumen in the presence of stenosis (**Figs. 6.11, 6.12,** and **6.13**) and may result in a false-positive diagnosis in the absence of stenosis (**Fig. 6.14**). In the presence of heavy coronary calcification, the diagnosis of significant coronary disease can sometimes be suggested on the basis of an adjacent noncalcified vascular segment (**Fig. 6.15**). Although the density of calcium may be similar to that of adjacent contrast media in the arterial lumen, use of wide window settings may be helpful to distinguish calcium from contrast material. Careful evaluation of CTA images with wide window settings using MIP and vessel tracking techniques allows accurate diagnosis of obstructive disease in greater than 90% of small and moderate-sized calcified coronary artery plaques.[11] Nonetheless, a calcium score above 1000 is frequently associated with reduced image quality and decreased accuracy in the assessment of coronary stenosis.[12]

Arterial size is another important issue that can limit the CTA evaluation of stenoses. The sensitivity for detection of stenosis is clearly superior in proximal arterial segments compared with more distal segments.[13] The left anterior descending and circumflex arteries may measure 3 to 4 mm in diameter proximally and then taper in caliber distally. Evaluation of diagonal and obtuse marginal branches may also be limited by their small caliber (**Fig. 6.16**). As arterial size decreases below 1 mm, the effect of volume averaging increases, thereby reducing vascular conspicuity and decreasing diagnostic accuracy. The right coronary artery does not taper significantly to the level of the posterior descending artery. However, the midportion of the right coronary artery is the most rapidly moving segment within the coronary tree and has the highest rate of nondiagnostic images attributable to motion artifact.

When reviewing published studies of coronary CTA, one should always note the methodologic differences of the studies. The severity of stenoses assessed by CTA is most often defined as severe or obstructive (>70%), moderate (50–70%), or mild (<50%). Studies that exclude patients who have rapid heart rate, arrhythmia, or an inability to take β-blockers will report higher diagnostic sensitivity and specificity. Many studies exclude patients with elevated calcium scores as well as patients with nondiagnostic examinations from the analysis. As with all tests, CTA's sensitivity and specificity affected by the population studied. CTA findings

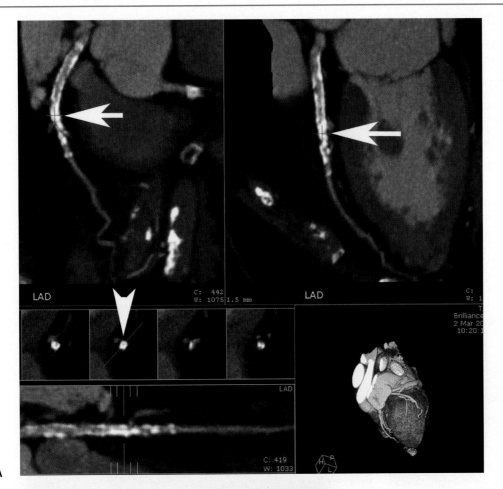

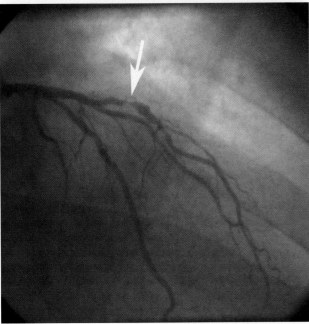

Fig. 6.11 Diffusely calcified proximal to mid left anterior descending artery (LAD) with focal high-grade narrowing. **(A)** Orthogonal curved maximum intensity projection images through the anterior descending artery demonstrate diffuse calcification in the proximal to midportion of the vessel. Although the calcium appears circumferential, the lumen is clearly visible in the proximal portion of the vessel. However, in the midportion of the LAD, there is dense calcification and the lumen is not visible (*arrow*). Cross-sectional images through the LAD at this level demonstrate circumferential calcification with severe narrowing of the lumen (*arrowhead*). **(B)** The findings of the CT angiogram are confirmed by conventional arteriography, demonstrating a severe narrowing in the midportion of the LAD (*arrow*).

Fig. 6.12 Densely calcified plaque in the proximal left anterior descending artery (LAD) with high-grade stenosis. **(A)** Globe maximum intensity projection (MIP) view demonstrates a densely calcified segment of the proximal LAD (*arrows*), just beyond the origin of the first diagonal branch. **(B)** Slab MIP of the LAD again demonstrates the densely calcified segment (*arrows*). The lumen of the LAD was not visible even with thin MIP images. **(C)** Conventional arteriogram demonstrates high-grade stenosis in the area of calcified plaque (*arrows*). The severity of stenosis cannot be adequately assessed by multislice–multidetector CT in the setting of densely calcified coronary vessels.

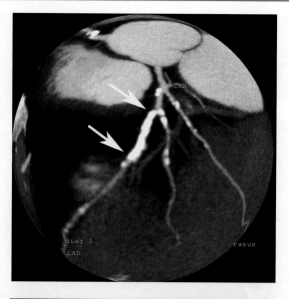

A

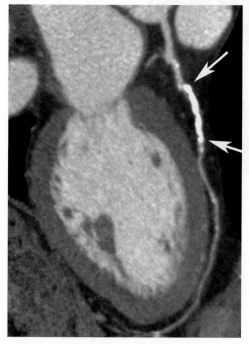

B

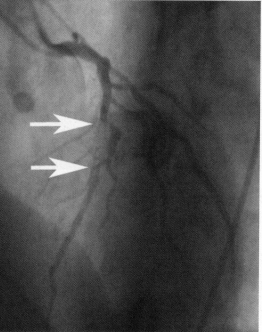

C

are also reported "by patient," "by artery," or "by segment." A "by patient" analysis will favor sensitivity over specificity, whereas a "by segment" analysis will favor specificity. These factors influence the "real-world" applicability of CTA.

The reported accuracy of CTA in detection of coronary artery stenosis is a moving target. Earlier studies using 16-detector multislice–multidetector (MDCT) technology often excluded smaller coronary segments from analysis. More recent studies using newer 64-row scanners generally include all coronary segments. A recent meta-analysis of 64-slice studies demonstrated a sensitivity of 99% (95% confidence interval [CI], 97–99%) and a specificity of 89% (95% CI, 83–94%) for the presence of significant coronary stenosis in a patient-based analysis.[14] In a by-segment analysis, CTA demonstrated a sensitivity of 90% (95% CI, 85–94%) and a specificity of 97% (95% CI, 95–98%). The median negative predictive value of CTA for patient-based detection of coronary disease was 100%.

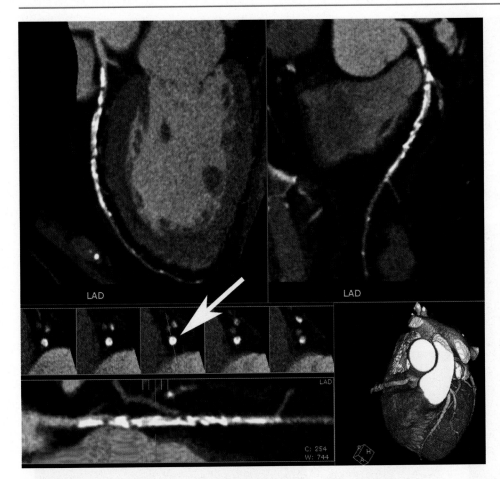

Fig. 6.13 Diffusely calcified left anterior descending artery (LAD) with high-grade stenosis. Orthogonal curved maximum intensity projection (MIP) views demonstrate a diffusely calcified proximal-to-mid LAD with mild focal calcification of the distal LAD. The straightened lumen view and associated cross-sectional images through the LAD demonstrate diffuse calcified plaque. The lumen of the LAD appears to be filled with calcium at several levels, but the excellent opacification of the distal vessel as well as the lack of collateral vessels suggest that the LAD is not occluded. The patient was referred for cardiac catheterization. High-grade disease was documented and angioplasty was performed.

There is good correlation between CTA and coronary angiography in the grading of stenoses, with a slight tendency to overestimate the degree of stenosis with CTA.[15] Current coronary CTA systems are capable of evaluating coronary vessels for the presence of stenosis with reasonable accuracy down to a vessel diameter of about 1 mm. The results of multicenter trials by Budoff and colleagues,[16] Meijboom et al,[17] and Miller and coworkers[18] are summarized in **Table 6.4** along with meta-analysis results from Mowatt et al,[14] Meijer and colleagues[19] and Vanhoenacker et al.[20] All these studies support the very high negative predictive value of a normal coronary CTA to exclude the presence of significant coronary stenosis. The use of new dose-reduction techniques for coronary CTA has generally been implemented without a significant loss of diagnostic image quality. However, large-scale studies of diagnostic accuracy are not available for new techniques such as prospective electrocardiographic (ECG) triggering and high-pitch flash spiral imaging (see Chapter 2).

◆ Prognostic Information Based on CT Angiographic Findings of Stenosis

The extent and severity of coronary artery stenosis have been demonstrated in several studies to provide important clinical and prognostic information. A study of 1127 patients examined by coronary CTA with average follow-up of 15.3 months demonstrated that the presence of severe stenosis, left main stenosis, proximal stenosis, three-vessel disease, and the number of involved coronary segments were all independent predictors of mortality.[21] A more recent study of coronary CTA patients with a mean follow-up of 16 months demonstrated an increasing frequency of cardiac events when patients are grouped by normal coronary arteries (no events), presence of coronary disease (30% events), obstructive coronary disease (63% events), and obstructive coronary disease in the proximal left coronary system (77% events).[22] These

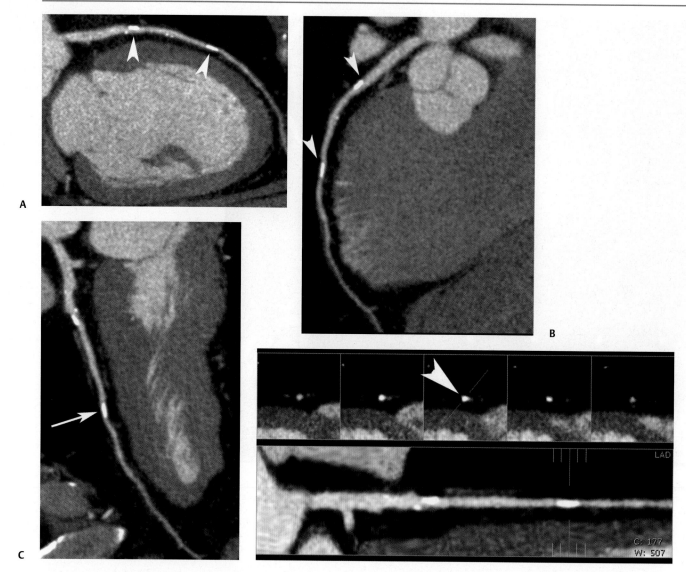

Fig. 6.14 Calcified atherosclerotic plaque within the left anterior descending artery (LAD), false-positive for significant stenosis. **(A,B)** Slab maximum intensity projection (MIP) images of the LAD demonstrate calcified plaque in the proximal and midportions of the vessel (*arrowheads*). The more proximal calcification is clearly eccentric with no more than 50% luminal narrowing. However, the more distal calcified plaque overlies the entire lumen. **(C)** Thin, curved MIP section obtained by vessel tracking once again demonstrates two calcified areas of atherosclerotic plaque. The more distal plaque again appears to overlie most of the LAD lumen (*arrow*). **(D)** Straightened lumen view with vessel tracking demonstrates that the more distal calcified plaque is present centrally within the lumen. Cross-sectional images through the LAD at the level of this plaque suggest that the calcium fills the vessel (*arrowhead*). Correlation with arteriography demonstrated only mild stenosis, suggesting that the calcified plaque is overestimated as a result of blooming artifact. A beaded appearance of isolated calcified plaques is generally not associated with significant stenosis, although this determination cannot be made with certainty when the calcium appears to fill the vessel lumen.

studies demonstrate that coronary CTA provides independent prognostic information beyond standard clinical risk factors.

A recent study compared the prognostic information in coronary CTA with the estimated risk based on the Framingham risk score.[23] A median follow-up of 18 months was obtained for 1256 consecutive patients with suspected CAD undergoing 64-slice coronary CTA. In 802 patients without obstructive CAD (<50% stenosis), four cardiac events occurred, of which one was severe. In 348 patients with obstructive CAD, 17 cardiac events occurred, of which five were severe. The difference between the groups was highly significant for severe events (odds ratio [OR] = 17.3) as well as for all cardiac events (OR = 16.1). The rate of all cardiac events in patients without obstructive CAD was significantly lower than that predicted by the Framingham risk score.

Another recent study compared the prognostic information in coronary CTA with that provided by nuclear scintigraphy in 541 patients referred for cardiac evaluation with a mean follow-up of almost 2 years.[24] The annualized rate of hard events was computed for patients with normal versus abnormal myocardial perfusion scans (1.1% versus 3.8%)

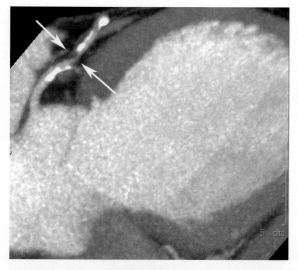

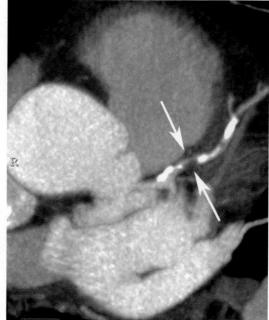

A

B

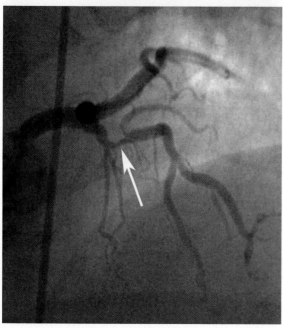

C

Fig. 6.15 Calcified proximal left anterior descending artery (LAD) with moderate stenosis. **(A,B)** Slab maximum intensity projection images through the proximal LAD demonstrate calcified plaque as well as focal noncalcified plaque (*arrows*). The lumen adjacent to the calcified plaque is obscured by artifact. However, there is a clear 50 to 70% narrowing of the vessel lumen associated with the noncalcified plaque. **(C)** Conventional arteriography confirms the presence of moderate stenosis in the proximal LAD (*arrow*).

and for patients with no significant coronary disease versus more than 50% stenosis on CTA (1.8% versus 4.8%). The presence of obstructive disease on CTA emerged as an independent predictor of events with an incremental prognostic value relative to nuclear perfusion imaging. The authors conclude that the anatomic information of coronary CTA and the functional information from perfusion imaging are complementary and that a combination of the two studies may allow improved risk stratification.

A common theme is present in all the above-cited studies: The absence of coronary disease on CTA suggests that a coronary event is unlikely. Conversely, the presence and severity of coronary disease on CTA are correlated with the risk of future coronary events.

◆ Prognostic Information Based on Plaque Characterization

Until recently, the morphology of atherosclerotic lesions could only be determined via direct examination of a specimen or inferred from the arterial silhouette obtained by selective coronary angiography. Angiographic features of CAD range from simple stenosis with a smooth contour to complex lesions with irregular outlines, ulceration, dissection, and filling defects indicating associated thrombus. Complex lesions are generally assumed to represent the "culprit lesions" of acute coronary syndromes. CTA demonstrates both the calcified and noncalcified components of atherosclerotic plaque (**Figs. 6.17, 6.18** and **6.19**). Furthermore,

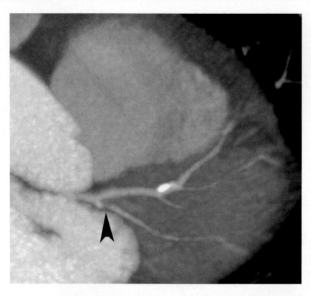
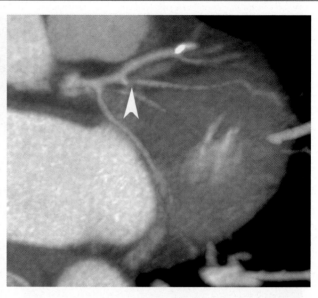

A

B

Fig. 6.16 High-grade stenosis of a small first diagonal branch. **(A,B)** Slab maximum intensity projection images through the left anterior descending artery and first diagonal branch demonstrate a high-grade stenosis at the origin of the first diagonal artery (*arrowhead*). The stenosis is clearly identified in this vessel with a diameter of about 1.5 mm. The flow-limiting nature of this lesion was confirmed by an anterior wall reversible defect on nuclear scintigraphy.

the presence of complex plaque with ulceration or dissection is clearly demonstrated with multiplanar CTA imaging (**Figs. 6.20, 6.21, 6.22, 6.23, 6.24,** and **6.25**). By analogy with conventional angiography, irregular or ulcerated plaques detected by CTA are more likely to represent ruptured, clinically unstable lesions.[25] However, in contrast to conventional angiography, which demonstrates only a lumen-gram of the coronary artery, coronary CTA provides the ability to visualize the plaque itself with new possibilities for plaque characterization.

The ability of intravascular ultrasound (IVUS) to visualize plaque within the arterial wall has led to a greater understanding of the evolution of atherosclerosis.[26] In addition to the degree of stenosis and the presence of plaque rupture, IVUS allows tomographic assessment of lumen area, plaque size, distribution, and composition. Features such as lipid

content, necrotic core, and the remodeling index are important IVUS markers for culprit lesions. The remodeling index (RI) describes the extent of positive remodeling as a ratio of a vessel's total cross-sectional area at the level of a plaque to the average vessel area in normal adjacent proximal and distal segments. Studies with IVUS have demonstrated that positive remodeling is associated with an unstable clinical presentation, whereas negative remodeling is more common in patients with a stable clinical presentation.[27] Virtual histology IVUS is an extension of IVUS to provide quantitative evaluation of coronary plaque components, including fibrotic tissue, fibrofatty tissue, necrotic core, and dense calcium.[28,29] Numerous recent publications have focused on the potential of coronary CTA to evaluate those characteristics of coronary atherosclerotic plaque that have been evaluated with IVUS.

Table 6.4 Accuracy of 64-Slice Coronary CT Angiography Compared with Catheter Angiography

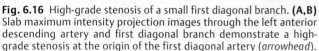

Author	Sensitivity (by patient)	Specificity (by patient)
Budoff et al	0.95	0.83
Miejboom et al	0.99	0.64
Miller et al	0.85	0.9
Mowatt et al	0.99	0.89
Meijer et al (40- and 64-slice)	0.98	0.91
Vanhoenacker et al	0.99	0.93

◆ Plaque Calcification

Although isolated case reports have described Mönckeberg sclerosis (medial calcification) of the coronary arteries related to renal dysfunction, coronary calcification is nearly always intimal in location and related to atherosclerotic disease.[30] It should be noted that CTA generally overestimates the amount of calcium compared with histology as a result of blooming artifact. Nonetheless, as discussed in Chapter 5, the aggregate amount of coronary calcium is related to the atherosclerotic burden and has prognostic significance.

In a study by Schuijf et al, patients with stable angina had a preponderance of calcified lesions, whereas those with ACS had more noncalcified and mixed lesions.[31] Accordingly, the mean of the signal intensities of all plaques in

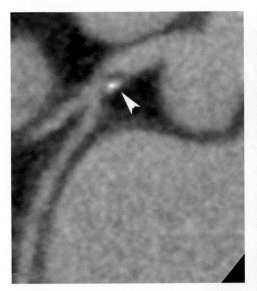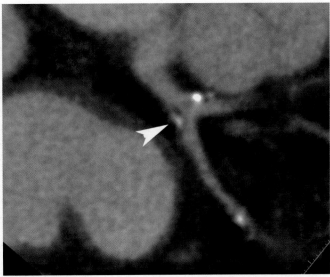

A   B

Fig. 6.17 Mild narrowing of the left main coronary artery. **(A)** Slab maximum intensity projection (MIP) image demonstrates centrally calcified plaque in the distal left main coronary artery (*arrowhead*). The vessel diameter is narrowed by about 50% at this level. **(B)** Slab MIP in a different projection demonstrates that this plaque also involves the origin of the left anterior descending artery (*arrowhead*) with greater than 50% diameter reduction at the origin of the left anterior descending artery. Cardiac catheterization was performed; the degree of narrowing was considered to be less than 50%.

patients with ACS was less than that in patients with stable angina. However, the signal intensity of the individual culprit lesions was not significantly different from that of the nonculprit lesions in the patients with ACS. This is an indication of the systemic nature of CAD and is illustrative as to how the differentiation of plaques can be meaningful when comparing groups of patients but not predictive in a single patient or a single plaque.

In a second study comparing coronary CTA with IVUS, the proportion of completely calcified plaques visualized at

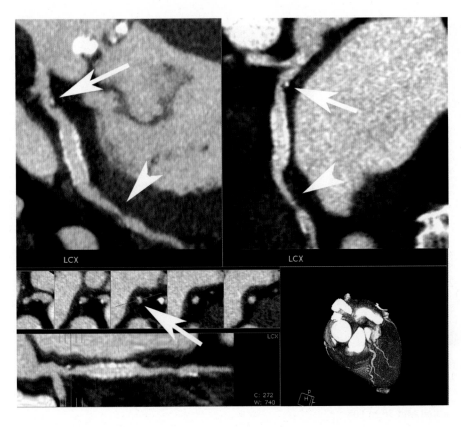

Fig. 6.18 Diseased left circumflex (LCX) artery status-post placement of a stent. Orthogonal curved maximum intensity projection (MIP) images demonstrate mild to moderate stenosis in the LCX proximal to the stent with minimally calcified plaque (*arrows*) and beyond the stent secondary to noncalcified plaque (*arrowheads*). Short-axis images derived from the straightened lumen view are presented at the bottom of the figure, demonstrating a 50% narrowing associated with the proximal plaque. The distal plaque results in a similar degree of narrowing.

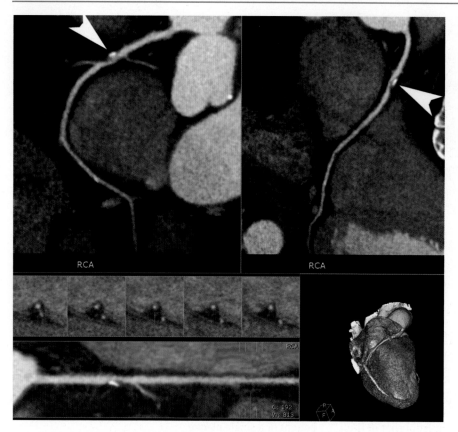

Fig. 6.19 Moderate stenosis of the right coronary artery (RCA). (A) Curved maximum intensity projections (MIPs) demonstrate focal narrowing in the proximal to midportion of the RCA related to plaque with associated calcification (arrowhead). The straightened lumen view at the bottom of the image suggests that the degree of diameter reduction in the proximal to mid RCA is about 60%. A second site of narrowing in the distal RCA is more obvious on the straightened lumen view. Cross-sectional views through the distal RCA demonstrate circumferential thickening of the vessel wall with 50 to 60% narrowing related to noncalcified plaque at this level.

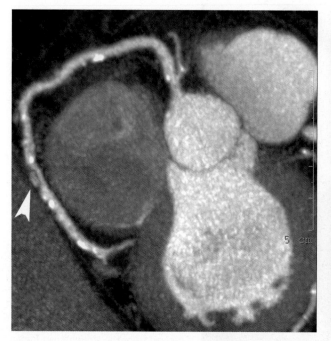

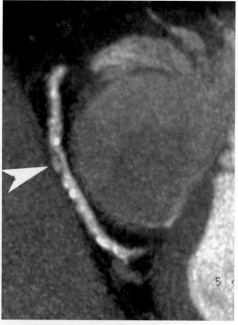

A   B

Fig. 6.20 Diffusely diseased right coronary artery (RCA) with ulcerated plaque in the distal RCA resulting in 50 to 60% luminal narrowing. (A,B) Slab maximum intensity projections (MIPs) demonstrate mild diffuse atherosclerotic disease throughout the RCA. In the mid to distal RCA, there is an ulcerated plaque (arrowhead) associated with 50 to 60% narrowing. The patient carried a diagnosis of unstable angina with a previous negative cardiac catheterization. The RCA ulcer was found on repeat catheterization and was treated with a stent. Anginal symptoms resolved after stent placement.

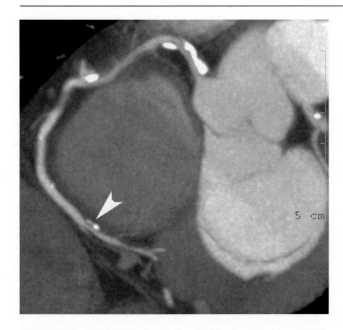

Fig. 6.21 Ulcerated plaque in the distal right coronary artery (RCA). Slab maximum intensity projection view of the RCA in a left anterior oblique projection demonstrates calcified plaque in the proximal and midportion of the vessel without significant stenosis. In the distal RCA there is a focal ulcerated plaque with 50% luminal narrowing (*arrowhead*).

coronary CTA was lower in patients with ACS, whereas noncalcified and mixed plaques were more prevalent in patients with stable CAD.[32] This observation corresponds with a larger amount of necrotic core and a higher prevalence of TCFA on virtual histology IVUS in the plaques of ACS patients. On the other hand, noncalcified and mixed plaques were present in both culprit and nonculprit vessels of patients presenting with ACS. Once again, this is an indication of the systemic nature of CAD and illustrates the difficulty in predicting whether an individual plaque will become a culprit lesion.

The association of calcification with stable plaque may be related to the development of calcification within a stable fibrotic plaque or to calcification that develops as a ruptured plaque heals. Although calcium is commonly associated with stable plaque, transitional lesions can develop microcalcifications that may contribute to their becoming a vulnerable plaque. A calcified nodule that develops on the fibrous cap of an atheroma can alter surface characteristics and lead to endothelial disruption and occlusive thrombosis. In these mechanisms of ACS, calcium appears to promote instability. Spotty calcifications smaller than 3 mm in diameter have been associated with ACS.

In summary, although calcification within a plaque is easily identified, the diverse mechanisms of coronary atherosclerosis complicate plaque characterization based simply on

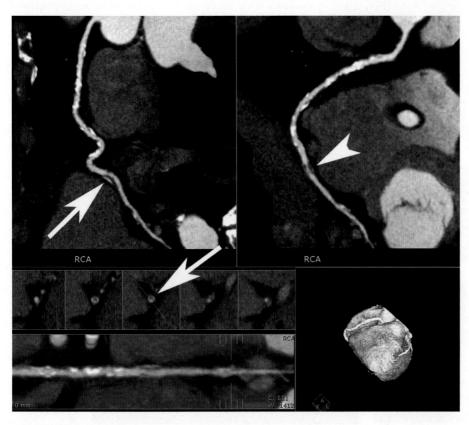

Fig. 6.22 Diffusely diseased right coronary artery (RCA) with false-positive ulcerated plaque proximal to the origin of the posterior descending artery. Orthogonal maximum intensity projections through the RCA demonstrate diffuse calcification without significant stenosis. In the distal portion of the vessel, there is noncalcified plaque (*arrowhead*) with apparent ulceration (*arrow*). Cross-sectional images through the distal RCA suggest a circumferential dissection of the vessel (*arrow*) that was interpreted as an ulcerated plaque. No ulcer was found at catheterization, but a small branch vessel was found at this level. The appearance of the branching vessel mimics a focal ulcer or dissection in the distal RCA.

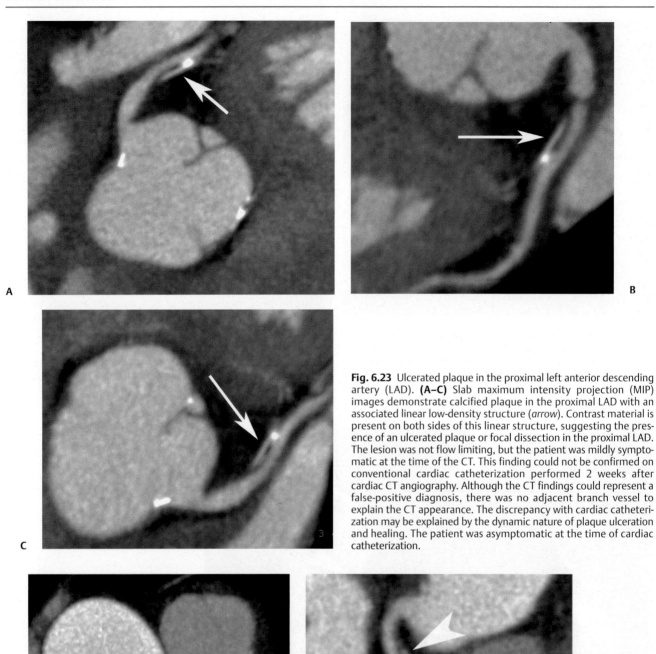

A

B

C

Fig. 6.23 Ulcerated plaque in the proximal left anterior descending artery (LAD). **(A–C)** Slab maximum intensity projection (MIP) images demonstrate calcified plaque in the proximal LAD with an associated linear low-density structure (*arrow*). Contrast material is present on both sides of this linear structure, suggesting the presence of an ulcerated plaque or focal dissection in the proximal LAD. The lesion was not flow limiting, but the patient was mildly symptomatic at the time of the CT. This finding could not be confirmed on conventional cardiac catheterization performed 2 weeks after cardiac CT angiography. Although the CT findings could represent a false-positive diagnosis, there was no adjacent branch vessel to explain the CT appearance. The discrepancy with cardiac catheterization may be explained by the dynamic nature of plaque ulceration and healing. The patient was asymptomatic at the time of cardiac catheterization.

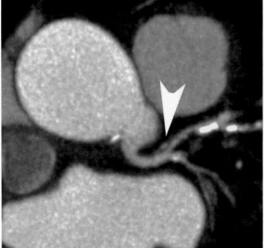

A

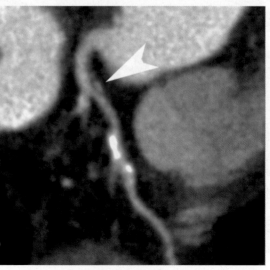

B

Fig. 6.24 Ulcerated plaques in the distal left main coronary artery and distal right coronary artery (RCA). **(A,B)** Slab maximum intensity projection (MIP) images through the left main coronary artery and proximal left anterior descending artery (LAD) demonstrate contrast on both sides of a noncalcified plaque that crosses the origin of the LAD (*arrowhead*). Additional areas of noncalcified and calcified plaque are identified within the proximal LAD beyond this lesion. The degree of diameter reduction at the level of the plaque is less than 50%.

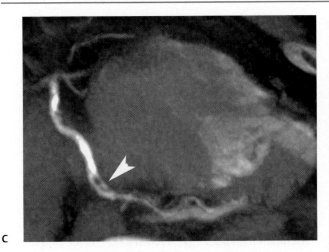

C

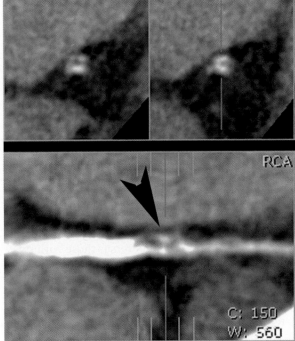

D

Fig. 6.24 (*Continued*) **(C)** Slab MIP image through the distal RCA demonstrates an ulcerated plaque (*arrowhead*) just beyond the calcified segment of the vessel. **(D)** Straightened lumen view of the distal RCA again demonstrates the focal ulcerated plaque (*arrowhead*). Cross-sectional images at this level confirm the presence of contrast on both sides of the plaque, confirming the diagnosis of an ulcerated arthrosclerotic plaque.

the presence or absence of calcium. Studies using both IVUS and CTA suggest that different patterns of calcification may be related to stable versus unstable "culprit" plaques as a group.[33] Completely calcified plaques are usually stable, whereas noncalcified plaques are more likely to represent

unstable plaques. Spotty calcifications have been associated with ACS. Finally, the overlap of imaging characteristics between stable and unstable plaques is too large to allow useful characterization of a single plaque based on its pattern of calcification.

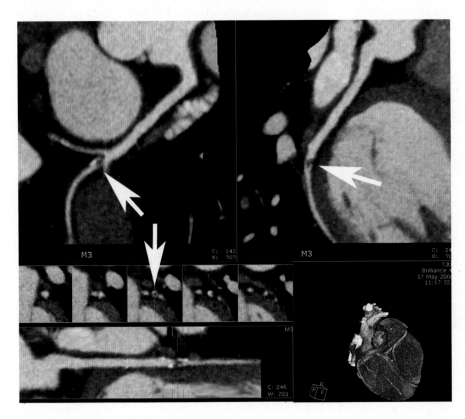

Fig. 6.25 Ulcerated plaque in the mid-circumflex artery. Orthogonal curved maximum intensity projections through the circumflex artery demonstrate an ulcerated plaque (*arrows*) just beyond the origin of the first obtuse marginal branch. The straightened lumen view at the bottom of the figure demonstrates a band-like low-density plaque crossing the vessel. The associated cross-sectional views demonstrate contrast material on both sides of the noncalcified plaque, confirming the presence of ulceration (*arrow*).

◆ Plaque Density and Composition

In theory, the ability to identify a lipid core within plaque should improve the detection of vulnerable coronary lesions. The wall thickness of a normal coronary artery is below the resolution of CT. The cap of a TCFA measures less than 0.065 mm and is also well below the spatial resolution of CT. However, large plaques associated with positive remodeling can be several millimeters thick and may be characterized by CT. Findings on coronary CT are strongly correlated with echogenicity and plaque composition on IVUS.[34] Several studies have evaluated the density of coronary plaque with IVUS correlation and have suggested that it may be possible to distinguish calcified plaque (>350 HU) from fibrous plaque (70–104 HU) and lipid-laden plaque (14–49 HU).[35–37] Clinical studies have demonstrated a difference in the CT density of coronary plaque between patients with ACS versus those with stable angina.[38] Although this type of plaque characterization appears promising, overlap in the CT density of different types of plaque limits the application of CT density to predict the vulnerability of an individual plaque.[39,40] When compared with IVUS, CTA can differentiate noncalcified, mixed, and calcified plaques, but it cannot reliably distinguish soft from fibrous plaques.

◆ Plaque Volume and Remodeling Index

The volume of noncalcified plaque and the presence of vascular remodeling are underestimated by conventional arteriography compared with IVUS. Larger plaque volumes are often associated with positive remodeling. As a plaque grows outward, the lesion can become large without significant visible stenosis on arteriography. Both larger plaque size and

a remodeling index greater than 10% are associated with acute coronary artery syndromes.

The presence of vascular remodeling is more obvious on CTA compared with conventional arteriography because the vessel wall is visible on CT. The diagnosis of coronary remodeling on coronary CTA is highly correlated with the remodeling index on IVUS ($r^2 = 0.82$).[41] A definite association is found between the presence of positive remodeling on coronary CTA and the presence of ACS.[42] In this study, positive remodeling was found by CTA in 19 of 31 patients with ACS, but it was not present in any of 26 patients with stable angina. A more recent study using coronary CTA demonstrated that positive remodeling of coronary atherosclerotic lesions correlates with lower CT attenuation of plaque.[43] The presence of positive remodeling with large-volume, low-attenuation plaque suggests increased risk for plaque rupture and should prove useful in defining vulnerable plaque (**Fig. 6.26**). Unfortunately, there is too much overlap in these measurements to allow reliable characterization of a single plaque as vulnerable versus stable.

◆ Plaque Characterization with Multiple Parameters

The prognostic utility of CTA can be improved by analyzing more than one plaque characteristic. The combination of positive-remodeling, low-attenuation plaque (using <30 HU as a cutoff value) and spotty calcification had a 97% specificity and 95% positive predictive value for ACS.[44] A more recent study of 1059 patients by the same group of researchers demonstrated that patients with plaques with both positive remodeling and low attenuation had a 22.2% incidence of developing an ACS over a mean of 27 months, those with one feature had a 3.7% incidence, and those with neither had

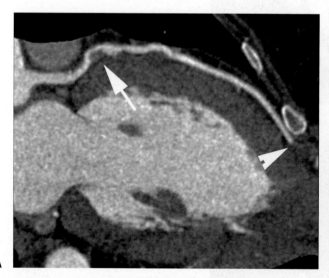
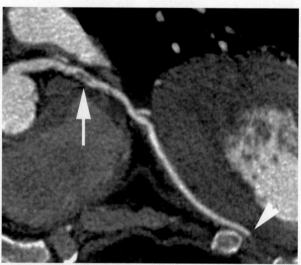

Fig. 6.26 Large low-density ulcerated plaque in the proximal left anterior descending artery (LAD) associated with an elevated remodeling index, thrombosis or occlusion of the distal LAD, and periapical infarct with thrombus. **(A,B)** Orthogonal curved maximum intensity projection images demonstrate a large noncalcified plaque in the proximal LAD associated with positive remodeling (*arrow*), and an abrupt occlusion of the distal LAD (*arrowhead*).

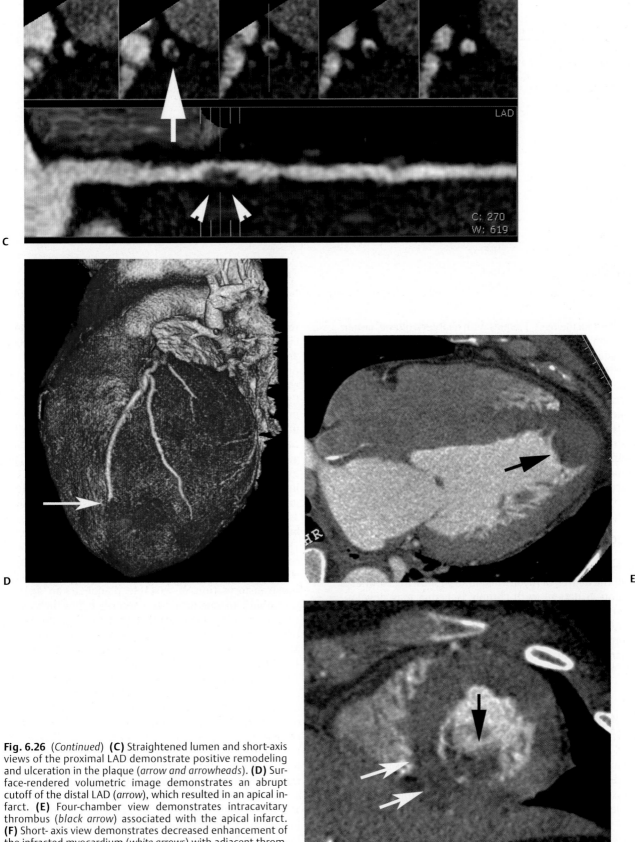

Fig. 6.26 *(Continued)* **(C)** Straightened lumen and short-axis views of the proximal LAD demonstrate positive remodeling and ulceration in the plaque *(arrow and arrowheads)*. **(D)** Surface-rendered volumetric image demonstrates an abrupt cutoff of the distal LAD *(arrow)*, which resulted in an apical infarct. **(E)** Four-chamber view demonstrates intracavitary thrombus *(black arrow)* associated with the apical infarct. **(F)** Short-axis view demonstrates decreased enhancement of the infracted myocardium *(white arrows)* with adjacent thrombus *(black arrow)*.

Table 6.5 Radiographic Characteristics of Plaque

		Significance
Location/ plaque burden	Proximal vs distal Multivessel vs single vessel	Most vulnerable lesions are proximal Frequency of events is related to plaque burden
Severity of stenosis	Severe < 50% Absent	More events occur in the setting of obstructive coronary artery disease
Calcification	Noncalcified Mixed/spotty calcification Dense calcification	Associated with acute coronary syndrome (ACS) Associated with ACS Associated with stable angina
Attenuation/ density	Low/soft Medium/mixed High/calcified	HU <30 associated with ACS Associated with stable plaque
Plaque volume	High Low	Potentially vulnerable plaque
Remodeling index	High Low	Potentially vulnerable plaque

only a 0.5% incidence.[45] Plaques with a larger-volume, larger low-attenuation plaque (LAP) volume, higher maximum LAP/plaque area, and higher remodeling index were associated with the development of an ACS within 1 year.

Important radiographic characteristics that may be used for risk stratification of coronary artery plaque are summarized in **Table 6.5**. Although these characteristics cannot be used to identify an individual plaque as a culprit lesion, these plaque characteristics will identify high-risk patients. The presence of multiple high-risk characteristics within an individual patient may warrant more aggressive treatment directed toward risk factor modification and plaque stabilization.

◆ Collateral Flow

Collateral flow in the myocardium is an important determinant of the degree of myocardial injury following coronary occlusion. A patient with chronic ischemia may develop collateral flow that limits the amount of myocardial injury with ACS. Much of the collateral circulation in the myocardium is at the sub-millimeter level and is not visible by coronary CTA (**Fig. 6.27**). Occasionally, larger tortuous collateral vessels can be identified (**Fig. 6.28**).

◆ Evaluation of Coronary Artery Disease: A Clinician's Viewpoint

The clinical assessment of an individual patient is based on an understanding of the pathophysiology of CAD and its expression in an individual patient. Although many clinical variables exist, some basic tenets can be applied:

◆ Patient care involves a hierarchy of decisions from generalized risk assessment to detailed decisions regarding

revascularization. As these decisions become more specific, testing needs to provide increasingly detailed anatomic information.

◆ Atherosclerosis is common. Coronary heart disease is the single largest cause of mortality in the United States.

◆ CAD usually occurs in patients with risk factors, but the presence of risk factors does not mean that the patient must have obstructive CAD. Some radiographic studies can provide prognostic information with similar, or even greater predictive value compared with clinical risk factor scores.

◆ In a patient with an intermediate or high risk of developing CAD, with known CAD, or with a CAD equivalent such as diabetes, aggressive treatment of risk factors reduces but does not eliminate the likelihood of a clinical event.

◆ The unpredictable growth of coronary artery plaques and coronary thrombotic occlusions causes an unpredictable clinical course for an individual patient. Mechanisms for the transformation of a stable plaque to an acutely thrombotic plaque have been described, but there is no clinical or radiographic test that can predict exactly when this might occur.

◆ Most acutely thrombotic or occlusive plaques were not significantly stenotic before their transformation.

◆ The clinical consequences of a coronary occlusion depend on its location, acuity, the inherent stability or instability of the occlusion, and the presence of collateral flow. Myocardial death begins within 1 hour (or less) of an acute coronary occlusion. A patient's long-term prognosis following myocardial infarction is in large part determined by the extent of myocardial damage.

◆ Depending on several factors, the consequence of an acute coronary occlusion can result in no clinical event, worsened angina, an ACS, an ST-elevation myocardial infarction, or sudden cardiac death.

◆ Despite the focus on a "culprit lesion," CAD is a systemic disease. There are differences throughout the coronary

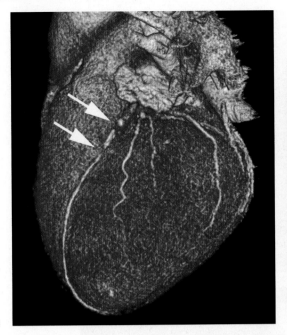

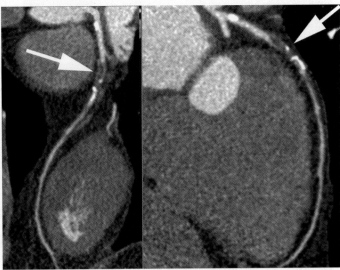

Fig. 6.27 Occlusion of the proximal left anterior descending artery (LAD) with reconstitution via small collateral vessels, which are not visible. **(A)** Volumetric surface rendering demonstrates focal occlusion of the proximal LAD (*arrows*) with distal reconstitution. **(B)** Tracked maximum intensity projection images of the LAD in orthogonal projections confirm occlusive plaque or thombus in the proximal or mid LAD (*arrows*) with reconstitution of the vessel beyond the plaque. The source of flow in the distal LAD is not identified and is assumed to be from small collateral vessels that are likely intramyocardial in location.

tree in patients with ACS as opposed to those with stable symptoms, including the presence of multiple "active" plaques.

♦ Chronic stable coronary artery stenoses may cause ischemia and angina, but usually do not cause infarctions unless there is an unusual physiologic stress. Nonstenotic atheroma cause neither angina nor ischemia, even on a stress test.

♦ Many patients with chest pain or dyspnea do not have CAD.

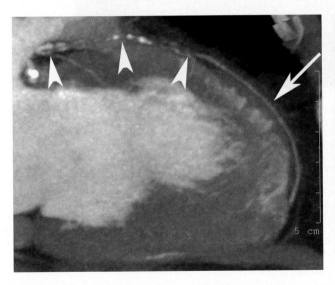

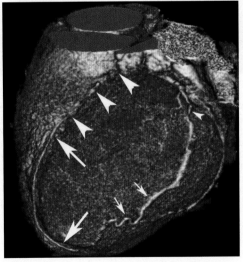

Fig. 6.28 Occlusion of the proximal to mid left anterior descending artery (LAD) with reconstitution of the distal LAD from the first obtuse marginal branch of the circumflex artery. Occlusion of the distal right coronary artery (RCA) with collateral flow to the inferior wall of the left ventricle (LV) and the posterior descending artery (PDA) from the second obtuse marginal branch. The myocardium of the LV is entirely supplied by the circumflex artery. **(A)** Slab maximum intensity projection (MIP) image demonstrates the calcified, occluded proximal to mid LAD (*arrowheads*) with reconstitution of the distal LAD (*arrow*). **(B)** Volumetric surface rendering demonstrates the calcified, occluded proximal to mid LAD (*arrowheads*) with reconstitution of the distal LAD (*large arrows*) via a tortuous collateral branch (*small arrows*) from the first obtuse marginal branch of the circumflex artery (*arrowhead*). (*Continued on page 134*)

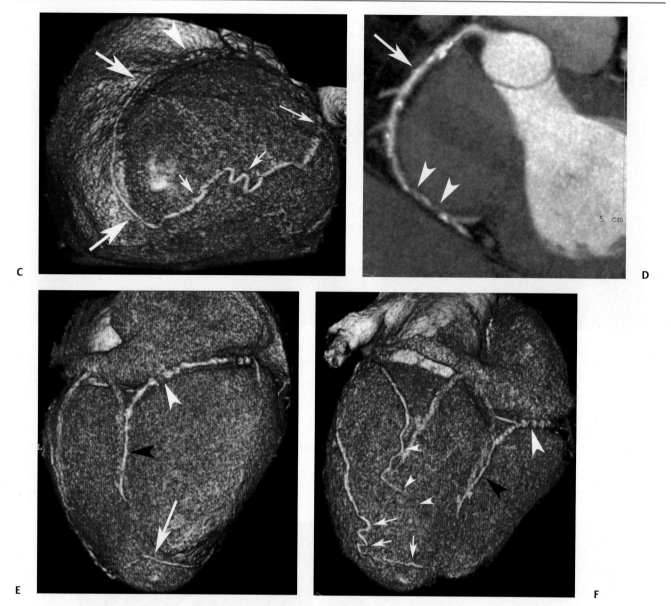

Fig. 6.28 (*Continued*) Occlusion of the proximal to mid left anterior descending artery (LAD) with reconstitution of the distal LAD from the first obtuse marginal branch of the circumflex artery. Occlusion of the distal right coronary artery (RCA) with collateral flow to the inferior wall of the left ventricle (LV) and the posterior descending artery (PDA) from the second obtuse marginal branch. The myocardium of the LV is entirely supplied by the circumflex artery. **(C)** A view from the apex demonstrates to better advantage the tortuous collateral vessel (*small arrows*) that reconstitutes the distal LAD (*arrows*). **(D)** Slab MIP image of the RCA demonstrates a diffusely diseased vessel (*arrow*) with distal occlusion (*arrowheads*). **(E)** Volumetric surface rendering of the heart again demonstrates occlusion of the distal RCA (*white arrowhead*) with reconstitution of the PDA (*black arrowhead*). The reconstituted distal LAD (*arrow*) wraps around the posterior aspect of the apex and likely provides some flow to the PDA. **(F)** Volumetric surface rendering of the crux rotated to demonstrate the inferior–posterior wall of the LV. The tortuous collateral branch from the first obtuse marginal is again demonstrated (*small arrows*). A collateral branch to the inferior LV wall (small *arrowheads*) arises from the second obtuse marginal artery. This collateral branch extends toward the posterior atrioventricular groove, and is responsible, in part, for reconstitution of the PDA (*black arrowhead*) beyond the distal RCA occlusion (*white arrowhead*). Compare the tortuous and poorly defined appearance of these acquired collateral vessels with the straight, extramural appearance of intracoronary communications that may represent a congenital pathway for collateral flow (see Fig. 4.20).

◆ Diagnostic Testing for Coronary Artery Disease: General Principles

◆ Proper testing begins with a clinical assessment of the risk of CAD based on a characterization of symptoms and physical findings referable to the cardiac and vascular system and an assessment of risk factors. Risk factor analysis can be formalized using one of several "risk scores," many of which have Internet-based calculators available.

◆ Patients with an intermediate or high probability of developing clinical CAD may benefit from testing for preclinical disease. Clarification of an individual's risk can help define appropriate goals for treatment.

Table 6.6 Common Tests for Coronary Artery Disease

Test	Functional information	Anatomic information	Comments
ECG exercise stress testing	Exercise tolerance Ischemic threshold	ECG localization of ischemia limited	Well-established clinical utility
Exercise stress with imaging (nuclear SPECT, stress echo)	Exercise tolerance Ischemic threshold Left ventricle (LV) and valve function	Myocardial perfusion Extent of ischemia	Well-established clinical utility + Radiation exposure (SPECT)
Pharmacologic stress with imaging (SPECT, dobutamine echo)	LV function	Myocardial perfusion Extent of ischemia	Well-established clinical utility + Radiation exposure (SPECT)
Intravascular Ultrasound (IVUS) Virtual histology		Luminal stenosis and cross-sectional area Intramural atheroma Plaque characterization Atherosclerotic burden	Invasive, clinically used to complement angio findings; significant research tool
Electron-Beam CT (EBCT)			Agatston score: atherosclerotic burden gives prognostic information
CT Angiography (CTA)	LV, right ventricle (RV), valve function (in future may quantify myocardial perfusion)	Luminal stenosis and cross-sectional area Intramural atheroma Plaque characterization Atherosclerotic burden	Noninvasive + radiation exposure + contrast medium exposure Calcium score, atherosclerotic burden, plaque characterization give prognostic information
Magnetic Resonance Imaging (MRI)	Excellent definition of LV, RV, and valve function Adenosine stress testing with Gd perfusion	Luminal stenosis and cross-sectional area Intramural atheroma Plaque characterization Atherosclerotic burden	No ionizing radiation With Gd perfusion, excellent sensitivity for small or late coronary events, noncoronary causes of LV dysfunction
Cardiac catheterization/ Selective coronary Angiography	Can measure hemodynamics Fractional flow reserve (FFR) can distinguish significance of angiographically borderline stenoses	"Gold standard" definition of coronary stenoses Essential for interventions	Invasive + contrast medium exposure + radiation exposure

Abbreviations: ECG, electrocardiographic; SPECT, single-photon emission CT.

◆ Testing can focus on the coronary anatomy (angiography), the functional adequacy of coronary blood flow or cardiac function (stress testing), or the prognosis (plaque morphology, calcium scoring). Though related, these three aspects of CAD are distinct from one another. Some tests evaluate more than one aspect (**Table 6.6**).

◆ The role of testing for coronary artery stenoses is to obtain information that will allow the physician to adjust treatment to improve a patient's survival or relieve symptoms.

◆ Occasionally "need to know" diagnostic testing must be performed, such as in a middle-aged man with an abnormal electrocardiogram who needs testing for insurance purposes or to maintain his pilot's license. "Preoperative cardiac clearance" can sometimes be included in this category.

◆ Not all clinically important processes related to cardiac vascular disease occur in the (visualized) epicardial coronary arteries (**Table 6.7**).

◆ Conclusion

Coronary CTA is a noninvasive test that can define the extent and severity of CAD with a high degree of accuracy and a negative predictive value that approaches 100%. Furthermore, coronary CTA can define subclinical CAD that would not be detected with routine stress testing. Although coronary CTA can characterize atherosclerotic plaques based on macroscopic characteristics, the radiographic overlap and biologic heterogeneity of different types of plaque limit this applicability. Characterization of plaque can stratify high- versus low-risk patients, but no findings have been reported at this time that are so directly predictive of plaque rupture that their discovery would warrant pre-emptive coronary intervention. Thus, at present, coronary CTA is most useful as a diagnostic test to exclude the presence of coronary disease. In the presence of CAD, plaque characterization with coronary

Table 6.7 Important Clinical Aspects of Coronary Artery Disease (CAD) Poorly Defined by Visualization

Myocardial O$_2$ demand	Ischemia caused by imbalance of O$_2$ supply vs demand Demand assessed indirectly by stress testing
Cross-sectional area of coronary stenosis	Angiography defines stenosis as a percent of an adjacent "normal" segment CTA, MRI, IVUS can define cross-sectional area; accuracy and utility to be determined
Coronary artery spasm	Dynamic process during acute coronary syndromes; changing degree of stenosis
Distal CAD Endothelial dysfunction Angina in women w/o epicardial disease "Syndrome X" "No reflow" phenomenon	Implicated cause of angina and ischemia w/o epicardial CAD Poorly defined syndrome of angina and ischemia w/o epicardial CAD Poorly defined syndrome of angina and ischemia w/o epicardial CAD Due to embolization of thrombus, vasoactive factors, ischemia–reperfusion injury Prognostically negative sign in PCI, AMI
Collateral circulation Changing flow due to arterial pressure Active growth of collaterals	Large collaterals may be visualized but remain insufficient for demand Angiographic opacification can change due to changing coronary blood flow Stimulated by ischemia or infarction, develop over weeks or months
Dynamic nature of CAD	Imaging a "snapshot" of a dynamic process, not giving the "whole picture"

Abbreviations: AMI, acute myocardial infarction; CTA, computed tomography angiography; IVUS, intravascular ultrasound; MRI, magnetic resonance imaging; PCI, percutaneous coronary intervention.

CTA may provide qualitative information to assist in risk stratification.

As CT technology continues to improve, the application of coronary CTA will likely expand beyond the exclusion of CAD into risk stratification and ultimately into the detection of vulnerable plaque. Improvements in spatial and temporal resolution will continue to improve plaque characterization. New technical innovations include evaluation of myocardial perfusion at rest and with stress and targeted contrast agents to identify inflammatory cells in atherosclerotic plaque (see Chapter 16). The radiation dose of coronary CTA continues to decrease, and it is likely that complete examinations will be performed with an exposure of no more than 1 to 2 mSv (see Chapter 2). Improvements in plaque characterization may provide a tool for directing interventions on specific "vulnerable" plaques before the development of an acute coronary occlusion. Finally, future improvements in diagnostic accuracy of coronary CTA, coupled with reductions in radiation exposure, may result in a cost-effective screening test for CAD.

References

1. Ridker PM, Rifai N, Rose L, Buring JE, Cook NR. Comparison of C-reactive protein and low-density lipoprotein cholesterol levels in the prediction of first cardiovascular events. N Engl J Med. 2002;347(20):1557–1565

2. Wang TJ, Gona P, Larson MG, et al. Multiple biomarkers for the prediction of first major cardiovascular events and death. N Engl J Med. 2006;355(25):2631–2639

3. Libby P. Current concepts of the pathogenesis of the acute coronary syndromes. Circulation. 2001;104(3):365–372

4. Stary HC, Chandler AB, Dinsmore RE, et al. A definition of advanced types of atherosclerotic lesions and a histological classification of atherosclerosis: a report from the Committee on Vascular Lesions of the Council on Arteriosclerosis, American Heart Association. Arterioscler Thromb Vasc Biol. 1995;15(9):1512–1531

5. Virmani R, Kolodgie FD, Burke AP, Farb A, Schwartz SM. Lessons from sudden coronary death: a comprehensive morphological classification scheme for atherosclerotic lesions. Arterioscler Thromb Vasc Biol. 2000;20(5):1262–1275

6. Fuster V, Moreno PR, Fayad ZA, Corti R, Badimon JJ. Atherothrombosis and high-risk plaque: part I: evolving concepts. J Am Coll Cardiol. 2005;46(6):937–954

7. Glagov S, Weisenberg E, Zarins CK, Stankunavicius R, Kolettis GJ. Compensatory enlargement of human atherosclerotic coronary arteries. N Engl J Med. 1987;316(22):1371–1375

8. Farb A, Burke AP, Tang AL, et al. Coronary plaque erosion without rupture into a lipid core. A frequent cause of coronary thrombosis in sudden coronary death. Circulation. 1996;93(7):1354–1363

9. Falk E. Pathogenesis of atherosclerosis. J Am Coll Cardiol. 2006;47(8, Suppl):C7–C12

10. Yusuf S, Sleight P, Pogue J, Bosch J, Davies R, Dagenais G; The Heart Outcomes Prevention Evaluation Study investigators. Effects of an angiotensin-converting-enzyme inhibitor, ramipril, on cardiovascular events in high-risk patients. N Engl J Med. 2000;342(3):145–153

11. Zhang S, Levin DC, Halpern EJ, Fischman D, Savage M, Walinsky P. Accuracy of MDCT in assessing the degree of stenosis caused by calcified coronary artery plaques. AJR Am J Roentgenol. 2008;191(6):1676–1683

12. Kuettner A, Trabold T, Schroeder S, et al. Noninvasive detection of coronary lesions using 16-detector multislice spiral computed tomography technology: initial clinical results. J Am Coll Cardiol. 2004;44(6):1230–1237

13. Hoffmann U, Moselewski F, Cury RC, et al. Predictive value of 16-slice multidetector spiral computed tomography to detect significant obstructive coronary artery disease in patients at high risk for coronary artery disease: patient-versus segment-based analysis. Circulation. 2004;110(17):2638–2643

14. Mowatt G, Cook JA, Hillis GS, et al. 64-Slice computed tomography angiography in the diagnosis and assessment of coronary artery disease: systematic review and meta-analysis. Heart. 2008;94(11):1386–1393

15. Leber AW, Knez A, von Ziegler F, et al. Quantification of obstructive and nonobstructive coronary lesions by 64-slice computed tomography: a comparative study with quantitative coronary angiography and intravascular ultrasound. J Am Coll Cardiol. 2005;46(1): 147–154

16. Budoff MJ, Dowe D, Jollis JG, et al. Diagnostic performance of 64-multidetector row coronary computed tomographic angiography for evaluation of coronary artery stenosis in individuals without known coronary artery disease: results from the prospective multicenter ACCURACY (Assessment by Coronary Computed Tomographic Angiography of Individuals Undergoing Invasive Coronary Angiography) trial. J Am Coll Cardiol. 2008;52(21):1724–1732

17. Meijboom WB, Meijs MF, Schuijf JD, et al. Diagnostic accuracy of 64-slice computed tomography coronary angiography: a prospective, multicenter, multivendor study. J Am Coll Cardiol. 2008; 52(25):2135–2144

18. Miller JM, Rochitte CE, Dewey M, et al. Diagnostic performance of coronary angiography by 64-row CT. N Engl J Med. 2008;359(22):2324–2336

19. Meijer AB, O YL, Geleijns J, Kroft LJ. Meta-analysis of 40- and 64-MDCT angiography for assessing coronary artery stenosis. AJR Am J Roentgenol. 2008;191(6):1667–1675

20. Vanhoenacker PK, Heijenbrok-Kal MH, Van Heste R, et al. Diagnostic performance of multidetector CT angiography for assessment of coronary artery disease: meta-analysis. Radiology. 2007;244(2): 419–428

21. Min JK, Shaw LJ, Devereux RB, et al. Prognostic value of multidetector coronary computed tomographic angiography for prediction of all-cause mortality. J Am Coll Cardiol. 2007;50(12):1161–1170

22. Pundziute G, Schuijf JD, Jukema JW, et al. Prognostic value of multislice computed tomography coronary angiography in patients with known or suspected coronary artery disease. J Am Coll Cardiol. 2007;49(1):62–70

23. Hadamitzky M, Freissmuth B, Meyer T, et al. Prognostic value of coronary computed tomographic angiography for prediction of cardiac events in patients with suspected coronary artery disease. JACC Cardiovasc Imaging. 2009;2(4):404–411

24. van Werkhoven JM, Schuijf JD, Gaemperli O, et al. Prognostic value of multislice computed tomography and gated single-photon emission computed tomography in patients with suspected coronary artery disease. J Am Coll Cardiol. 2009;53(7):623–632

25. Ambrose JA, Winters SL, Arora RR, et al. Angiographic evolution of coronary artery morphology in unstable angina. J Am Coll Cardiol. 1986;7(3):472–478

26. Nissen SE, Yock P. Intravascular ultrasound: novel pathophysiological insights and current clinical applications. Circulation. 2001;103(4): 604–616

27. Schoenhagen P, Ziada KM, Kapadia SR, Crowe TD, Nissen SE, Tuzcu EM. Extent and direction of arterial remodeling in stable versus unstable coronary syndromes: an intravascular ultrasound study. Circulation. 2000;101(6):598–603

28. Nair A, Kuban BD, Tuzcu EM, Schoenhagen P, Nissen SE, Vince DG. Coronary plaque classification with intravascular ultrasound radiofrequency data analysis. Circulation. 2002;106(17):2200–2206

29. Philipp S, Böse D, Wijns W, et al. Do systemic risk factors impact invasive findings from virtual histology? Insights from the international virtual histology registry. Eur Heart J. 2010;31(2):196–202

30. Qiao JH, Doherty TM, Fishbein MC, et al. Calcification of the coronary arteries in the absence of atherosclerotic plaque. Mayo Clin Proc. 2005;80(6):807–809

31. Schuijf JD, Beck T, Burgstahler C, et al. Differences in plaque composition and distribution in stable coronary artery disease versus acute coronary syndromes; non-invasive evaluation with multi-slice computed tomography. Acute Card Care. 2007;9(1):48–53

32. Pundziute G, Schuijf JD, Jukema JW, et al. Evaluation of plaque characteristics in acute coronary syndromes: non-invasive assessment with multi-slice computed tomography and invasive evaluation with intravascular ultrasound radiofrequency data analysis. Eur Heart J. 2008;29(19):2373–2381

33. Ehara S, Kobayashi Y, Yoshiyama M, Ueda M, Yoshikawa J. Coronary artery calcification revisited. J Atheroscler Thromb. 2006;13(1):31–37

34. Leber AW, Knez A, Becker A, et al. Accuracy of multidetector spiral computed tomography in identifying and differentiating the composition of coronary atherosclerotic plaques: a comparative study with intracoronary ultrasound. J Am Coll Cardiol. 2004;43(7):1241–1247

35. Nikolaou K, Sagmeister S, Knez A, et al. Multidetector-row computed tomography of the coronary arteries: predictive value and quantitative assessment of non-calcified vessel-wall changes. Eur Radiol. 2003;13(11):2505–2512

36. Schroeder S, Kopp AF, Baumbach A, et al. Noninvasive detection and evaluation of atherosclerotic coronary plaques with multislice computed tomography. J Am Coll Cardiol 2001;37(5):1430–1435

37. Schroeder S, Kuettner A, Leitritz M, et al. Reliability of differentiating human coronary plaque morphology using contrast-enhanced multi-slice spiral computed tomography: a comparison with histology. J Comput Assist Tomogr. 2004;28(4):449–454

38. Hoffmann U, Moselewski F, Nieman K, et al. Noninvasive assessment of plaque morphology and composition in culprit and stable lesions in acute coronary syndrome and stable lesions in stable angina by multidetector computed tomography. J Am Coll Cardiol. 2006;47(8):1655–1662

39. Ferencik M, Chan RC, Achenbach S, et al. Arterial wall imaging: evaluation with 16-section multidetector CT in blood vessel phantoms and ex vivo coronary arteries. Radiology. 2006;240(3):708–716

40. Pohle K, Achenbach S, Macneill B, et al. Characterization of non-calcified coronary atherosclerotic plaque by multi-detector row CT: comparison to IVUS. Atherosclerosis. 2007;190(1):174–180

41. Achenbach S, Ropers D, Hoffmann U, et al. Assessment of coronary remodeling in stenotic and nonstenotic coronary atherosclerotic lesions by multidetector spiral computed tomography. J Am Coll Cardiol. 2004;43(5):842–847

42. Imazeki T, Sato Y, Inoue F, et al. Evaluation of coronary artery remodeling in patients with acute coronary syndrome and stable angina by multislice computed tomography. Circ J. 2004;68(11):1045–1050

43. Schmid M, Pflederer T, Jang IK, et al. Relationship between degree of remodeling and CT attenuation of plaque in coronary atherosclerotic lesions: an in-vivo analysis by multi-detector computed tomography. Atherosclerosis. 2008;197(1):457–464

44. Motoyama S, Kondo T, Sarai M, et al. Multislice computed tomographic characteristics of coronary lesions in acute coronary syndromes. J Am Coll Cardiol. 2007;50(4):319–326

45. Motoyama S, Sarai M, Harigaya H, et al. Computed tomographic angiography characteristics of atherosclerotic plaques subsequently resulting in acute coronary syndrome. J Am Coll Cardiol. 2009;54(1):49–57

7

Coronary Stents

David L. Fischman and Aaron M. Giltner

◆ Percutaneous Coronary Interventions

The introduction of percutaneous transluminal coronary angioplasty (PTCA) to clinical practice by Grüntzig in 1977 offered a less invasive alternative to conventional bypass surgery for patients in need of coronary artery revascularization.[1] Early comparative studies suggested that even in cases of multivessel coronary artery disease long-term mortality rates of patients treated by PTCA were similar to those undergoing more invasive surgical bypass procedures.[2,3] Enthusiasm for these results was tempered by high rates of restenosis following PTCA, often resulting in a need for repeat revascularization procedures.

Implantation of metal stents during PTCA, first performed by Sigwart and Puel in 1986, became standard during the 1990s as a result of the associated improvements in procedural and clinical outcomes. Despite this advance, restenosis occurred in 22.0 to 31.6% of stented patients, often resulting in a need for repeat invasive procedures.[4,5] Even with the dramatically reduced rates of restenosis for newer drug-eluting stents, many patients require repeat catheterization. Recent data suggest that late thrombosis of drug-eluting stents occurs more frequently than initially reported, often with devastating consequences.[6] Acute thrombosis invariably presents with signs of epicardial injury that is best treated by urgent catheterization, but restenosis usually presents subacutely. CT has emerged as a diagnostic alternative to invasive coronary angiography for assessment of coronary artery disease and can often provide interpretable images of stented coronary vessels (**Fig. 7.1**). CT imaging of stented segments remains subject to technical limitations.

◆ Electron Beam Versus Multidetector CT

Early electron-beam computed tomography (EBCT) studies imaged coronary calcium and used quantitative calcium scoring to predict restenosis following angioplasty. In a study of 28 coronary arteries treated by PTCA, there was a 71% three-month restenosis rate among 17 vessels with moderate or heavy calcification but not a single case of restenosis among 11 noncalcified or only mildly calcified vessels.[7] A calcium score of 27 or greater predicts restenosis within 6 months (sensitivity 73%, specificity 67%).[8] Furthermore, an increase in the incidence of periprocedural complications has been described for angioplasty of calcified vessels.

Visualization of the stent lumen with EBCT is limited. EBCT protocols have relied on coronary flow distal to stents to determine patency.[9–12] This technique is subject to several limitations. Foremost, resting coronary flow is not significantly diminished in the post-stenotic segment until obstruction exceeds 85%, even when lesser degrees of stenosis are clinically important. Furthermore, collateral blood flow may result in opacification of a vessel beyond an occlusion. In vitro studies have highlighted the tendency of EBCT to underestimate stent length and overestimate diameter, with resulting poor sensitivity (65%) and positive predictive value (69%) for in-stent stenosis.[11] Although multislice–multidetector computed tomography (MDCT) offers improvements in spatial and temporal resolution, imaging of stents with this newer technology is also limited by technical issues related to stent architecture and CT imaging.

◆ Stent Characteristics

CT imaging of stents is complicated by variations in stent composition and structure that result in differences in radiopacity and CT appearance.[13] Most stents in use today are made of 316L surgical stainless steel, an alloy composed primarily of iron with a small amount of nickel.[14,15] Other metals, including cobalt alloys, nitinol, and tantalum, are used in a smaller percentage of commercially available stents.[13] Many stents are coated with compounds—most commonly heparin, gold, phosphorylcholin, carbon, or chromium oxide—intended to reduce biological activity and improve biocompatibility.[15,16] In addition, there is considerable variability between stents with respect to size, mesh design, and radiopacity.[14]

Stent materials result in variable degrees of CT artifact. Radiopaque metals, although helpful to the cineangiographer in the cardiac catheterization laboratory, result in artifact and decreased visibility of the stent lumen when imaged by CT

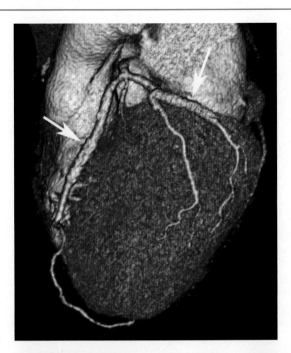

A

Fig. 7.1 Patent left anterior descending artery (LAD) and circumflex stents. **(A)** Volume-rendered surface display demonstrates the presence of stents in the LAD and circumflex arteries (*arrows*) but does not provide an evaluation of the internal stent lumen. **(B)** Curved maximum intensity projection images based on vessel tracking in the LAD clearly demonstrate a patent stent (*arrows*) with mild overexpansion of the LAD.

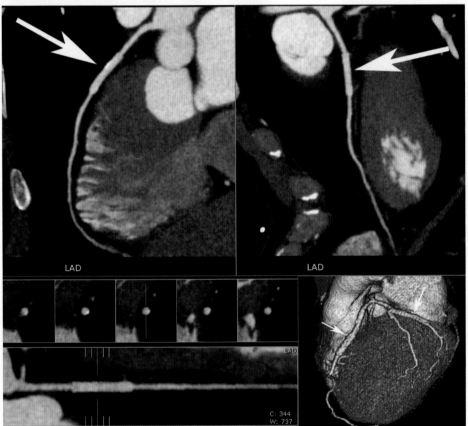

B

(**Fig. 7.2**). Stent densities, when imaged by CT, range from 600 to more than 1500 Hounsfield units (HU).[14,15,17] Higher attenuation values are associated with greater CT artifact, limiting visualization of the internal stent lumen. Tantalum in particular results in a greater amount of artifact than stainless steel or nitinol.[13,16] Stent weight and strut diameter have been shown to correlate with artifactual luminal narrowing on CT.[16] Radiopaque markers at stent margins, intended to aid cineangiographic visualization, significantly decrease lumen visibility.[18,19] Mahnken and colleagues examined, in vitro, 10

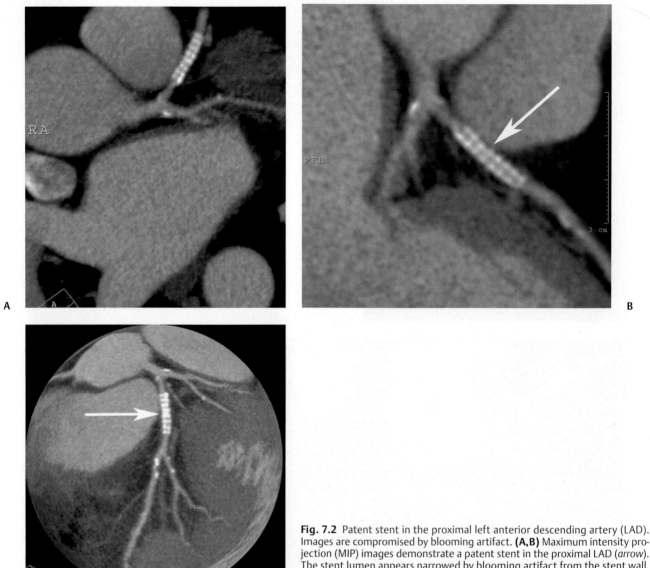

A

B

C

Fig. 7.2 Patent stent in the proximal left anterior descending artery (LAD). Images are compromised by blooming artifact. **(A,B)** Maximum intensity projection (MIP) images demonstrate a patent stent in the proximal LAD (*arrow*). The stent lumen appears narrowed by blooming artifact from the stent wall. **(C)** Globe MIP with thin-section depiction of the LAD. The internal lumen is obscured by ridges from blooming artifact (*arrow*). RA, right atrium.

different coronary artery stents, including a novel biodegradable stent made from polylactide with a microcellular foam structure.[18] No beam hardening occurred with the polylactide stent because of its construction from a low-attenuation material. As a result, the polylactide stent showed greater luminal visibility than the metal stents. A more recent in vitro evaluation of 29 different stent types with dual-source CT demonstrated magnesium to be a more favorable stent material compared with more common materials, including steel, cobalt–chromium, or tantalum. In this analysis a magnesium stent exhibited the least artifacts, with a lumen visibility of 90%. Most other stents exhibited a lumen visibility of 50 to 59%.[20]

Stent size plays a particularly important role, as the blooming effect created by high-density stent material tends to be a relatively static phenomenon, resulting in greater degrees of luminal obscuration with smaller stents.[17] Artifact from high-density stent material leads to increased intraluminal density, overestimation of stent outer diameters, and underestimation of inner lumen diameters. As a result, the lumen of larger stents may appear artifactually smaller, whereas the lumen of smaller stents may appear to be occluded.[17] CT-generated artifical luminal narrowing in stainless steel stents may be as great as 62 to 94.3%, depending on stent size.[16]

In clinical practice, most coronary stents are 3 mm or smaller.[4] In vitro studies have tended to include a disproportionate number of larger-diameter stents, thus overestimating the ability of MDCT to characterize stent lumens and detect in-stent restenosis.[17,21] Schuijf and colleagues imaged 68 stents in 22 patients using 16-slice MDCT. Of 15 uninterpretable stents, 13 had diameters 3 mm or smaller, whereas only 2 of 19 larger stents were uninterpretable. Additionally, stent strut thickness of 140 μm or greater was associated with significantly decreased lumen interpretability. Another study reported that only 50% of stents 3 mm or smaller were interpretable, compared with 81% of larger stents.[22] In a study of left main coronary artery stents, 27 of 29 (93%) stents with a mean diameter of 3.9 mm were of sufficient quality to permit lumen visualization.[23]

◆ CT Technical Factors

Number of Detectors and Z-Axis Resolution

The progression from 4- to 64-slice MDCT has been accompanied by progressive improvements in spatial and temporal resolution.[16,17] Early case reports suggested that even with lower-resolution scanners (1.25-mm slice thickness), MDCT has utility to visualize the lumens of stents in larger coronary arteries, such as the left main and proximal left anterior descending.[24-26] However, visualization of the stent lumen is limited by partial volume effects and beam hardening.[27] Comparisons of 4- and 16-slice MDCT have demonstrated only a modest improvement in stent lumen visualization with 16-slice collimation.[18,28]

Newer 64-detector row CT scanners provide improved z-axis resolution with isotropic pixels (resolution about 0.5–0.6 mm in all directions). Isotropic imaging minimizes the importance of stent orientation, and improved resolution minimizes blooming artifact. In one study, stent lumen diameter imaged by 64-slice CT at multiple stent orientations averaged 53.4% of the true lumen as confirmed by standardized caliper measurements, representing a 10% improvement over 16-slice CT.[19] Seifarth and colleagues compared 16- and 64-slice scanning of 15 different coronary stents at various orientations. The 64-slice scanner provided better overall images, with decreased artificial luminal narrowing and similar luminal attenuation values for stented and unstented segments (**Figs. 7.3** and **7.4**). Images obtained with the 64-slice scanner did not appear to be significantly affected by stent orientation.[29]

A more recent investigation focused on imaging of coronary stents with a prototype flat-panel detector computed tomography (FPCT). Isotropic images with slice thickness of 0.25 mm resulted in artificial lumen narrowing of only

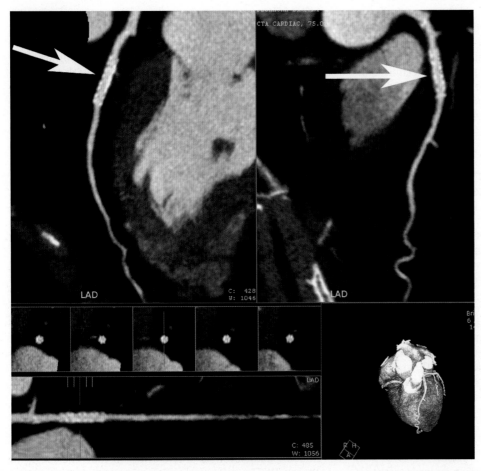

Fig. 7.3 Proximal left anterior descending artery (LAD) stent. Two orthogonal curved maximum intensity projection views demonstrate a stent within the proximal LAD. The stent is widely patent without narrowing (*arrow*). At the bottom of the figure, there is a straightened lumen view of the LAD with short-axis (cross-sectional) views through the stent demonstrating the patent lumen.

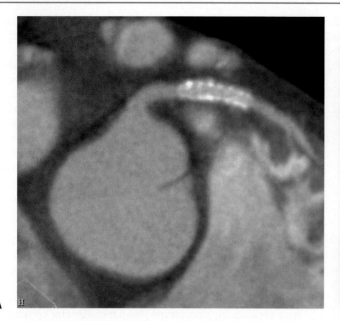
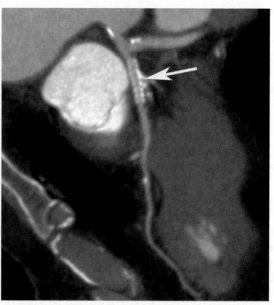

Fig. 7.4 Proximal left anterior descending artery (LAD) stent. Slab maximum intensity projection (MIP) versus curved reformat with tracking. **(A)** MIP image demonstrates patency of the proximal LAD stent. **(B)** Curved reformat image obtained by automated tracking of the LAD. This image demonstrates excellent visualization of the stent lumen because the tracked image depicts a thin section through the center of the stent (*arrow*).

16.1% compared with standardized caliper measurements. The superior spatial resolution of FPCT allowed for delineation of stent struts with minimal blooming artifact. Currently, FPCT remains subject to significant technical limitations, including poor temporal resolution, which does not allow in vivo cardiac imaging. Application of this technology to clinical patients remains a future consideration.[30]

Viewing Technique

Thin-section images are required to view the lumen of a coronary stent. Slab maximum intensity projection images with a slab thickness of 0.5 to 1.0 mm may be centered within the stent lumen. However, the lumen of a stented segment, particularly the lumen of a long stented segment, may not be optimally visualized in a single plane. In many patients, tracked reconstructions with thin-section curved reformats may be useful to visualize optimally vessel lumen within a stent (**Fig. 7.4**).

The use of an extended CT scale technique (ECTS) has been shown to improve visualization adjacent to cobalt screws and steel plates in porcine femur specimens.[27] Most in vitro coronary stent imaging studies have used a standardized window width of 700 HU. Increasing window width to 1500 HU clearly decreases blooming artifact (**Figs. 7.5** and **7.6**), but clinical improvements in accuracy of stent assessment with ECTS have not yet been evaluated in a controlled study.[29]

Reconstruction Kernel

Dedicated sharp-kernel reconstruction improves stent imaging by MDCT. A sharp kernel (B46) used in a phantom study with 16-slice MDCT increased mean visible lumen diameter from 31% to 54% of caliper-obtained measurements and decreased average luminal attenuation from 349 to 250 HU.[28] Visualization and classification of artificial stenoses were poor using a standard kernel, with more than half of all stents either uninterpretable or interpreted with low certainty. Reconstruction with the sharp kernel significantly increased diagnostic accuracy; all stents were correctly classified as stenosed or nonstenosed, and 75 to 85% were classified with high certainty. Similar findings have been reported with 64-slice MDCT stent images, including significantly improved visualization of stent lumen and decreased overall lumen attenuation with the addition of a high-resolution kernel (**Fig. 7.7**).[13] Patient-based protocols have reported decreases in artificial luminal narrowing from 27 to 37% down to 16 to 29% with a dedicated sharp reconstruction kernel.[31,32]

Both subcentimeter collimation and the use of a sharp kernel reconstruction result in increased image noise.[13] Image noise may be reduced to levels approaching those associated with standard reconstruction kernels by use of noise-reduction filters.[32] Improvements in stent lumen visualization and decreases in attenuation with the sharp kernel are maintained after processing with a noise-reduction filter.

Dual Energy

Dual-energy CT (DECT) is a promising technology that may improve the differentiation of tissues based on synchronous CT data obtained at two different tube energies.[33] In theory, DECT can be used to perform tissue decomposition and to create monoenergetic images that can reduce artifact related to beam hardening (Chapter 16). At least one in

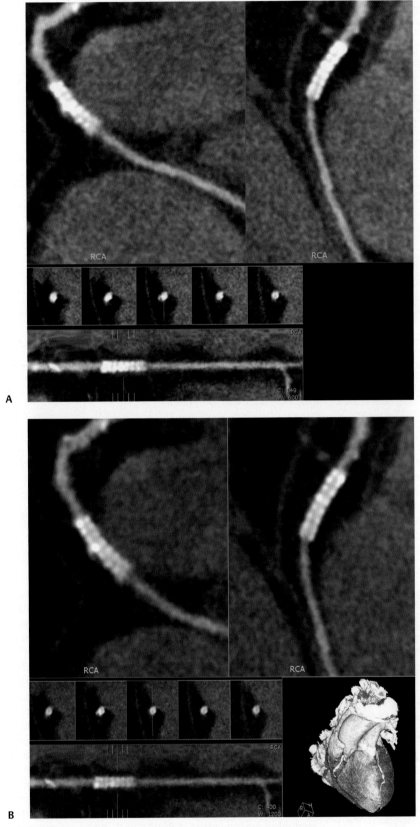

Fig. 7.5 Patent right coronary artery (RCA) stent with blooming artifact. The stent lumen is more clearly visualized with an extended window width. **(A)** The stent lumen is difficult to appreciate with a window width of 600. **(B)** When the window width is doubled to 1200, the internal stent lumen is clearly patent.

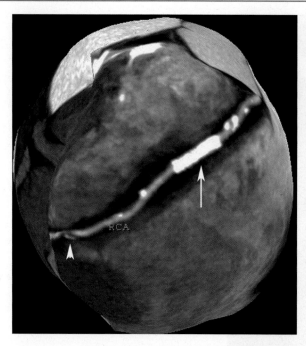

A

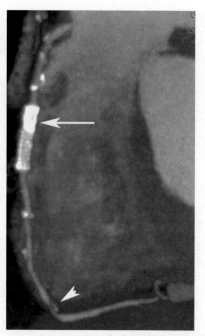

B

Fig. 7.6 Patent stent in the midportion of the right coronary artery (RCA). Impact of windowing with an extended CT scale technique. **(A)** Globe maximum intensity projection (MIP) with narrow window width demonstrates marked blooming of the stent wall that precludes evaluation of the stent lumen (*arrow*). Vascular calcifications are seen along the RCA. The distal RCA demonstrates an area of noncalcified plaque undermined by contrast (*arrowhead*). This appearance is diagnostic of an ulcerated plaque in the distal RCA. **(B)** Slab MIP image with a wide window setting allows visualization of patency in the mid to distal portion of the stent. Even with the extended CT scale, vascular calcification around the proximal portion of the stent (*arrow*) precludes visualization of the lumen at this level. Once again, ulcerated plaque is identified in the more distal RCA (*arrowhead*).

vitro study has suggested that DECT can be used to reduce beam hardening and blooming artifact and improve visualization of the lumen inside a coronary stent.[34] A recent study by our group, however, failed to demonstrate improved visualization of the lumen inside a coronary stent with dual-energy imaging.[35] Full width at half maximum measurements in our study suggest that there is no significant objective improvement in CT assessment of stent lumen diameter and strut thickness with images reconstructed from the higher-energy portion of the radiographic spectrum. Further studies are needed to determine whether DECT projection data can be processed to improve visualization of the stent lumen.

◆ Clinical Applications

In vivo imaging of stents is complicated by artifacts resulting from vessel calcification (**Figs. 7.6** and **7.8**), overlapping stents (**Figs. 7.9, 7.10,** and **7.11**), incompletely expanded stents (**Figs. 7.12, 7.13,** and **Fig. 7.14**) and cardiac motion (**Figs. 7.14** and **7.15**). Stents are often placed within calcified segments of the coronary circulation. The high CT density of calcium approaches that of stent material, compounding the blooming and partial volume effects of the stent and limiting the interpretability of images.[22,36] A similar effect is demonstrated by the increased density and blooming associated with overlapping stents and incompletely expanded stents. Arrhythmias and elevated heart rates result in motion artifact in all coronary vessels, but this artifact is even more pronounced in stented segments. Interpretability has been strongly linked to heart rate. In one study, five of six uninterpretable stents were in patients with heart rates greater than 70 beats per minute, and 13 of 14 interpretable stents were in patients with heart rates less than 70.[31]

Fig. 7.7 Impact of reconstruction kernel on imaging a 3.5-mm Cypher stent expanded within a plastic tube containing dilute intravenous contrast. Images of the same stent obtained at two different slice thicknesses and with various reconstruction kernels (filters). The stent filter provides the sharpest detail, with slightly increased image noise. The true thickness of this paper-thin stent is overestimated, even with the sharpest filter.

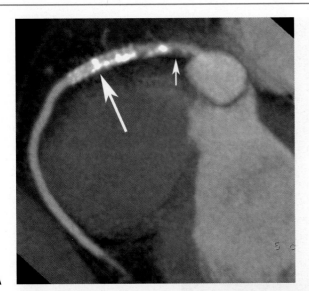

Fig. 7.8 Patent right coronary artery (RCA) stent with surrounding calcification. **(A)** Maximum intensity projection image of the RCA demonstrates a patent stent in the proximal RCA with calcification of the surrounding vessel wall (*arrow*). Calcification around the stent contributes to substantial blooming artifact. Calcified and noncalcified plaque are present within the RCA proximal to the stent. Mild to moderate stenosis is associated with the noncalcified plaque (*small arrow*). **(B)** Curved reformatted images through the RCA and stent provide a thinner section that allows better visualization of the stent lumen (*arrow*), but visualization is still limited by adjacent calcified plaque. Stenosis in the proximal RCA is again demonstrated (*small arrow*).

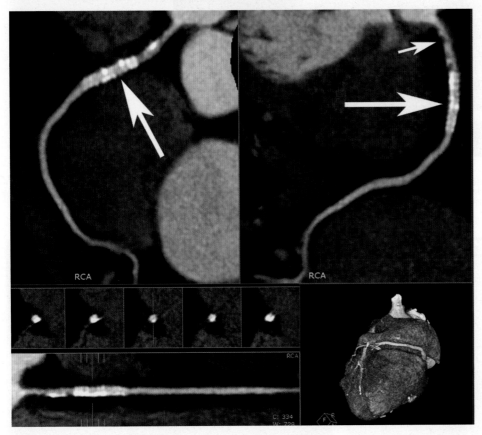

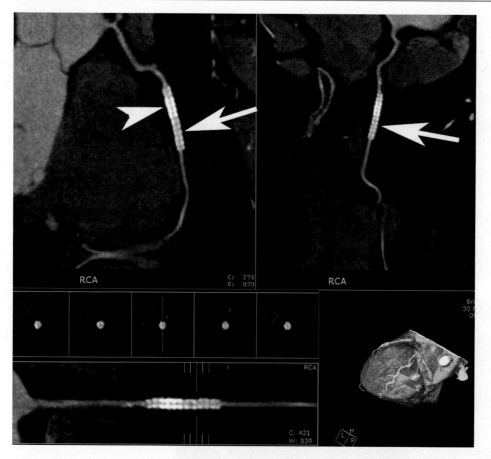

Fig. 7.9 Overlapping right coronary artery (RCA) stents. Orthogonal views of RCA with a patent stent (*arrow*). The stent appears thicker in its proximal portion (*arrowhead*). This actually represents the overlap of two stents. The lumen is more difficult to visualize within this area of overlap because of increased metallic density of the overlapped stents.

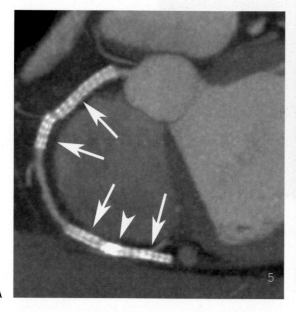

A

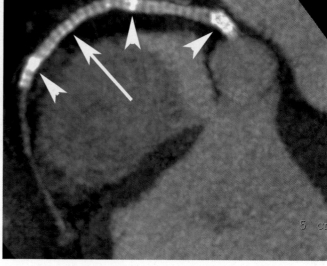

B

Fig. 7.10 Multiple stents within the right coronary artery (RCA). **(A)** Four stents within the RCA (*arrows*). Area of overlap between the two distal stents demonstrates increased density (*arrowhead*). **(B)** Multiple overlapping RCA stents (*arrows*) in another patient. Areas of overlap demonstrate increased density (*arrowheads*). Although the stents are patent, it is not possible to assess the lumen in the areas of overlap because of artifact from the dense metal. The RCA beyond the stent appears diffusely diseased and small in caliber.

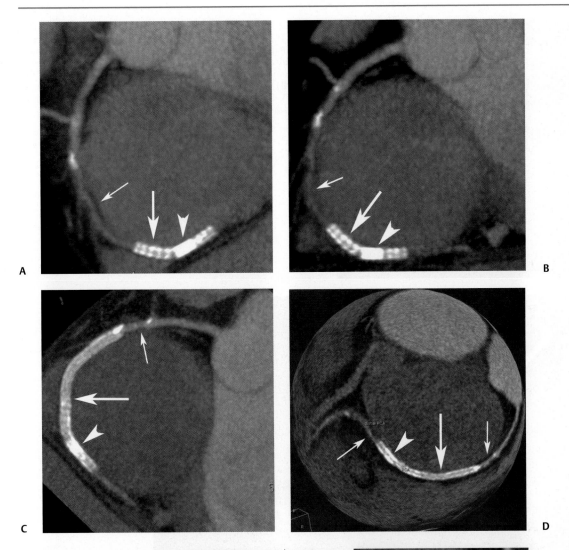

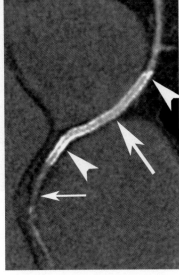

Fig. 7.11 Distal right coronary artery (RCA) stents with persistent chest pain. Initial evaluation: **(A,B)** A diseased segment of the RCA is present just proximal to the stent (*small arrow*). Maximum intensity projection (MIP) images through the RCA demonstrate the presence of stents in the distal RCA (*arrow*) with overlap of the two stents (*arrowhead*). The area of overlap is obscured by blooming artifact. In addition, the mid to distal portion of the RCA just proximal to the stents demonstrates diffuse disease with noncalcified plaque resulting in moderate stenosis (*small arrow*). Additional stents were placed within this segment, and a 1-year follow-up was obtained when the patient returned with chest pain (C–E). **(C)** MIP image demonstrates patent RCA stents (*arrow*) with blooming artifact in the area of overlap of stents in the distal RCA (*arrowhead*). There is new mild disease within the RCA just proximal to the stent (*small arrow*). **(D)** Globe view demonstrates a similar appearance with a long stented segment of the RCA, which is patent. Low-density plaque is identified both proximal and distal to the stented segment. **(E)** Vessel tracking demonstrates a patent RCA (*arrow*). An area of calcified plaque along the proximal aspect of the stent, as well as the area of stent overlap distally (*arrowheads*), demonstrates increased stent density, which makes it more difficult to evaluate the internal lumen. Again noted is the diseased segment of RCA just beyond the stent (*small arrow*).

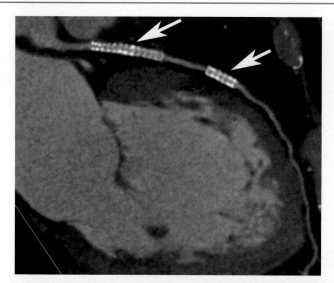

A

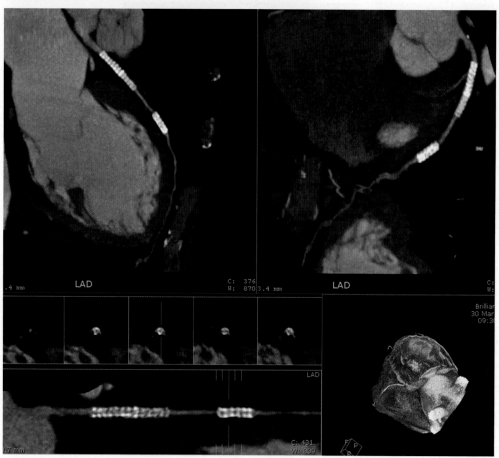

B

Fig. 7.12 Tandem stents within the left anterior descending artery (LAD). The proximal third of the more proximal stent is incompletely expanded. **(A)** Maximum intensity projection (MIP) image demonstrates two patent stents within the proximal LAD (*arrows*). The internal lumen is obscured by blooming of the dense stent material. **(B)** Vessel tracking is used to create two orthogonal views of the LAD. The blooming artifact within the proximal stent is most obvious in the underexpanded stent segment.

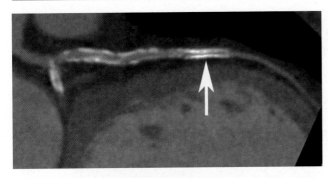

Fig. 7.13 Calcified left anterior descending artery (LAD) with incompletely expanded stent. Maximum intensity projection image through the LAD demonstrates diffuse calcification along the LAD with a patent lumen. There is a stent in the midportion of the LAD (*arrow*). The stent is patent, but the stent wall appears thickened in the midportion of the stent, with apparent narrowing of the LAD lumen. The apparent thickening of the stent is related to relative underdistention of the midportion of this stent.

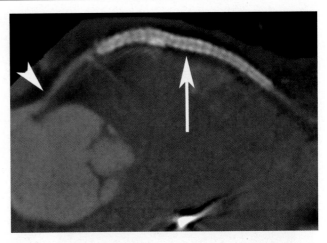

Fig. 7.14 Long stented segment within the proximal left anterior descending artery (LAD) with motion artifact. Motion artifact is demonstrated as linear streaking below the stent and as blurring of the stent itself. The stent is clearly patent in its midportion (*arrow*). However, patency of the stent is more difficult to judge at its proximal and distal ends because of underexpansion of the stent in these areas. Incomplete distention of the stent results in increased blooming artifact related to increased local density of stent material. Mild arthrosclerotic disease with noncalcified plaque is identified at the junction of the left main coronary artery with proximal LAD (*arrowhead*).

The goal of MDCT after stent placement is the determination of patency and characterization of restenosis. Determination of stent patency cannot be based solely on assessment of downstream coronary flow because clinically significant stenosis may not impede resting coronary blood flow and because collateral flow may provide enhancement beyond an occluded segment (**Figs. 7.16 and 12.7**). Mean in-stent attenuation values are significantly lower in

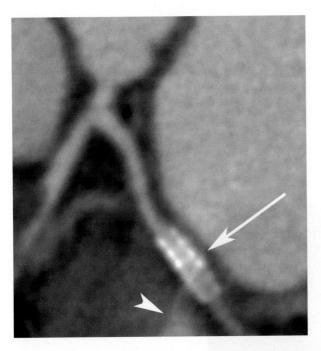

Fig. 7.15 Stent within the circumflex artery with blurring of the distal stent and linear streak artifact related to cardiac motion and adjacent high-density material in the mitral annulus. Although this stent is patent, there is a lower level of internal enhancement in the distal portion of the stent related to the artifact.

stenosed than in nonstenosed stents[22,36] and are clearly reduced in the setting of stent occlusion. However, evaluation of mean in-stent attenuation is limited by the artifactual increase in luminal density secondary to blooming artifact within stented segments and cannot be used to quantify the extent of narrowing within a stent. Ultimately, evaluation of stent patency and in-stent stenosis must be based on a combination of direct visual assessment of the stent lumen and quantification of downstream coronary flow (**Figs. 7.17, 7.18, and 7.19**).[37,38] Evaluation of coronary segments just proximal and distal to the stent is also important because these segments may represent the cause of a patient's symptoms (**Fig. 7.9**).

A small, patient-based 4-slice MDCT study successfully identified two cases of total stent occlusion but failed to identify any of five cases in which stents were shown by invasive angiography to have lesser degrees of restenosis.[27] In general, only stenoses greater than 50% are consistently detectable by 16-slice MDCT.[23] One study demonstrated the ability of 16-slice MDCT to detect neointimal hyperplasia to a lower limit of 1 mm, as measured by intravascular ultrasound. This corresponded to approximately 30% stenosis in 3-mm stents.[39] As with in vitro studies, stent-specific features (stent size and strut thickness) strongly correlate with lumen visibility, and better results have been reported for larger (ie, left main coronary artery) stents.[22,36]

Gaspar and colleagues imaged 111 stents, 18 of which were determined by invasive angiography to have at least 60% restenosis, using 40-slice MDCT.[40] The MDCT protocol used combinations of visual and quantitative analyses to

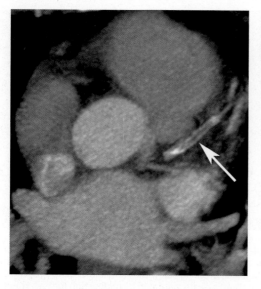 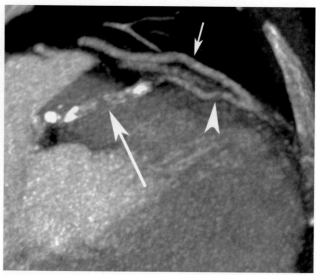

Fig. 7.16 Occluded proximal left anterior descending artery (LAD) stent with reconstitution of the distal vessel via a subsequently placed left internal mammary artery (LIMA) bypass graft just beyond the stent. **(A)** Maximum intensity projection (MIP) view through the proximal LAD demonstrates an occluded stent with internal low-density material (*arrow*). **(B)** Orthogonal MIP demonstrates the patent LIMA bypass graft (*small arrow*) with anastomosis to the LAD (*arrowhead*). Retrograde flow within the diseased LAD is present proximal to this anastomosis (*arrowhead*). However, the proximal LAD stent (*arrow*) is occluded.

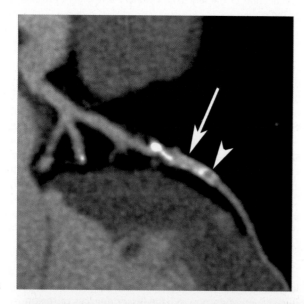

Fig. 7.17 Left anterior descending artery (LAD) stent with in-stent stenosis. **(A)** Maximum intensity projection (MIP) image through the LAD demonstrates a patent stent (*arrow*). However, at the distal aspect of the stent, there is a focal filling defect (*arrowhead*). **(B)** The straightened lumen view of the LAD once again demonstrates the stent with a focal filling defect in its distal aspect. Short-axis views through the LAD at this level again demonstrate the filling defect (*arrowhead*). It is not possible to distinguish focal high-grade stenosis from thrombosis based on this CT image.

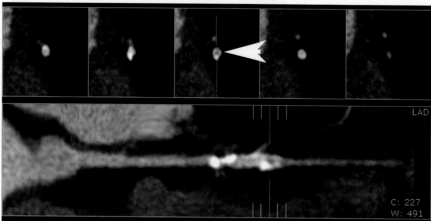

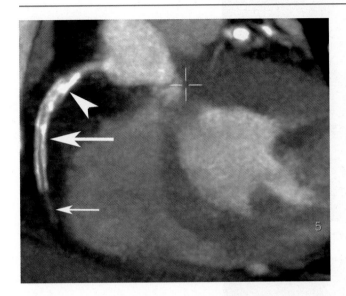

Fig. 7.18 Long stented segment in the proximal right coronary artery (RCA) with occlusion. A stent is present in the proximal RCA (*arrow*). Vascular calcification along the proximal aspect of the stent (*arrowhead*) results in blooming that obscures the adjacent lumen. The mid-distal stent lumen demonstrates low density, compatible with occlusion. There is a small segment of reconstituted distal RCA visible just beyond the stent (*small arrow*).

determine stent patency with a sensitivity of 88.9% and specificity of 80.6%.

Recent advances in MDCT technology—including a greater number of slices per rotation, improved temporal resolution, increased sampling rates, and faster detector response times—have resulted in improved visualization of the lumen within stents (**Fig. 7.20**), often allowing definitive visualization of in-stent stenosis (**Fig. 7.21**). Nonetheless, results of studies with 64-slice MDCT have been mixed with respect to differences in the overall accuracy when comparing 16-slice with 64-slice scanners.[41] Despite improvements in image quality, stent accessibility for determination of stent restenosis has been variable, ranging from 58 to 100%.[42,43] In an early, small meta-analysis on stent evaluation in studies using only 64-slice MDCT (270 stents), a sensitivity of 80%, a specificity of 95%, and positive predictive value of 80% were observed.[44] A larger meta-analysis of stent restenosis studies by Kumbhani et al identified 14 studies, which included 1447 stents in 895 patients.[45] Of these, 91% (1231 stents) were accessible. In accessible stents, the overall sensitivity was 91%, specificity 91%, and positive predictive value 68% in the evaluation for

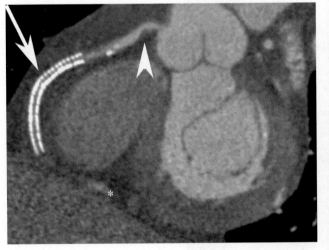

A

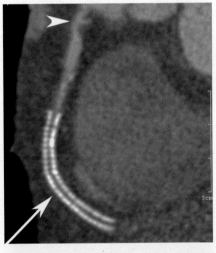

B

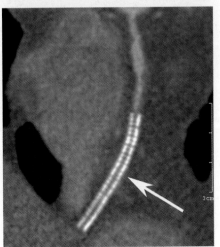

C

Fig. 7.19 Heavily diseased proximal right coronary artery (RCA) with occluded stent in the mid-RCA. The RCA is occluded beyond the stent. **(A)** Slab maximum intensity projection (MIP) in the left anterior oblique projection demonstrates irregular, noncalcified plaque in the proximal RCA (*arrowhead*) with an occluded stent in the mid-RCA (*arrow*). Minimal segmental reconstitution of the distal RCA is demonstrated at the crux of the heart (*). **(B,C)** Orthogonal curved MIP images have been tracked through the center of the stent and more clearly demonstrate the occluded stent lumen (*arrow*).

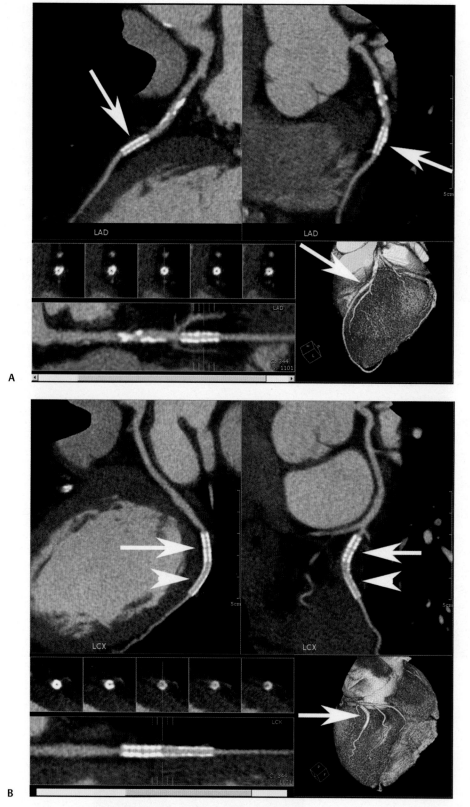

Fig. 7.20 Multislice–multidetector CT with 256-slice scanner technology and 270-msec gantry rotation time clearly demonstrates patent stents in the left anterior descending artery (LAD) and circumflex arteries. The patent lumen is clearly visualized, even within the overlapping stents in the distal circumflex artery. **(A)** Tracked maximum intensity projection (MIP) images of the LAD demonstrate calcified plaque in the proximal to midportion of the vessel, with less than 50% narrowing, and a patent stent in the mid-LAD (*arrow*). The patent lumen is clearly visualized in orthogonal curved MIP images as well as in the straightened lumen view. **(B)** Tracked MIP images of the circumflex artery demonstrate stents in the distal circumflex artery, extending into a posterolateral brach (*arrow* and *arrowhead*). The more proximal stented segment is of higher density because there are two overlapping stents in this segment (*arrow*); the distal segment has only a single stent (*arrowhead*). The patent lumen is clearly visualized within both stents.

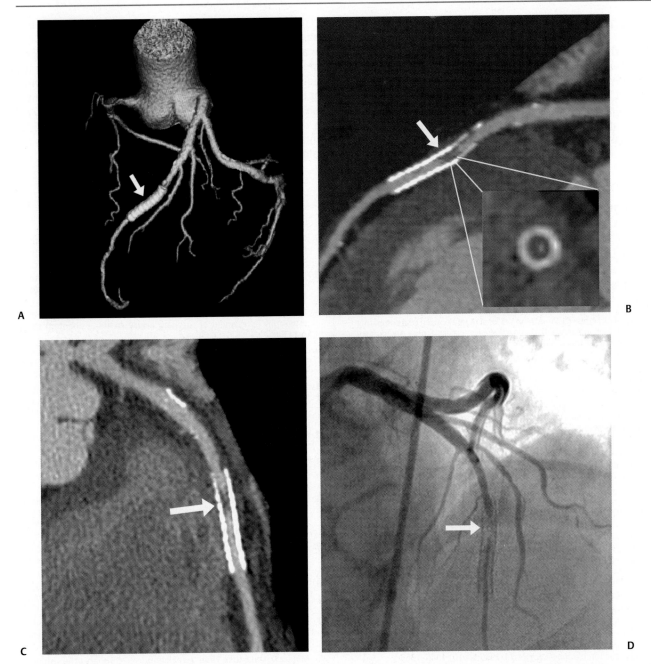

Fig. 7.21 High-definition CT with a 64-slice scanner using an increased sampling rate and new detector technology with a faster response time demonstrates focal high-grade stenosis within a 3-mm stent in the mid left anterior descending artery (LAD) with enhancement of the LAD proximal and distal to the stent. **(A)** Volumetric rendering of the coronary tree demonstrates the presence of a stent in the midportion of the LAD (*arrow*). **(B)** Thin-slab curved MIP reconstruction demonstrates the stented segment of the LAD with mild atherosclerotic disease in the LAD just proximal to the stent and a focal high-grade stenosis within the stent (*arrow*). **Inset** demonstrates a cross-section of the stent at the level of the stenosis, suggesting that there is a small amount of residual flow centrally. **(C)** Orthogonal thin-slab curved maximum intensity projection again demonstrates the focal high-grade stenosis of the stent (*arrow*). **(D)** Conventional arteriogram confirms the presence of high-grade stenosis within the stent, with a string sign of minimal flow through the stent. The high-resolution mode of this scanner provides exquisite detail to demonstrate the thrombus and tiny residual lumen within the stent. (Images courtesy of James P. Earls, MD, Fairfax Radiological Consultants, Fairfax, Virginia.)

stent restenosis. These performance measures were significantly decreased when all stents were included in the analysis. Overall, sensitivity and specificity decreased to 87% and 84%, respectively, with a positive predictive value of 53%. Presently, most stents implanted are drug-eluting stents. In a study specifically assessing the utility of 64-slice MDCT for detecting in-stent restenosis in this population, the sensitivity was moderate at 84%.[46]

◆ Conclusion

Published results using MDCT for imaging of stents have been mixed because of the large numbers of uninterpretable stents. Despite advances in CT technology with 64- and 256-slice MDCT, inconsistent visualization of clinically significant stenoses persists as a result of "beam hardening," blooming artifact, and image acquisition influenced by heart rate, arrhythmias, calcification, and overlapping stents. With the current state of MDCT technology, evaluation of in-stent stenosis should be limited to stents that are at least 3 to 4 mm in diameter in patients with easily controlled heart rates. Smaller stents may be evaluated only for patency. Additional improvements in MDCT resolution and image quality are required before this technology can be applied successfully for the routine clinical evaluation of the currently implanted coronary stents. Future improvement in stent design may aid in the utility of this technology to assess coronary stents. Until such time, invasive coronary angiography remains the gold-standard for assessment of stent restenosis.

References

1. Grüntzig AR, Senning A, Siegenthaler WE. Nonoperative dilatation of coronary-artery stenosis: percutaneous transluminal coronary angioplasty. N Engl J Med. 1979;301(2):61–68
2. Frye R; The Bypass Angioplasty Revascularization Investigation (BARI) investigators. Comparison of coronary bypass surgery with angioplasty in patients with multivessel disease. N Engl J Med. 1996;335(4):217–225
3. King SB III, Lembo NJ, Weintraub WS, et al. A randomized trial comparing coronary angioplasty with coronary bypass surgery. Emory Angioplasty versus Surgery Trial (EAST). N Engl J Med. 1994;331(16):1044–1050
4. Fischman DL, Leon MB, Baim DS, et al; Stent Restenosis Study investigators. A randomized comparison of coronary-stent placement and balloon angioplasty in the treatment of coronary artery disease. N Engl J Med. 1994;331(8):496–501
5. Serruys PW, de Jaegere P, Kiemeneij F, et al; Benestent Study Group. A comparison of balloon-expandable-stent implantation with balloon angioplasty in patients with coronary artery disease. N Engl J Med. 1994;331(8):489–495
6. Pfisterer MD. Late clinical events related to late stent thrombosis after stopping clopidogral (BASKET LATE trial). Cardiosource: Presented at the March, 2006 ACC Annual Scientific Sessions, Atlanta, GA
7. Takahashi M, Takamoto T, Aizawa T, Shimada H. Severity of coronary artery calcification detected by electron beam computed tomography is related to the risk of restenosis after percutaneous transluminal coronary angioplasty. Intern Med. 1997;36(4):255–262
8. Sinitsyn V, Belkind M, Matchin Y, Lyakishev A, Naumov V, Ternovoy S. Relationships between coronary calcification detected at electron beam computed tomography and percutaneous transluminal coronary angioplasty results in coronary artery disease patients. Eur Radiol. 2003;13(1):62–67
9. Pump H, Moehlenkamp S, Sehnert C, et al. Electron-beam CT in the noninvasive assessment of coronary stent patency. Acad Radiol. 1998;5(12):858–862
10. Schmermund A, Haude M, Baumgart D, et al. Non-invasive assessment of coronary Palmaz-Schatz stents by contrast enhanced electron beam computed tomography. Eur Heart J. 1996;17(10):1546–1553
11. Möhlenkamp S, Pump H, Baumgart D, et al. Minimally invasive evaluation of coronary stents with electron beam computed tomography: in vivo and in vitro experience. Catheter Cardiovasc Interv. 1999;48(1): 39–47
12. Pump H, Möhlenkamp S, Sehnert CA, et al. Coronary arterial stent patency: assessment with electron-beam CT. Radiology 2000;214(2):447–452
13. Maintz D, Seifarth H, Raupach R, et al. 64-slice multidetector coronary CT angiography: in vitro evaluation of 68 different stents. Eur Radiol. 2006;16(4):818–826
14. Colombo A, Stankovic G, Moses JW. Selection of coronary stents. J Am Coll Cardiol. 2002;40(6):1021–1033
15. Stone G. Coronary stenting. In: Baim D, ed. Grossman's Cardiac Catheterization, Angiography, and Intervention. 7th ed. Philadelphia: Lippincott Williams & Wilkins; 2006:492–542
16. Maintz D, Juergens KU, Wichter T, Grude M, Heindel W, Fischbach R. Imaging of coronary artery stents using multislice computed tomography: in vitro evaluation. Eur Radiol. 2003;13(4):830–835
17. Nieman K, Cademartiri F, Raaijmakers R, Pattynama P, de Feyter P. Noninvasive angiographic evaluation of coronary stents with multislice spiral computed tomography. Herz. 2003;28(2):136–142
18. Mahnken AH, Buecker A, Wildberger JE, et al. Coronary artery stents in multislice computed tomography: in vitro artifact evaluation. Invest Radiol. 2004;39(1):27–33
19. Mahnken AH, Mühlenbruch G, Seyfarth T, et al. 64-slice computed tomography assessment of coronary artery stents: a phantom study. Acta Radiol. 2006;47(1):36–42
20. Maintz D, Burg MC, Seifarth H, et al. Update on multidetector coronary CT angiography of coronary stents: in vitro evaluation of 29 different stent types with dual-source CT. Eur Radiol. 2009;19(1):42–49
21. Suzuki S, Furui S, Kaminaga T, et al. Evaluation of coronary stents in vitro with CT angiography: effect of stent diameter, convolution kernel, and vessel orientation to the z-axis. Circ J 2005;69(9): 1124–1131
22. Gilard M, Cornily JC, Pennec PY, et al. Assessment of coronary artery stents by 16 slice computed tomography. Heart. 2006;92(1):58–61
23. Gilard M, Cornily JC, Rioufol G, et al. Noninvasive assessment of left main coronary stent patency with 16-slice computed tomography. Am J Cardiol. 2005;95(1):110–112
24. Funabashi N, Komiyama N, Yanagawa N, Mayama T, Yoshida K, Komuro I. Images in cardiovascular medicine: coronary artery patency after metallic stent implantation evaluated by multislice computed tomography. Circulation. 2003;107(1):147–148
25. Shaohong Z, Yongkang N, Zulong C, Hong Z, Li Y. Images in cardiovascular medicine. Imaging of coronary stent by multislice helical computed tomography. Circulation. 2002;106(5):637–638
26. Nieman K, Ligthart JM, Serruys PW, de Feyter PJ. Images in cardiovascular medicine. Left main rapamycin-coated stent: invasive versus noninvasive angiographic follow-up. Circulation. 2002;105(18):e130–e131
27. Krüger S, Mahnken AH, Sinha AM, et al. Multislice spiral computed tomography for the detection of coronary stent restenosis and patency. Int J Cardiol. 2003;89(2–3):167–172
28. Maintz D, Seifarth H, Flohr T, et al. Improved coronary artery stent visualization and in-stent stenosis detection using 16-slice computed-tomography and dedicated image reconstruction technique. Invest Radiol. 2003;38(12):790–795
29. Seifarth H, Ozgün M, Raupach R, et al. 64- Versus 16-slice CT angiography for coronary artery stent assessment: in vitro experience. Invest Radiol. 2006;41(1):22–27
30. Mahnken AH, Seyfarth T, Flohr T, et al. Flat-panel detector computed tomography for the assessment of coronary artery stents: phantom study in comparison with 16-slice spiral computed tomography. Invest Radiol. 2005;40(1):8–13
31. Hong C, Chrysant GS, Woodard PK, Bae KT. Coronary artery stent patency assessed with in-stent contrast enhancement measured at multi-detector row CT angiography: initial experience. Radiology. 2004;233(1):286–291
32. Seifarth H, Raupach R, Schaller S, et al. Assessment of coronary artery stents using 16-slice MDCT angiography: evaluation of a dedicated reconstruction kernel and a noise reduction filter. Eur Radiol. 2005;15(4):721–726

33. Yeh BM, Shepherd JA, Wang ZJ, Teh HS, Hartman RP, Prevrhal S. Dual-energy and low-kVp CT in the abdomen. AJR Am J Roentgenol. 2009;193(1):47–54

34. Boll DT, Merkle EM, Paulson EK, Fleiter TR. Coronary stent patency: dual-energy multidetector CT assessment in a pilot study with anthropomorphic phantom. Radiology. 2008;247(3):687–695

35. Halpern EJ, Halpern DJ, Yanof JH, et al. Is coronary stent assessment improved with spectral analysis of dual energy CT? Acad Radiol. 2009;16(10):1241–1250

36. Watanabe M, Uemura S, Iwama H, et al. Usefulness of 16-slice multislice spiral computed tomography for follow-up study of coronary stent implantation. Circ J. 2006;70(6):691–697

37. Schuijf JD, Bax JJ, Jukema JW, et al. Feasibility of assessment of coronary stent patency using 16-slice computed tomography. Am J Cardiol. 2004;94(4):427–430

38. Ohnuki K, Yoshida S, Ohta M, et al. New diagnostic technique in multislice computed tomography for in-stent restenosis: pixel count method. Int J Cardiol. 2006;108(2):251–258

39. Van Mieghem CA, Cademartiri F, Mollet NR, et al. Multislice spiral computed tomography for the evaluation of stent patency after left main coronary artery stenting: a comparison with conventional coronary angiography and intravascular ultrasound. Circulation 2006;114(7):645–653

40. Gaspar T, Halon DA, Lewis BS, et al. Diagnosis of coronary in-stent restenosis with multidetector row spiral computed tomography. J Am Coll Cardiol. 2005;46(8):1573–1579

41. Sun Z, Davidson R, Lin CH. Multi-detector row CT angiography in the assessment of coronary in-stent restenosis: a systematic review. Eur J Radiol. 2009;69(3):489–495

42. Rixe J, Achenbach S, Ropers D, et al. Assessment of coronary artery stent restenosis by 64-slice multi-detector computed tomography. Eur Heart J. 2006;27(21):2567–2572

43. Pugliese F, Weustink AC, Van Mieghem C, et al. Dual source coronary computed tomography angiography for detecting in-stent restenosis. Heart. 2008;94(7):848–854

44. Abdulla J, Abildstrom SZ, Gotzsche O, Christensen E, Kober L, Torp-Pedersen C. 64-multislice detector computed tomography coronary angiography as potential alternative to conventional coronary angiography: a systematic review and meta-analysis. Eur Heart J. 2007; 28(24):3042–3050

45. Kumbhani DJ, Ingelmo CP, Schoenhagen P, Curtin RJ, Flamm SD, Desai MY. Meta-analysis of diagnostic efficacy of 64-slice computed tomography in the evaluation of coronary in-stent restenosis. Am J Cardiol. 2009;103(12):1675–1681

46. Carrabba N, Bamoshmoosh M, Carusi LM, et al. Usefulness of 64-slice multidetector computed tomography for detecting drug eluting in-stent restenosis. Am J Cardiol. 2007;100(12):1754–1758

8

Bypass Grafts

Linda J. Bogar, Stephanie Fuller, and James T. Diehl

In addition to its application for the evaluation of native coronary vessels, cardiac CT is an increasingly valuable technique for pre-operative and post-operative evaluation of coronary bypass patients. Pre-operative evaluation of the ascending aorta, native coronary arteries, and cardiac function is critical to the planning of bypass surgery. Post-operative confirmation of bypass graft patency is important for the diagnosis and management of recurrent anginal symptoms as well as in operative planning for repeat surgical revascularization or valve surgery after coronary bypass.

◆ Arterial Versus Venous Coronary Bypass Grafts

Traditionally, coronary artery bypass grafting (CABG) has been performed with vein grafts that extend from the ascending aorta to a target vessel on the epicardial surface of the heart (**Figs. 8.1, 8.2,** and **8.3**). The saphenous vein (SV) is comparable in size to major coronary arteries and is easily harvested from the lower extremity without significant consequences. The SV has good early patency, but it has been noted that up to 10% of vein grafts may be closed by the time the patient is discharged from the hospital. Accelerated graft atheroma has contributed to saphenous graft failure at 5 to 10 years after coronary bypass. By 10 years about 40% of grafts have failed because of thrombosis, intimal hyperplasia, or accelerated atherosclerosis.[1]

As bypass surgery has evolved, arterial revascularization has become more popular. The right and left internal mammary arteries (RIMA and LIMA), inferior epigastric artery, right gastroepiploic artery, and radial artery (RA) have all been used (**Fig. 8.4, 8.5, 8.6,** and **8.7**). Although vein grafts are much larger than arterial grafts (3–4 mm versus 1.5–2 mm) and vein grafting may be technically easier than arterial grafting, recent literature supports the use of all-arterial conduits when possible because of their longer patency rates compared with venous grafts.[2] Coronary arteries that

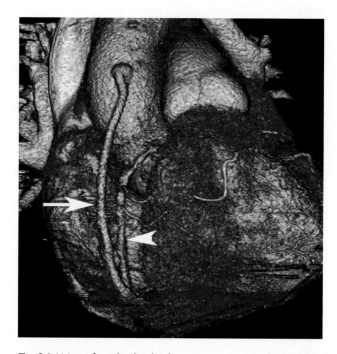

Fig. 8.1 Vein graft to the distal right coronary artery. Surface-rendered volumetric projection demonstrates a vein graft (*arrow*) extending from the proximal aorta to the right coronary artery (*arrowhead*). The course of the graft is clearly demonstrated, but it is not possible to evaluate for stenosis on surface-rendered images.

are suitable as target sites for bypass grafts are usually 1 to 2 mm in diameter. These include the left anterior descending (LAD) and its diagonal branches, the right coronary artery (RCA) and its posterior descending artery (PDA), and posterolateral (PL) branches and obtuse marginal (OM) branches of the circumflex artery.

Early thrombosis of vein grafts following surgery can be related to technical factors, anatomic factors causing poor distal runoff, or hemodynamic factors causing sluggish flow, whereas mid- to long-term vein graft occlusion is related to proliferative intimal fibroplasia with concentric narrowing

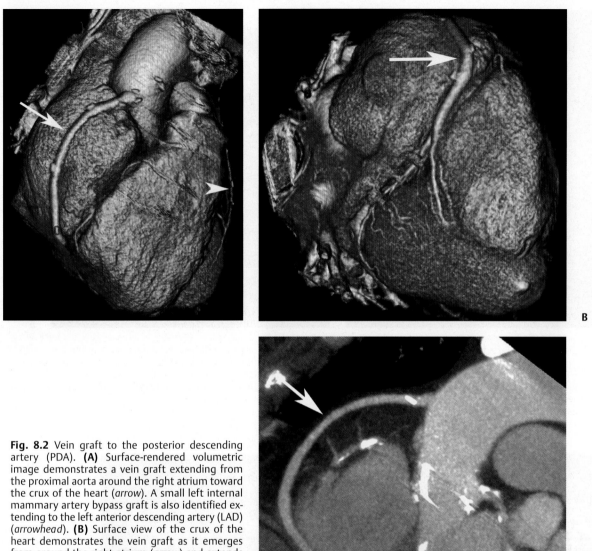

Fig. 8.2 Vein graft to the posterior descending artery (PDA). **(A)** Surface-rendered volumetric image demonstrates a vein graft extending from the proximal aorta around the right atrium toward the crux of the heart (*arrow*). A small left internal mammary artery bypass graft is also identified extending to the left anterior descending artery (LAD) (*arrowhead*). **(B)** Surface view of the crux of the heart demonstrates the vein graft as it emerges from around the right atrium (*arrow*) and extends toward the posterior interventricular groove. The anastomosis of the graft is not with the right coronary artery, but rather in the posterior interventricular groove with the posterior descending artery. **(C)** Slab maximum intensity projection demonstrates patency of this bypass graft as it courses around the right atrium (*arrow*). The distal anastomosis of the graft is not visualized on this image, although the graft is seen to course adjacent to the PDA at the crux of the heart.

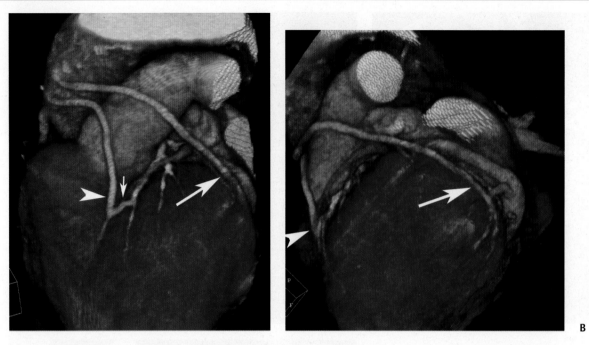

A   B

Fig. 8.3 Venous bypass grafts to the left anterior descending artery (LAD) and circumflex territories. **(A)** Two venous bypass grafts are identified. The more superior graft (*arrow*) extends to the circumflex territory. The second graft (*arrowhead*) extends to the proximal LAD. In addition, there is a jump graft segment (*small arrow*) to a diagonal branch of the LAD. **(B)** The anastomosis of the more superior venous bypass graft to an obtuse marginal branch of the circumflex is more clearly defined on this projection (*arrow*). The second anastomosis to the LAD is not as clearly visualized (*arrowhead*). The native coronary arteries are heavily diseased beyond the graft anastomoses and are patent for only a short distance.

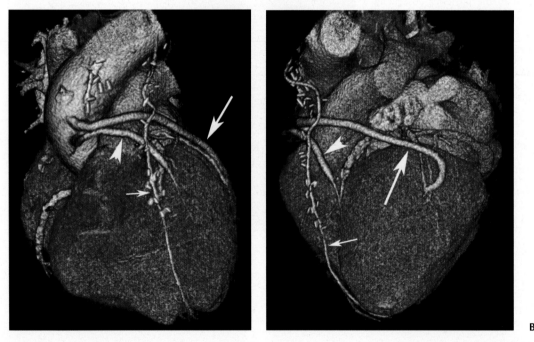

A   B

Fig. 8.4 Venous bypass grafts to an obtuse marginal branch and a diagonal branch of the left anterior descending artery (LAD). Left internal mammary artery (LIMA) bypass graft to the distal LAD. **(A)** Two large venous grafts are identified. The more superior graft extends across the free wall of the left ventricle to an obtuse marginal (OM) branch of the circumflex (*arrow*). The proximal portion of this obtuse marginal artery fills in a retrograde fashion, but the distal OM beyond the anastomosis is not well filled. A second venous graft crosses over the LAD (*arrowhead*) into a small diagonal branch. The LIMA courses anterior to the venous bypass grafts (*small arrow*) into the distal LAD. **(B)** Left anterior oblique image demonstrates the anastomosis of the upper vein graft (*arrow*) to the OM branch more clearly. The more inferior vein graft is identified (*arrowhead*). The anastomosis of the LIMA to the proximal LAD is clearly identified (*small arrow*).

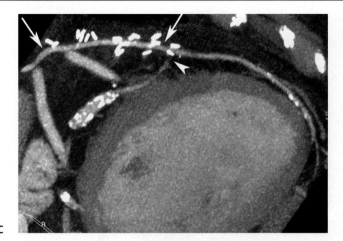

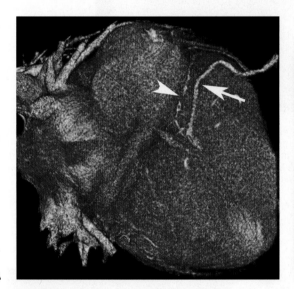

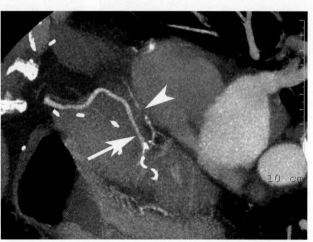

Fig. 8.4 (*Continued*) **(C)** Slab maximum intensity projection demonstrates the LIMA graft (*arrows*) anastomosis to the native LAD. The native LAD is occluded just proximal to this anastomosis (*arrowhead*).

Fig. 8.5 Gastroepiploic artery bypass to the posterior descending artery (PDA). **(A)** Surface-rendered volumetric image of the crux of the heart demonstrates the distal segment of a gastroepiploic graft to the PDA (*arrow*). The native right coronary artery (RCA) is diseased, with a segmental occlusion just proximal to the anastomosis (*arrowhead*).

(B) Slab maximum intensity projection image demonstrates the gastroepiploic bypass graft (*arrow*). The anastomosis with the PDA is obscured by overlying surgical clips. The diseased distal RCA is just to the right of the graft, with a focal occlusion in its distal segment (*arrowhead*).

of the inner lumen (**Fig. 8.8**). Vein graft atherosclerosis mimics fibroplasia but is more eccentric and associated with mural thrombus (**Fig. 8.9**). As stated previously, atherosclerosis is typically a late process seen more than 5 to 10 years after surgery, and up to 50 to 70% of vein grafts are occluded or have a significant stenosis by 10 years after surgery. These results seem to be improving in recent years as a result of the addition of aggressive antilipid therapy in all post-bypass patients.

Arterial grafts exhibit a longer patency, up to and beyond 20 years. It is well established that the graft exhibiting the longest patency and survival benefit is the LIMA to the LAD graft.[3] The 10-year patency of the LIMA to LAD exceeds 90%. Most failures of arterial grafts are attributable to technical

errors at the graft anastomosis or a failure of the graft to mature because of insufficient runoff to the distal vessel (**Fig. 8.10**). Arterial grafts develop intimal hyperplasia but are highly resistant to atherosclerosis. Recent studies have advocated the use of bilateral internal mammary bypass grafts with excellent results (**Figs. 8.11** and **8.12**).[4,5]

When multiple bypass grafts are required, arterial grafts are generally preferred because of their longer patency rates. Currently the prospective single-center Radial Artery Patency and Clinical Outcome (RAPCO) Study is conducting a 10-year comparison of angiographic patency and outcome among RA, internal mammary artery (IMA), and SV grafts. Interim results of this study at 5 years demonstrated similar patency rates for all three types of grafts.[6] The results of this

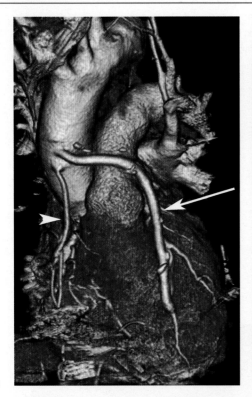

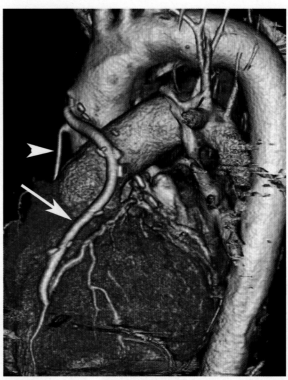

Fig. 8.6 Vein graft to the left anterior descending artery (LAD); radial bypass graft to the right coronary artery (RCA). **(A)** A vein bypass graft extends from the aorta to the midportion of the LAD *(arrow)*. Just below the origin of the vein bypass graft, a smaller radial artery bypass graft originates from the aorta and extends to the RCA *(arrowhead)*.

(B) Left lateral view demonstrates the vein graft to the LAD *(arrow)*. The more proximal LAD and diagonal branches are better visualized on this projection. Only the most proximal portion of the radial artery graft is identified *(arrowhead)*. Note the discrepancy in size between the venous graft, which is much larger, and the radial artery graft.

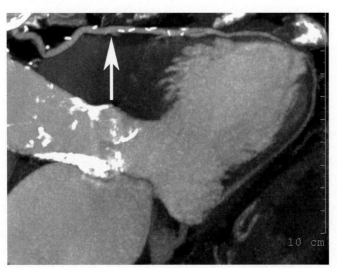

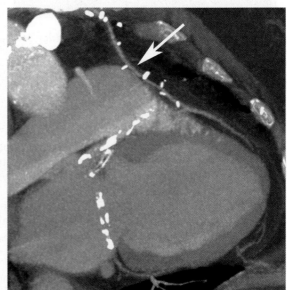

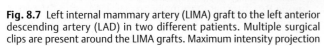

Fig. 8.7 Left internal mammary artery (LIMA) graft to the left anterior descending artery (LAD) in two different patients. Multiple surgical clips are present around the LIMA grafts. Maximum intensity projection images. **(A)** Patent LIMA bypass graft *(arrow)* to the mid-distal LAD. **(B)** Patent LIMA bypass graft *(arrow)* to the LAD. The more proximal LAD is calcified and occluded.

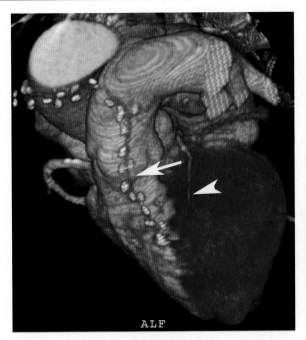

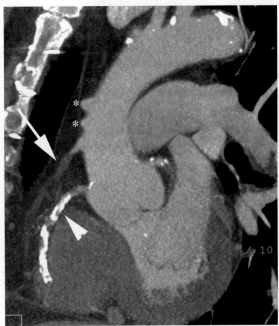

Fig. 8.8 Venous bypass graft occlusion. **(A)** Occlusion of a venous bypass graft to the left anterior descending artery (LAD). Multiple surgical clips mark the course of a bypass graft extending from the aorta down to the LAD (*arrow*). The graft itself is not enhanced by contrast and is not visible. The native LAD is a small vessel that terminates just proximal to the anastomosis (*arrowhead*). **(B)** Occlusion of a venous bypass graft to the distal right coronary artery (RCA). The bypass graft is occluded just beyond its origin from the ascending aorta (*arrow*). The calcified and occluded RCA is identified just caudal to the bypass graft (*arrowhead*). Origins of two other patent bypass grafts are identified just superior to the origin of the occluded graft (*).

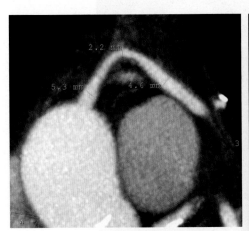

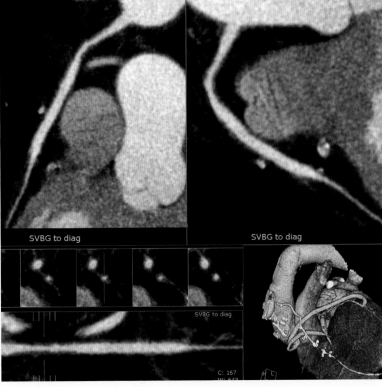

Fig. 8.9 Saphenous vein bypass graft with stenosis (SVBG). **(A)** Slab maximum intensity projection (MIP) image through the proximal portion of the vein graft demonstrates mild narrowing of the lumen from 5 to 2 mm. **(B)** Orthogonal curved MIP images again demonstrate narrowing of the proximal portion of the graft. The straightened lumen view at the bottom of the figure demonstrates approximately 50% narrowing.

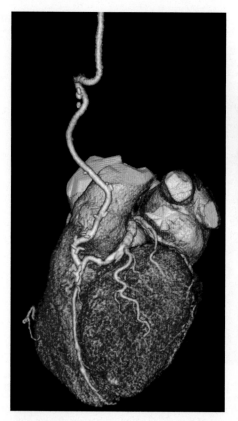

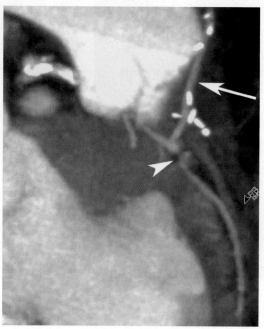

A

B

Fig. 8.10 Left internal mammary artery (LIMA) bypass graft to the left anterior descending artery (LAD). **(A)** Volumetric rendering demonstrates a LIMA graft to the LAD but does not allow assessment of the vessels for stenosis. **(B)** Slab maximum intensity projection (MIP) of the distal LIMA (*arrow*) demonstrates a high-grade stenosis within the LAD just beyond the anastomosis (*arrowhead*).

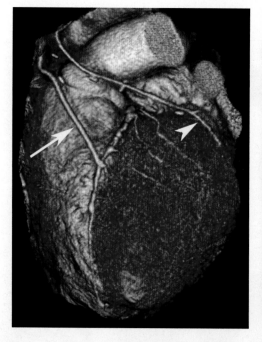

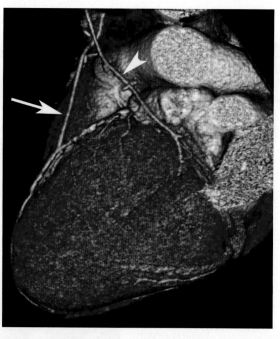

A

B

Fig. 8.11 Right internal mammary artery (RIMA) graft to the left anterior descending artery (LAD) and left internal mammary artery (LIMA) graft to an obtuse marginal (OM) branch of the circumflex artery. **(A)** Surface-rendered volumetric image in the left anterior oblique (LAO) projection demonstrates a RIMA graft to the LAD (*arrow*), as well as a LIMA graft to the circumflex distribution (*arrowhead*). **(B)** Surface-rendered image along the long axis of the left ventricle again demonstrates the two arterial bypass grafts. The calcified and diseased nature of the LAD is apparent, but the internal degree of vessel narrowing cannot be assessed on a surface-rendered image. The LIMA graft is anastomosed to a proximal OM branch as it exits the left atrioventricular (AV) groove. Grafts are typically placed into OM branches of the circumflex rather than directly into the circumflex artery within the AV groove.

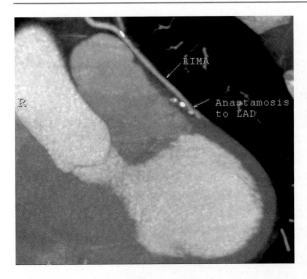

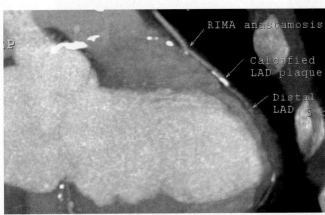

C

D

Fig. 8.11 (*Continued*) **(C)** Slab maximum intensity projection (MIP) demonstrates the RIMA down to the level of its anastomosis with the LAD. The anastomosis is widely patent, but the LAD is not visualized in this projection. **(D)** Slab MIP in a slightly different projection demonstrates the distal LAD beyond the anastomosis of the RIMA. The presence of calcified plaque is identified, as well as marked narrowing or occlusion of the distal LAD related to noncalcified plaque near the cardiac apex.

study should help to clarify the extent to which RA grafts may be superior to RIMA and SV grafts.

RA bypass grafting was almost completely abandoned after early reports of high occlusion rates.[7] More recently, the RA has been used with increased frequency with excellent short- and long-term patency.[8] Some of the early failures may have been due to spasm of the RA, a feature more commonly seen in RAs compared with IMAs. For this reason, most surgeons place patients who undergo bypass grafting with the RA on oral nitrates or calcium channel blockers for several months postoperatively. A recent 6-year study with angiographic correlation demonstrated improved survival and greater patency of RA grafts compared with SV grafts as the second conduit in LIMA to LAD CABG.[9] A similar study of 90 consecutive patients demonstrated an 88% long-term angiographic patency of RA grafts to an OM or PDA. Although

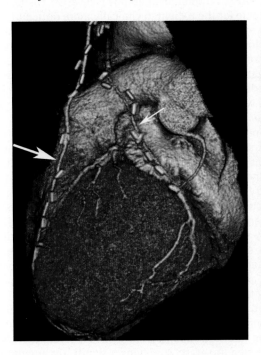

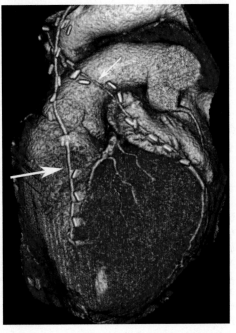

A

B

Fig. 8.12 Left internal mammary artery (LIMA) bypass graft to the left anterior descending artery (LAD); right internal mammary artery (RIMA) graft to the circumflex; radial artery bypass graft to the right coronary artery (RCA). **(A)** Left lateral view demonstrates a LIMA bypass graft to the distal LAD (*arrow*), as well as the RIMA bypass graft (*small arrow*) to a large obtuse marginal branch of the circumflex. **(B)** Left anterior oblique projection demonstrates that the LIMA bypass graft (*large arrow*) crosses anterior to the RIMA bypass graft (*small arrow*) proximal to their anastomoses with the coronary arteries. (*Continued on page 164*)

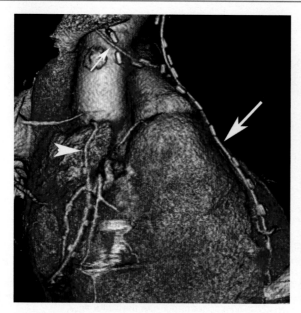

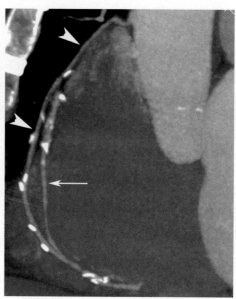

C

D

Fig. 8.12 (*Continued*) Left internal mammary artery (LIMA) bypass graft to the left anterior descending artery (LAD); right internal mammary artery (RIMA) graft to the circumflex; radial artery bypass graft to the right coronary artery (RCA). **(C)** Right anterior oblique projection demonstrates a third arterial bypass graft extending from the aorta to the distal RCA (*arrowhead*). The LIMA bypass graft to the LAD is again identified (*arrow*). **(D)** Slab maximum intensity projection image demonstrates the radial artery bypass graft (*arrowhead*) to the distal RCA (*arrow*). The proximal RCA is occluded. The RCA is reconstituted from the bypass graft. (Also see Cine 8.4.)

this rate was lower than the patency rate for IMA grafts (96.3%), it was significantly higher than the rate for SV grafts (53.4%).[10] There has been some question as to the reliability of RA grafting to the right-sided coronary system. A follow-up study to the previously mentioned RAPCO study looked at differences between RA and SV grafting to the RCA or its branches. The authors found no significant differences in patency between the SV or RA to the right-sided vessels, with a trend toward greater RA patency.[11]

◆ The Post-Bypass Patient

The likelihood of reoperation after a primary coronary bypass procedure is dependent on many variables, including patient symptoms, comorbidities, primary operation-related variables, and other available treatment options. Time since revascularization is an important predictor of reoperation: reoperation rates for coronary bypass have been approximated to be 3% at 5 years, 10% at 10 years, and 25% by 20 years. Factors associated with longer survival and increased likelihood of reoperation include young age at first operation, normal left ventricular function, and disease limited to only one or two coronary vessels. Improvements in surgery, including use of all-arterial conduits and hybrid procedures combining bypass surgery with percutaneous coronary interventions, have improved survival and lengthened the time to repeat intervention.

When a patient experiences anginal symptoms after revascularization, an abnormal electrocardiogram (ECG) is typically followed by stress testing, radionuclide ventriculography, and myocardial perfusion scintigraphy. These noninvasive examinations provide an indirect assessment of graft patency via evaluation of myocardial perfusion and function. In contrast to these methods, conventional selective catheter angiography provides direct images of bypass graft patency and remains the gold standard after CABG. Unfortunately, catheter angiography is invasive, costly, uncomfortable for the patient, technically more difficult than for native vessels, requires multiple skilled personnel, and poses a low but real risk of serious complications. Risks of angiography include conduit dissection, conduit spasm, embolization down the venous grafts, myocardial infarction, arrhythmia, stroke, and death. Given these risks, patients who are asymptomatic or have minimal symptoms after operation are reluctant to undergo catheterization.

Treatment options for the symptomatic post-operative patient include medical therapy, percutaneous intervention, or repeat bypass surgery. The choice of management is determined by the severity of disease and symptoms, the feasibility of each procedure, the procedure's risk, and patient choice. Percutaneous intervention may be performed if vessels are accessible and large enough to accommodate coronary stents (**Fig. 8.13**). In the setting of graft conduit stenosis, early lesions are usually more amenable to angioplasty and stenting. Native coronary stenoses in bypass patients are also eligible for percutaneous intervention, particularly if the myocardium in the coronary distribution is protected by a patent graft. Reoperation may be indicated when there is increased risk of substantial myocardial injury, including late stenosis in a vein graft supplying the LAD, multiple stenotic grafts supplying a significant amount of myocardium, or multivessel disease with reversible ischemia and worsening left ventricular function.

In performing a "re-do" sternotomy, great care must be used in opening the sternum so as not to injure grafts traveling

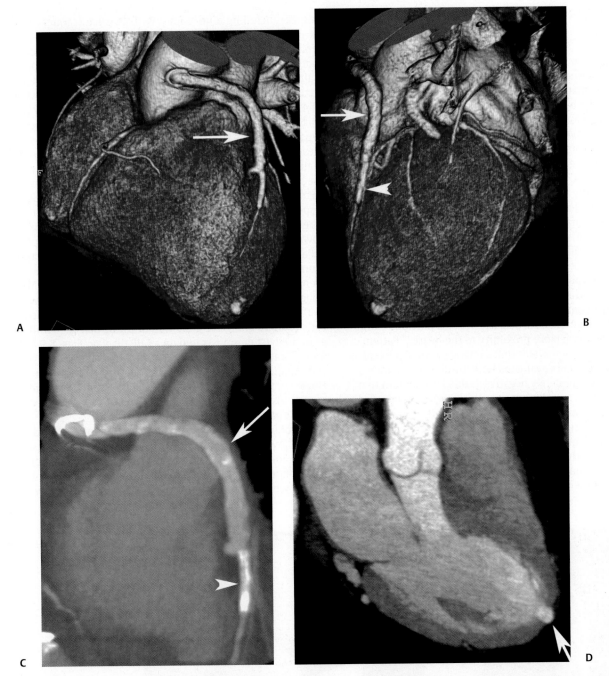

Fig. 8.13 Vein bypass graft to the left anterior descending artery (LAD) with a stent in the LAD beyond the anastomosis. **(A)** Surface-rendered volumetric image in the anteroposterior (AP) projection demonstrates a large vein bypass graft (*arrow*) to the midportion of the LAD. The distal LAD is small and diseased. **(B)** Left lateral projection demonstrates the vein bypass graft again (*arrow*) as well as a mildly distended segment of the LAD just beyond the anastomosis (*arrowhead*). **(C)** Slab maximum intensity projection through the graft (*arrow*) and the LAD (*arrowhead*) demonstrates that the distended segment of the LAD is related to a stent just beyond the anastomosis (*arrowhead*). The stent is patent, although the distal portion of the stent is obscured by calcification. The calcification was outside the stent on an orthogonal view. **(D)** Long-axis view of the left ventricle demonstrates a focal pseudoaneurysm at the ventricular apex (*arrow*), corresponding to the site of a venting cannula placed at the time of surgery.

immediately below the posterior plate. Typically, grafts within 0 to 3 mm of the sternum are at risk for direct injury on opening the chest. Injury may also occur by stretching and direct traction maneuvers used to spread the sternum before releasing the heart and underlying structures from the underside of the sternum. In addition to the risk of injury to bypass grafts, the thin-walled right ventricle is often directly adherent to the underside of the sternum in post-bypass patients and can be injured during reopening.

◆ CT Evaluation of the Post-Bypass Patient

Precise anatomic information is critical to obtain before planning a reoperation coronary bypass surgery. The required information includes the location, patency, and condition of the bypass grafts and native coronary arteries as well as an assessment of cardiac chamber sizes and function. Less invasive imaging techniques have emerged as alternatives to cardiac catheterization for the assessment of previous bypass grafts as well as native coronary arteries. CT angiography (CTA) of the heart and coronary arteries has advanced rapidly from the earliest 4-detector scan to the current 64-detector systems.

Early studies of post-bypass patients with 4-detector CT systems had difficulty with visualization of grafts and reported a 38% rate of nonevaluable grafts.[12] Improvements that have been noted with 16-detector scanners include better visualization and improved sensitivity and specificity.[13–18] Although visualization is improved in 16-detector scanners, some studies continue to report a substantial number of nonevaluable segments, particularly in those portions of the conduits that are in close proximity to the heart.[19] Patient-based analysis demonstrates that a relatively small percentage of bypass patients evaluated with 16-detector scanners demonstrate a completely negative graft CT angiogram that spares them from invasive angiography.[20] This has improved with currently available 64-section CT scanners.

More recent studies with 64-detector systems demonstrate a marked improvement in the rate of evaluable grafts (94 to 100%) with high sensitivity (100%) and specificity (94%) for occlusion and stenosis.[21,22] The most recent review of newer scanner results, a meta-analysis of 15 recent studies—including nine studies with 16-slice scanners and six studies with 64-slice scanners—reports that only 7.6% of bypass grafts are currently not fully assessable. This meta-analysis concludes that multislice CT scanning for bypass graft occlusion (sensitivity 99.3%, specificity 98.7%) is more accurate than detection of bypass graft stenoses (sensitivity 94.4%, specificity of 98.0%) and confirms the previously reported excellent results of cardiac CT scanning for post-bypass patient.[23] However, the native coronary vessels in these patients are often small, calcified, and not as well evaluated by CTA. One study found the sensitivity and specificity of nongrafted segments of coronary arteries in post-bypass patients evaluated by CTA to be 97% and 86%, respectively.[24] Additional studies are needed to determine whether 64-detector CTA will provide sufficient diagnostic power to spare bypass patients from invasive angiography.

Patency of grafts is assessed in a two-dimensional maximum intensity projection (MIP) image based on enhancement of the graft with contrast material (**Fig. 8.13C**). MIP images demonstrate the internal lumen of the graft as well as the graft wall and surrounding structures. Atherosclerotic changes along the graft wall or filling defects within a graft are best demonstrated on a MIP display (**Figs. 8.9** and **8.14**). Graft assessment is more difficult with smaller arterial conduits compared with the larger venous grafts.[25] However, for patients in whom all graft segments are adequately visualized, the predictive value of a negative CT scan for graft patency is close to 100%.

CT volumetric data acquisition throughout the cardiac cycle allows three-dimensional reconstruction of complex bypass anatomy along with evaluation of cardiac anatomy and function. Bypass grafts are visualized from their point of origin (whether from the aorta, native subclavian artery, or

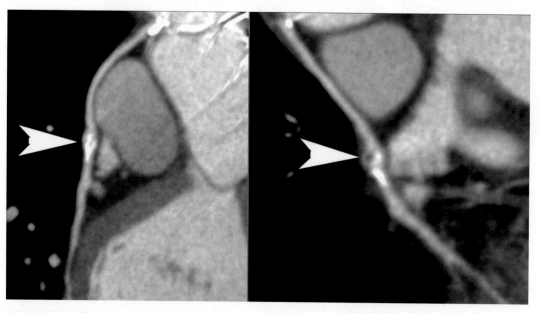

Fig. 8.14 Venous bypass graft with internal thrombus. Orthogonal curved maximum intensity projection images demonstrate the internal architecture of a bypass graft. An area of slight dilatation is related to the site of a venous valve that has been removed (*arrowhead*). A small filling defect associated with this dilatation (in the image on the right) represents thrombus. A calcification is visible within the graft just beyond the thrombus.

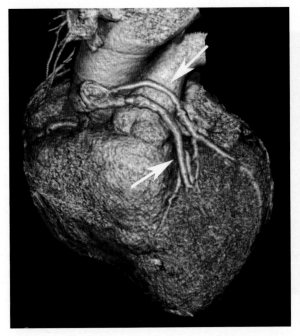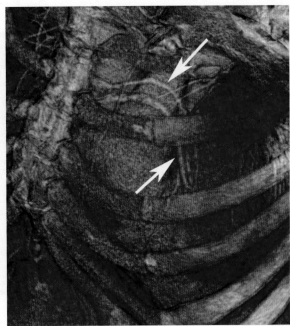

A   B

Fig. 8.15 Relationship of bypass grafts to the overlying bones. **(A)** Surface-rendered volumetric image in the left anterior oblique projection demonstrates two bypass grafts (*arrows*). The more superior graft extends to an obtuse marginal branch of the circumflex artery. The second graft extends to a diagonal branch of the left anterior descending artery. **(B)** Surface-rendered volumetric image in the identical projection demonstrates the relationship of the bypass grafts to the overlying rib cage.

another bypass graft) to their target site on a native coronary artery.[26] Grafts that cross each other or grafts that are adherent to the heart may be at increased risk during reoperation (**Fig. 8.12B**). Volumetric images clearly demonstrate bypass conduit anatomy in relation to the topical anatomy of the heart and surrounding structures, including the overlying rib cage (**Fig. 8.15**), and may be useful to avoid graft injury.[27] Assessment of complex graft anatomy generally requires a combination of MIP and volumetric images (**Figs. 8.16** and **8.17**). The presence of any bypass graft crossing the midline

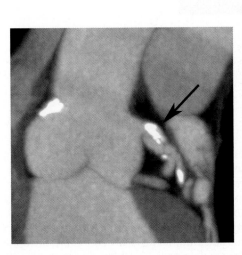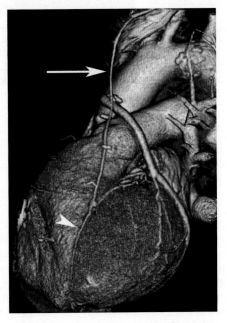

A   B

Fig. 8.16 Maximum intensity projection (MIP) and volumetric images demonstrating left main and proximal right coronary artery (RCA) disease with triple bypass. **(A)** MIP of the left main coronary artery demonstrates ulcerated plaque (*black arrow*). **(B)** Volumetric surface projection demonstrates a left internal mammary artery (LIMA) bypass (*white arrow*) with anastomosis to the left anterior descending artery (LAD) (*white arrowhead*).   (*Continued on page 168*)

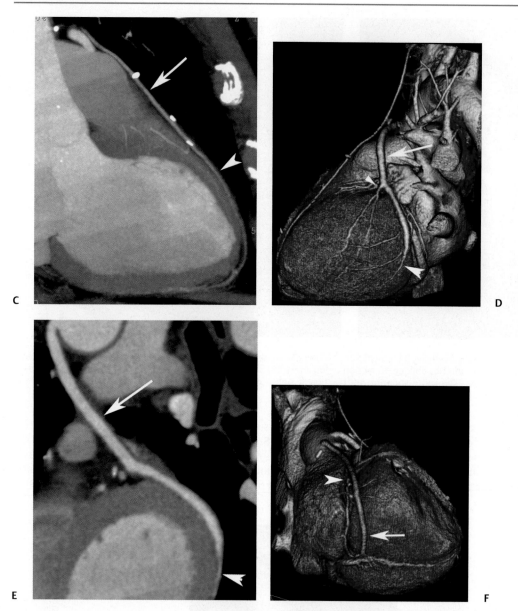

Fig. 8.16 (*Continued*) Maximum intensity projection (MIP) and volumetric images demonstrating left main and proximal right coronary artery (RCA) disease with triple bypass. **(C)** MIP confirms the patency of the LIMA (*arrow*) and LAD (*arrowhead*). **(D)** Vein graft (*arrow*) with anastomosis to a ramus intermedius (*small arrowhead*) and a second anastomosis to a distal obtuse marginal branch (*large arrowhead*). **(E)** Curved MIP confirms the patency of the vein graft (*arrow*) down to the obtuse marginal artery (*arrowhead*). **(F)** Volumetric surface image in a right anterior oblique projection with caudal angulation demonstrates the distal RCA (*arrowhead*) as well as a vein graft (*arrow*) to the proximal posterior descending artery (PDA).

within 1 cm of the sternum in a post-bypass patient must be reported because this may alter the surgical approach (**Fig. 8.18**). Adherence of a bypass graft, the right ventricle, the RCA, pulmonary artery, or aorta to the sternum may result in severe injury and hemorrhage during sternotomy. In one study, pre-operative volumetric information provided by cardiac CT resulted in a modification of the surgical strategy in 7 of 33 patients studied before "re-do" CABG.[28]

During conventional open bypass surgery, each target vessel is visually identified on the epicardial surface. Nonetheless, a site of stenosis or mural calcification in the target vessel may not be apparent at the time of surgery. Pre-operative CTA can provide this information to determine the most appropriate target site for bypass grafting. With the advent of total endoscopic coronary bypass surgery, CT may be used to define whether a target vessel is on the surface of the epicardium and easily accessible, intramural, or deep within the epicardial fat.[29] Pre-operative identification of accessible epicardial target vessels is critical for a successful endoscopic bypass procedure.

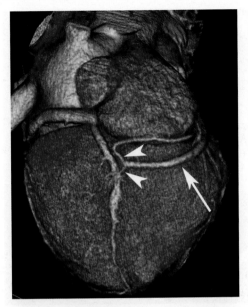

G

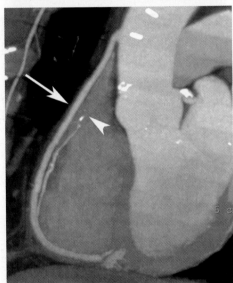

H

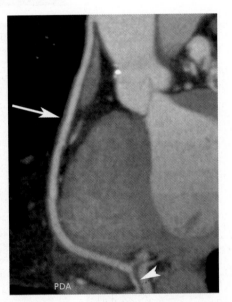

I

Fig. 8.16 (*Continued*) **(G)** Volumetric image of the crux of the heart clearly demonstrates the anastomosis of the vein graft (*arrow*) to the proximal posterior descending artery (PDA) (*arrowheads*). **(H)** MIP in the left anterior oblique projection demonstrates a proximal occlusion of the native RCA (*arrowhead*). The vein graft (*arrow*) courses parallel to the native RCA to the crux of the heart. The RCA is filled in a retrograde fashion from the vein graft to the PDA. (Also see Cine 8.3.) **(I)** MIP of the same graft in a slightly different projection demonstrates patency of the vein graft (*arrow*) as well as patency of its anastomosis to the PDA (*arrowhead*). (Also see Cine 8.5.)

The location of bypass graft origins along the ascending aorta should be visualized to avoid injury in exposing the aorta for cannulation or proximal anastomosis. The amount of free aorta available for graft anastomosis should also be evaluated. Severe calcification or atherosclerosis in the ascending aorta may preclude anastomosis of bypass grafts to the aorta or cross-clamping of the aorta for standard cardiopulmonary bypass. New bypass grafts may need to be anastomosed to existing patent grafts in such patients.

When aortic valve surgery is performed after CABG, the aorta must be transected, and occasionally grafts must be transected to achieve proper exposure of the valve. Pre-operative imaging should be used to select the optimal site for transection and to determine whether bypass grafts will need to be transected.

◆ Advantages of CT

Conventional pre-operative imaging of previous bypass patients includes a chest radiograph and coronary angiogram. These modalities provide a limited two-dimensional assessment of mediastinal anatomy. In planning for repeat bypass or valve surgery on a previous CABG, it is critical to have a three-dimensional sense of the operative field. Cardiac CT can provide volumetric images of the ascending aorta, native coronary anatomy, and bypass graft anatomy as needed. Other advantages of CT scanning include the ability to visualize difficult-to-catheterize areas such as gastroepiploic artery grafts (**Fig. 8.5**) and sequential bypass grafts, especially those originating from an IMA. CT can clearly visualize ostial lesions that may be difficult to demonstrate on conventional angiogram because of difficulty in positioning the catheter tip to visualize

Fig. 8.17 Maximum intensity projection (MIP) and volumetric images demonstrating aneurismal dilatation of a vein graft to the posterior descending artery (PDA). **(A)** Volumetric rendering demonstrates a graft extending from the aorta, just superior to the right coronary artery (RCA). A large aneurysm is present along the proximal aspect of the graft (*arrow*) with a bi-lobed aneurysm adjacent to the distal graft anastomosis (*arrowheads*). **(B)** Slab MIP demonstrates a stent within the graft, just proximal to a focus of aneurismal dilatation (*arrow*). Extensive thrombus is present in the aneurysm adjacent to the distal graft anastomosis (*arrowheads*). **(C)** Globe MIP demonstrates a large aneurysm (*arrow*) extending from the proximal aspect of a vein graft that runs parallel to the RCA. The relationship of the graft aneurysms to adjacent structures and the presence of thrombus within the aneurysms are clearly depicted on MIP and volumetric views.

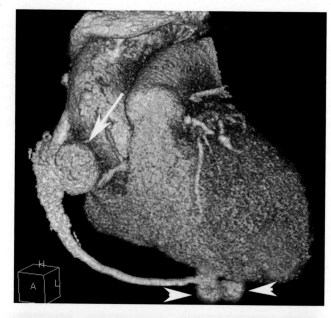

A

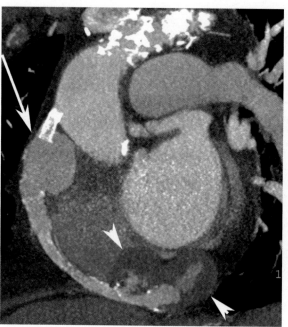

B

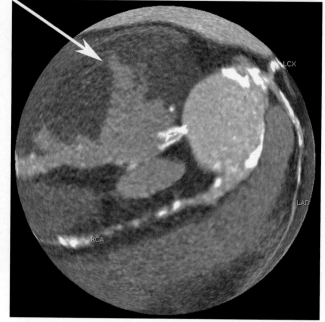

C

adequately an ostial lesion. Finally, CT imaging offers the unique ability to visualize ancillary or incidental findings in the thorax.

◆ Limitations of CT

To achieve quality coronary artery images with many current CT systems, it is ideal to have a stable heart rate in the range of 50 to 65 beats per minute. Patients with heart

failure may not tolerate β-blockers to reduce the heart rate. Patients who experience atrial fibrillation or frequent ectopy may have suboptimal study results. The latest generation of CT scanners with dual-source technology and faster gantry rotation times now provide improved temporal resolution that allows high-quality imaging in patients with mild tachycardia or arrhythmia.

Additional patient characteristics that limit CT imaging include allergy or intolerance to contrast medium, renal failure prohibiting the administration of contrast, and

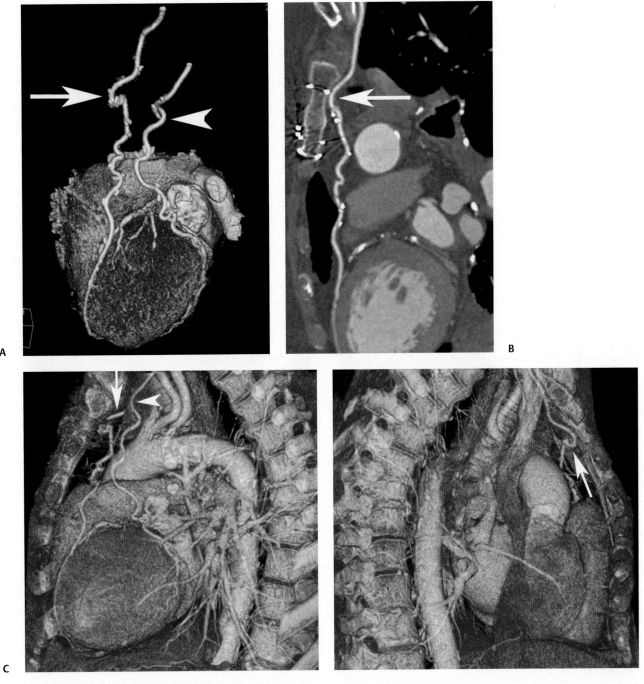

Fig. 8.18 Right internal mammary artery (RIMA) graft to the left anterior descending artery (LAD) and left internal mammary artery (LIMA) to an obtuse marginal branch of the circumflex. The RIMA graft courses immediately adjacent to the upper portion of the sternum, representing a significant risk for injury on "re-do" sternotomy. The surgical plan was changed based on this finding. **(A)** Volumetric image demonstrates the RIMA graft to the LAD (*arrow*) and the LIMA graft to the circumflex territory (*arrowhead*). **(B)** Tracked MIP image of the RIMA demonstrates the proximity of the RIMA to the upper sternum (*arrow*) at the level of the first sternal wire. **(C)** Volumetric image from the left side demonstrates both grafts. The RIMA graft (*arrow*) courses anteriorly in the upper chest and lies on the undersurface of the sternum. The LIMA graft (*arrowhead*) has a more posterior course. **(D)** Volumetric rendering from the right side demonstrates the proximity of the RIMA (*arrow*) to the undersurface of the sternum more clearly.

severe respiratory disease or heart failure. To obtain a complete coronary CT examination, including bypass grafts, patients must be able to hold their breath for about 15 seconds. Metallic clips associated with previous bypass surgery may result in streak artifact. These clips are often placed immediately adjacent to grafts, rendering evaluation of the graft lumen impossible. Finally, although cardiac CT is an excellent diagnostic modality, a separate procedure is needed for percutaneous intervention if an amenable lesion is found as opposed to a single procedure in the case of diagnostic catheterization with immediate angioplasty or stenting.

◆ Conclusion

Post-operative imaging is essential to the management of cardiac surgery patients. Cardiac CT provides a noninvasive modality for pre-operative planning of bypass surgery as well as post-operative evaluation of the symptomatic patient.[30] Cardiac CT provides the unique advantage of imaging flow within the coronary bypass grafts and native vessels as well as imaging the relationship between these vessels and surrounding structures. As the field of cardiac surgery advances, especially as the quest for improved minimally invasive techniques continues, it will be important for coronary imaging to provide the anatomic roadmap for these techniques. This is especially true as new and improved anastomotic devices are developed and as surgical procedures are performed with limited visual exposure.

Cine 8.1   Single bypass graft. Left internal mammary artery (LIMA) bypass to the left anterior descending artery (LAD). Surface-rendered cine begins in the anterior projection, demonstrating a LIMA bypass graft to the LAD. The heart rotates into an right anterior oblique projection to demonstrate the LIMA-LAD anastomosis and the dominant right coronary artery. Further rotation of the heart demonstrates small native circumflex branches. The larger proximal diagonal branches of the LAD are filled by retrograde flow from the LIMA bypass graft.

Cine 8.2   Single bypass graft. Left internal mammary artery (LIMA) bypass to the left anterior descending artery (LAD), diagonal branch, and distal right coronary artery (RCA). Surface-rendered cine begins in the anterior projection, demonstrating a LIMA bypass graft to the LAD. The heart is rotated into an left anterior oblique projection to demonstrate a jump graft from the LAD to the first (and only visible) diagonal branch. Further rotation of the heart demonstrates an additional jump graft that continues around the left ventricle to the crux, where it is anastomosed to the distal RCA.

Cine 8.3   Double bypass. Right internal mammary artery (RIMA) bypass to the left anterior descending artery (LAD) and the left internal mammary artery (LIMA) bypass to the obtuse marginal branch of the left circumflex artery (LCX). Surface-rendered cine begins in the anterior projection, demonstrating a RIMA bypass graft to the LAD. The heart then rotates into an left anterior oblique projection, demonstrating that the LIMA graft courses along the anterolateral wall of the left ventricle. The LIMA courses over the visible first obtuse marginal branch and terminates in an anastomosis with a poorly opacified (nonvisualized) second obtuse marginal branch. A normal right coronary artery is also visualized.

Cine 8.4   Triple bypass (see Fig. 8.12). Surface-rendered cine begins in the right anterior oblique projection, demonstrating a radial artery bypass graft. The heart is rotated to demonstrate the anastomosis of the radial artery to the distal right coronary artery near the crux. The heart is next rotated into an anterior projection, demonstrating a left internal mammary artery LIMA graft that crosses anterior to a right internal mammary artery (RIMA) graft to its anastomosis with the left anterior descending artery. Further rotation into the left anterior oblique projection demonstrates the anastomosis of the RIMA to a large obtuse marginal branch of the circumflex.

Cine 8.5   Triple bypass (see Fig. 8.16). Surface-rendered cine begins in the left lateral projection and demonstrates a vein graft to a ramus intermedius and to a distal obtuse marginal branch. As the heart turns, a left internal mammary artery bypass is seen to pass anterior to the vein graft with an anastomosis to the left anterior descending artery. As the heart turns into a right anterior oblique projection, a second vein graft is identified coursing along the right atrioventricular groove. The heart then rotates to demonstrate the crux. The second vein graft is anastomosed to the proximal posterior descending artery at the crux of the heart.

Cine 8.6   Triple bypass. Surface-rendered cine begins in an anterior projection and rotates into a left anterior oblique projection to demonstrate both a vein graft to the left anterior descending artery (LAD) and a left internal mammary artery (LIMA) graft to a small proximal diagonal branch from the LAD. An additional vein graft is demonstrated to course around the pulmonary artery just behind the LIMA and to continue to course around the left heart to the posterior descending artery.

References

1. Lau GT, Lowe HC, Kritharides L. Cardiac saphenous vein bypass graft disease. Semin Vasc Med. 2004;4(2):153–159

2. van Brussel BL, Voors AA, Ernst JM, Knaepen PJ, Plokker HW. Venous coronary artery bypass surgery: a more than 20-year follow-up study. Eur Heart J. 2003;24(10):927–936

3. Mack MJ, Osborne JA, Shennib H. Arterial graft patency in coronary artery bypass grafting: what do we really know? Ann Thorac Surg. 1998;66(3):1055–1059

4. Lytle BW, Blackstone EH, Loop FD, et al. Two internal thoracic artery grafts are better than one. J Thorac Cardiovasc Surg. 1999;117(5):855–872

5. Lytle BW, Blackstone EH, Sabik JF, Houghtaling P, Loop FD, Cosgrove DM. The effect of bilateral internal thoracic artery grafting on survival during 20 postoperative years. Ann Thorac Surg. 2004;78(6):2005–2012, discussion 2012–2014

6. Buxton BF, Raman JS, Ruengsakulrach P, et al. Radial artery patency and clinical outcomes: five-year interim results of a randomized trial. J Thorac Cardiovasc Surg. 2003;125(6):1363–1371

7. Carpentier A, Guermonprez JL, Deloche A, Frechette C, DuBost C. The aorta-to-coronary radial artery bypass graft: a technique avoiding pathological changes in grafts. Ann Thorac Surg. 1973;16(2):111–121

8. Nezić DG, Knezević AM, Milojević PS, et al. The fate of the radial artery conduit in coronary artery bypass grafting surgery. Eur J Cardiothorac Surg. 2006;30(2):341–346

9. Zacharias A, Habib RH, Schwann TA, Riordan CJ, Durham SJ, Shah A. Improved survival with radial artery versus vein conduits in coronary bypass surgery with left internal thoracic artery to left anterior descending artery grafting. Circulation. 2004;109(12):1489–1496

10. Possati G, Gaudino M, Prati F, et al. Long-term results of the radial artery used for myocardial revascularization. Circulation. 2003;108(11):1350–1354

11. Hadinata IE, Hayward PA, Hare DL, et al. Choice of conduit for the right coronary system: 8-year analysis of Radial Artery Patency and Clinical Outcomes trial. Ann Thorac Surg. 2009;88(5):1404–1409

12. Ropers D, Ulzheimer S, Wenkel E, et al. Investigation of aortocoronary artery bypass grafts by multislice spiral computed tomography with electrocardiographic-gated image reconstruction. Am J Cardiol. 2001;88(7):792–795

13. Gurevitch J, Gaspar T, Orlov B, et al. Noninvasive evaluation of arterial grafts with newly released multidetector computed tomography. Ann Thorac Surg. 2003;76(5):1523–1527

14. Chiurlia E, Menozzi M, Ratti C, Romagnoli R, Modena MG. Follow-up of coronary artery bypass graft patency by multislice computed tomography. Am J Cardiol. 2005;95(9):1094–1097

15. Martuscelli E, Romagnoli A, D'Eliseo A, et al. Evaluation of venous and arterial conduit patency by 16-slice spiral computed tomography. Circulation. 2004;110(20):3234–3238

16. Moore RK, Sampson C, MacDonald S, Moynahan C, Groves D, Chester MR. Coronary artery bypass graft imaging using ECG-gated multislice computed tomography: comparison with catheter angiography. Clin Radiol. 2005;60(9):990–998

17. Burgstahler C, Beck T, Kuettner A, et al. Non-invasive evaluation of coronary artery bypass grafts using 16-row multi-slice computed tomography with 188 ms temporal resolution. Int J Cardiol. 2006; 106(2):244–249

18. Salm LP, Bax JJ, Jukema JW, et al. Comprehensive assessment of patients after coronary artery bypass grafting by 16-detector-row computed tomography. Am Heart J. 2005;150(4):775–781

19. Wintersperger BJ, Bastarrika G, Nikolaou K, et al. [ECG-gated bypass CT angiography-application in imaging arterial bypasses]. Radiologe. 2004;44(2):140–145

20. Anders K, Baum U, Schmid M, et al. Coronary artery bypass graft (CABG) patency: assessment with high-resolution submillimeter 16-slice multidetector-row computed tomography (MDCT) versus coronary angiography. Eur J Radiol. 2006;57(3):336–344

21. Pache G, Saueressig U, Frydrychowicz A, et al. Initial experience with 64-slice cardiac CT: non-invasive visualization of coronary artery bypass grafts. Eur Heart J. 2006;27(8):976–980

22. Ropers D, Pohle FK, Kuettner A, et al. Diagnostic accuracy of noninvasive coronary angiography in patients after bypass surgery using 64-slice spiral computed tomography with 330-ms gantry rotation. Circulation. 2006;114(22):2334–2341, quiz 2334

23. Hamon M, Lepage O, Malagutti P, et al. Diagnostic performance of 16- and 64-section spiral CT for coronary artery bypass graft assessment: meta-analysis. Radiology. 2008;247(3):679–686

24. Malagutti P, Nieman K, Meijboom WB, et al. Use of 64-slice CT in symptomatic patients after coronary bypass surgery: evaluation of grafts and coronary arteries. Eur Heart J. 2007;28(15):1879–1885

25. Nieman K, Pattynama PM, Rensing BJ, Van Geuns RJ, De Feyter PJ. Evaluation of patients after coronary artery bypass surgery: CT angiographic assessment of grafts and coronary arteries. Radiology. 2003;229(3):749–756

26. Schlosser T, Konorza T, Hunold P, Kühl H, Schmermund A, Barkhausen J. Noninvasive visualization of coronary artery bypass grafts using 16-detector row computed tomography. J Am Coll Cardiol. 2004; 44(6):1224–1229

27. Aviram G, Mohr R, Sharony R, Medalion B, Kramer A, Uretzky G. Open heart reoperations after coronary artery bypass grafting: the role of preoperative imaging with multidetector computed tomography. Isr Med Assoc J. 2009;11(8):465–469

28. Gasparovic H, Rybicki FJ, Millstine J, et al. Three dimensional computed tomographic imaging in planning the surgical approach for redo cardiac surgery after coronary revascularization. Eur J Cardiothorac Surg. 2005;28(2):244–249

29. Herzog C, Dogan S, Diebold T, et al. Multi-detector row CT versus coronary angiography: preoperative evaluation before totally endoscopic coronary artery bypass grafting. Radiology. 2003;229(1): 200–208

30. Song MH, Ito T, Watanabe T, Nakamura H. Multidetector computed tomography versus coronary angiogram in evaluation of coronary artery bypass grafts. Ann Thorac Surg. 2005;79(2):585–588

9

Cardiac Morphology and Function

Ethan J. Halpern and Alyson N. Owen

Quantitative analysis of cardiac chamber geometry and ventricular function is an essential component of a complete cardiac evaluation. Many cardiac imaging studies—including echocardiography, nuclear scintigraphy, and cardiac magnetic resonance (MR) imaging—evaluate cardiac morphology and function. As part of a comprehensive cardiac imaging study, gated cardiac CT can provide an anatomically precise evaluation of chamber morphology and function, along with a detailed assessment of coronary anatomy and valves. With respect to chamber size, assessment of chamber enlargement is optimally performed with measurements indexed to body size.[1] As cardiac CT is a relatively young technology, however, there are few published studies that quantify CT measurements for the assessment of cardiac morphology and function. Most of the criteria provided in this chapter are based on accepted echocardiographic standards.[2]

Is it appropriate to use echocardiographic standards when interpreting cardiac CT? Linear measurements of cardiac wall thickness and chamber size, as well as global measures of left ventricular (LV) function by electrocardiographically (ECG)-gated CT demonstrate a high correlation with echocardiography.[3] However, several studies suggest that left atrial volume may be substantially underestimated by echocardiography compared with both CT[4,5] and MR.[6] Our own analysis suggests that volume measurements of the left atrium obtained during ECG-gated CT are approximately twice as large as the corresponding volumes calculated from transthoracic echocardiography with apical four-chamber and two-chamber measurements.[7] Although the discrepancy can be explained in part by geometric assumptions used for echocardiographic calculations, much of the discrepancy persists when the same echocardiographic formulas are applied to CT data. Our findings therefore suggest that underestimation of left atrial volume by transthoracic echocardiography is related primarily to foreshortening of the left atrium and suboptimal definition of the back wall of the atrium when visualized from the cardiac apex.

Based on our experience with cardiac CT and echocardiography, we believe that linear measurements of chamber size and wall thickness on CT correspond very well to conventional echocardiographic measurements obtained in the parasternal three-chamber view. There is no substantial foreshortening of anterior–posterior echocardiographic measurements in the parasternal view. CT measurements of ejection fraction also seem to correlate well with echocardiography.[8] Although we provide additional echocardiographic standards for chamber area and volume in **Table 9.1** that are generally calculated from apical views, the reader is cautioned that normative values for chamber area and volume on CT will be much larger than those defined by echocardiography. Further studies are needed to establish normative data for cardiac chamber volumes with ECG-gated CT and MR studies.

◆ Standard Imaging Views

To assess cardiac chamber morphology, size, and function, standard views that should be obtained include the four-chamber view, three-chamber view, two-chamber view, and short-axis projection. The three-chamber and five-chamber views are useful to assess the LV outflow tract (LVOT) and aortic valve. All of these views are typically created with a maximum intensity projection (MIP) technique with 2- to 5-mm slab MIPs. Normal values are available for chamber measurements obtained from these views (see **Table 9.1**). LV function should be reviewed in long axis (four-chamber view, three-chamber view, and two-chamber view) as well as short axis. Accurate calculation of LV volume and ejection fraction should be performed in two orthogonal long-axis planes or with short-axis views through the entire LV.

◆ Four-Chamber View

The four-chamber view provides an overview of all four cardiac chambers and allows a side-by-side comparison of the right-sided and left-sided chambers (**Fig. 9.1**). To obtain a four-chamber MIP, the heart is rotated along its short axis so that both the mitral and tricuspid valves are visible. Once both valves are optimally imaged, the image is rotated into the long axis of the heart to extend the

Table 9.1 Normal Values for Left-Sided Cardiac Measurements by Echocardiography

	Women	Men
LA dimension (systole)	2.7–3.8 cm	3.0–4.0 cm
LA area	≤20 cm³	≤20 cm³
LV dimension (diastole)	3.9–5.3 cm	4.2–5.9 cm
LV volume	56–104 cm³	67–155 cm³
LV volume/BSA	35–75 mL/m³	35–75 mL/m³
Ejection fraction	≥55%	≥55%
LV wall thickness (diastole)	0.6–0.9 cm	0.6–1.0 cm
LV mass	66–150 g	96–200 g
LV mass/BSA	44–88 g/m³	50–102 g/m³

Abbreviations: BSA, body surface area; LA, left atrium; LV, left ventricle.

Source: Adapted from Neilan TG, Pradhan AD, King ME, Weyman AE. Derivation of a size-independent variable for scaling of cardiac dimensions in a normal paediatric population. Eur J Echocardiogr 2009;10(1):50–55.

cardiac chambers and visualize the cardiac apex. The plane of this image is different from the standard axial image obtained on CT. A four-chamber view of the normal heart demonstrates that the cardiac apex is formed by the LV

and that the right-sided chamber diameters are smaller than the corresponding left-sided chamber diameters. In the four-chamber projection, the lateral wall of the LV is observed as the free wall, whereas the interventricular septum separates the two ventricles. The interatrial septum and interventricular septum may be evaluated in this view by scrolling superiorly and inferiorly. Diastolic and systolic frames in the four-chamber projection demonstrate normal motion of the atrioventricular valves, as well as normal thickening and contraction of the ventricular walls.

◆ Three-Chamber View

The three-chamber view demonstrates the LV, left atrium, and aortic root in one image (**Fig. 9.2**). As discussed in Chapter 10, the three-chamber view is required to assess for mitral valve prolapse. It is also the standard view (from the parasternal window) for echocardiographic M-mode assessment of the size of the LV, left atrium, and aortic root. This view is most easily obtained by identifying the shared portion of the annulus between the aortic and mitral valves—the mitral–aortic intervalvular fibrosa—on an axial image. The intervalvular fibrosa is selected as a fixed center of rotation. The heart is rotated around this point such that both the aortic and mitral valves are visualized, and the LV is elongated to image the apex of the heart. The aorta and left atrium are demonstrated above the LV. The anteroseptal wall is ipsilateral to the aortic valve; the inferolateral wall

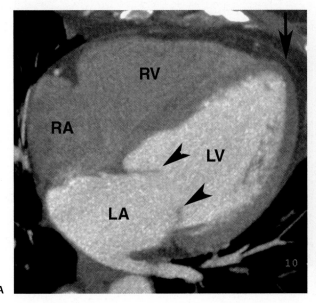
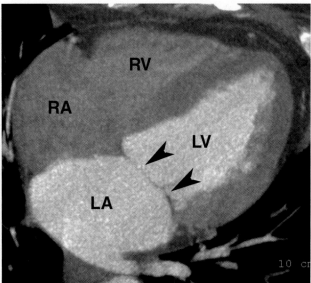

A   B

Fig. 9.1 Four-chamber view of the heart. **(A)** Four-chamber view in diastole. The four-chamber view is obtained in a plane that passes through both the mitral and tricuspid valves and demonstrates the cardiac apex. The open mitral valve (*arrowheads*) is identified between the left atrium (LA), and left ventricle (LV). The tricuspid valve is present between the right atrium (RA), and right ventricle (RV) but is not well visualized because a saline flush was used to clear contrast out of the

right side of the heart. The cardiac apex is formed by the tip of the left ventricle (*arrow*). Although the RV volume is slightly greater than the LV volume, the width of the LV appears greater on the four-chamber view. **(B)** Four-chamber view in systole. The ventricles have contracted and appear smaller. The mitral valve is in a closed position (*arrowheads*). The atria appear larger at end systole because atrial filling occurs during systole.

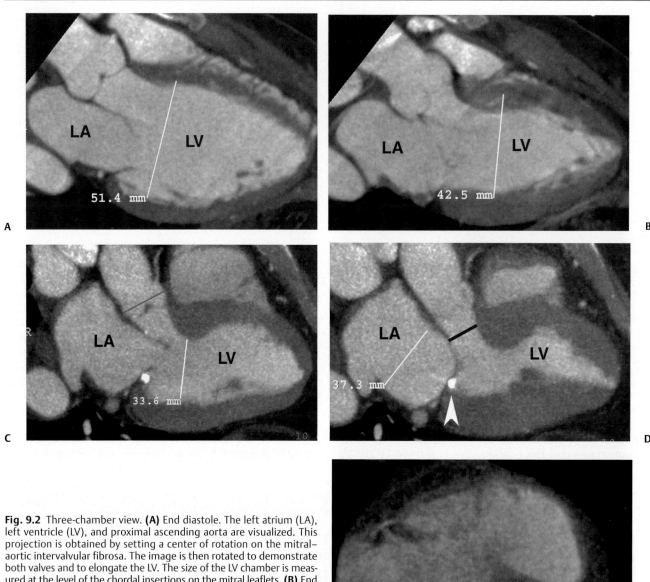

Fig. 9.2 Three-chamber view. **(A)** End diastole. The left atrium (LA), left ventricle (LV), and proximal ascending aorta are visualized. This projection is obtained by setting a center of rotation on the mitral–aortic intervalvular fibrosa. The image is then rotated to demonstrate both valves and to elongate the LV. The size of the LV chamber is measured at the level of the chordal insertions on the mitral leaflets. **(B)** End systole. The LV has contracted. The LA is slightly larger during systole, but it is clearly within normal limits. The aortic and mitral valves are suboptimally visualized because of systolic heart motion. **(C)** End diastole in a second individual. Once again, the LV chamber size is measured just below the open mitral valve. The aortic valve is in a closed position. The aortic root is measured above the level of the aortic valve (*bar*). **(D)** End systole. The LV has now contracted, and the mitral valve is in the closed position. A calcification is identified in the posterior mitral annulus (*arrowhead*). Posterior mitral annular calcification is a common finding. LA size is measured in the three-chamber view at end systole at the level of the aortic root. The LV outflow tract (LVOT) is marked below the level of the aortic valve (*bar*). **(E)** Short-axis view of the LVOT with anteroposterior and transverse measurement (*bars*). The LVOT often has a mildly oval shape.

(formerly known as the posterior wall) is ipsilateral to the left atrium.

The LV diameter is measured on the three-chamber view at the level of the chordal attachments just below the tips of the mitral leaflets (**Fig. 9.2**). The aortic root is typically measured at the level of the sinuses of Valsalva,

just above the aortic valve, although measurement of the diameter at the sinotubular junction may also be useful. The left atrium is measured along its minor axis (anteroposterior dimension), in a plane that is roughly parallel to the aortic root. This convention derives from M-mode data, although now measurements will frequently be performed on the two-dimensional image. The maximum diameters of the LV and the aortic root are measured at end diastole; the maximum diameter of the left atrium is measured at end systole. Normal values for the left atrium and ventricle are presented in **Table 9.1**. The expected aortic root diameter is slightly smaller than the left atrium diameter. Published equations are available that relate the precise limits of normal aortic root diameter to age and body surface area.[9]

The LVOT diameter is traditionally measured at midsystole in the (parasternal) three-chamber view, just below the plane of the aortic valve, at the level of the insertion points of the aortic valve leaflets (**Fig. 9.2D**). This measurement is used for echocardiographic calculation of aortic valve area with the continuity equation. Measurement errors in the echocardiographic assessment of LVOT diameter are a common cause of errors in calculation of aortic valve area, particularly because any measurement error is compounded by its squaring to obtain area. A more accurate estimate of the true LVOT area may be obtained with a two-dimensional CT cross-section of the LVOT. To visualize the LVOT in cross-section, an MIP is created in the short axis of the aortic valve and stepped caudally to demonstrate the short axis of the LVOT (**Fig. 9.2E**).

◆ Two-Chamber View

The two-chamber projection demonstrates only the left atrium and LV, with the mitral valve separating these two chambers (**Fig. 9.3**). The right-sided chambers and the aorta are not visible in this projection. Starting with a four-chamber or a three-chamber view, the two-chamber view is obtained by setting the center of rotation at the center of the mitral valve and rotating the image so that the right–sided chambers and aorta are no longer visible. As with the four-chamber and three-chamber views, the imaging plane is adjusted to maximize the length of the LV and to demonstrate the LV apex. The two-chamber projection demonstrates the inferior wall of the LV along the diaphragm. The anterior wall is opposite the inferior wall.

◆ Five-Chamber View

The four-chamber, three-chamber, and two-chamber views are obtained by rotating the imaging plane in the true long axis of the LV. Each of these views is rotated about 60 degrees from the adjacent view to provide a complete picture of the LV walls for assessment of function. The five-chamber projection is tilted away from the true long axis of the four-chamber view to provide an additional assessment of the LVOT and aortic valve (**Fig. 9.4**). The five-chamber view is obtained from the four-chamber view by setting the center of rotation on the cardiac apex and tilting the base of the heart in a cranial direction to demonstrate the aortic root. As with the four-chamber view, this view demonstrates the septum and the lateral walls of the LV, although the portion of the septum that is demonstrated is more anterior than that seen in the four-chamber view.

◆ Atrial Anatomy

The two atria serve as antechambers for blood entering into their respective ventricles. The left atrium is the most superior and the most posterior of all four cardiac chambers. Inflow from the left atrium to the LV is directed in an anterior–inferior–leftward direction through the mitral valve into the LV. The right atrium is anterior, to the right, and inferior relative to the left atrium. A thin septum separates the right and left atria. The tricuspid valve is located on the anterior or left aspect of the right atrium. The right ventricular inflow (tricuspid valve) and right ventricular outflow (infundibulum to pulmonic valve) form an arc anterior to the aortic valve, perpendicular to the long axis of aortic outflow; both the tricuspid and pulmonic valves are visible along this arc on a short-axis image through the aortic valve.

Atrial diastole, the time during which the two atria fill with blood, corresponds to ventricular systole. In normal sinus rhythm, the atria distend to their maximum volume

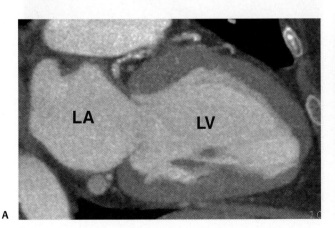
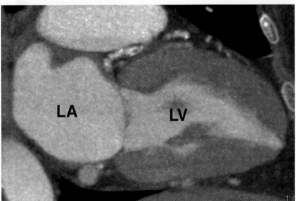

A   B

Fig. 9.3 Two-chamber view obtained by setting a center of rotation on the mitral valve and rotating the heart so that the right ventricle and aorta are no longer visible. As with the four-chamber and three-chamber views, rotation is performed to elongate the left ventricle (LV) and display the apex of the heart. **(B)** Two-chamber view in systole. The mitral valve is now closed. LA, left atrium.

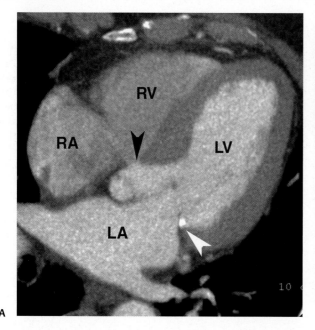

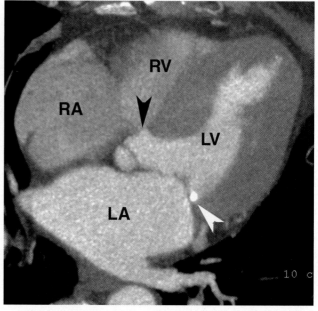

Fig. 9.4 (A) Five-chamber view in diastole. The four-chamber view is angled cranially to display the root of the aorta (*black arrowhead*) in addition to the four cardiac chambers. Posterior mitral annular calcification is identified (*white arrowhead*). **(B)** Five-chamber view in systole. RV, right ventricle; RA, right atrium; LA, left atrium; LV, left ventricle.

during ventricular systole. Rapid ventricular filling in early diastole results from active relaxation of the ventricles, as well as elastic recoil from the force of systolic contraction. Additional ventricular filling in late diastole is related to active contraction of the atria (atrial systole). To obtain a consistent and accurate measurement of atrial size, atrial measurements should be obtained at end systole (**Fig. 9.2**).

The right and left atria demonstrate narrow anterior extensions, the atrial appendages, which are visible on the surface of the heart (**Figs. 9.5** and **9.6**). The right atrial appendage is a relatively flat triangular structure that

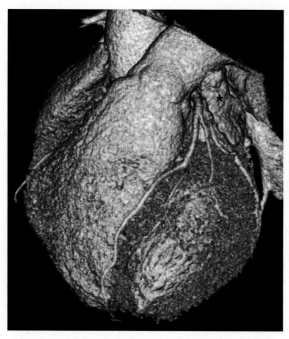

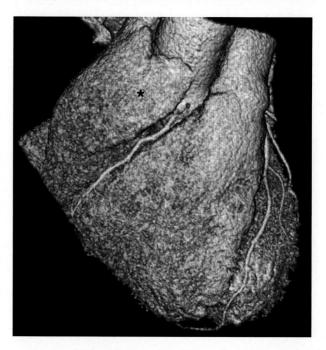

Fig. 9.5 Atrial appendages. **(A)** Surface-rendered image in the left anterior oblique projection demonstrates the left atrial appendage (*). The left atrial appendage often obscures the underlying proximal circumflex and left main coronary arteries. **(B)** Surface-rendered view in the anterior projection demonstrates the right atrial appendage (*). The right coronary artery is clearly visible in this case just below the atrial appendage.

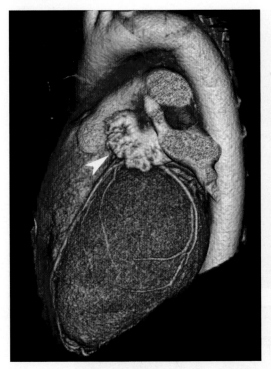
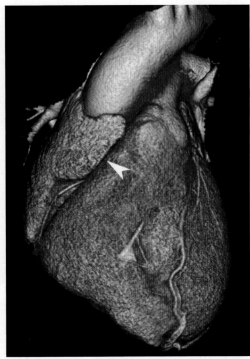

A   B

Fig. 9.6 Atrial appendages. **(A)** Left anterior oblique surface-rendered image demonstrates the left atrial appendage (*arrowhead*), which overlies the origin of both the circumflex and left anterior descending arter- ies. **(B)** Anterior surface rendered projection demonstrates the right atrial appendage (*arrowhead*), which overlies the origin of the right coronary artery.

extends anteriorly over the right anterior surface of the heart. The anterior margin of this appendage often covers the proximal right coronary artery in the right atrioventricular (AV) groove. The left atrial appendage is a crescent-shaped structure that extends anteriorly from the left atrium, covering the left AV groove, and terminating over the junction of the left AV groove with the anterior interventricular groove. The left atrial appendage often covers the left main coronary artery, as well as the origin of the circumflex and left anterior descending artery. The left atrial appendage may have a more complex configuration with accessory lobes. Both atrial appendages contain trabecular fibers known as pectinate muscles.

◆ Right Atrium

As the antechamber for the right ventricle, the right atrium receives inflow from the superior vena cava (SVC), the inferior vena cava (IVC), and the coronary sinus. The SVC enters the roof of the right atrium between the base of the right atrial appendage and the superior margin of the interatrial septum. The IVC enters the posterolateral portion of the floor of the right atrium along the inferior margin of the interatrial septum. The smooth-walled sinus venosus portion of the right atrium extends between the orifices of the SVC and IVC. The coronary sinus crosses the crux of the heart from the left AV groove to enter the inferior aspect of the right atrium adjacent to the inferior

margin of the interatrial septum. Although both the IVC and coronary sinus enter the right atrium along the inferior margin of the interatrial septum, the orifice of the coronary sinus is slightly more anterior and to the left, closer to the tricuspid annulus and to the crux of the heart.

Anatomic variations of normal right atrial anatomy can mimic the presence of a mass. A ridge of muscle along the right side of the right atrium, the crista terminalis, extends from the IVC orifice up to the SVC orifice. The crista terminalis separates the smooth sinus venosus portion of the right atrium from the more anterior trabeculated right atrial appendage (**Fig. 9.7**). The crista terminalis has a variable thickness and can appear masslike within the right atrium.[10] The sulcus terminalis is a subtle groove on the epicardial surface of the heart corresponding to the crista terminalis. The sinoatrial node is located in the sulcus terminalis.

The Chiari network consists of long fibers that extend from the crista terminalis to the eustachian valve. These fibers may interfere with device placement during a percutaneous interventional procedure and are a potential, although infrequent, site of right atrial thrombus or attachment of an embolus in transit. Pectinate muscles along the right atrial appendage and along the free wall of the right atrium can appear prominent and can mimic the presence of thrombus. Lipomatous hypertrophy of the interatrial septum (see below) bulges preferentially into the right atrium and may be associated with thickening of the crista terminalis. The typical location, shape, and density of these

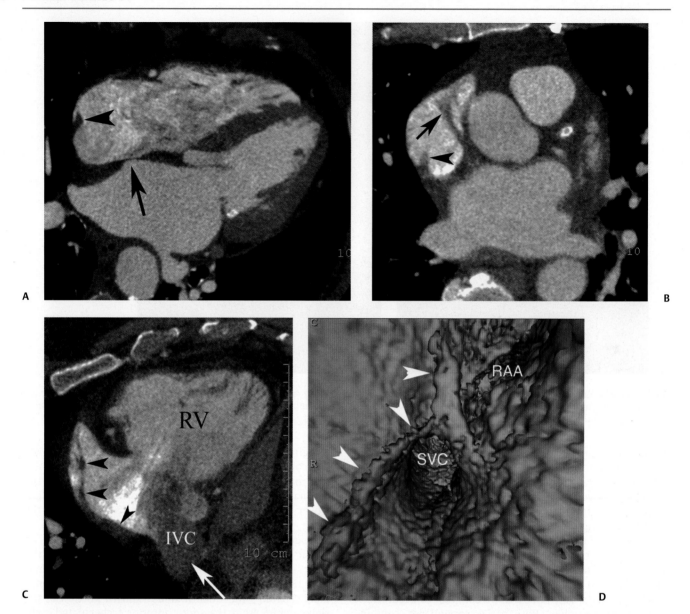

Fig. 9.7 Right atrial anatomy: crista terminalis and pectinate muscles. **(A)** Four-chamber view at the level of the fossa ovalis (*arrow*) demonstrates the crista terminalis as a ridge along the right side of the right atrium (*arrowhead*). **(B)** Axial maximum intensity projection through the superior right atrium and atrial appendage demonstrates continuation of the crista terminalis (*arrowhead*) to the level of the appendage as well as pectinate muscle bundles (*arrow*) within the appendage. **(C)** Right ventricular (RV) inflow view demonstrates continuity of the crista terminalis (*arrowheads*) from the lower portion of the right atrium adjacent to the inferior vena cava (IVC) orifice up to the atrial appendage. Unopacified blood enters the right atrium from the IVC (*arrow*). **(D)** Endoluminal view demonstrates the crista terminalis (*arrowheads*) as it passes adjacent to the superior vena cava (SVC) and passes into the base of the right atrial appendage (RAA).

anatomic structures distinguish them from intracardiac tumor or thrombus (**Fig. 9.8**).[11]

The eustachian valve is an embryologic remnant that presents as a flap of variable thickness and mobility along the orifice of the IVC and may continue as a ridge along the right atrium. The cavotricuspid isthmus is the part of the right atrium between the ostium of the IVC, the eustachian ridge, and the tricuspid valve. This area is important in the management of certain arrhythmias, most notably atrial flutter. In theory the eustachian valve or ridge might present as a small defect along the right atrium.

In practice, however, the eustachian valve and ridge are not easily identified by CT because of the inflow of unopacified blood from the IVC.

◆ Left Atrium

As the antechamber for the LV, the left atrium receives inflow from the pulmonary veins. Anatomic variation in the drainage of the pulmonary veins into the left atrium is discussed in detail in Chapter 11. Left atrial size has been

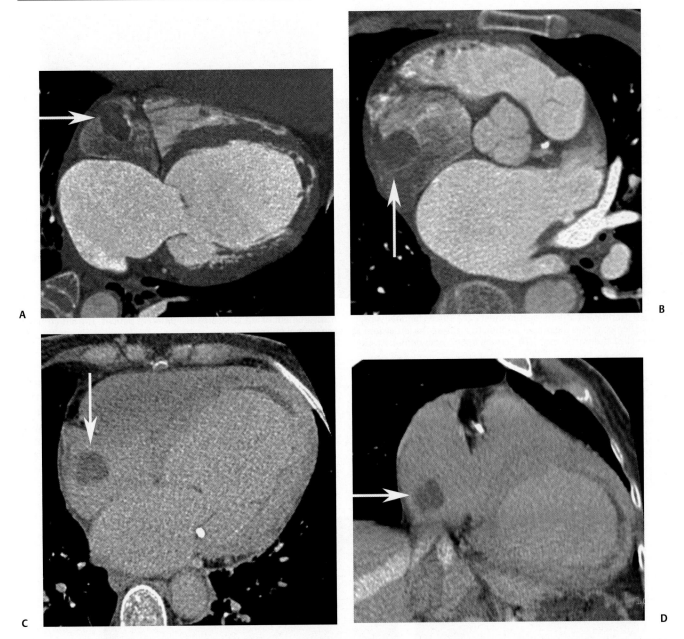

Fig. 9.8 Right atrial thrombus. **(A)** Four-chamber view in the arterial phase demonstrates a hypodense mass attached to the low anterior wall of the right atrium and outlined by contrast (*arrow*). **(B)** Short-axis image again demonstrates the right atrial mass (*arrow*). **(C)** Four-chamber view in a delayed phase demonstrates that there is no enhancement of the mass (*arrow*). **(D)** Delayed view demonstrates that the mass is just above the insertion of the inferior vena cava into the right atrium. Right atrial thrombus is often related to the presence of a catheter in the superior vena cava. This patient had a right atrial catheter recently removed. Follow-up magnetic resonance imaging demonstrated shrinkage of the mass with anticoagulation, confirming that it represented a thrombus.

traditionally reported by a single diameter measurement on the three-chamber view. More recent echocardiographic studies suggest that atrial volumes, calculated from four-chamber and two-chamber views, provide a more clinically relevant estimate of chamber size compared with one-dimensional measurements of atrial diameter or two-dimensional measurements of atrial area.[12,13] Area measurements of the left atrium can be quantified on the four-chamber view (**Fig. 9.9**) and on the two-chamber view. These areas can be converted to a volume measurement via the area-length equation: $8/3\pi\,[(A1)(A2)/L]$, where A1 and A2 are the areas from the four- and two-chamber views, respectively, and L is the shortest inferior–superior length from the annular plane to the back wall of the atrium. However, as noted in the introduction to this chapter, normative values for atrial volumes computed from apical four-chamber and two-chamber views by echocardiography underestimate the volumes measured by cardiac CT. Thus, although we believe it is

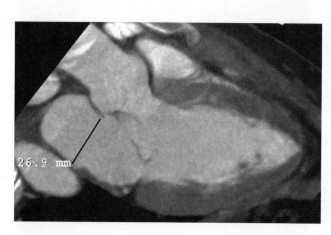

A

B

Fig. 9.9 Normal left atrium measurements. **(A)** Three-chamber view in systole demonstrates the proper position to measure the left atrium at the level of the aortic root. **(B)** Four-chamber view demonstrating measurement of left atrial area in a different patient. The left atrium is top normal in size.

important to assess chamber morphology on CT in standard echocardiographic projections, one must be careful not to overcall chamber enlargement based on published echocardiographic standards for chamber volume. Enlargement of the left atrium may be suggested when the atrium appears larger than the adjacent aortic root in the three-chamber view (**Fig. 9.10A**) or when the left atrium appears large relative to the LV on the four-chamber view (**Fig. 9.10B**).

Left atrial dilatation is associated with many disease processes, including LV failure, hypertension, and mitral valve disease. A dilated left atrium may be present in association with atrial fibrillation, both as a contributing cause and as a consequence of atrial fibrillation. Clot may form in a dilated left atrium, most commonly within the left atrial appendage (**Fig. 9.11**). Left atrial thrombus may result in embolic complications, including stroke.

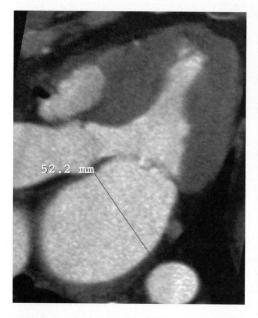

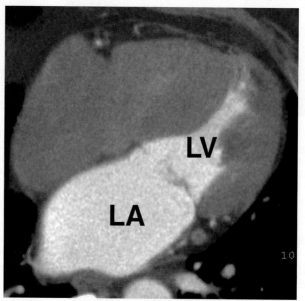

A

B

Fig. 9.10 Left atrial (LA) enlargement. **(A)** Three-chamber view in systole demonstrates measurement of the LA at the level of the aortic root. LA size of 5.2 cm suggests at least moderate dilatation of the LA. **(B)** Four-chamber view through the heart in systole again demonstrates enlargement of the LA. The LA area can be measured in the four-chamber view, but there are no established criteria for a single linear measurement of the left atrium in this projection. LV, left ventricle.

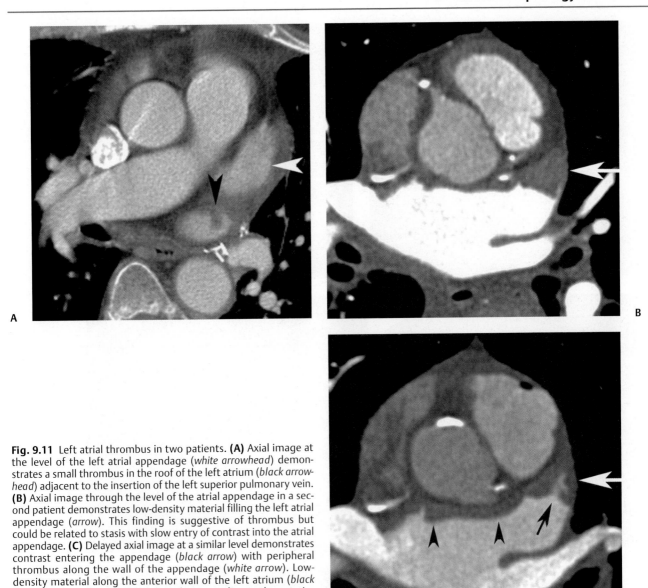

Fig. 9.11 Left atrial thrombus in two patients. **(A)** Axial image at the level of the left atrial appendage (*white arrowhead*) demonstrates a small thrombus in the roof of the left atrium (*black arrowhead*) adjacent to the insertion of the left superior pulmonary vein. **(B)** Axial image through the level of the atrial appendage in a second patient demonstrates low-density material filling the left atrial appendage (*arrow*). This finding is suggestive of thrombus but could be related to stasis with slow entry of contrast into the atrial appendage. **(C)** Delayed axial image at a similar level demonstrates contrast entering the appendage (*black arrow*) with peripheral thrombus along the wall of the appendage (*white arrow*). Low-density material along the anterior wall of the left atrium (*black arrowheads*) represents mural thrombus extending to the anterior wall of the left atrium. When there is uncertainty about whether the low density represents thrombus versus stagnant flow, a delayed scan may be useful to clarify the diagnosis.

◆ Atrial Septum

The interatrial septum is a thin-walled structure between the right and left atria. The interatrial septum develops from two separate structures, the septum primum and the septum secundum. The septum primum develops first and extends toward the AV junction. The gap that is present during development between the septum primum and the AV junction is called the *ostium primum*. As the septum primum closes this gap, a series of fenestrations within the septum primum coalesce into the ostium secundum. The septum secundum then grows to the right of the septum primum to cover this ostium secundum. During fetal life, a connection between the atria remains as an oblique pathway that courses between the septum primum and septum secundum and through the ostium secundum, taking oxygenated blood from the placenta to the systemic circulation, bypassing the pulmonary circuit. This pathway, the foramen ovale, generally closes after birth. However, the resultant fossa ovalis may be visible as an area of thinning within the interatrial septum (**Fig. 9.12A**). In patients with incomplete fusion of the septum primum to the septum secundum, the residual space between the septum primum and septum secundum may be visible on imaging (**Fig. 9.12B**). A redundancy of the interatrial septum is often present at the level of the fossa ovalis (**Fig. 9.12C**). When this redundancy is large, the finding is called an *interatrial septal aneurysm* (**Fig. 9.12D,E**). Atrial septal aneurysms are

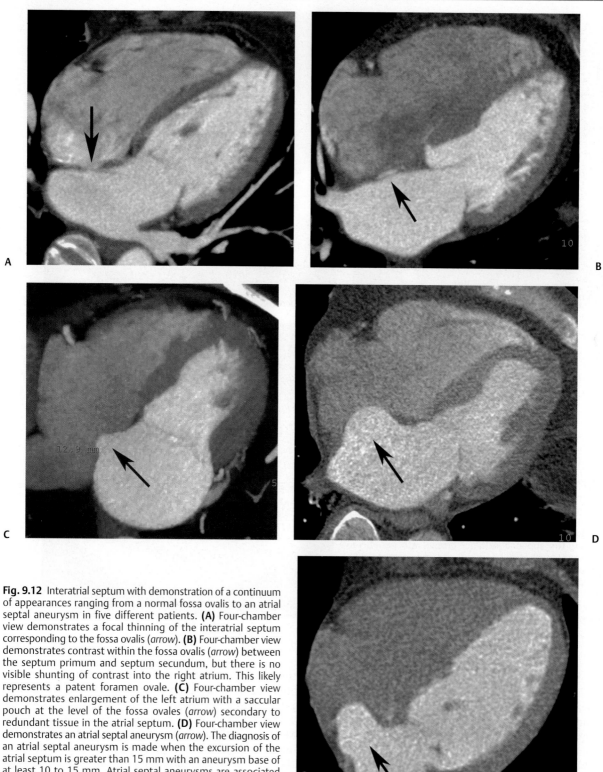

Fig. 9.12 Interatrial septum with demonstration of a continuum of appearances ranging from a normal fossa ovalis to an atrial septal aneurysm in five different patients. **(A)** Four-chamber view demonstrates a focal thinning of the interatrial septum corresponding to the fossa ovalis (*arrow*). **(B)** Four-chamber view demonstrates contrast within the fossa ovalis (*arrow*) between the septum primum and septum secundum, but there is no visible shunting of contrast into the right atrium. This likely represents a patent foramen ovale. **(C)** Four-chamber view demonstrates enlargement of the left atrium with a saccular pouch at the level of the fossa ovales (*arrow*) secondary to redundant tissue in the atrial septum. **(D)** Four-chamber view demonstrates an atrial septal aneurysm (*arrow*). The diagnosis of an atrial septal aneurysm is made when the excursion of the atrial septum is greater than 15 mm with an aneurysm base of at least 10 to 15 mm. Atrial septal aneurysms are associated with acquired and congenital heart disease, as well as with cardioembolic events. **(E)** Four-chamber view demonstrates an atrial septal aneurysm (*arrow*).

diagnosed when the septum protrudes 11 mm off the midline or demonstrates a total excursion of 15 mm during the cardiac cycle.[14] Atrial septal aneurysms are associated with an increased incidence of thromboembolic events, with the presence of a patent foramen ovale (PFO) (**Fig. 9.13**), and with small perforations in the atrial septum associated with interatrial shunting (see **Fig. 14.3**).

Lipomatous hypertrophy of the interatrial septum is increasingly recognized with CT of the heart (**Fig. 9.14**) and can present as an area of increased 2-fluoro-2-deoxyglucose (FDG) uptake during positron emission tomography (**Fig. 9.15**).[15] Lipomatous hypertrophy consists of unencapsulated mature adipose cells that proliferate within the

interatrial septum. This entity was first described in 1964.[16] In a prospective study using CT, lipomatous hypertrophy was identified in 2.2% of the patients.[17] Lipomatous hypertrophy is associated with obesity and is seen more frequently in older patients. The diagnosis of lipomatous hypertrophy of the interatrial septum is based on a characteristic fat density with thickening of the interatrial septum in a dumb-bell shape that spares the fossa ovalis. Lipomatous hypertrophy is generally a benign entity, although it may be associated with supraventricular arrhythmia and, in singular cases, with sudden death.[18] Rarely, lipomatous hypertrophy may present with SVC obstruction or intractable arrhythmia (**Fig. 9.14D**).[19]

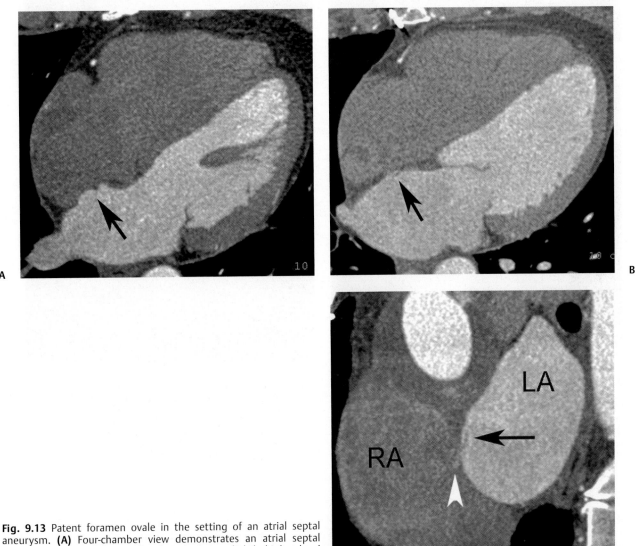

Fig. 9.13 Patent foramen ovale in the setting of an atrial septal aneurysm. **(A)** Four-chamber view demonstrates an atrial septal aneurysm (*arrow*). **(B)** Four-chamber view at a slightly higher level demonstrates a small flap related to the unfused end of the septum primum (*arrow*). **(C)** Oblique sagittal view of the left atrium (LA) and right atrium (RA) demonstrates the flap of the septum primum (*arrow*) as well as a small jet of contrast entering the RA (*arrowhead*). IVC, inferior vena cava.

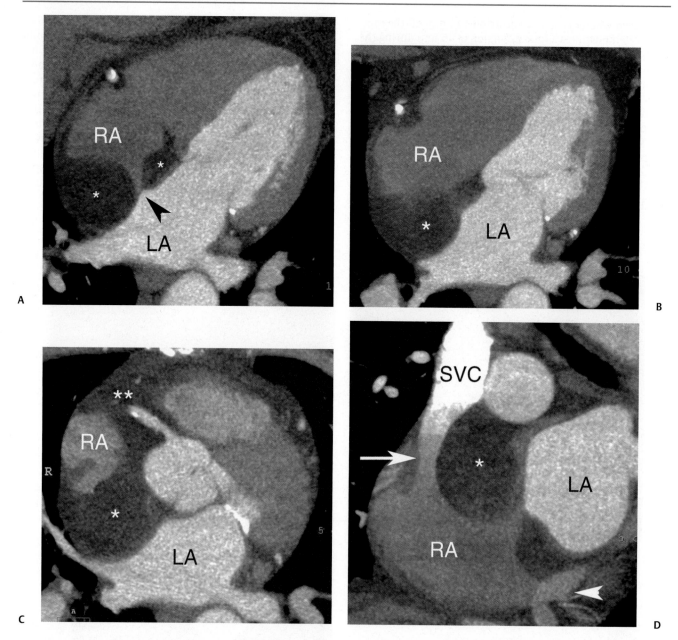

Fig. 9.14 Lipomatous hypertrophy of the interatrial septum with mass effect. **(A)** Four-chamber view at the level of the fossa ovalis demonstrates lipomatous tissue infiltrating the septum (*) between the right (RA) and left atria (LA) with sparing of the fossa ovalis (*arrow*head). **(B)** Four-chamber view above the level of the fossa ovalis demonstrates low-density material infiltrating the entire interatrial septum (*). **(C)** Slab maximum intensity projection (MIP) at a higher level demonstrates extensive lipomatous infiltration around the RA (*) extending into the right atrioventricular groove around the right coronary artery (**). The RA is compressed by the lipomatous tissue. **(D)** Sagittal MIP demonstrates lipomatous infiltration (*) that narrows the lumen of the superior vena cava (SVC) (*arrow*). However, the infiltration respects the fossa ovalis, which is not involved. The coronary veins are seen to enter the inferior aspect of the RA via the coronary sinus (*arrowhead*).

◆ Foramen Ovale

The patent foramen ovale is a hemodynamically insignificant communication between the right and left atria at the level of the fossa ovalis. The foramen ovale normally closes spontaneously after birth. However, a probe PFO may be present in upward of 25% of the adult population.[20] A probe PFO is not generally associated with an intracardiac shunt,[21] but it may be detected echocardiographically with a Valsalva maneuver during injection of agitated saline. A PFO is prone to serve as a conduit for paradoxical right-to-left embolization. Paradoxical embolism is often cited as one possible cause of ischemic stroke.[22] Clinical studies suggest an increased prevalence of migraine headaches with aura in

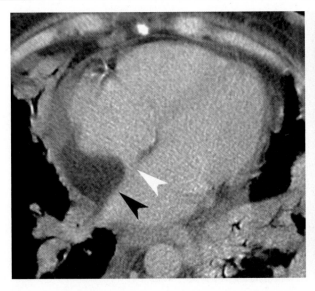

A

Fig. 9.15 Lipomatous hypertrophy within the interatrial septum. **(A)** The lipomatous tissue (*black arrowhead*) in the septum has a characteristic appearance of a low-density area of infiltration within the septum, respecting the fossa ovalis (*white arrowhead*). **(B)** 2-Fluoro-2-deoxyglucose

B

(FDG)-positron emission tomography demonstrates the presence of increased metabolic activity corresponding to the site of lipomatous hypertrophy (*arrow*). It is important to recognize this finding to avoid false-positive interpretations related to lipomatous hypertrophy.

patients with a PFO.[23] Trials are currently under way to evaluate the efficacy of PFO closure for prevention of migraine headaches and for secondary prevention of embolic stroke. The site of a PFO may be visible on cardiac CT (**Fig. 9.16**), but interatrial shunting is uncommonly demonstrated. PFO can be differentiated from an atrial septal defect (ASD) based on its tunneled intraseptal course (**Fig. 9.12B**) or the presence of a flap valve on the left atrial side of the foramen, representing the free margin of the septum primum that overlaps the septum secundum

(**Figs. 9.13** and **9.16**).[24,25] The shunt from a PFO is generally directed toward the orifice of the IVC (**Fig. 9.16C** and see **Fig. 16.1E**).

◆ Intracardiac Shunts

Intracardiac shunts found in the adult include ASDs, ventricular septal defects (VSDs), partial anomalous pulmonary venous return (PAPVR), and patent ductus arteriosus (PDA).

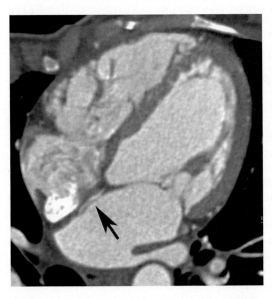

A

B

Fig. 9.16 Patient foramen ovale (PFO). **(A)** Four-chamber view in diastole demonstrates a patent tunnel within the interatrial septum between the septum primum and septum secundum (*arrow*).

(B) Oblique sagittal view of the left atrium (LA) and right atrium (RA) demonstrates the flap of the septum primum on the LA side of the PFO (*arrow*). (*Continued on page 188*)

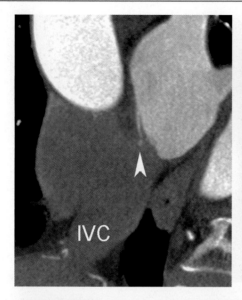

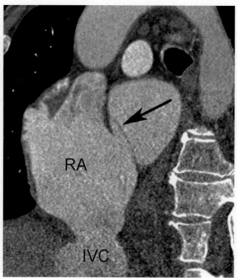

C

D

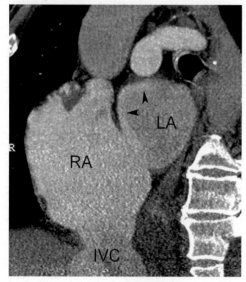

E

Fig. 9.16 (*Continued*) Patient foramen ovale (PFO). **(C)** Oblique sagittal view in a second patient demonstrates that the left-to-right shunt through the PFO is directed inferiorly (*arrowhead*) toward the orifice of the inferior vena caval (IVC). **(D)** Oblique sagittal view in a third patient with elevation of right-sided pressures (Eisenmenger physiology) demonstrates the flap of the septum primum on the LA side of the PFO (*arrow*) as well as a dilated RA. **(E)** Similar view during reinjection of contrast into the RA demonstrates right-to-left shunting of contrast through the foramen ovale and along the superior aspect of the LA (*arrowheads*).

Intracardiac shunts generally result in flow from the high (systemic) pressure left-sided circulation into the lower (pulmonary) pressure right-sided circulation. Increased flow related to intracardiac shunts results in volume overload and dilatation of the right side of the heart (**Figs. 9.18, 9.19, 9.20, 9.21, 9.22, 9.23, 9.24, 9.25, 9.26, 9.27, 9.28, 9.29, 9.30,** and **9.31**). PDA is associated with increased blood flow through both sides of the heart and results in dilatation of the LV along with right-sided chamber dilatation. Elevation of pulmonary pressure is initially related to increased volume without a change in pulmonary resistence; but when a shunt of sufficient volume persists for an extended period, increased pulmonary resistance may result as well. Once right-sided pressures are elevated beyond the left-sided pressures, Eisenmenger physiology develops with reversal of shunt flow from the right-sided circulation into the left-sided circulation and an associated decrease in left-sided oxygen saturation.

◆ Atrial Septal Defect

ASDs are present in about 10% of newborns with congenital heart disease and are also encountered in adults. Most small ASDs (<8 mm in diameter) diagnosed in the first 3 months of life will close spontaneously before 18 months of age.[26] Larger ASDs do not generally close spontaneously and may persist into adult life.

ASDs are classified based on location. The ostium secundum defect, located in the midportion of the interatrial septum, accounts for 50 to 75% of ASDs (**Figs. 9.17, 9.18, 9.19,** and **9.20**). An ostium primum defect, located adjacent to the AV valve plane, accounts for about 15 to 30% of defects. This type of defect is often associated with endocardial cushion defects and may be associated with abnormalities of the AV valves, including cleft anterior mitral leaflet and mitral regurgitation. Ostium primum ASD is a cardiac anomaly associated with Down syndrome. The

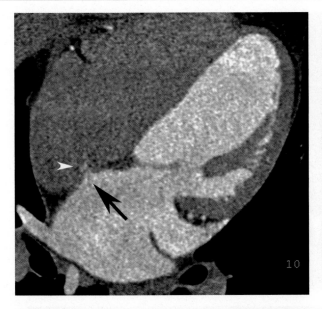

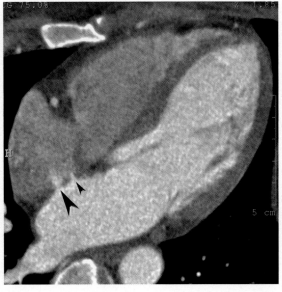

Fig. 9.17 Small ostium secundum atrial septal defects (ASDs). **(A)** Four-chamber view demonstrates thinning of the atrial septum at the level of the foramen ovale (*black arrow*). Subtle left-to-right shunting of contrast is visible through this portion of the septum (*white arrow*). **(B)** Four-chamber view in a second patient demonstrates normal-sized cardiac chambers with two defects in the atrial septum (*arrowheads*). The recognition of multiple defects or a fenestrated ASD can be important if the patient is to have successful percutaneous repair of the ASD (Chapter 12).

next most common subtype of ASD is the sinus venosus ASD. Most sinus venosus ASDs are located in the upper septum adjacent to the entrance of the SVC (**Figs. 9.21, 9.22, and 9.23**). These superior sinus venosus defects are often associated with a superior SVC that overrides both atria and

anomalous drainage of the superior right pulmonary vein into the SVC. Rarely, a sinus venosus ASD may be located in the inferior portion of the interatrial septum, adjacent to the IVC (**Fig. 9.24**). An inferior sinus venosus ASD is not generally associated with anomalous pulmonary venous

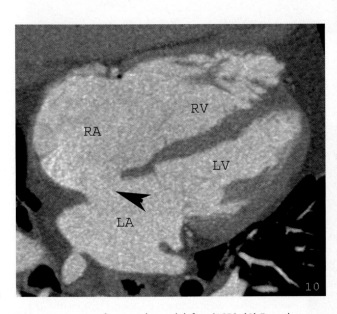

Fig. 9.18 Ostium secundum atrial septal defect (ASD). **(A)** Four-chamber view of the heart demonstrates a normal-sized left side of the heart (left atrium [LA] and left ventricle [LV]), mild enlargement of the right side of the heart (right atrium [RA] and right ventricle[RV]) and an obvious ASD (*arrowhead*). **(B)** Coronal view through the atria demonstrates a wide communication between the RA and LA. The superior vena cava (SVC) and inferior vena cava (IVC) are seen to empty into the RA.

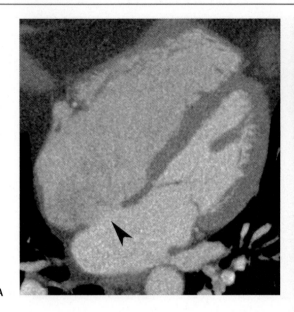

A

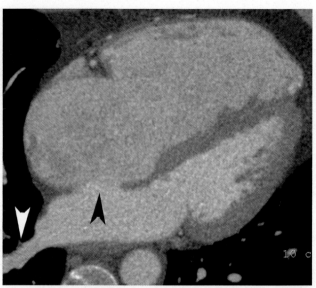

B

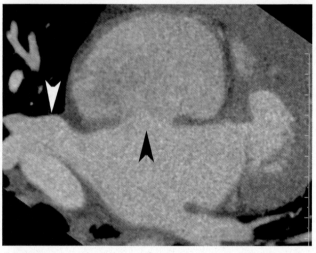

C

Fig. 9.19 Ostium secundum atrial septal defect (ASD) with right-sided heart enlargement. **(A)** Four-chamber view of the heart demonstrates enlargement of the right side of the heart. The apex of the heart is formed by the right ventricle. A large secundum ASD defect is present (*arrowhead*). Right-sided heart enlargement in this patient is related to right-sided volume overload secondary to shunting through the ASD. **(B)** Angled four-chamber view at a slightly more caudal level again demonstrates the ASD (*black arrowhead*). In addition, the right inferior pulmonary vein (*white arrowhead*) is identified as it enters the left atrium. **(C)** Image through the left atrium at the level of the right superior pulmonary vein (*white arrowhead*). The ostium secundum ASD is again identified (*black arrowhead*). The right superior pulmonary vein enters the left atrium. The left superior pulmonary vein is also visualized entering the left atrium at the bottom of the image. Ostium secundum-type ASDs are associated with normal pulmonary venous anatomy.

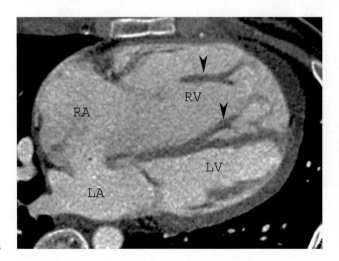

A

Fig. 9.20 Ostium secundum atrial septal defect (ASD) with right-sided heart enlargement and hypertrophy. **(A)** Four-chamber view of the heart demonstrates a large atrial septal defect with contrast shunting (*) from the left atrium (LA) to the right atrium (RA). In addition to enlargement of the right side of the heart (RA and right ventricle [RV]), there are prominent trabeculations in the RV (*arrowheads*) suggesting hypertrophy.

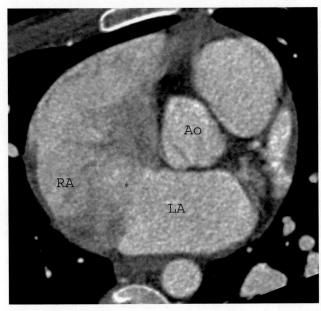

B

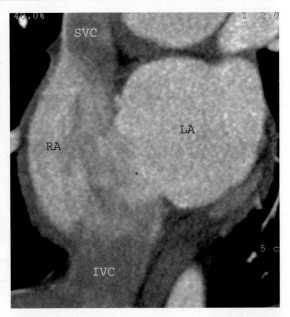

C

Fig. 9.20 (*Continued*) **(B)** Short-axis view again demonstrates dense contrast shunting from the left atrium (LA) to the right atrium (RA). **(C)** Coronal view through the atria demonstrates a wide communication between the RA and LA (*). The superior vena cava (SVC) and inferior vena cava (IVC) are seen to empty into the RA.

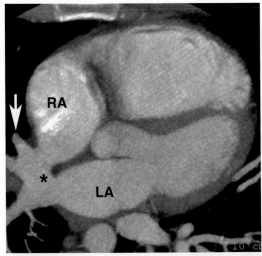

A

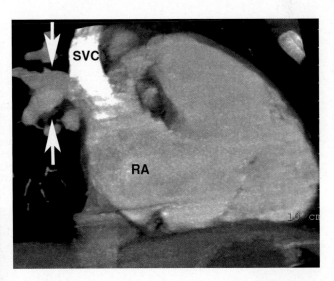

B

C

Fig. 9.21 Sinus venosus atrial septal defect (ASD). **(A)** Five-chamber view demonstrates a high ASD linking the right and left atria (*). The sinus venosus ASD affects the portion of the interatrial septum adjacent to the superior vena cava (SVC) insertion. Several pulmonary veins empty directly into the ASD (*arrow*). A superior sinus venosus ASD is often associated with anomalous pulmonary venous return. **(B)** Coronal maximum intensity projection demonstrates a right-sided superior pulmonary vein emptying directly into the superior vena cava. **(C)** Four-chamber view at a slightly lower level demonstrates an inferior pulmonary vein emptying into the left atrium (*arrow*). A normal appearance is identified at the level of a closed foramen ovale (*arrowhead*). The right side of the heart is dilated, secondary to the presence of shunting through the ASD and anomalous pulmonary venous return.

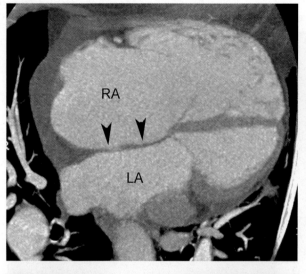

A

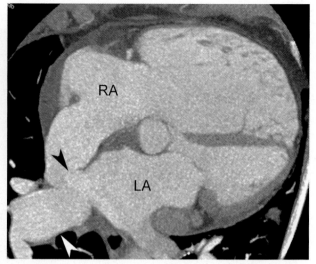

B

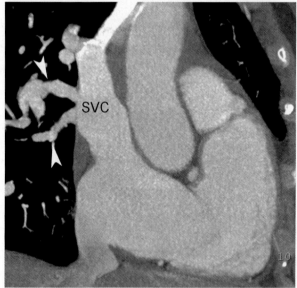

C

Fig. 9.22 Sinus venosus atrial septal defect (ASD). **(A)** Four-chamber view demonstrates an intact atrial septum (*arrowheads*) at the level of the foramen ovale. The left atrium (LA) is normal in size, but the right atrium (RA) is markedly dilated. **(B)** Five-chamber view demonstrates an ASD in the more superior portion of the atrial septum (*black arrowhead*) between the LA and RA. A large pulmonary vein (*white arrowhead*) communicates with both atria at the level of the defect. **(C)** Oblique coronal maximum intensity projection demonstrates two right-sided superior pulmonary veins (*arrowheads*) emptying directly into the superior vena cava.

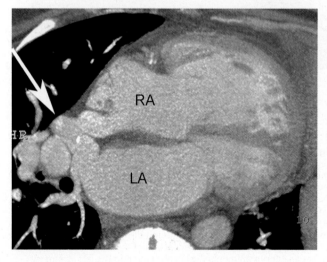

A

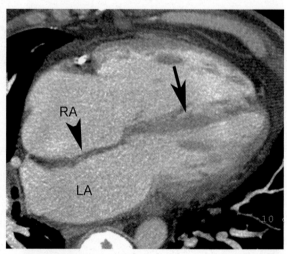

B

Fig. 9.23 Sinus venosus atrial septal defect (ASD) with pressure or volume overload of the right side of the heart. **(A)** Four-chamber view at a superior level demonstrates a complex communication between the left atrium (LA) and right atrium (RA) via an overriding vessel (*arrow*).

(B) Four-chamber view at a more caudal level demonstrates bowing of the atrial septum (*arrowhead*) toward the LA and straightening of the interventricular septum (*arrow*).

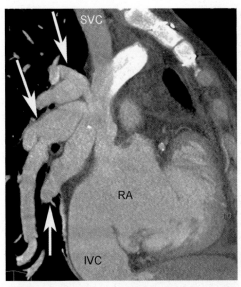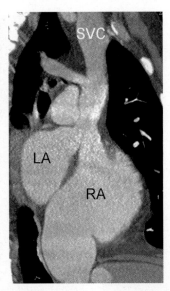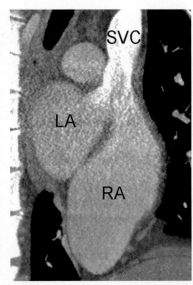

C–E

Fig. 9.23 *(Continued)* **(C)** Sagittal view demonstrates multiple pulmonary veins *(arrows)* entering the superior vena cava (SVC). A dilated inferior vena cava (IVC) is also noted. **(D)** Oblique sagittal view demonstrates that the SVC overrides both the RA and LA at the level of the sinus venosus ASD. **(E)** Oblique sagittal view during the early venous phase of the study demonstrates contrast from the SVC entering both the RA and the LA. The right-sided heart enlargement, bowing of the atrial septum, flattening of the interventricular septum, and dilated IVC are all indicators of severe right-sided pressure or volume overload.

drainage. Finally, a rare form of ASD is the unroofed coronary sinus that communicates with the left atrium. Unroofed coronary sinus is frequently associated with other forms of congenital heart disease and is also frequently associated with a persistent left SVC. When treatment of an ASD is required, both surgical and percutaneous treatment options are available for closure.[27]

◆ Ventricular Septal Defect

The interventricular septum consists of a thin upper membranous portion immediately below the aortic valve and a larger muscular septum. The muscular septum is further divided into the inlet septum, the trabecular septum, and the outlet septum. A VSD is the most common cardiac

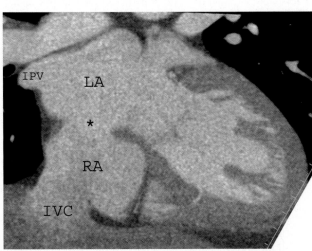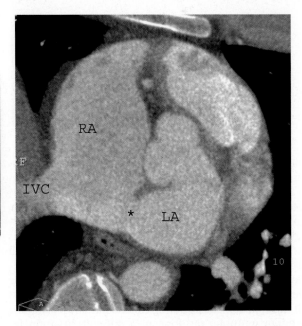

A
B

Fig. 9.24 Inferior sinus venosus atrial septal defect (ASD). **(A)** Sagittal maximum intensity projection (MIP) demonstrates an ASD (*) in the inferior aspect of the atrial septum, between the orifice of the inferior pulmonary veins (IPV) and the inferior vena cava (IVC). The pulmonary veins enter the left atrium (LA). **(B)** Short-axis MIP again demonstrates the proximity of the ASD (*) to the IVC. An inferior sinus venosus ASD is not generally associated with anomalous insertion of the pulmonary veins.

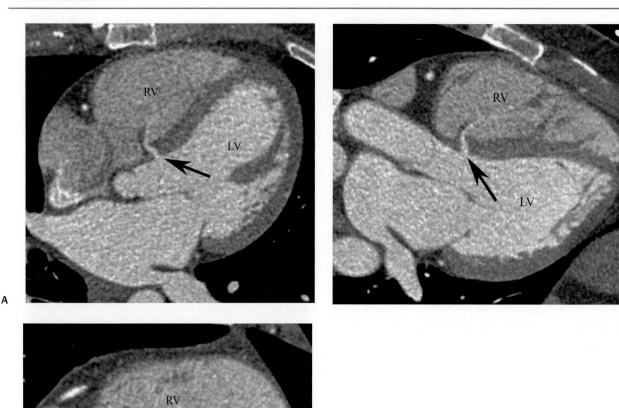

A

B

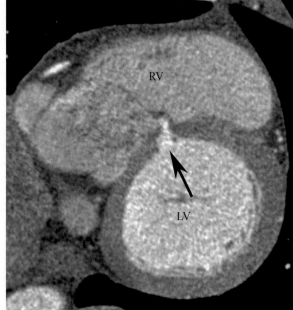

C

Fig. 9.25 Low perimembranous ventral septal defect (VSD). **(A)** Five-chamber view demonstrates a VSD just below the left ventricular outflow tract (*arrow*) involving the superior portion of the muscular septum. **(B)** Three-chamber view again demonstrates the perimembranous VSD (*arrow*) with shunting of dense contrast material from the left ventricle (LV) toward the right ventricle (RV). **(C)** Short-axis view again demonstrates the VSD (*arrow*) between the LV and RV. This image could also be interpreted as a high muscular VSD.

malformation. The most common form of VSD, the perimembranous VSD, involves the membranous septum and a varying amount of muscular tissue adjacent to the membranous septum (**Figs. 9.25** and **9.26**). A defect in the outlet septum, also called a supracristal, conal, subpulmonary, or subarterial defect, may be associated with tetralogy of Fallot and is more common in Far Eastern countries (**Fig. 9.27**).[28] A small percentage of patients with a VSD will develop aortic insufficiency as a result of prolapse of aortic valve cusps into the defect, particularly with an outlet septum VSD. Many VSDs will close spontaneously during childhood.[29] Muscular VSDs are often multiple, resulting in a difficult situation for percutaneous or surgical repair. The reader is referred to Chapter 14 for a more detailed discussion of ASD and VSD pathophysiology.

◆ Partial Anomalous Pulmonary Venous Return

As discussed in the section on ASDs, anomalous pulmonary venous drainage is frequently associated with a sinus venosus ASD (**Figs. 9.21, 9.22,** and **9.23**). Isolated PAPVR occurs in 0.4% of adult autopsy patients without known congenital heart disease (**Fig. 9.28**).[30] Anomalous pulmonary venous return to the right side of the cardiac circulation results in a left-to-right side shunt of oxygenated blood back to the right heart. Although PAPVR is classified as a left-to-right shunt, all of the shunt flow is through the right side of the heart, with resulting volume overload of the right side of the heart. The most common form of PAPVR is from the right upper lobe to the SVC, but other

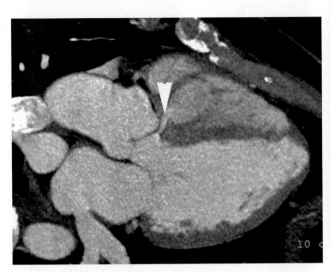

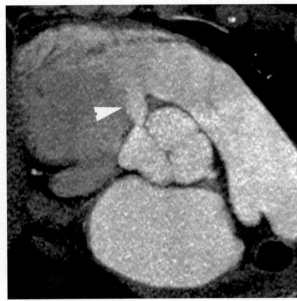

A

B

Fig. 9.26 High perimembranous or membranous ventral septal defect (VSD). **(A)** Long-axis image demonstrates a VSD just below the aortic valve (*arrowhead*). Prolapse of aortic leaflets into this type of VSD may result in aortic insufficiency. **(B)** Short-axis image demonstrates that the VSD communicates with the right ventricular outflow tract just below the pulmonary infundibulum (*arrowhead*).

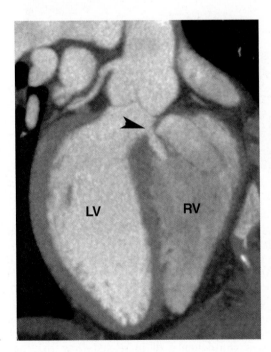

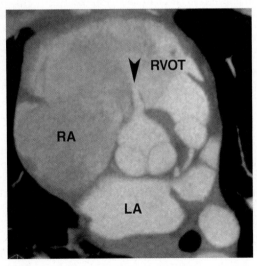

A

B

Fig. 9.27 Perimembranous–outlet septum ventral septal defect (VSD). **(A)** Long-axis image demonstrates the presence of a VSD in the subaortic portion of the interventricular septum, with communication between the left ventricular outflow tract (LVOT) and the right ventricle (RV; *arrowhead*). **(B)** Short-axis image at the level of the aortic valve demonstrates that the VSD communicates with the dilated right ventricular outflow tract (RVOT; *black arrowhead*) immediately below the pulmonic valve. The proximity of the defect to the pulmonic valve could be interpreted as an outlet septum VSD. LA, left atrium; RA, right atrium.

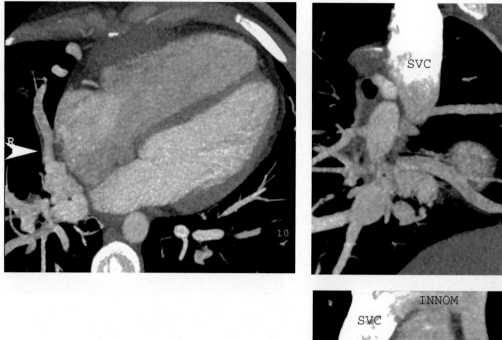

Fig. 9.28 Bilateral anomalous pulmonary venous return. **(A)** Four-chamber view demonstrates a confluence of pulmonary veins along the right side of the heart border (*) that does not communicate with either atrium. Instead, an anomalous vessel courses anteriorly from the confluence (*arrowhead*). **(B)** Sagittal maximum intensity projection demonstrates that the anomalous vessel from the right pulmonary venous confluence (*arrowhead*) has a tortuous course through the right lung and ultimately drains into the superior vena cava (SVC). **(C)** The superior pulmonary vein on the left side (*arrowhead*) drains superiorly into the innominate vein. Thus there is partial anomalous venous return from both lungs.

anomalous connections have been described, including drainage into an innominate vein (**Fig. 9.28C**), into the coronary sinus (**Fig. 9.29**), into a vein below the diaphragm, or directly into the right atrium.[31] Although most patients are asymptomatic, surgical correction is recommended when the pulmonary-to-systemic blood flow ratio exceeds 1.5 because of the likelihood of progression to pulmonary hypertension.[32]

◆ Patent Ductus Arteriosus

PDA is the persistence of a normal fetal communication—the ductus arteriosus—between the upper thoracic descending aorta and the roof of the main pulmonary artery near the origin of the left pulmonary artery.[33] The ductus

normally closes within 24 to 48 hours after birth and is completely sealed in the first few weeks of life. Although PDA is generally detected soon after birth based on a characteristic murmur or clinical symptoms, a small PDA may persist undetected into adulthood. The morbidity of PDA is directly related to the size of the communication and the flow volume through the ductus. A PDA may cause congestive heart failure and elevated pulmonary arterial resistance as a consequence of increased flow that passes through both the left and right sides of the heart. The diagnosis of PDA by CT is based on visualization of a communication between the upper descending thoracic aorta and the proximal left pulmonary artery, with associated shunting of flow into the pulmonary artery.[34] Cardiac CT is an excellent modality to define the location and size of a

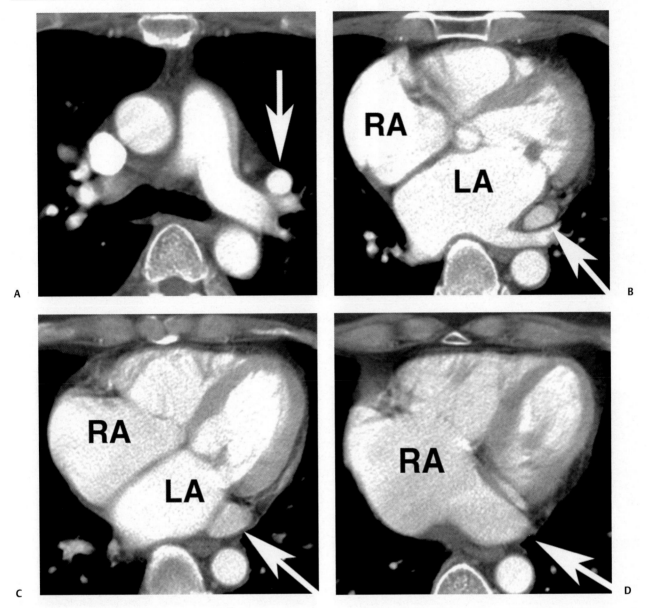

Fig. 9.29 Anomalous pulmonary venous return to the coronary sinus. **(A)** Axial image at the level of the pulmonary arteries demonstrates the left superior pulmonary vein (*arrow*). **(B)** Axial image at the level of the atria demonstrates the left superior pulmonary vein (*arrow*) as it crosses anterior to the left inferior pulmonary vein. The left inferior pulmonary vein empties into the left atrium (LA) at this level. **(C)** Axial image at a slightly lower level demonstrates a left superior pulmonary vein as it continues caudally around the left atrium (*arrow*). **(D)** At a slightly more inferior level, the left superior pulmonary vein enters a dilated coronary sinus (*arrow*). The right atrium (RA) is clearly dilated, likely secondary to volume overload due to shunting of pulmonary blood flow.

PDA (**Fig. 9.30**) and may be used for preprocedure planning of PDA closure.

◆ Other Left-to-Right Shunts

A communication between a left-sided cardiac structure and a right-sided structure will generally result in right-sided volume overload. Fistulous communications, whether congenital, post-traumatic, or iatrogenic, may result in volume overload of the right side of the heart and secondary pulmonary hypertension (**Fig. 9.31**). Cardiac CT is a useful technique to distinguish between right-sided volume or pressure overload that results from cardiac anomalies (intracardiac shunts, valvular disease, myocardial failure) versus pulmonary parenchymal pathology or primary pulmonary arterial disease.[35]

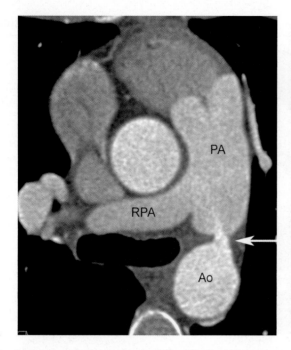
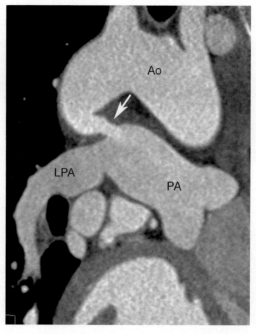

Fig. 9.30 Patent ductus arteriosus. **(A)** Axial image demonstrates the main pulmonary artery (PA) with the right pulmonary artery (RPA) branching off behind the ascending aorta. A patent ductus (*arrow*) is present between the PA and the descending aorta (Ao). **(B)** Oblique sagittal view demonstrates the patent ductus arteriosus extending from the distal PA to the undersurface of the aortic arch (Ao).

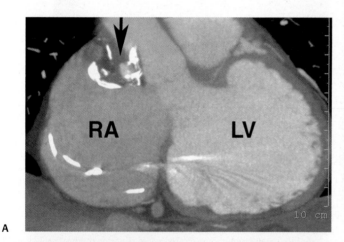

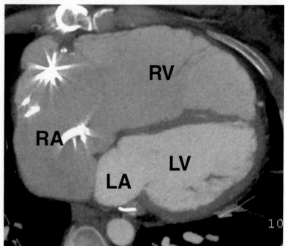

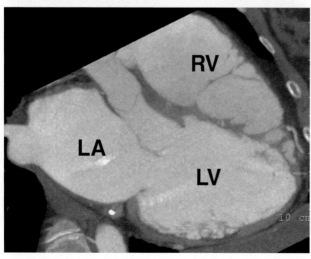

Fig. 9.31 Dilated right side of the heart as a result of a fistula between the aorta and right atrium. **(A)** Oblique maximum intensity projection demonstrates the left ventricle (LV) and the aortic outflow tract. An enlarged right atrium (RA) is identified adjacent to the root of the aorta with post-surgical changes related to closure of a fistula between the aorta and right atrium (*arrow*). **(B)** Four-chamber view demonstrates marked enlargement of the right side of the heart, secondary to a long-standing shunt between the aorta and right atrium. **(C)** Three-chamber view demonstrates an enlarged right ventricle (RV) with increased trabeculation. Only a small portion of the right ventricle is generally visible on the three-chamber view. LA, left atrium.

◆ Right-Sided Heart Volume or Pressure Overload

In a morphologically normal heart imaged in the four-chamber view, the apex of the LV forms the cardiac apex. In the setting of increased volume or pressure in the right side of the heart, the right ventricle may dilate and become the apex-forming chamber (**Figs. 9.18, 9.19, 9.20, 9.21, 9.22** and **9.31**). In theory, volume overload of the right side of the heart results in enlargement of the right atrium and right ventricle, whereas pressure overload will result in right ventricular hypertrophy. In practice, however, volume and pressure overload are often present in the same patient.

In addition to changes in the right side of the heart, elevated right-sided heart pressures may present with changes in the structures leading into and out of the right-sided heart. A dilated IVC and hepatic veins suggest elevated right atrial pressure (**Fig. 9.32**). Failure to collapse with inspiration suggests even greater elevation of right atrial pressure, but changes with respiration are not generally visible on CT. An increased diameter of the main pulmonary artery,[36] or enlargement of the proximal right and left pulmonary arteries, suggests the possibility of pulmonary hypertension.[37]

◆ Ventricular Morphology and Function

The LV cavity is bullet-shaped with the tip of the bullet corresponding to the apex of the ventricle. In the short-axis projection, the LV appears round and the right ventricle has a crescent shape, wrapping around the anterior and right side of the LV. Although the volume of the right ventricle is usually slightly greater than that of the left ventricle, the normal diameter of the mid-right ventricle on a four-chamber view (2.7–3.3 cm) is smaller than the normal diameter of the LV (4.2–5.9 cm). This apparent contradiction is explained by the very different geometries of the two ventricular chambers.

◆ Normal Right Ventricle

The wall of the right ventricle is thinner than the wall of the LV, but the chamber interior is more trabeculated. The moderator band, also known as the *septomarginal trabecula*, is a prominent band of tissue near the apex of the right ventricle extending from the base of the anterior papillary muscle to the interventricular septum (**Fig. 9.32**). The moderator band is responsible for electrical conduction to the right ventricular

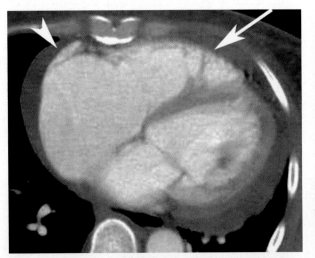

A

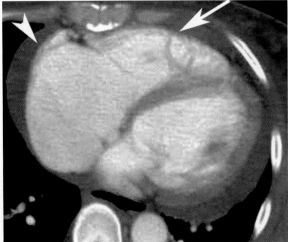

B

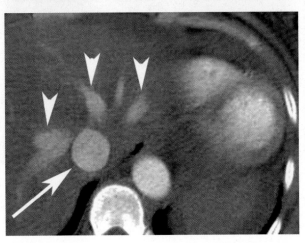

C

Fig. 9.32 Right atrial enlargement with volume overload. **(A)** Four-chamber view demonstrates marked enlargement of the right atrium (*arrowhead*). Prominent trabeculae at the right ventricular apex correspond to the moderator band (*arrow*). **(B)** Axial view at a slightly lower level demonstrates persistent right atrial enlargement. **(C)** Axial image just below the level of the heart demonstrates a dilated inferior vena cava (IVC) (*arrow*), as well as dilated hepatic veins (*arrowheads*). Dilatation of these vessels is related to volume overload and elevated right-sided heart pressure.

free wall. The papillary muscles associated with the tricuspid valve may also present as prominent bands of tissue. These bands may be identified by their attachments and course.

Right ventricular function may have prognostic significance in several disease states, including congestive heart failure, chronic pulmonary disease, and pulmonary embolism. Unlike the LV, which has a relatively cylindrical shape in the short axis, the right ventricle has a more complex geometric shape that is wrapped around the LV in short axis. The lack of a simple geometric model for the right ventricle is a complicating factor in the computation of a right ventricular ejection fraction. The lack of uniform contrast enhancement in the right ventricular cavity can also present a technical problem for functional evaluation with cardiac CT.[38] Nonetheless, early studies suggest that CT may be useful in evaluation of right ventricular function and estimation of right ventricular ejection fraction.[39] Patients with pulmonary embolism demonstrate increased right ventricular end diastolic volume along with reduced right ventricular ejection fraction on cardiac CT.[40]

◆ Arrhythmogenic Right Ventricular Cardiomyopathy

Arrhythmogenic right ventricular cardiomyopathy (ARVC) is a rare disorder of heart muscle characterized by mechanical dysfunction and arrhythmias. Imaging findings include dilatation of the right ventricle with conspicuous, fatty replaced trabeculations, especially along the anterior, inferior, and apical right ventricular walls. There is also a scalloped appearance to the right ventricular wall (**Figs. 9.33** and **9.34**).[41] Deposition of adipose tissue around a normal right ventricle is associated with obesity and

must be distinguished from the much less common disorder of ARVC.

◆ Normal Left Ventricle

The myocardium of the LV is the most well-developed muscle in the heart. Although the endocardial surface of the LV is smoother than that of the right ventricle, trabeculations and papillary muscles are observed along the wall of the LV. Normal values for LV dimensions, wall thickness, and mass are provided in **Table 9.1**. An LV end diastolic wall thickness of 0.6 to 1.0 cm is generally considered normal. Focal thinning of the myocardium at the ventricular apex is a normal variation when associated with normal myocardial function (**Figs. 9.2** and **9.3**).

◆ Myocardial Morphology

Normal LV myocardium is uniform in thickness. Deviations of the LV myocardium from its normal morphology may be characterized as thinning or hypertrophy in a segmental or global distribution. Evaluation of LV wall motion is the key to assessing morphologic changes in LV myocardium.

Thinning of the myocardium associated with a segmental wall motion abnormality suggests an area of infarction or scaring. Segmental myocardial infarcts may appear lower in density relative to normally enhancing adjacent myocardium (**Fig. 9.35**). Areas of infarct may atrophy and demonstrate myocardial thinning with fatty replacement (**Fig. 9.36**). With time, infracted regions of myocardium may calcify (**Fig. 9.37**).

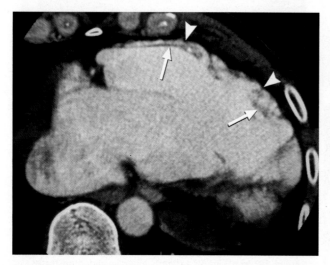 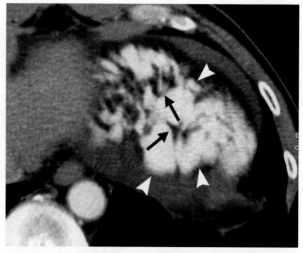

Fig. 9.33 Arrhythmogenic right ventricular cardiomyopathy (ARVC). **(A)** Axial image demonstrates low-density trabeculation in the free wall of the right ventricle (*arrows*). There is also a scalloped appearance to the free wall of the right ventricle (*arrowheads*). **(B)** Axial image through the inferior right ventricle. Low-density trabeculations (*black arrows*) are identified, as well as a scalloped border of the wall (*arrowheads*). Low-density trabeculations and scalloping of the right ventricular wall are characteristic of ARVC. (From Kimura F, Sakai F, Sakomura Y, et al. Helical CT features of arrhythmogenic right ventricular cardiomyopathy. Radiographics. 2002;22:1111–1124. Reprinted with permission.)

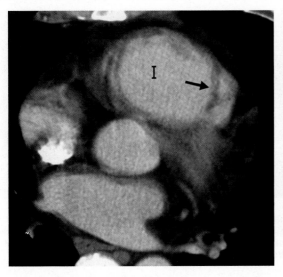

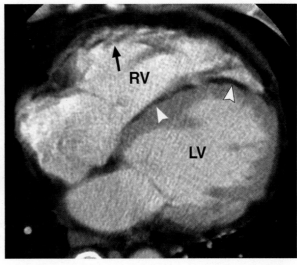

A

B

Fig. 9.34 Arrhythmogenic right ventricular cardiomyopathy. **(A)** Axial image through the right ventricular outflow tract demonstrates a low-density trabeculation in the infundibulum (*arrow*). **(B)** Axial image at a lower level demonstrates low density trabeculations along the right ventricular free wall (*black arrow*), as well as deposition of fatty material along the interventricular septum (*arrowheads*). Deposition of fat within trabeculations along the infundibulum, free wall, and inferior wall of the right ventricle (RV), as well as along the septum are characteristic of ARVC. LV, left ventrical. (From Kimura F, Sakai F, Sakomura Y, et al. Helical CT features of arrhythmogenic right ventricular cardiomyopathy. Radiographics. 2002;22:1111–1124. Reprinted with permission.)

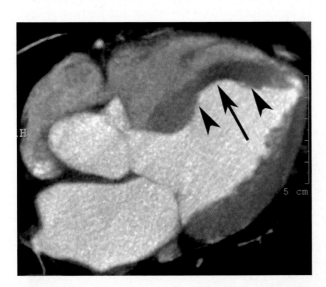

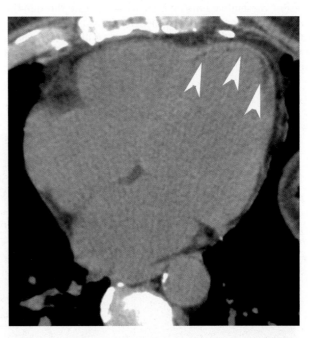

Fig. 9.35 Anteroseptal infarct. Five-chamber view demonstrates focal thinning of the anterior septum (*arrow*) which bulges into the right ventricle. There is a clear hinge point at the proximal and distal ends of this area of thinning (*arrowheads*), characteristic of a focal infarct. Decreased myocardial enhancement is also demonstrated at the site of the infarct.

Fig. 9.36 Apical infarct with myocardial thinning and fatty replacement. Four-chamber view on this noncontrast scan demonstrates thinning of the left ventricular apex with subendocardial fat presenting as a low-density line (*arrowheads*).

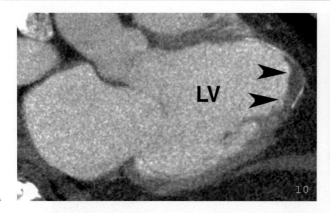

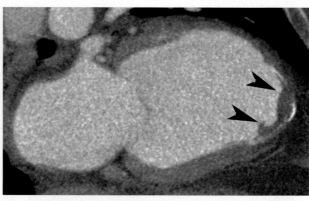

A

B

Fig. 9.37 Apical infarct with associated calcification and thrombus. **(A)** Three-chamber view demonstrates thinning of the apical walls with a fine linear calcification, suggesting an old infarct. Low-density material along akinetic apex (*arrowheads*) represents thrombus and does not enhance with adjacent viable myocardium. **(B)** Two-chamber view demonstrates the thrombus to better advantage (*arrowheads*). Contrast material can be seen extending under the thrombus into the ventricular apex.

Mural thrombus may develop along areas of infarction because of stasis associated with decreased contractility (**Fig. 9.37**). Apical infarcts often result in true aneurysmal dilatation of the cardiac apex. (**Fig. 9.38**). Pseudoaneurysms of the LV develop more frequently at sites of infarction in the inferior or inferolateral walls (**Fig. 9.39**). Unlike a true aneurysm in which all three layers of the cardiac wall are present, a pseudoaneurysm is an actual rupture through the myocardium contained by either the pericardium or extracardiac tissue. Whereas a true aneurysm will generally have a wide neck, a pseudoaneurysm is characterized by a thin neck and a markedly thin wall.

Myocardial rupture is a potentially life-threatening condition that may present as a complication of myocardial infarction. The diagnosis of myocardial rupture is suggested when a focal defect in the myocardium is associated with coronary artery disease and abnormal function (**Fig. 9.40**).

Patients with poor LV function may be supported with a ventricular assist device. These devices are often used as a temporary measure in the setting of a massive acute myocardial infarction or severe cardiomyopathy. Cardiac CT may be useful to image the inflow and outflow of these devices for obstruction or thrombosis that can lead to dysfunction (**Figs. 9.41** and **9.42**), as well as for any site of

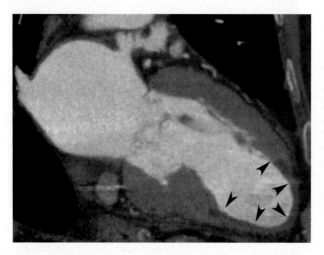

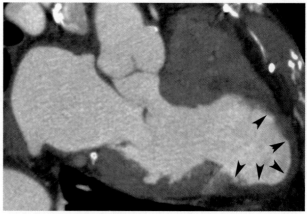

A

B

Fig. 9.38 Apical infarct with aneurysm. **(A)** Two-chamber view demonstrates thinning of the left ventricular periapical walls with associated low density, compatible with an infarct. The apex bulges out, and was completely akinetic, diagnostic of an apical aneurysm. **(B)** Similar findings of periapical thinning and akinesis are identified in the three chamber view.

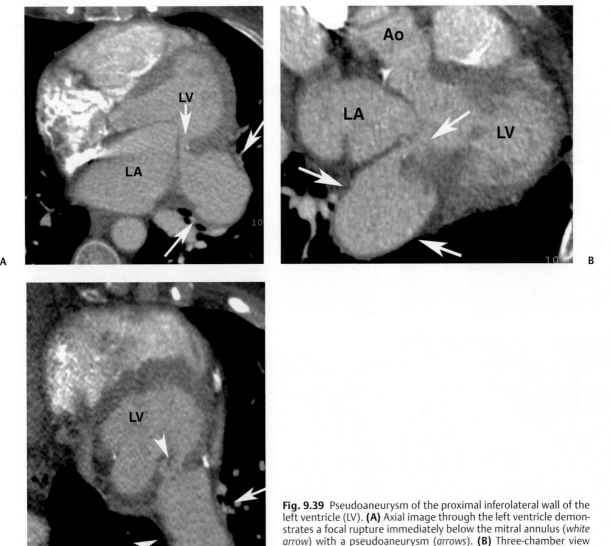

Fig. 9.39 Pseudoaneurysm of the proximal inferolateral wall of the left ventricle (LV). **(A)** Axial image through the left ventricle demonstrates a focal rupture immediately below the mitral annulus (*white arrow*) with a pseudoaneurysm (*arrows*). **(B)** Three-chamber view demonstrates rupture of the proximal inferolateral wall with associated pseudoaneurysm (*arrows*). **(C)** Short-axis image through the left ventricle confirms the location of rupture (*arrowhead*) and associated pseudoaneurysm (*arrows*). LA, left atrium; Ao, aorta.

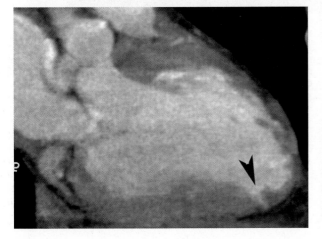

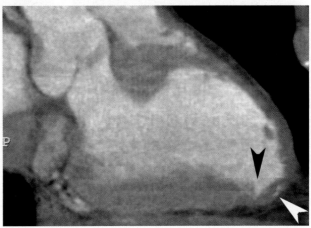

Fig. 9.40 Subepicardial aneurysm (ie, a partial myocardial rupture) with impending cardiac rupture. **(A)** Three-chamber view during diastole demonstrates thinning of the anterior and periapical walls (area of a known infarction), as well as a focal breach in the myocardium in the distal inferolateral wall adjacent to the apex (*arrowhead*). **(B)** Three-chamber view in a slightly different plane again demonstrates the near full-thickness rupture of the distal inferolateral wall (*black arrowhead*), as well as extravasation of contrast into the subepicardial space along the cardiac apex (*white arrowhead*). At surgery this patient was found to have a focal disruption of the myocardium with impending cardiac rupture.

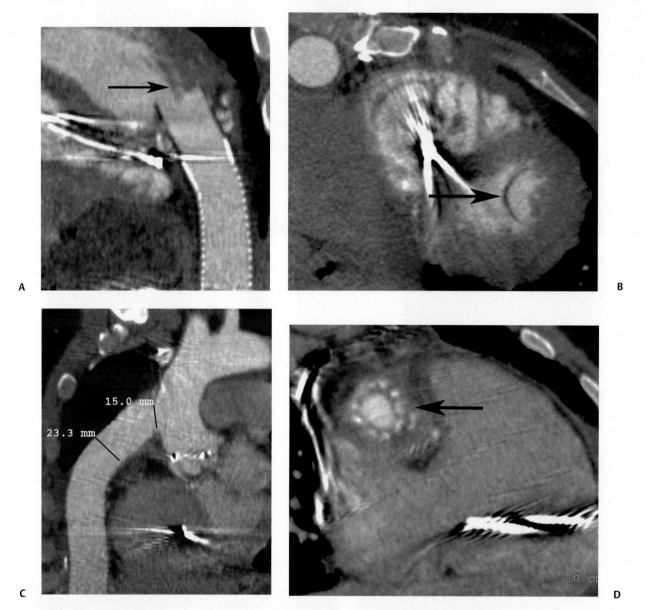

Fig. 9.41 Left ventricular assist device (LVAD) with decreased pressures related to obstruction of LV inflow. **(A)** Sagittal image through the LV apex demonstrates the presence of a large cannula from the LVAD. This cannula removes blood from the LV so that it can be pumped into the ascending aorta. Of note, a papillary muscle (*arrow*) narrows the lumen of the cannula by 50%. **(B)** Short-axis image through the cannula at the apex of the left ventricle (*arrow*) again demonstrates narrowing of the lumen of the cannula by residual papillary muscle. **(C)** Sagittal image of the ascending aorta with anastomosis of the LVAD. The outflow cannula of the LVAD is connected to the ascending aorta. There is a mild narrowing at this anastomosis that was not hemodynamically significant. **(D)** Short-axis view of the cannula at the level of the anastomosis with the ascending aorta.

leak that could result in blood loss or a fluid collection (**Fig. 9.43**).

A diverticulum of the LV may be distinguished from a partial rupture of the myocardium by the presence of normal thickness and function in the surrounding myocardium. The incidence of LV diverticula is reported to be about 0.26% in patients who undergo cardiac catheterization.[42] With increased use of CT imaging, small diverticula are more commonly identified in the wall of the left ventricle (**Figs. 9.44, 9.45, 9.46,** and **9.47**).

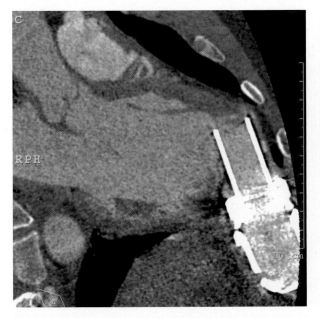

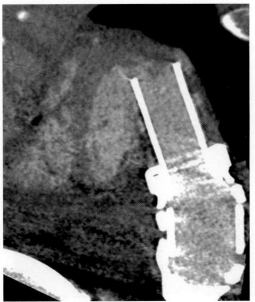

Fig. 9.42 Left ventricular assist device (LVAD) with decreased pressures related to obstruction of LV inflow. **(A)** Three-chamber view demonstrates an apical cannula that provides inflow for a LVAD. The tip of the cannula is directed up into the distal anterior wall, resulting in partial obstruction of inflow to the cannula. **(B)** Short-axis view of the distal LV again demonstrates that the cannula is up against the anterior wall of the LV, resulting in obstruction of inflow to the LVAD.

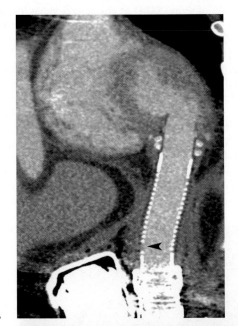

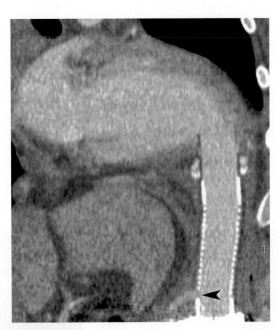

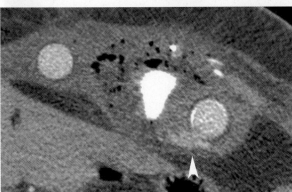

Fig. 9.43 Fracture of the inflow cannula to a left ventricular assist device (LVAD). **(A)** Coronary image demonstrates a cannula extending down from the LV apex. A missing ring is identified in the lower portion of the cannula (*arrowhead*). **(B)** Oblique image of the cannula demonstrates contrast extravasation from the cannula. **(C)** Axial image just above the LVAD pump demonstrates contrast extravasation (*arrowhead*) with a fluid/air collection around the LVAD cannulas.

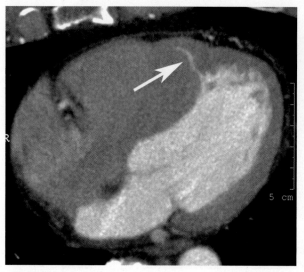

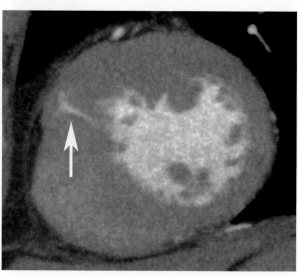

Fig. 9.44 Left ventricular diverticulum of the interventricular septum. **(A)** Four-chamber image demonstrates a thin diverticulum in the interventricular septum (*arrow*). **(B)** Short-axis image confirms the diverticulum (*arrow*). The dense contrast that is present in the left ventricle fills the diverticulum, but it does not communicate with the right ventricle. Cine images demonstrated normal contraction of the left ventricle.

◆ Hypertrophic Cardiomyopathy

LV hypertrophy (LVH) is most commonly associated with hypertension, although there may be other contributing metabolic factors. LVH can also be related to a primary hypertrophic cardiomyopathy. Hypertrophy that develops secondary to hypertension generally presents as concentric hypertrophy with normal or dynamic function. LV function may deteriorate in the late stages of hypertrophic cardiomyopathy. Although outflow tract obstruction is most commonly associated with primary hypertrophic cardiomyopathy, other causes of LVH may be associated dynamic systolic function and may result in systolic obstruction of the LVOT related to

systolic anterior motion (SAM) of the mitral valve leaflets (**Fig. 9.48**) or of the mitral chordal structures (**Fig. 9.49**). Concentric hypertrophy may also present with systolic obstruction of the LV midcavity (**Fig. 9.50**).

Primary hypertrophic cardiomyopathy is a morphologic and functional anomaly of the myocardium related to genetic mutations that affect the sarcomeric proteins. Primary hypertrophic cardiomyopathy may be diffuse or localized and is usually associated with hyperdynamic function. Hypertrophic cardiomyopathy is a relatively common genetic cardiac disease with a frequency of 1:500 in the general population and an annual mortality rate of about 1%.[43] The vast majority of patients with hypertrophic cardiomyopathy

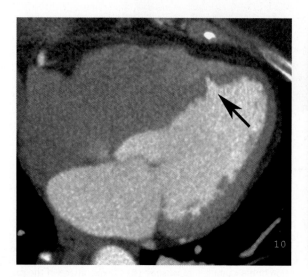

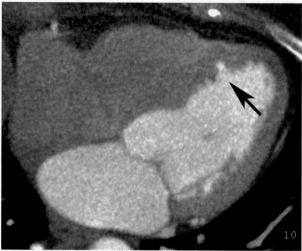

Fig. 9.45 Left ventricular diverticulum with normal systolic function. **(A)** Four-chamber view in diastole demonstrates a diverticulum of the interventricular septum (*arrow*). **(B)** Systolic view in the same projection demonstrates normal contraction of the wall containing the diverticulum, confirming that this is a benign process, unrelated to ischemic coronary disease.

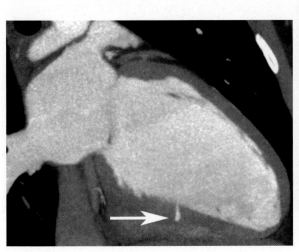

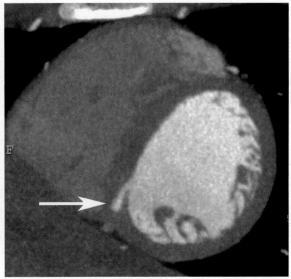

A   B

Fig. 9.46 Diverticulum of the inferior wall. **(A)** Angled two-chamber view demonstrates a diverticulum of the inferior wall in the midportion of the left ventricle (*arrow*). **(B)** Short-axis image through the mid-ventricle again demonstrates the presence of a diverticulum (*arrow*). Functional images demonstrated normal left ventricular contraction.

present with asymmetrical hypertrophy (95%), most commonly involving the interventricular septum (90%).[44] Most patients with hypertrophic cardiomyopathy do not have a sizable resting outflow tract gradient. However, asymmetric septal hypertrophy (ASH) can be associated with LVOT obstruction (**Figs. 9.51** and **9.52**). ASH should be distinguished from discrete hypertrophy of the upper septum, which may be considered a normal variation in older patients, although more recent data suggest that this may represent a late presentation of a true genetic abnormality in some patients.

Doppler echocardiography in ASH may demonstrate an elevated outflow velocity associated with dynamic LVOT obstruction. Although the LVOT gradient cannot be measured by CT, the diameter of the LVOT and the presence of SAM may be described.

Hypertrophy of the apical or mid-ventricular portions of the LV is distinctly less common than ASH. Asymmetric hypertrophy is often diagnosed by echocardiography or MRI, but the morphology is equally well defined on CT. Apical hypertrophy presents with a characteristic spade-shaped

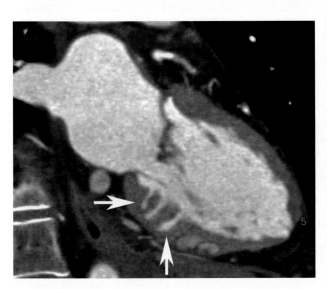

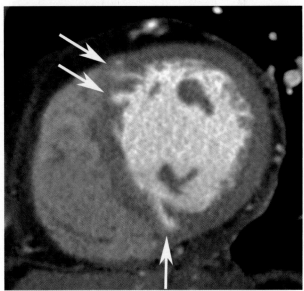

A   B

Fig. 9.47 Multiple diverticula of the septum and inferior walls. **(A)** Two-chamber view demonstrates three diverticula of the proximal inferior wall (*arrows*). **(B)** Short-axis view demonstrates one of the three inferior-wall diverticula (*bottom arrow*) as well as two additional diverticula in the anterior septum (*upper arrows*).

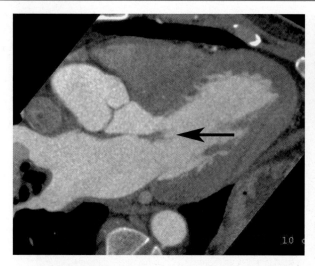

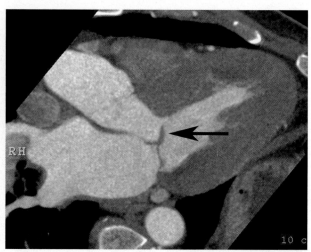

Fig. 9.48 Left ventricular hypertrophy with systolic anterior motion of thickened mitral leaflet tips and associated chordal attachments. **(A)** Three-chamber view in diastole demonstrates left ventricular hypertrophy (wall thickness: 15–17 mm) with a thickened anterior mitral leaflet (*arrow*). **(B)** Systolic frame demonstrates anterior motion of the mitral leaflet tips (*arrow*) and associated chordal attachments into the left ventricular outflow tract.

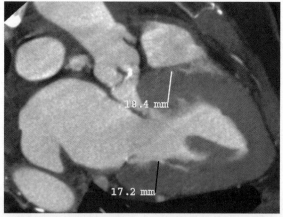

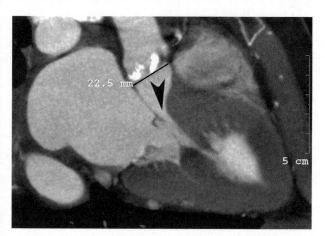

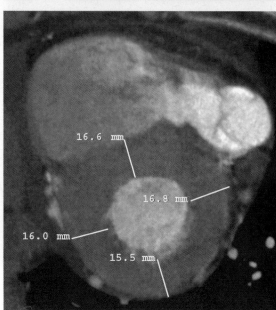

Fig. 9.49 Left ventricular hypertrophy secondary to aortic stenosis, with systolic anterior motion of chordal structures resulting in left ventricular outflow tract (LVOT) obstruction and mitral insufficiency. **(A)** Three-chamber view in diastole demonstrates thickening of the left ventricular wall, measuring 18 mm at the level of the septum and 17 mm in the proximal posterior wall. Note the presence of calcification in the aortic valve in this patient with aortic stenosis. **(B)** Three-chamber view during systole demonstrates systolic anterior motion of mitral chordal structures into the LVOT with incomplete coaptation of the mitral valve. There is narrowing of the LVOT between a chordal structure attached to the anterior mitral leaflet and the thickened left ventricular wall (*black arrowhead*). Although the outflow tract measures 22.5 mm at the level of the aortic valve, it is markedly narrowed below this level by the presence of left ventricular hypertrophy as well as systolic anterior motion of chordal structures. **(C)** Short-axis image of the left ventricle in diastole confirms the presence of concentric hypertrophy.

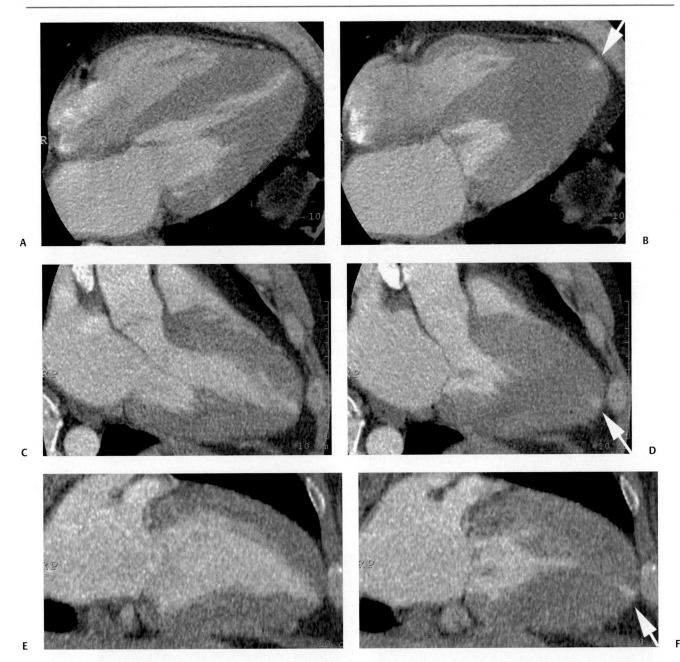

Fig. 9.50 Concentric left ventricular (LV) hypertrophy with intracavitary obstruction. **(A)** Four-chamber view in diastole demonstrates symmetric hypertrophy of the septum and lateral walls. **(B)** Four-chamber view in systole demonstrates obliteration of most of the left ventricular cavity with a small residual lumen associated with an obstructed, akinetic apex (*arrow*). **(C)** Three-chamber view in diastole, **(D)** three-chamber view in systole, **(E)** two-chamber view in diastole, and **(F)** two-chamber view in systole all confirm the symmetric nature of the concentric hypertrophy and apical cavity obstruction (*arrow*). There is no evidence of LV outflow tract obstruction. Coronary CT angiography demonstrated no significant narrowing in the left anterior descending artery. Apical thinning and akinesis in this hypertensive patient are presumed to be secondary to longstanding LV cavity obstruction with elevated apical wall tension, resulting in a relative ischemic state of the apex. Alternatively, this could represent a primary hypertrophic cardiomyopathy with an apical myocardial abnormality.

ventricular cavity and may be associated with apical obstruction (**Fig. 9.53**). Gated cardiac CT can demonstrate both the morphologic abnormality and functional abnormalities associated with hypertrophic cardiomyopathy.

The mortality of primary hypertrophic cardiomyopathy is directly related to the magnitude of LVH, although there are other factors, such as family history, that also impact estimation of the risk of death.[45] The description and prognosis of the usual forms of LVH may be further refined based on the LV mass index, as well as the relative wall thickness. Computation of the LV mass index from linear measurements with two-dimensional echocardiography is

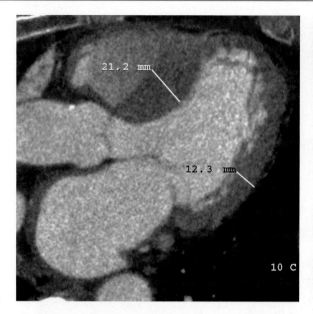

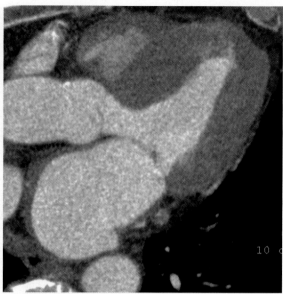

A

B

Fig. 9.51 Left ventricular hypertrophy, most pronounced in the septum. **(A)** Three-chamber view in diastole demonstrates thickening of the left ventricular walls, which is more pronounced in the septum (21 mm) compared with the posterior wall (12 mm). **(B)** Three-chamber view in systole is more suggestive of concentric hypertrophy. The LV outflow tract is clearly visualized with no evidence of outflow tract obstruction.

based on diastolic measurements of the septum (SWTd), posterior wall (PWTd), and left ventricular internal diameter (LVIDd) and on the assumption of a prolate ellipse model.[46] Relative wall thickness is calculated from the thickness of the posterior wall and the LV internal diameter in diastole.

$$LVmass = 0.8x\{1.04[(LVIDd + PWTd + SWTd)^3 \qquad \text{Eq 9.1}$$
$$- (LVIDd)^3]\} + 0.6\,g$$

$$Relative\ Wall\ Thickness = (2xPWTDd)/LVIDd \qquad \text{Eq 9.2}$$

Echocardiographic computation of LV mass is subject to large interobserver variation as well as error related to

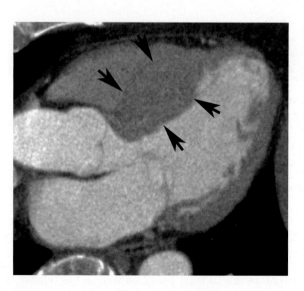

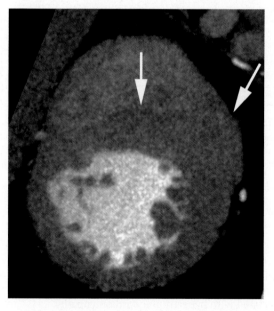

A

B

Fig. 9.52 Asymmetric septal hypertrophy. **(A)** Three-chamber view in diastole demonstrates septal hypertrophy (*arrows*). The remaining walls are normal in thickness. **(B)** Short-axis view demonstrates marked thickening of the septum relative to the remaining walls, particularly the anterior portion of the septum.

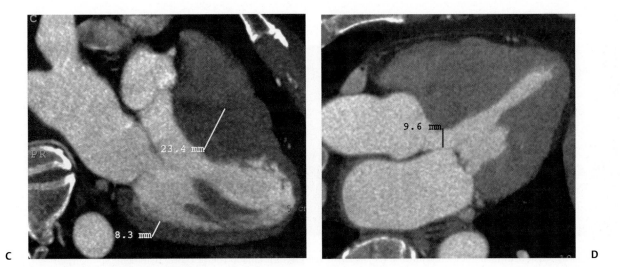

Fig. 9.52 (*Continued*) **(C)** Three-chamber view in diastole demonstrates a septal measurement of 23 mm with a posterior wall measurement of 8 mm. **(D)** Three-chamber view in systole demonstrates narrowing of the left ventricular outflow tract to just under 1 cm in diameter secondary to septal hypertrophy. Correlation with echocardiography demonstrated asymmetric septal hypertrophy with a mild gradient in the left ventricular outflow tract.

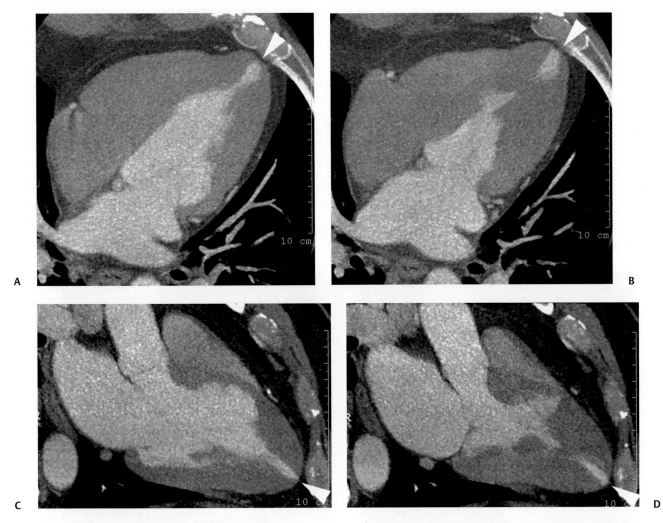

Fig. 9.53 Asymmetric mid-distal left ventricular (LV) hypertrophy with apical obstruction. Long-axis images demonstrate the classic spade-shaped LV cavity associated with a rare form of asymmetric left ventricular hypertrophy called apical hypertrophy. **(A)** Four-chamber view in diastole demonstrates asymmetric hypertrophy of the mid and distal ventricular walls with apical thinning and a small apical aneurysm (*arrowhead*). **(B)** Four-chamber view in systole demonstrates obliteration of the mid-distal LV cavity with a small, akinetic apical aneurysm (*arrowhead*). **(C)** Three-chamber view in diastole, **(D)** three-chamber view in systole, (*Continued on page 212*)

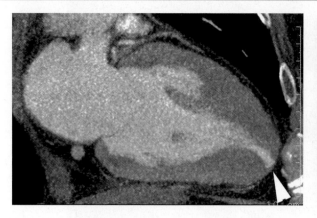

E   F

Fig. 9.53 (*Continued*) Asymmetric mid-distal left ventricular (LV) hypertrophy with apical obstruction. Long-axis images demonstrate the classic spade-shaped LV cavity associated with a rare form of asymmetric left ventricular hypertrophy called apical hypertrophy. **(E)** two-chamber view in diastole, and **(F)** two-chamber view in systole all confirm the classic spade-shaped LV cavity associated with apical hypertrophy. This case represents a variation of the classic asymmetric apical hypertrophy with apical thinning. Coronary CT angiography demonstrated no significant narrowing in the left anterior descending artery. Apical thinning and akinesis are presumed to be secondary to longstanding LV cavity obstruction or a primary apical myocardial abnormality.

inadequacy of the prolate ellipse model and the dependence of the formula on LV volume status.

When the heart is imaged by cardiac CT and software is available for automated contour detection, the LV mass may be computed directly from CT determination of the LV myocardial volume. Computation of LV mass directly from the measured volume will be more accurate because it does not depend on modeling the ventricle as a prolate ellipse of revolution. Normal values for LV mass are provided in **Table 9.1**. A normal LV mass index with a relative wall thickness less than or equal to 0.42 suggests normal geometry of the left ventricle. A normal LV mass index with an elevated relative wall thickness suggests concentric remodeling, whereas an elevated LV mass index with an elevated relative wall thickness suggests concentric hypertrophy. When the LV mass index is increased with a normal relative wall thickness, the process is classified as eccentric hypertrophy.

◆ Left Ventricular Noncompaction

Left ventricular noncompaction (LVNC), also known as LV hypertrabeculation or spongy myocardium, is a rare disorder that is characterized by increased trabeculation of the LV myocardium and may be confused with hypertrophic cardiomyopathy or other dilated cardiomyopathies that demonstrate apical trabeculation on imaging studies. LVNC is usually associated with decreased LV systolic function. LVNC is diagnosed echocardiographically in 0.05 to 0.24% of studies by the presence of a noncompacted layer of myocardium that is more than twice the thickness of the compact layer.[47] Other diagnostic criteria that have been used include the presence of more than three visible trabeculations within one imaging plane below the insertion of the papillary muscles. Hypertrabeculation is most frequently present in the LV apex and along adjacent portions of the lateral and inferior walls (**Fig. 9.54**).

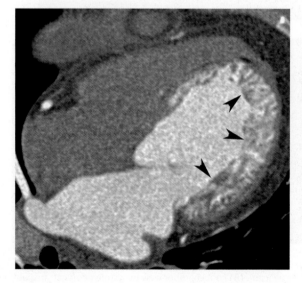

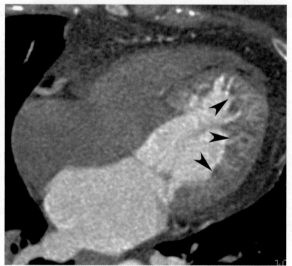

A   B

Fig. 9.54 Left ventricular noncompaction. Diastolic images demonstrate a clear distinction between the inner hypertrabeculated myocardium (*arrowheads*) and the thin layer of outer compact myocardium. The spongy inner layer is more than twice the thickness of the compact layer. The trabeculations are more difficult to visualize during systole. **(A)** Four-chamber view in diastole and **(B)** systole.

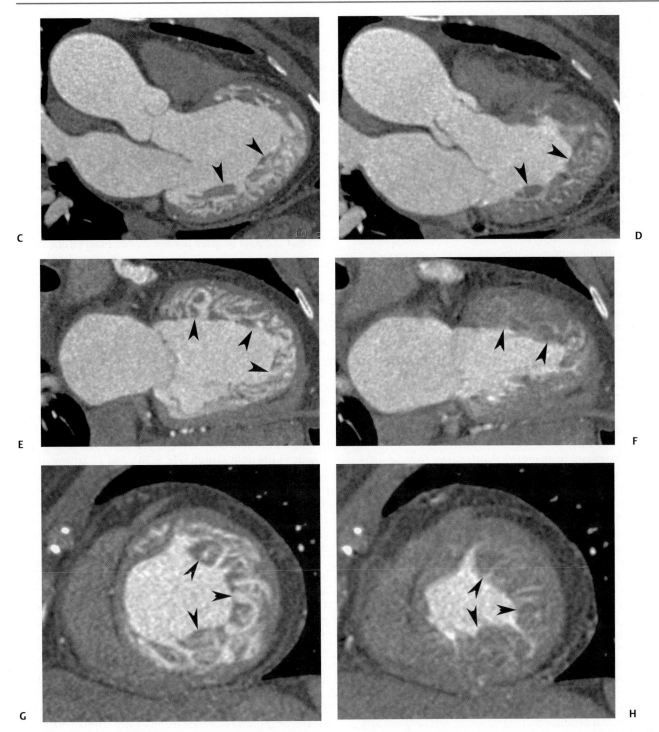

C

D

E

F

G

H

Fig. 9.54 (*Continued*) **(C)** Three-chamber view in diastole and **(D)** systole **(E)** Two-chamber view in diastole and **(F)** systole. **(G)** Short-axis view in diastole and **(H)** systole. The left ventricle is mildly globular in shape during diastole with an elevated end diastolic volume calculated at 200 mL. Left ventricular function was low normal. Although the diagnosis of noncompaction is obvious on CT, it was missed on the initial echocardiograms.

Numerous case reports have demonstrated a large variety of cardiac and extracardiac abnormalities in individual cases of LVNC. Associated clinical issues reported most commonly with LVNC include electrocardiographic abnormalities, LV dysfunction, heart failure, palpitations, and sudden death. LVNC can present in isolation or in association with other structural cardiac abnormalities and may develop in previously normal myocardium.[48] LVNC may be associated with chromosomal abnormalities, but the relationship of LVNC to these disorders is unclear.[49] Although therapy is often required for the abnormalities associated with LVNC, clinical characteristics, outcomes, and appropriate therapy for LVNC remain poorly defined.[50]

Ventricular trabeculation and compaction are two essential steps in the development of a functionally competent LV. Although LVNC is thought to be related to an arrest of myocardial development,[51] recent evidence suggests that some cases may actually be acquired, whereas other cases have regressed with time. Increased trabeculations associated with LVNC are clearly visualized by CT imaging during the diastolic phase of the cardiac cycle but are less apparent during systole (**Figs. 9.54B,D,F,H**). It is possible that apparent progression or regression of LVNC on echocardiographic studies may be related to the impact of cardiac function because the trabeculated myocardial appearance of LVNC may be masked by improved systolic function.

◆ Cine Evaluation of Ventricular Function

The CT diagnosis of myocardial infarction may be suggested on the basis of LV morphology but is based primarily on a cine analysis of function. Normal myocardium demonstrates both thickening and centripetal motion in systole, with an overall ejection fraction greater than 55%. An area of infarction will demonstrate reduced or absent thickening and a lack of normal contraction. Often a "hinge point" is identified between normally contracting myocardium and infarcted tissue. Cine analysis of ventricular function is also useful in evaluation of cardiomyopathy and dynamic outflow tract obstruction. When myocardial function is diffusely depressed, it might not be possible to distinguish multiple infarctions from cardiomyopathy. Perfusion imaging and delayed myocardial enhancement may be helpful in this distinction (see Chapter 16). In the distinction between a LV diverticulum versus pseudoaneurysm, cine function should be normal with a diverticulum, whereas a pseudoaneurysm is generally present within an area of abnormally functioning myocardium and should appear dyskinetic during systole. Finally, cine evaluation of right ventricular function may be useful for evaluation of right-sided pressure or volume overload based on paradoxical motion of the interventricular septum and for the diagnosis of pulmonary embolism based on the McConnell sign (hypokinesis of the right ventricle with preservation of function in the right ventricular apex). The interested reader is encouraged to review the numerous cine clips provided with this chapter that demonstrate normal and abnormal function of the LV.

◆ Left Ventricular Ejection Fraction

An ejection fraction may be estimated visually from cine CT images of the LV throughout the cardiac cycle or calculated from a tracing of the LV cavity contour in systole and diastole. Reconstruction of cardiac CT in multiple phases is mandatory to obtain an ejection fraction from cardiac CT. Various geometric models have been tested to optimize the accuracy of automated ejection fraction calculations.[52] In our experience, reconstruction of 10 phases throughout the cardiac cycle with application of a biplane Simpson's algorithm appears to be adequate for determination of ejection fraction (**Fig. 9.55**). Correlation with echocardiography is relatively good, with r^2 approximately 0.8. Other groups have also demonstrated good correlation between ejection fraction obtained by cardiac CT and that obtained by gated nuclear studies[53] and cardiac MR.[54]

◆ Cardiac Neoplasms

Neoplasms in the heart are relatively uncommon, and apparent cardiac tumors are often related to normal anatomic structures.[55] True cardiac neoplasms are classified as primary or metastatic. Approximately 75% of primary cardiac tumors are benign.[56] Myxomas are the most common benign primary cardiac neoplasm, accounting for 30% of primary cardiac neoplasms. Most myxomas arise from the area of the fossa ovalis (**Fig. 9.56 and 9.57**), with 75% arising in the left atrium (**Figs. 9.5, 9.57, and 9.58**), 23% arising in the right atrium (**Fig. 9.59**), and 2% arising in the ventricles.[57] Although myxomas are benign neoplasms, they may present with serious complications resulting from intracardiac obstruction or embolization. Myxomas are usually round with a heterogeneous texture and occasional calcification. They are typically connected to the atrial septum by a stalk.

Lipomas account for 10% of primary benign cardiac neoplasms. They may arise in the LV, in the right atrium, or along the interatrial septum, and they range in size from 1 to 15 cm. CT can provide a specific diagnosis by identification of fatty tissue.[58] Cardiac lipomas should be distinguished from lipomatous hypertrophy of the interatrial septum, which is not a true neoplasm.

Papillary fibroelastoma is a small tumor, generally less than 1 cm in diameter, that is most commonly identified on the mitral or aortic valve (see **Fig. 10.16**). A characteristic mobility of this finger-like tumor may be visualized by transesophageal echocardiography. Unlike valvular vegetations, these tumors are most frequently found on the downstream side of the valve and are rarely associated with valvular dysfunction. Fibroelastomas are difficult to visualize with CT because of their small size and vibratory motion related to their valvular attachment and adjacent blood flow. Papillary fibroelastomas are surgically removed because of their association with embolic events.

Other rare benign cardiac tumors include rhabdomyomas and fibromas, most frequently found in children. Almost all

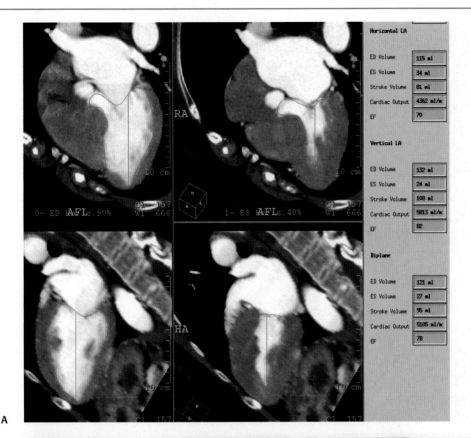

A

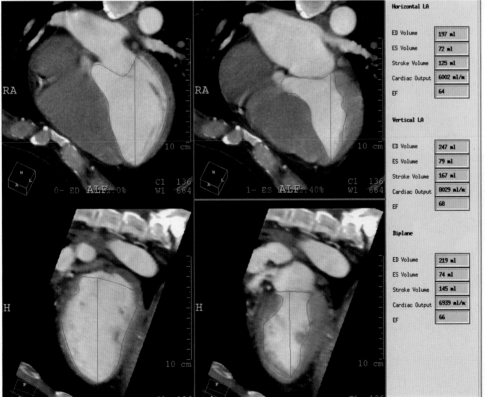

B

Fig. 9.55 Cardiac function and estimation of ejection fraction with biplane Simpson's method. **(A)** Dynamic left ventricular function with an estimated ejection fraction of 78%. **(B)** Normal left ventricular function with an estimated ejection fraction of 56%.   (*Continued on page 216*)

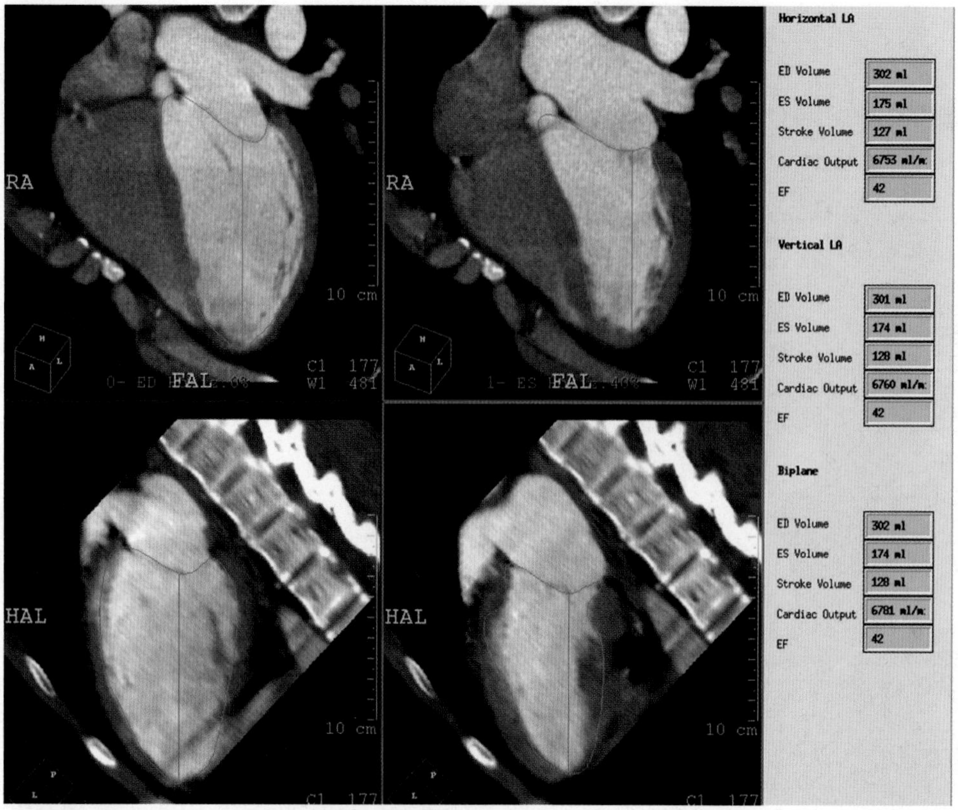

Horizontal LA

ED Volume	302 ml
ES Volume	175 ml
Stroke Volume	127 ml
Cardiac Output	6753 ml/m
EF	42

Vertical LA

ED Volume	301 ml
ES Volume	174 ml
Stroke Volume	128 ml
Cardiac Output	6760 ml/m
EF	42

Biplane

ED Volume	302 ml
ES Volume	174 ml
Stroke Volume	128 ml
Cardiac Output	6781 ml/m
EF	42

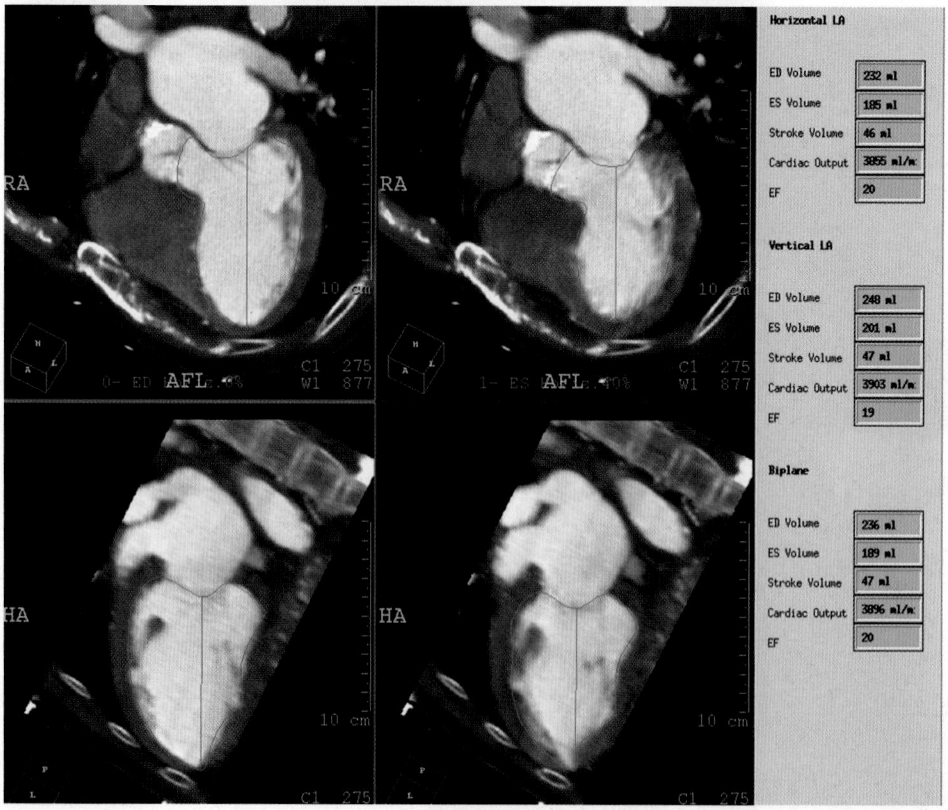

Horizontal LA

ED Volume	232 ml
ES Volume	185 ml
Stroke Volume	46 ml
Cardiac Output	3855 ml/m
EF	20

Vertical LA

ED Volume	248 ml
ES Volume	201 ml
Stroke Volume	47 ml
Cardiac Output	3903 ml/m
EF	19

Biplane

ED Volume	236 ml
ES Volume	189 ml
Stroke Volume	47 ml
Cardiac Output	3896 ml/m
EF	20

Fig. 9.55 (*Continued*) Cardiac function and estimation of ejection fraction with biplane Simpson's method. **(C)** Mild to moderate global hypokinesis with an estimated ejection fraction of 42%. **(D)** Severe hypokinesis with an estimated ejection fraction of 20%. In all cases, orthogonal long axis views of the left ventricle are traced in diastole and in systole. The biplane Simpson's algorithm is used to compute the ejection fraction.

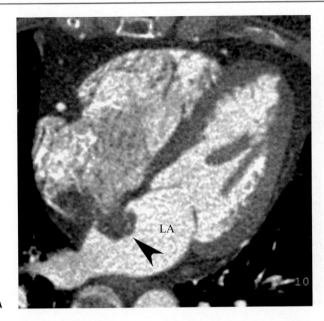

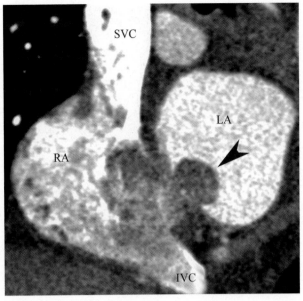

Fig. 9.56 Left atrial myxoma along the atrial septum. **(A)** Four-chamber image demonstrates a mass adherent to the left atrial (LA) side of the interatrial septum (*arrowhead*). **(B)** Coronal image again demonstrates the mass within the LA attached to the interatrial septum (*arrowhead*).

The superior vena cava (SVC) and inferior vena cava (IVC) are seen to empty into the right atrium (RA). Left atrium myxoma is the most common primary tumor of the heart. The interatrial septum is the most common site for a left atrial myxoma.

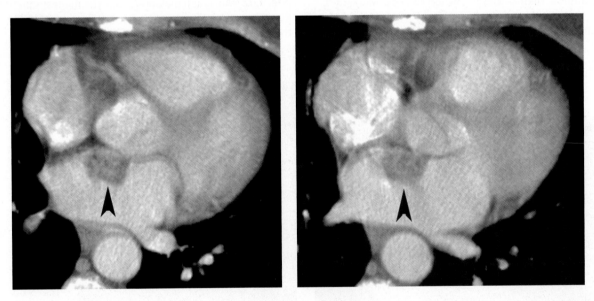

Fig. 9.57 Left atrial myxoma. **(A)** Axial image at the level of the aortic root demonstrates an enhancing mass within the anterior aspect of the left atrium (*arrowhead*). **(B)** Axial image at a slightly lower level demonstrates that this mass (*arrowhead*) is contiguous with the interatrial septum.

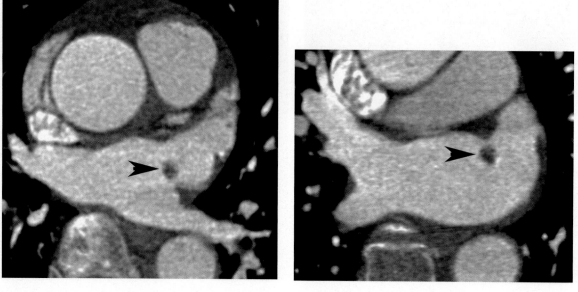

A   B

Fig. 9.58 Left atrial myxoma attached to the warfarin ridge. **(A)** Axial image demonstrates a round low-density mass at the base of the left atrial appendage (*arrowhead*). **(B)** Coronary image again demonstrates the mass at the base of the left atrial appendage (*arrowhead*).

malignant primary cardiac neoplasms are sarcomas, and most are angiosarcomas or rhabdomyosarcomas.

Metastatic neoplasms of the heart are about 20 times more common than primary cardiac tumors. Metastatic tumors that most commonly involve the heart include direct invasion of breast cancer (**Fig. 9.60**) or lung cancer

(**Fig. 9.61**) and hematogenous or lymphatic spread from lymphoma and melanoma. Renal cell carcinoma may spread to the right side of the heart via direct invasion up the IVC (**Fig. 9.62**). Although melanoma has the highest rate of cardiac metastases of any neoplasm, metastatic involvement of the heart by lung or breast cancer is more common.[59]

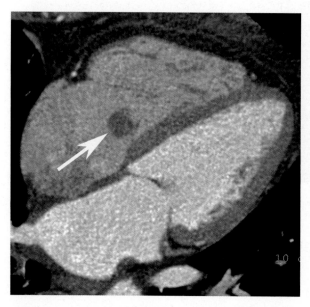

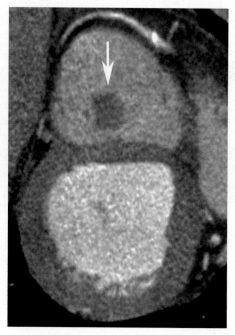

A   B

Fig. 9.59 Right atrial myxoma. **(A)** Four-chamber view demonstrates a round mass that appears to be attached to the atrial surface of the tricuspid valve, adjacent to the atrial septum (*arrow*). **(B)** Short-axis image confirms the location of the mass within the right atrium and slightly removed from the atrial septum (*arrow*).

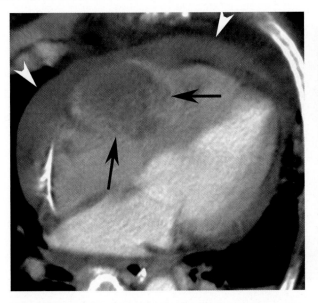

Fig. 9.60 Right ventricular (RV) mass in a patient with metastatic adenocarcinoma of the breast. **(A)** Four-chamber view demonstrates a large mass within the RV (*black arrows*), as well as a pericardial effusion (*white arrowheads*) anterior to the RV. **(B)** Short-axis view confirms the mass within the right ventricle (*black arrows*) and the anterior pericardial effusion (*arrowheads*). Given the presence of normal cardiac function, the mass was most likely related to metastatic disease.

◆ Pericardium

Evaluation of the pericardium for cysts, pericardial effusion, and masses should be a component of every cardiac CT examination. Pericardial cysts represent focal accumulations

of fluid loculated by pericardium (**Fig. 9.63**). Pericardial cysts are of little clinical significance unless they result in mass effect.

Pericardial effusion may be secondary to a variety of etiologies. CT evaluation of pericardial fluid may demonstrate

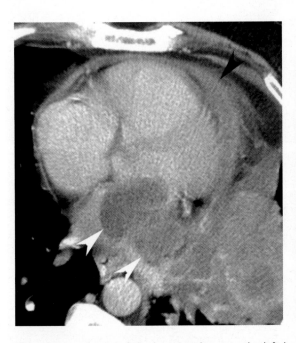

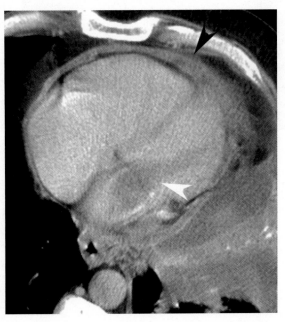

Fig. 9.61 Adenocarcinoma of the lung invading into the left heart through the inferior left pulmonary vein with associated malignant pericardial effusion. **(A)** Axial image at the level of the inferior left pulmonary vein demonstrates a lobulated mass (*white arrowheads*) invading into the left atrium from the pulmonary vein. High-density fluid within the pericardial space (*black arrowhead*) represents malignant effusion or hematoma. **(B)** Four-chamber view demonstrates a low-density mass crossing the mitral valve from the left atrium into the left ventricle (*white arrowhead*), representing either tumor or thrombus. High-density pericardial effusion is again identified (*black arrowhead*).

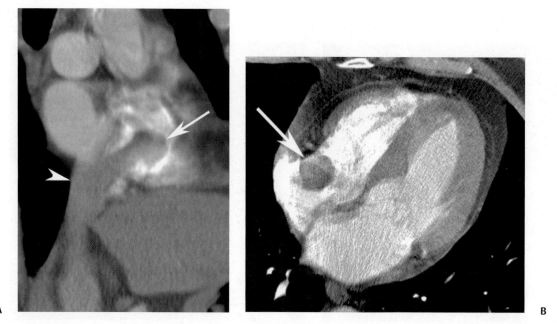

Fig. 9.62 Renal cell carcinoma with extension into the right atrium, and resulting in pulmonary embolism. **(A)** Sagittal image demonstrates thrombus extending up the inferior vena cava (*arrowhead*) into the right atrium (*arrow*). **(B)** Four-chamber view demonstrates the presence of tumor thrombus within the right atrium (*arrow*), along the atrial side of the tricuspid valve.

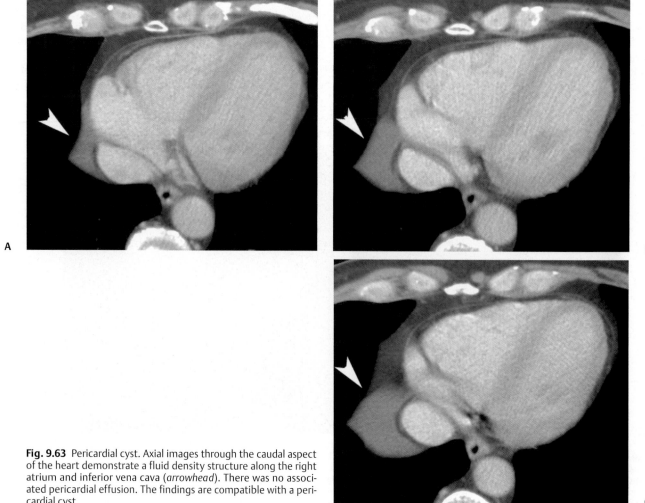

Fig. 9.63 Pericardial cyst. Axial images through the caudal aspect of the heart demonstrate a fluid density structure along the right atrium and inferior vena cava (*arrowhead*). There was no associated pericardial effusion. The findings are compatible with a pericardial cyst.

simple or complex fluid and may suggest an etiology based on the characteristics of the fluid (**Figs. 9.63** and **9.64**). During the workup of chest pain with coronary CTA, the diagnosis of pericarditis may present as a pericardial effusion (**Fig. 9.65**). The diagnosis of tamponade is usually confirmed by echocardiographic demonstration of increased respiratory variation of mitral inflow along with evidence of compression of cardiac chambers. This diagnosis can also be suggested based on changes in septal motion with respiration, but such respiratory evaluation cannot be observed with CT performed in a single breath-hold. The diagnosis of tamponade can be suggested by CT based on compression and collapse of the cardiac chambers, especially by the presence of diastolic collapse of the right or left ventricle (**Fig. 9.66**).

Restrictive or constrictive physiology may be related to intrinsic disease within the heart muscle or to pericardial constriction. Calcification of the pericardium may be visible by CT and is associated with constrictive pericarditis

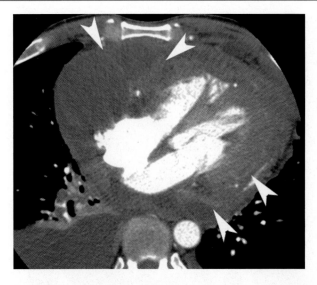

Fig. 9.64 Malignant pericardial effusion in a patient with diffuse metastatic disease. There is a moderate to large effusion with associated septations and enhancement (*arrowheads*). The presence of enhancing tissue within the pericardial fluid is diagnostic of malignant effusion.

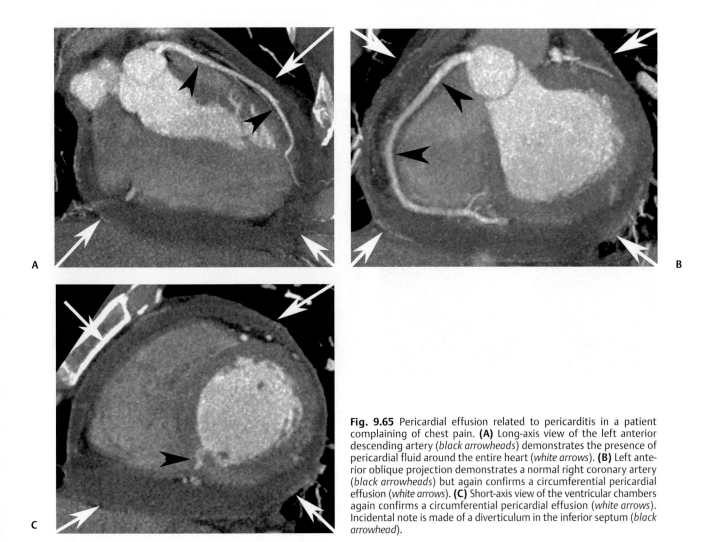

Fig. 9.65 Pericardial effusion related to pericarditis in a patient complaining of chest pain. **(A)** Long-axis view of the left anterior descending artery (*black arrowheads*) demonstrates the presence of pericardial fluid around the entire heart (*white arrows*). **(B)** Left anterior oblique projection demonstrates a normal right coronary artery (*black arrowheads*) but again confirms a circumferential pericardial effusion (*white arrows*). **(C)** Short-axis view of the ventricular chambers again confirms a circumferential pericardial effusion (*white arrows*). Incidental note is made of a diverticulum in the inferior septum (*black arrowhead*).

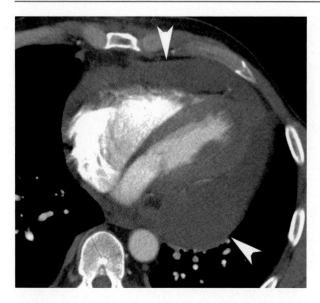

Fig. 9.66 Simple pericardial effusion with tamponade physiology. Note the low-density, homogeneous attenuation of the pericardial fluid (*arrowheads*). There was diastolic narrowing of both ventricles, related to compression by the pericardial fluid. Echocardiography demonstrated Doppler evidence for tamponade physiology.

(**Fig. 9.67**). However, the diagnosis of restrictive or constrictive physiology should be based on hemodynamics observations with Doppler echocardiography or during catheterization because constrictive physiology might be present in the absence of pericardial calcification (**Fig. 9.68**). When surgical stripping of the pericardium is indicated, cardiac CT can be used to demonstrate the relationship of the thickened pericardium to the cardiac surface and coronary arteries (**Fig. 9.69**).

◆ Conclusion

Normal cardiac morphology is essential to normal functioning of the heart. The superb spatial and temporal resolution provided by state-of-the-art multidetector CT provides an excellent tool for evaluation of cardiac anatomy. Many pathologic processes—including intracardiac shunts, infarcts, and neoplasms—demonstrate characteristic morphologic changes in the heart. Evaluation of cardiac motion adds another dimension to the diagnostic capability of CT that may help to explain morphologic abnormalities. The evaluation of cardiac valves discussed in Chapter 10 completes the comprehensive diagnostic examination of the heart by CT.

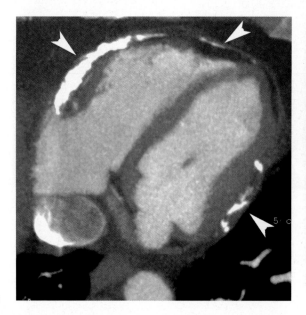

A

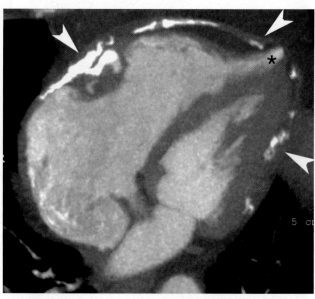

B

Fig. 9.67 Constrictive pericarditis with pericardial calcification in a patient with right ventricle (RV) pressure or volume overload. **(A,B)** Axial and four-chamber views demonstrate diffuse pericardial calcification (*arrowheads*). The four-chamber view demonstrates an elongated appearance to the RV apex (*). The RV apex does not properly distend because of pericardial constriction.

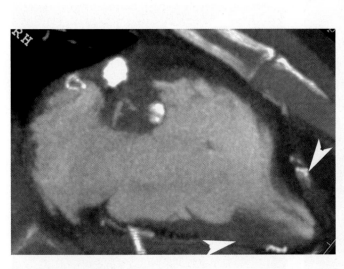

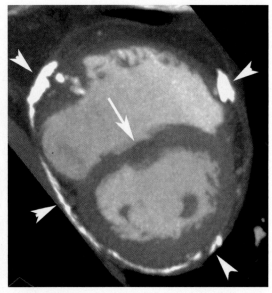

C

D

Fig. 9.67 (*Continued*) **(C)** Long-axis view of the RV demonstrates distortion of the right ventricular apex (*arrowheads*), related to constrictive pericarditis. **(D)** Short-axis view demonstrates diffuse pericardial calcification (*arrowheads*). Septal flattening (*arrow*) is related to right-sided pressure or volume overload.

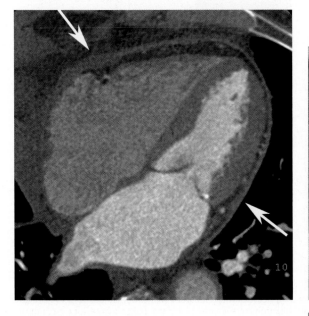

A

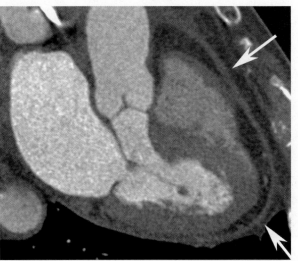

B

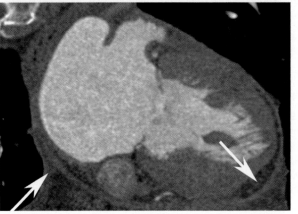

C

Fig. 9.68 Constrictive physiology in a patient with a long history of pericarditis. Diffuse mild thickening of the pericardium (*arrows*) is indistinguishable from pericardial fluid on **(A)** four-chamber view, **(B)** three-chamber view, and **(C)** two-chamber view. Even though there was no calcification of the pericardium, this patient was treated with pericardial stripping on the basis of constrictive physiology demonstrated by echocardiography and pressure measurements during catheterization.

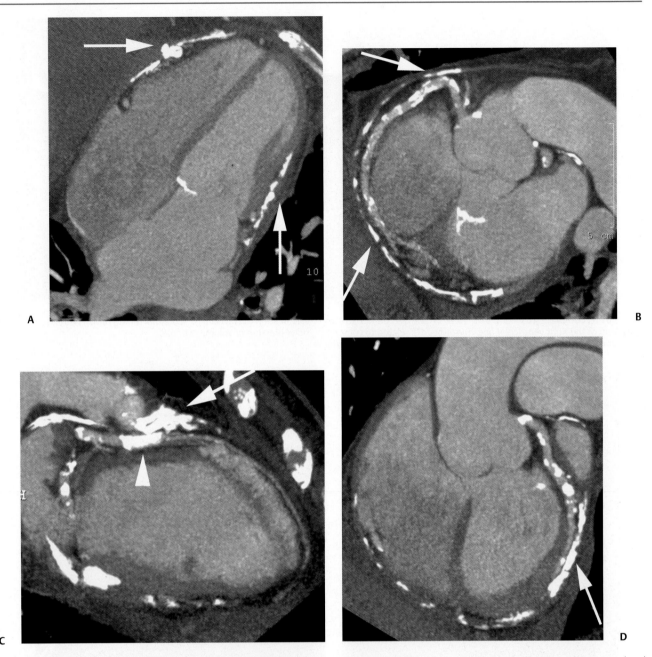

Fig. 9.69 Constrictive pericarditis. Coronary CT angiography was performed as a pre-operative study before pericardial stripping. **(A)** Four-chamber view demonstrates thickened or calcified pericardium along the free walls of the right and left ventricles (*arrows*) with an elongated appearance of the left ventricle related to restriction of diastolic expansion along the proximal to mid left ventricle. **(B)** Right coronary artery with pericardial thickening or calcification adjacent to the proximal and midportions of the vessel (*arrows*). **(C)** Left anterior descending artery with pericardial calcification (*arrow*) immediately adjacent to a stent in the proximal LAD (*arrowhead*). **(D)** Circumflex artery with thick calcified pericardium extending adjacent to a large obtuse marginal branch (*arrow*).

Normal Left Ventricular Function

Cine 9.1   Normal left and right ventricular function. The four projections include a four-chamber view (top left), five-chamber view (top right), two-chamber view (bottom left), and short axis (bottom right). Normal function is characterized by symmetric thickening of the ventricular walls as well as normal wall motion and ejection fraction.

Cine 9.2   Normal left and right ventricular function. Incidental note is made of calcification of the anterior mitral annulus.

Cine 9.3   Normal left and right ventricular function. The right side of the heart is enlarged, with moderate to severe enlargement of the right atrium.

Cine 9.4 Normal left ventricular function with a dilated, hypokinetic right ventricle. The four-chamber view (top left) and short-axis view (top right) demonstrate an enlarged right ventricle. The three-chamber view (bottom left) demonstrates normal motion of the arotic and mitral valves.

Cine 9.5 Low normal left ventricular function with paradoxical motion of the interventricular septum related to right ventricular pressure or volume overload. Note the presence of a pacing catheter in the right ventricle, which appears dilated and hypokinetic.

Cine 9.6 High normal left ventricular function. Estimated ejection fraction of 75%. Although the function is dynamic, the three-chamber view clearly demonstrates that the outflow tract is not obstructed during systole.

Cine 9.7 Low normal left ventricular function. Estimated ejection fraction of 50 to 55%.

Global Left Ventricular Dysfunction

Cine 9.8 Mild global hypokinesis. Estimated ejection fraction of 45%.

Cine 9.9 Mild to moderate global hypokinesis. Estimated ejection fraction of 40%.

Cine 9.10 Mild to moderate global hypokinesis. Estimated ejection fraction of 40%.

Cine 9.11 Mild to moderate global hypokinesis. Estimated ejection fraction of 40%. The left ventricular contour is slightly rounded in the long-axis projections, compatible with dilatation of this chamber.

Cine 9.12 Severe global hypokinesis. Estimated ejection fraction of 15 to 20%. Note the calcification and lack of motion in the aortic valve on the five-chamber view, compatible with the diagnosis of aortic stenosis. There is no evidence of left ventricular hypertrophy, as might be expected with chronic aortic stenosis.

Cine 9.13 Severe global hypokinesis related to ischemic cardiomyopathy. Estimated ejection fraction of 5 to 10%. Slow mixing of contrast is identified within the left ventricular chamber. The aortic and mitral valves open incompletely (low-profile motion) as a result of the reduced cardiac output.

Segmental Left Ventricular Dysfunction

Cine 9.14 Midseptal infarct. The midportion in the interventricular septum is akinetic on the four-chamber, five-chamber, and short-axis views. The remaining walls are hypokinetic.

Cine 9.15 Mid-distal anteroseptal infarct. The mid and distal portions of the anterior portion of the septum and the adjacent anterior wall are akinetic on the three-chamber and short-axis views. The remainder of the septum is hypokinetic; the lateral, inferolateral, and inferior walls demonstrate normal contraction.

Cine 9.16 Anteroseptal infarct. The distal anteroseptal wall is akinetic on the three-chamber, four- chamber, and short-axis views. The remaining walls contract normally.

Cine 9.17 Anteroseptal infarct. The mid to distal anteroseptal wall is akinetic on the four-chamber, five-chamber, and short-axis views. The remaining walls are mildly hypokinetic.

Cine 9.18 Septal contraction abnormality. The segmental wall motion abnormality is apparent on the four-chamber and short-axis views as a paradoxical motion of the septum in early systole, resulting in a septal bounce. Contraction of the remaining left ventricular walls appears normal. The septum demonstrates normal thickening, suggesting that the wall motion abnormality is related to a conduction abnormality rather than an infarct (compare with previous two cases).

Cine 9.19 Distal septal and apical infarct. The distal portion of the septum and apex are akinetic on the five-chamber view. The distal septum appears hypokinetic on the short-axis view. The apex appears to contract normally on the four-chamber and two-chamber views because these views are foreshortened and do not demonstrate the true cardiac apex. The myocardium of the distal septum and apex appears thin on the five-chamber and short-axis views, compatible with an infarct.

Cine 9.20 Mid-distal anteroseptal hypokinesis. There is reduced thickening and motion of the mid-distal anteroseptal wall on the four-chamber and three-chamber projections.

Cine 9.21 Basal inferoseptal infarct. The basal portion of the inferior septum appears thin and akinetic on the four-chamber view (top left) and short axis (top right). Normal wall motion is observed in the two-chamber and three-chamber projections.

Cine 9.22 Proximal inferior–inferolateral infarct. The proximal inferior and inferolateral walls are akinetic on the short-axis, three-chamber, and two-chamber views. This proximal portion of the ventricle appears aneurysmal during systole when the remainder of the left ventricle contracts.

Cine 9.23 Distal inferior–inferolateral and apical akinesis. Moderate hypokinesis of the remaining walls. Low-density infiltrating of the periapical myocardium, particularly in the distal inferolateral wall (short-axis and three-chamber views) and distal inferior wall (two-chamber view), suggests a prior infarct.

Cine 9.24 Severe global hypokinesis with segmental-wall motion abnormalities. Akinesis of the septum and periapical walls is demonstrated on the four-chamber, short-axis, and three-chamber views. The remaining walls demonstrate severe hypokinesis. A pacemaker–defibrillator catheter is identified in the right ventricle.

Cine 9.25 Severe global hypokinesis with segmental-wall motion abnormalities and calcified infarct in the lateral–posterolateral wall. Anteroseptal akinesis is best appreciated on the three-chamber view. Calcification of the lateral–inferolateral walls is present on the four-chamber and short-axis views and is accompanied by calcification of the posterolateral papillary muscles on the two- and three-chamber views. The remaining walls are severely hypokinetic in this patient with ischemic cardiomyopathy.

Cine 9.26 Severe global hypokinesis with septal contraction abnormality in another patient with ischemic cardiomyopathy. Note the presence of calcification in the posterior mitral annulus with a normally functioning mitral valve.

Cine 9.27 Severe global left ventricular hypokinesis with relative sparing of the proximal lateral wall. The septum appears thin and akinetic on the five-chamber and short axis-views. The periapical area is akinetic on all the long-axis views. The remaining walls are severely hypokinetic.

Cine 9.28 Hypokinesis to akinesis of the distal third of the left ventricle with mild to moderate hypokinesis of the proximal–mid walls. A pacemaker–defibrillator is present in the right ventricle.

(Continued on page 226)

Segmental Left Ventricular Dysfunction with Aneurysm

Cine 9.29   Focal myocardial thinning with akinesis–dyskinesis of the midportion of the anteroseptum, representing a focal infarct, which may have been related to a post-surgical complication. Myocardial thinning is clearly visible in the anteroseptum on the short-axis view. The thinned segment appears to bulge toward the right ventricle in systole. This dyskinetic area is visible on the three-chamber long axis and, to a lesser degree, on the four-chamber view.

Cine 9.30   Aneurysm of the mid-inferior wall related to a prior infarct. Dyskinesis of the mid-inferior wall is demonstrated on the two-chamber and short-axis views. The remaining walls demonstrate normal contraction.

Cine 9.31   (A,B) Apical infarct. Small apical aneurysm. The apical-wall motion abnormality is not identified on the foreshortened four-chamber view. However, the apex is clearly akinetic–dyskinetic on the five-chamber and two-chamber views.

Cine 9.32   Apical infarct with aneurysm. The left ventricular apex is dyskinetic and appears to balloon outward during systole on all the long-axis projections, representing a true aneurysm following an infarction. The distal septum is also dyskinetic on the four-chamber view. The remaining walls demonstrate mild hypokinesis.

Cine 9.33   Apical infarct. Large apical aneurysm. The distal third of the ventricle is akinetic or slightly dyskinetic. Image quality is limited by streak from a pacemaker–defibrillator in the right ventricle.

Left Ventricular Dysfunction with Thrombus

Cine 9.34   Dilated left ventricle with severe global left ventricular hypokinesis, periapical akinesis, and apical clot. Long-axis images demonstrate hypokinesis of the proximal walls with akinesis of the distal left ventricle. Apical thrombus is most obvious on the two-chamber view.

Cine 9.35   Distal anteroseptal and apical infarct with apical thrombus. A pacing catheter is present in the right ventricle. The apex appears akinetic on all the long-axis projections. The distal anteroseptal wall is also akinetic on the three-chamber projection.

Cine 9.36   Global left ventricular hypokinesis with thinning of the distal inferior wall, periapical akinesis, and a small amount of clot in the ventricular apex. The diagnosis of partial myocardial rupture was suggested after conventional left ventriculography in the cardiac catheter laboratory. The appearance on the two-chamber view (bottom right) is similar to the appearance of the ventriculogram and suggests a possible perforation of the myocardium. However, short-axis views through the distal portion of the left ventricle demonstrate that this appearance is related to contrast extending between the thrombus and the thinned inferior wall.

Cine 9.37   (A,B) Apical infarct. Large apical aneurysm identified on five-chamber and two-chamber views. Apical thrombus is identified on the five-chamber view.

Focal Defects in the Left Ventricular Wall

Cine 9.38   Inferolateral infarct with large aneurysm or pseudoaneurysm containing thrombus. Although the aneurysm appears to have a wide neck, it was suspected of being a pseudoaneurysm because of the lack of visible myocardium under the thrombus.

Cine 9.39   (A,B) Mid-distal septal and periapical akinesis with subepicardial aneurysm in the distal inferolateral wall (see Fig. 9.40). There is thinning of the distal anteroseptal wall and apex, as well as thinning and irregularity of the distal inferior and inferolateral walls. Contrast appears to extend through the myocardium of the distal inferior wall on the two-chamber views. The diagnosis of subepicardial aneurysm was confirmed at surgery.

Cine 9.40   (A,B) Small pseudoaneurysm along the margin of an apical ventricular patch following apical resection for myxoma. Normal function of the proximal left ventricle with an apical patch. Two-chamber view demonstrates an outward bulge of contrast during systole at the anterior and posterior apex along the margins of a patch.

Cine 9.41   (A) Normal left ventricular function with diverticulum in the inferoposterior left ventricular wall. (B) Normal left ventricular function with diverticulum in the septum. Contrast material extends into the myocardium. However, the normal myocardial thickness and function confirm that the findings represent diverticula rather than subepicardial aneurysms or pseudoaneurysms.

Septal Motion Abnormalities Unrelated to Coronary Disease

Cine 9.42   Post-infarct ventricular septal defect in the inferior septum following a large RCA infarct. Four chamber and short axis views demonstrate a 2×1 cm VSD in the mid-distal portion of the inferior septum. The inferolateral, inferior, and inferoseptal walls are akinetic. A myocardial patch is present in the inferior-inferolateral walls.

Cine 9.43   Normal left ventricular function with septal contraction abnormality. The septum has a biphasic motion or "bounce" during diastole but demonstrates a normal increase in wall thickness during systolic contraction. This finding is most often related to a conduction abnormality and is frequently observed after cardiac surgery.

Cine 9.44   (A,B) Dilated right side of the heart with normal left and right ventricular function. The right ventricular volume is normally slightly larger than the left ventricular volume. In this patient, however, the right ventricle is clearly volume overloaded. Flattening of the septum is observed on the short-axis view and is often associated with right ventricular volume or pressure overload. The right atrium is also dilated, appearing larger than the left atrium.

Cine 9.45   Dilated right side of the heart with paradoxical septal motion related to right-sided pressure or volume overload. Global left ventricular hypokinesis. A pacemaker–defibrillator is present in the right ventricle (short-axis view). The right ventricle demonstrates mildly increased trabeculation related to chronic pressure overload. "Pulmonary hypertension." Paradoxical septal motion with severe pulmonary hypertension.

Cine 9.46   Focal upper septal hypertrophy. Older patient with focal thickening of the basal septum demonstrated on four chamber, short axis, and three chamber views. Overall depressed left ventricular function with segmental hypokinesis involving the proximal inferolateral wall, representing an area of infarction. Focal upper septal hypertrophy can be considered a normal variation in older patients.

Hypertrophic Cardiomyopathy

Cine 9.47 Asymmetric septal hypertrophy with normal left ventricular function. Young patient with focally thickened myocardium in the proximal to mid-interventricular septum visible on four-chamber, short-axis, and three-chamber views. This form of asymmetric hypertrophic cardiomyopathy can lead to left ventricular outflow tract obstruction. However, the three-chamber view demonstrates no evidence of outflow tract obstruction during systole.

Cine 9.48 Mild concentric left ventricular hypertrophy with normal left ventricular function. The five-chamber view demonstrates no evidence of outflow tract obstruction.

Cine 9.49 Moderate concentric left ventricular hypertrophy with dynamic left ventricular function. The combination of left ventricular hypertrophy with dynamic function and systolic anterior motion of the mitral apparatus can lead to outflow tract obstruction, although outflow obstruction was not observed in this patient.

Cine 9.50 Concentric left ventricular hypertrophy with mid-distal left ventricular cavity obstruction during systole. There is no evidence of left ventricular outflow tract obstruction on the three-chamber view. The apex appears thin and akinetic; this can represent a developmental anomaly, or it could be related to apical ischemia or infarction. Increased wall stress at the apex related to left ventricular cavity obstruction may contribute to apical thinning and dysfunction.

Cine 9.51 Apical hypertrophy is a form of asymmetric hypertrophic cardiomyopathy. This patient demonstrates mid-distal left ventricular cavity obstruction during systole. The apex appears thin and akinetic; this can represent a developmental anomaly associated with apical hypertrophy, or it could be related to apical ischemia/infarction.

Cine 9.52 Apical hypertrophy with distal cavity obstruction during systole.

Cine 9.53 Apical hypertrophy with a classic spade shape of the left ventricular cavity.

Other Forms of Nonischemic Cardiomyopathy

Cine 9.54 Noncompaction of the left ventricle (LVNC). **(A,B)** The inner trabeculated portion of the left ventricular wall is more than twice the thickness of the outer compact portion. This patient demonstrates relative sparing of the septum in this process. Although left ventricular wall thickness is increased, LVNC may be distinguished from hypertrophic cardiomyopathy by the increased trabeculation. Although LVNC is often associated with reduced ventricular function, left ventricular function is relatively preserved in this patient with only mild mid-distal septal hypokinesis. **(C)** Six-month follow-up demonstrates similar findings with slight improvement in septal function.

Cine 9.55 Noncompaction of the left ventricle (LVNC) associated with a dilated cardiomyopathy with severe global hypokinesis (LVEF ~15%). The inner trabeculated portion of the left ventricular wall is more than twice the thickness of the outer compact portion, with relative sparing of the septum. Dilated, hypokinetic right heart with septal flattening and mild paradoxical septal motion likely related to pulmonary hypertension.

Cine 9.56 Global ventricular dysfunction with acute myocarditis–pericarditis. Previously healthy young man presents with acute global left ventricular dysfunction, an ejection fraction of 35%, and pericardial effusion with normal coronary arteries.

Cine 9.57 Dilated cardiomyopathy with overall ejection fraction of 20% in a patient with normal coronary arteries but with a history of cocaine use and chronic hypertension.

Cine 9.58 Dilated cardiomyopathy of undefined etiology in a patient with normal coronary arteries.

Right-Sided Pressure and Volume Overload

Cine 9.59 McConnell sign in pulmonary embolism. Dilated right ventricle with akinesis of the basal to midportions of the right ventricle but normal contraction of the right ventricular apex (best seen on the four-chamber view). This sign is considered relatively specific for pulmonary embolism on echocardiography. This patient had a saddle embolus diagnosed on CT.

Cine 9.60 McConnell sign in pulmonary embolism. Mildly dilated right side of the heart with right ventricular hypokinesis. The right ventricular apex demonstrates normal function on the three-chamber long-axis projection.

Cine 9.61 Right ventricular enlargement and septal flattening during systole secondary to pulmonary hypertension.

Cine 9.62 Right ventricular enlargement and septal flattening in a patient with D-transposition status post Jatene procedure (arterial switch). Right-sided pressures are elevated secondary to pulmonary hypertension, resulting in septal flattening.

Cine 9.63 Right ventricular volume overload related to partial anomalous pulmonary venous return.

Cine 9.64 Right ventricular volume overload related to a large secundum atrial septal defect. Marked enlargement of the right side of the heart with relative preservation of right ventricular function. Diastolic flattening of the interventricular septum is most apparent on the short-axis projection.

Cine 9.65 Right ventricular volume overload related to a secundum atrial septal defect. Enlargement of the right side of the heart is accompanied by relative preservation of right ventricular function and diastolic flattening of the interventricular septum.

Cine 9.66 Right ventricular volume overload related to a secundum atrial septal defect. Enlargement of the right side of the heart is accompanied by preservation of right ventricular function and diastolic flattening of the interventricular septum.

Cine 9.67 Right ventricular volume overload related to a secundum atrial septal defect with left-to-right shunting. Enlargement of the right side of the heart is accompanied by preservation of right ventricular function and diastolic flattening of the interventricular septum. Left-to-right shunting is visible at the atrial level on the four-chamber view.

Cine 9.68 Right ventricular volume overload related to a secundum atrial septal defect (ASD) with left-to-right shunting. Enlargement of the right side of the heart with compression of the left side. Mildly decreased right ventricular function is accompanied by diastolic flattening of the interventricular septum. The large ASD is visible in the four-chamber view.

(Continued on page 228)

Atrial Septal Aneurysm

Cine 9.69 Atrial septal aneurysm bulging into the right atrium. Although these aneurysms often swing back and forth between the atria, they are typically bowed into the right atrium because of greater left atrial pressures.

Cine 9.70 Atrial septal aneurysm bulging into the right atrium.

Cine 9.71 Patent foramen ovale with left-to-right shunt. Dense contrast is seen to track from the enhanced left atrium to the unenhanced right atrium. The shunt is directed toward the inferior vena cava orifice at the inferior aspect of the right atrium.

Cine 9.72 **(A)** Long-axis and short-axis images demonstrate normal left and right ventricular function. **(B)** Although right-sided heart function is normal, there is increased right ventricular trabeculation related to elevated right-sided pressure. **(C)** Four-chamber view demonstrates an atrial septal aneurysm that bulges into the left atrium, suggesting that right atrial pressure is greater than left atrial pressure. **(D)** Sagittal image through the atrial septum as well as the superior and inferior vena cava demonstrates a patent foramen ovale, which presents as a mobile flap in the upper portion of the septum. **(E)** Early imaging following reinjection of contrast demonstrates increased contrast density in the right atrium with right-to-left shunting of the dense contrast, which swirls along the roof of the left atrium. This sagittal image is optimized to visualize the inferior vena cava. **(F)** Early imaging following reinjection of contrast demonstrates increased contrast density in the right atrium with right-to-left shunting of the dense contrast, which swirls along the roof of the left atrium. This sagittal image is optimized to visualize the superior vena cava.

Atrial Myxoma

Cine 9.73 Right atrial myxoma adjacent to the tricuspid annulus. The myxoma presents as a mobile hypodensity moving across the tricuspid valve during the cardiac cycle.

Cine 9.74 Left atrial myxoma along the atrial septum. This is the most common location for a left atrial myxoma.

Cine 9.75 Huge left atrial myxoma filling the left atrium and obstructing mitral valve flow.

Pericardial Defects

Cine 9.76 Partial absence of the pericardium with herniation of the left atrial appendage. The left atrial appendage is enlarged (8 × 7 cm) with mass effect upon the basal anterior and lateral walls of the left ventricle. Delayed filling of the atrial appendage is observed with dependent layering of contrast material. Direct communication with the left atrium is observed in the two chamber view (bottom left).

Left Ventricular Assist Devices

Cine 9.77 Left ventricular failure with a left ventricular assist device. The cannula in the left ventricular apex serves as the intake for the device. Blood is pumped back through a second cannula, which may be placed in the ascending or descending thoracic aorta.

Cine 9.78 Left ventricular assist device with obstructed inflow cannula. The inflow cannula is angled superiorly such that it is partially obstructed by the anterior wall of the left ventricle.

Cine 9.79 **(A,B)** Severe left ventricular dysfunction with a Jarvik ventricular assist device. The aortic valve demonstrates reduced motion because little blood is pumped by the heart through the left ventricular outflow tract.

References

1. Neilan TG, Pradhan AD, King ME, Weyman AE. Derivation of a size-independent variable for scaling of cardiac dimensions in a normal paediatric population. Eur J Echocardiogr. 2009;10(1):50–55

2. Lang RM, Bierig M, Devereux RB, et al; Chamber Quantification Writing Group; American Society of Echocardiography's Guidelines and Standards Committee; European Association of Echocardiography. Recommendations for chamber quantification: a report from the American Society of Echocardiography's Guidelines and Standards Committee and the Chamber Quantification Writing Group, developed in conjunction with the European Association of Echocardiography, a branch of the European Society of Cardiology. J Am Soc Echocardiogr. 2005;18(12):1440–1463

3. Stolzmann P, Scheffel H, Trindade PT, et al. Left ventricular and left atrial dimensions and volumes: comparison between dual-source CT and echocardiography. Invest Radiol. 2008;43(5):284–289

4. Kircher B, Abbott JA, Pau S, et al. Left atrial volume determination by biplane two-dimensional echocardiography: validation by cine computed tomography. Am Heart J. 1991;121(3 Pt 1):864–871

5. Christiaens L, Lequeux B, Ardilouze P, et al. A new method for measurement of left atrial volumes using 64-slice spiral computed tomography: comparison with two-dimensional echocardiographic techniques. Int J Cardiol. 2009;131(2):217–224

6. Rodevan O, Bjornerheim R, Ljosland M, Maehle J, Smith HJ, Ihlen H. Left atrial volumes assessed by three- and two-dimensional echocardiography compared to MRI estimates. Int J Card Imaging. 1999;15(5):397–410

7. Koka AR, Yau J, Van Why C, Cohen IS, Halpern EJ. Underestimation of left atrial size measured with transthoracic echocardiography compared with 3D MDCT. AJR Am J Roentgenol. 2010;194(5):W375–W381

8. Ko SM, Kim YJ, Park JH, Choi NM. Assessment of left ventricular ejection fraction and regional wall motion with 64-slice multidetector CT: a comparison with two-dimensional transthoracic echocardiography. Br J Radiol. 2010;83(985):28–34

9. Roman MJ, Devereux RB, Kramer-Fox R, O'Loughlin J. Two-dimensional echocardiographic aortic root dimensions in normal children and adults. Am J Cardiol. 1989;64(8):507–512

10. Pharr JR, West MB, Kusumoto FM, Figueredo VM. Prominent crista terminalis appearing as a right atrial mass on transthoracic echocardiogram. J Am Soc Echocardiogr. 2002;15(7):753–755

11. Peters PJ, Reinhardt S. The echocardiographic evaluation of intracardiac masses: a review. J Am Soc Echocardiogr. 2006;19(2):230–240

12. Lester SJ, Ryan EW, Schiller NB, Foster E. Best method in clinical practice and in research studies to determine left atrial size. Am J Cardiol. 1999;84(7):829–832

13. Tsang TS, Abhayaratna WP, Barnes ME, et al. Prediction of cardiovascular outcomes with left atrial size: is volume superior to area or diameter? J Am Coll Cardiol. 2006;47(5):1018–1023

14. Hanley PC, Tajik AJ, Hynes JK, et al. Diagnosis and classification of atrial septal aneurysm by two-dimensional echocardiography: report of 80 consecutive cases. J Am Coll Cardiol. 1985;6(6):1370–1382

15. Fan CM, Fischman AJ, Kwek BH, Abbara S, Aquino SL. Lipomatous hypertrophy of the interatrial septum: increased uptake on FDG PET. AJR Am J Roentgenol. 2005;184(1):339–342

16. Prior JT. Lipomatous hypertrophy of cardiac interatrial septum. A lesion resembling hibernoma, lipoblastomatosis and infiltrating lipoma. Arch Pathol. 1964;78:11–15

17. Heyer CM, Kagel T, Lemburg SP, Bauer TT, Nicolas V. Lipomatous hypertrophy of the interatrial septum: a prospective study of incidence, imaging findings, and clinical symptoms. Chest. 2003;124(6): 2068–2073

18. Shirani J, Roberts WC. Clinical, electrocardiographic and morphologic features of massive fatty deposits ("lipomatous hypertrophy") in the atrial septum. J Am Coll Cardiol. 1993;22(1):226–238

19. Christiansen S, Stypmann J, Baba HA, Hammel D, Scheld HH. Surgical management of extensive lipomatous hypertrophy of the right atrium. Cardiovasc Surg. 2000;8(1):88–90

20. Homma S, Sacco RL. Patent foramen ovale and stroke. Circulation. 2005;112(7):1063–1072

21. Khairy P, O'Donnell CP, Landzberg MJ. Transcatheter closure versus medical therapy of patent foramen ovale and presumed paradoxical thromboemboli: a systematic review. Ann Intern Med. 2003;139(9): 753–760

22. Chong JY, Homma S, Mohr JP. Stroke as a complication of congenital heart disease. Curr Atheroscler Rep. 2005;7(4):263–267

23. Schwedt TJ, Dodick DW. Patent foramen ovale and migraine—bringing closure to the subject. Headache. 2006;46(4):663–671

24. Saremi F, Channual S, Raney A, et al. Imaging of patent foramen ovale with 64-section multidetector CT. Radiology. 2008;249(2):483–492

25. Kim YJ, Hur J, Shim CY, et al. Patent foramen ovale: diagnosis with multidetector CT—comparison with transesophageal echocardiography. Radiology. 2009;250(1):61–67

26. Radzik D, Davignon A, van Doesburg N, Fournier A, Marchand T, Ducharme G. Predictive factors for spontaneous closure of atrial septal defects diagnosed in the first 3 months of life. J Am Coll Cardiol. 1993;22(3):851–853

27. Wahl A, Windecker S, Meier B. Evaluation and treatment of abnormalities of the interatrial septum. Catheter Cardiovasc Interv. 2004; 63(1):94–103

28. Hoffman JI, Kaplan S. The incidence of congenital heart disease. J Am Coll Cardiol. 2002;39(12):1890–1900

29. Mehta AV, Goenka S, Chidambaram B, Hamati F. Natural history of isolated ventricular septal defect in the first five years of life. Tenn Med. 2000;93(4):136–138

30. Healey JE Jr. An anatomic survey of anomalous pulmonary veins: their clinical significance. J Thorac Surg. 1952;23(5):433–444

31. Kiseleva IP, Malsagov GU. Differential diagnosis of anomalous pulmonary venous return. A clinical-roentgenological study. Cor Vasa. 1984;26(2):140–146

32. Toyoshima M, Sato A, Fukumoto Y, et al. Partial anomalous pulmonary venous return showing anomalous venous return to the azygos vein. Intern Med. 1992;31(9):1112–1116

33. Schneider DJ, Moore JW. Patent ductus arteriosus. Circulation. 2006;114(17):1873–1882

34. Ito N, Tsujino I, Nishimura M. Enhanced computed tomography unveiling the underlying cause of pulmonary hypertension. Int J Cardiovasc Imaging. 2010;26(3):257–258

35. Filipek MS, Gosselin MV. Multidetector pulmonary CT angiography: advances in the evaluation of pulmonary arterial diseases. Semin Ultrasound CT MR. 2004;25(2):83–98

36. Tan RT, Kuzo R, Goodman LR, Siegel R, Haasler GB, Presberg KW; Medical College of Wisconsin Lung Transplant Group. Utility of CT scan evaluation for predicting pulmonary hypertension in patients with parenchymal lung disease. Chest. 1998;113(5):1250–1256

37. O'Callaghan JP, Heitzman ER, Somogyi JW, Spirt BA. CT evaluation of pulmonary artery size. J Comput Assist Tomogr. 1982;6(1):101–104

38. Raman SV, Shah M, McCarthy B, Garcia A, Ferketich AK. Multi-detector row cardiac computed tomography accurately quantifies right and left ventricular size and function compared with cardiac magnetic resonance. Am Heart J. 2006;151(3):736–744

39. Coche E, Vlassenbroek A, Roelants V, et al. Evaluation of biventricular ejection fraction with ECG-gated 16-slice CT: preliminary findings in acute pulmonary embolism in comparison with radionuclide ventriculography. Eur Radiol. 2005;15(7):1432–1440

40. Doğan H, Kroft LJ, Huisman MV, van der Geest RJ, de Roos A. Right ventricular function in patients with acute pulmonary embolism: analysis with electrocardiography-synchronized multi-detector row CT. Radiology. 2007;242(1):78–84

41. Kimura F, Sakai F, Sakomura Y, et al. Helical CT features of arrhythmogenic right ventricular cardiomyopathy. Radiographics. 2002;22(5): 1111–1124

42. Yazici M, Demircan S, Durna K, Yasar E. Left ventricular diverticulum in two adult patients. Int Heart J. 2005;46(1):161–165

43. Maron BJ. Hypertrophic cardiomyopathy: a systematic review. JAMA. 2002;287(10):1308–1320

44. Wigle ED, Rakowski H, Kimball BP, Williams WG. Hypertrophic cardiomyopathy. Clinical spectrum and treatment. Circulation. 1995; 92(7):1680–1692

45. Spirito P, Bellone P, Harris KM, Bernabo P, Bruzzi P, Maron BJ. Magnitude of left ventricular hypertrophy and risk of sudden death in hypertrophic cardiomyopathy. N Engl J Med. 2000;342(24): 1778–1785

46. Devereux RB, Alonso DR, Lutas EM, et al. Echocardiographic assessment of left ventricular hypertrophy: comparison to necropsy findings. Am J Cardiol. 1986;57(6):450–458

47. Stöllberger C, Finsterer J. Left ventricular hypertrabeculation/noncompaction. J Am Soc Echocardiogr. 2004;17(1):91–100

48. Hofer M, Stöllberger C, Finsterer J. Acquired noncompaction associated with myopathy. Int J Cardiol. 2007;121(3):296–297

49. Finsterer J. Cardiogenetics, neurogenetics, and pathogenetics of left ventricular hypertrabeculation/noncompaction. Pediatr Cardiol. 2009;30(5):659–681

50. Stanton C, Bruce C, Connolly H, et al. Isolated left ventricular noncompaction syndrome. Am J Cardiol. 2009;104(8):1135–1138

51. Chen H, Zhang W, Li D, Cordes TM, Mark Payne R, Shou W. Analysis of ventricular hypertrabeculation and noncompaction using genetically engineered mouse models. Pediatr Cardiol. 2009;30(5): 626–634

52. Dulce MC, Mostbeck GH, Friese KK, Caputo GR, Higgins CB. Quantification of the left ventricular volumes and function with cine MR imaging: comparison of geometric models with three-dimensional data. Radiology. 1993;188(2):371–376

53. Schepis T, Gaemperli O, Koepfli P, et al. Comparison of 64-slice CT with gated SPECT for evaluation of left ventricular function. J Nucl Med. 2006;47(8):1288–1294

54. Sugeng L, Mor-Avi V, Weinert L, et al. Quantitative assessment of left ventricular size and function: side-by-side comparison of real-time three-dimensional echocardiography and computed tomography with magnetic resonance reference. Circulation. 2006;114(7): 654–661

55. Ragland MM, Tak T. The role of echocardiography in diagnosing space-occupying lesions of the heart. Clin Med Res. 2006;4(1):22–32

56. Shapiro LM. Cardiac tumours: diagnosis and management. Heart. 2001;85(2):218–222

57. Meng Q, Lai H, Lima J, Tong W, Qian Y, Lai S. Echocardiographic and pathologic characteristics of primary cardiac tumors: a study of 149 cases. Int J Cardiol. 2002;84(1):69–75

58. Araoz PA, Mulvagh SL, Tazelaar HD, Julsrud PR, Breen JFCT. CT and MR imaging of benign primary cardiac neoplasms with echocardiographic correlation. Radiographics. 2000;20(5):1303–1319

59. Gibbs P, Cebon JS, Calafiore P, Robinson WA. Cardiac metastases from malignant melanoma. Cancer. 1999;85(1):78–84

10

Valve Assessment

Ethan J. Halpern and Donna R. Zwas

Assessment of the cardiac valves is an integral part of a comprehensive cardiac CT assessment. Valve dysfunction may be related to coronary disease and can be the cause or the consequence of alterations in cardiac morphology and function. The aortic and mitral valves are well visualized with coronary CT angiography (CTA) because there is ample contrast in the left heart. CTA often provides complementary information to echocardiography for the evaluation of normal and diseased valves.[1] When the examination is performed with an appropriate infusion of contrast material to assess right-sided cardiac structures, the pulmonic and tricuspid valves may also be evaluated. Most recently, CTA has been applied to planning and post-procedure evaluation of transcatheter valve implantation.[2,3]

◆ Aortic Valve Anatomy

The aortic valve consists of three leaflets of equal size attached along the aortic annulus at the proximal margin of the aortic root (**Fig. 10.1**). In the closed, diastolic position, the three commissures that separate the leaflets intersect at the center of the annulus at 120-degree angles. During systole the valve leaflets swing superiorly into the sinuses of Valsalva, revealing the triangular orifice of the aortic valve. Normal aortic valve motion is documented by demonstration of complete coaptation of the leaflets in diastole and unrestricted leaflet motion in systole to form an equilateral triangle whose vertices extend to the walls of the aortic root.

The annulus of the aortic valve is located between the left ventricular outflow tract (LVOT) and the aortic root. A short-axis image through the aortic annulus demonstrates that the annulus and aortic valve are related to the pulmonic valve, which is located anterior and to the left of the aortic valve. The commissure between the right and left cusps of the aortic valve is aligned with the posterior commissure of the pulmonic valve (see discussion of aortic root in Chapter 3). The posterior aspect of the aortic annulus is in direct fibrous continuity with the anterior wall of the left atrium and the anterior mitral leaflet, as demonstrated on the long-axis view of the heart (**Fig. 10.2**).

The aortic valve is imaged with little motion artifact because the leaflets remain in a fixed, closed position throughout diastole and in a relatively stable open position throughout most of systole. The open aortic valve is best visualized during mid-systole, at about 20 to 30% of the RR interval. The closed aortic valve is best visualized in mid-diastole, at about 70 to 80% of the RR interval. The precise phase at which the valve is best imaged depends on the patient's heart rate and may be vendor specific, depending on the method used to define percentage of the RR interval. The individual aortic valve cusps are best imaged in the short axis (**Fig. 10.2A**), whereas valve motion is best visualized in the long axis (**Fig. 10.2B**).

Echocardiography is the noninvasive standard for assessment of aortic valve function. Aortic valve morphology and function are evaluated echocardiographically in both the short and long axis. Aortic valve area is estimated with a hemodynamic calculation based on the continuity equation[4] or by direct planimetry.[5] Assessment of the aortic valve with CT is based on evaluation of the aortic leaflet morphology, aortic leaflet motion, and direct planimetry. Hemodynamic measurements are not possible with CT. Several studies suggest that planimetric measurements of the narrowest aortic valve orifice observed in midsystole demonstrate high correlation with aortic valve area calculated with the continuity equation using transesophageal echocardiography.[6–8] Our own experience suggests that planimetric measurements on CT are slightly larger than aortic valve area calculated from the continuity equation with echocardiography. The lower estimates of aortic valve area by echocardiography are likely related to the elliptical shape of the LVOT (see **Fig. 9.2**), which results in echocardiographic underestimation of the LVOT area.[9]

◆ Aortic Stenosis

The most common causes for aortic stenosis in adults include degenerative calcification of a normal trileaflet valve, rheumatic aortic valvulitis, and congenital bicuspid valve. Calcific aortic stenosis is a process characterized by accumulation of calcium that resembles ectopic bone formation.

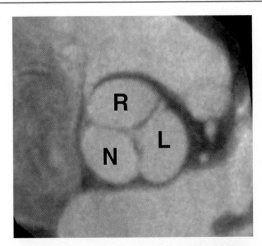

A

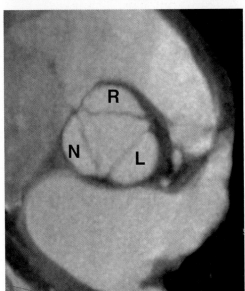

B

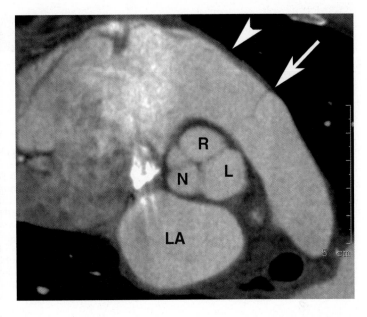

C

Fig. 10.1 **(A)** Short-axis view of the aortic valve during diastole. The three cusps of the aortic valve are defined by the commissures that separate the right (R), left (L), and noncoronary (N) cusps. **(B)** Short-axis image of the tricuspid aortic valve during systole demonstrates a triangular opening as the three cusps separate along their commissures. The right ventricular outflow tract crosses anterior to the aorta at the level of the aortic valve. **(C)** Using a slightly different angulation, the right ventricular outflow tract is demonstrated (*arrowhead*) with the pulmonic valve (*arrow*). The left atrium (LA) is posterior to the aortic valve.

This process may share a pathophysiologic pathway with atherosclerosis of the coronary arteries.[10] Renal dysfunction and abnormal calcium metabolism may accelerate aortic valve calcification. Calcific aortic sclerosis is present in about 25% of adults over the age of 65 and is associated with a 50% increased risk of myocardial infarction and cardiovascular death compared with age-matched controls with a normal aortic valve.[11,12] Rheumatic heart disease was once a common cause of aortic stenosis but is now much less common and almost invariably accompanied by mitral valve disease. Other less common causes of aortic stenosis include homozygous hypercholesterolemia and systemic lupus.

Because the area of aortic valve varies with patient body habitus, a fixed lower threshold value for aortic valve area cannot be provided. Several studies suggest that the valve area measured by CT planimetry correlates well with echocardiographic measurements in aortic stenosis.[13] In our experience using direct planimetry of the aortic valve with CTA, the mean normal adult aortic valve area is 4.2 cm^2 with a range from about 2.5 to 6 cm^2.[14] The 2006

American College of Cardiology (ACC)/American Heart Association (AHA) guidelines for normal aortic and mitral valve areas are summarized in **Table 10.1**.[15] Mild aortic stenosis demonstrates a valve area greater than 1.5 cm^2 with a mean gradient less than 25 mm Hg. When the valve motion appears restricted but the CT planimetric measurement is greater than 1.5 cm^2, the stenosis is classified as mild (**Fig. 10.2C**). A valve area of about 1.5 cm^2 is classified as mild to moderate stenosis (**Fig. 10.3**). Moderate aortic stenosis demonstrates a valve area in the range of 1.0 to 1.5 cm^2 with a mean gradient in the range of 25 to 40 mm Hg (**Figs. 10.4, 10.5,** and **10.6**). Severe aortic stenosis demonstrates a valve area of less than 1 cm^2 with a mean gradient greater than 40 mm Hg (**Fig. 10.7**). When the aortic valve area is less than 0.7 cm^2, aortic stenosis is classified as critical (**Fig. 10.8**). As noted, our experience suggests that aortic valve area measured at coronary CTA is slightly larger than the area suggested by echocardiography.[9] Because the ACC/AHA guidelines are based on echocardiographic measurements, allowances should be made for a slightly greater area on CTA.

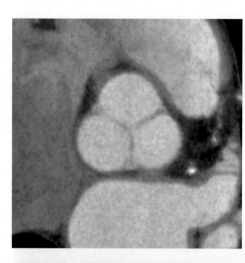

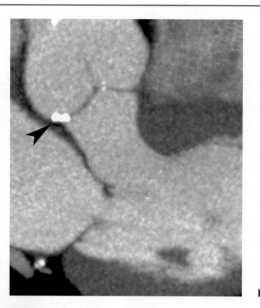

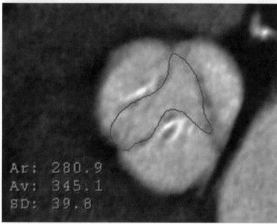

Fig. 10.2 Calcified aortic valve without significant stenosis. **(A)** Short-axis image of the aortic valve demonstrates normally placed commissures of a trileaflet valve. **(B)** Three-chamber view through the aortic valve demonstrates the presence of calcification at the margin of the valve leaflets (*arrowhead*). **(C)** Short-axis image through the valve in systole demonstrates a trileaflet opening with valve area of 2.8 cm² by planimetry, suggesting that there is only minimal restriction of valve motion.

Although the classification of aortic stenosis is based on valve area, absolute valve area might not correlate with symptoms. Valve area indexed to body surface area may provide a better estimate of the true severity of stenosis, and clinical management of patients with aortic stenosis must be based on the patient's symptoms. As a general rule, however, the rate of progression of aortic stenosis and clinical outcome can be predicted based on hemodynamic factors and the aortic valve area.[16]

Bicuspid aortic valve is easily diagnosed by cardiac CTA. The bicuspid valve demonstrates a characteristic "fish-mouth" opening, which is distinct from the normal triangular opening of the trileaflet aortic valve. A bicuspid valve may demonstrate a fused commissure, known as a pseudoraphae,

Table 10.1 Grading of Aortic and Mitral Stenosis

	Aortic valve area (cm²)	Aortic valve gradient (mm Hg)	Mitral valve area (cm²)	Mitral valve gradient (mm Hg)
Normal value	2.5–6.0	<15	4.0–5.0	<5
Mild stenosis	>1.5	<25	1.5–2.5	5–10
Moderate stenosis	1.0–1.5	25–40	1.0–1.5	
Severe stenosis	<1.0	>40	<1.0	>10

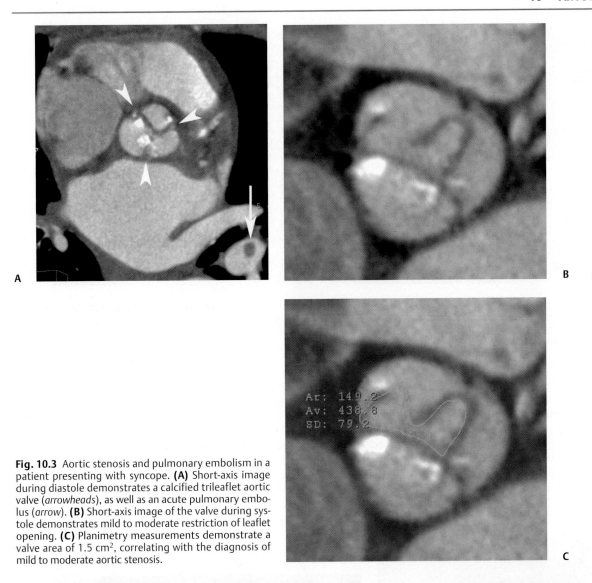

Fig. 10.3 Aortic stenosis and pulmonary embolism in a patient presenting with syncope. **(A)** Short-axis image during diastole demonstrates a calcified trileaflet aortic valve (*arrowheads*), as well as an acute pulmonary embolus (*arrow*). **(B)** Short-axis image of the valve during systole demonstrates mild to moderate restriction of leaflet opening. **(C)** Planimetry measurements demonstrate a valve area of 1.5 cm², correlating with the diagnosis of mild to moderate aortic stenosis.

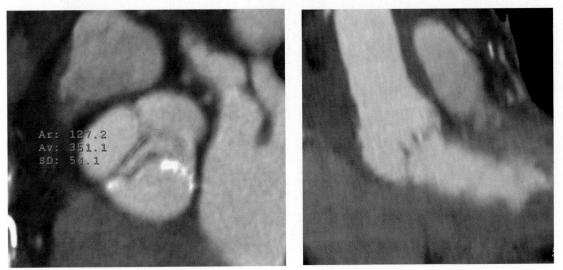

Fig. 10.4 Calcified aortic valve with moderate stenosis. **(A)** Short-axis image during systole demonstrates restricted opening of the valve with a valve area of 1.3 cm² by planimetry. **(B)** Long-axis view during systole confirms restriction of leaflet motion.

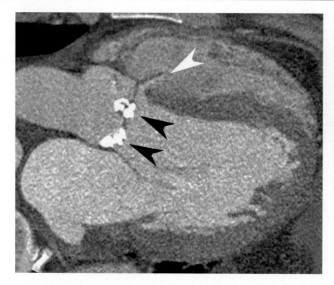
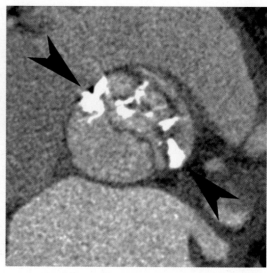

Fig. 10.5 Calcified aortic valve with moderate stenosis and subvalvular perimembranous ventricular septal defect (VSD). **(A)** Three-chamber image during diastole demonstrates the calcified aortic valve (*black arrowheads*) as well as an anterior subvalvular VSD (*white arrowhead*).

(B) Short-axis image during systole demonstrates restricted opening of the calcified valve with a valve area of 1.3–1.4 cm², suggesting moderate aortic stenosis.

or absence of an expected commissure (**Figs. 10.9** and **10.10**). CT grading of stenosis for a bicuspid valve is based on planimetry (**Figs. 10.10** and **10.11**). When performing planimetry of a bicuspid aortic valve, particular care is required to measure the narrowest orifice observed in midsystole. Patients with bicuspid aortic valve often have a disorder of vascular connective tissue that can result in aortic root dilatation, even in the absence of a hemodynamically

significant stenosis of the aortic valve.[17–19] The recommended threshold for elective replacement of a dilated ascending aorta is lower in patients with bicuspid aortic valve because of an increased risk of dissection or rupture. When a bicuspid valve demonstrates normal function, elective replacement is recommended when the diameter of the aorta exceeds 5 cm (**Fig. 10.9**). In a patient with a bicuspid valve that must be replaced, replacement of the ascending aorta is

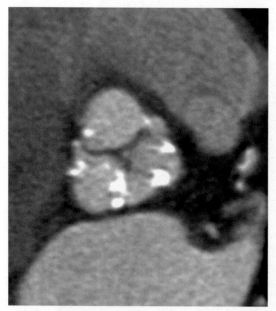
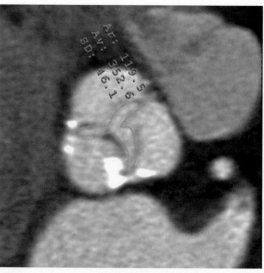

Fig. 10.6 Calcified aortic valve with moderate stenosis and mild insufficiency. **(A)** Short-axis image during diastole demonstrates incomplete coaptation at the center of the valve, consistent with the diagnosis of

aortic insufficiency. **(B)** Short-axis image during systole demonstrates restricted opening of the calcified valve with a valve area of 1.2 cm² by planimetry.

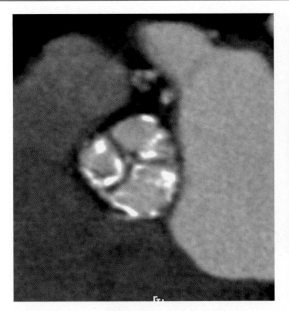

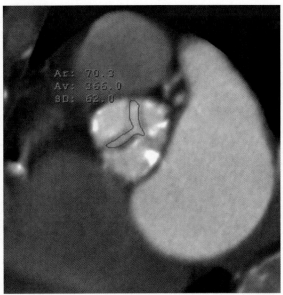

Fig. 10.7 Calcified aortic valve with severe stenosis. **(A)** Short-axis image during diastole demonstrates diffuse calcification of the aortic valve, as well as thickening of the commissures and a small regurgitant orifice at the center of the valve. **(B)** Short-axis image of the valve during systole demonstrates severe stenosis with a valve area of 0.7 cm².

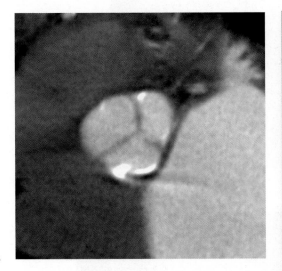

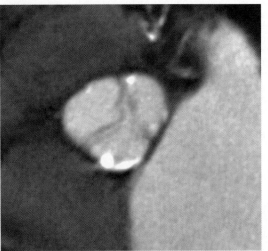

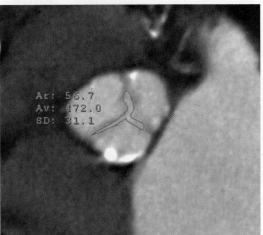

Fig. 10.8 Critical aortic stenosis. **(A)** Short-axis image through the aortic valve demonstrates minimally thickened commissures of a trileaflet valve with calcification around the aortic annulus. **(B)** Short-axis image through the aortic valve during systole demonstrates severe restriction of motion in this trileaflet valve. **(C)** Valve area of 0.56 cm² by planimetry is compatible with critical aortic stenosis.

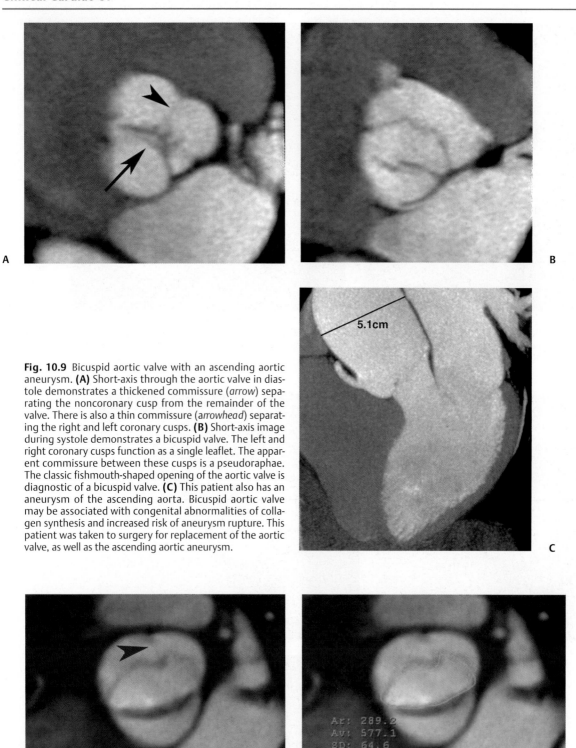

Fig. 10.9 Bicuspid aortic valve with an ascending aortic aneurysm. **(A)** Short-axis through the aortic valve in diastole demonstrates a thickened commissure (*arrow*) separating the noncoronary cusp from the remainder of the valve. There is also a thin commissure (*arrowhead*) separating the right and left coronary cusps. **(B)** Short-axis image during systole demonstrates a bicuspid valve. The left and right coronary cusps function as a single leaflet. The apparent commissure between these cusps is a pseudoraphae. The classic fishmouth-shaped opening of the aortic valve is diagnostic of a bicuspid valve. **(C)** This patient also has an aneurysm of the ascending aorta. Bicuspid aortic valve may be associated with congenital abnormalities of collagen synthesis and increased risk of aneurysm rupture. This patient was taken to surgery for replacement of the aortic valve, as well as the ascending aortic aneurysm.

Fig. 10.10 Bicuspid aortic valve. **(A)** Short-axis image of the aortic valve during systole demonstrates the classic fishmouth-shaped opening of a bicuspid valve with a pseudoraphae between the right and left coronary cusps (*arrowhead*). **(B)** Planimetry of the bicuspid valve demonstrates a valve area of 2.9 cm², suggesting that there is no significant stenosis.

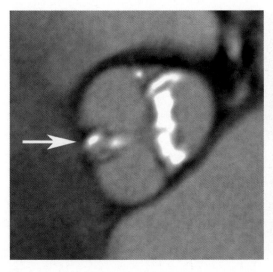
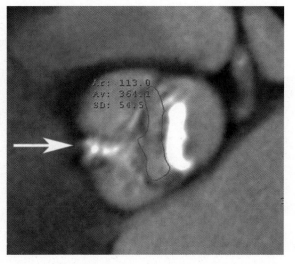

Fig. 10.11 Bicuspid aortic valve with moderate to severe stenosis. **(A)** Short-axis image of the aortic valve during diastole demonstrates calcified commissures. **(B)** Short-axis image during systole demonstrates fusion of the commissure between the right coronary and noncoronary cusps (*arrow*). The aortic valve area by planimetry measures 1.1 cm^2, compatible with moderate to severe aortic stenosis.

recommended when the diameter is greater than 4.5 cm.[20] Aortic root and ascending aorta replacement is also suggested when the rate of increase in diameter is greater than 0.5 cm per year.

In a rare variation, a trileaflet aortic valve may present as a functionally bicuspid valve secondary to fusion of an aortic valve leaflet to the wall of the aorta. Fusion of the free margin of an aortic valve leaflet to the aortic wall at the sinotubular junction likely represents failure of normal embryologic cavitation of endocardial cushion tissue in the LVOT.[21] We recently encountered a case of a trileaflet aortic valve with the left coronary cusp congenitally fixed in an open position and blocking the flow of blood into the left sinus of Valsalva (**Fig. 10.12**). Although there are three independent leaflets, only two of the leaflets demonstrated normal motion, resulting in a functionally bicuspid valve. In our patient, this anomaly was associated with aortic insufficiency as well as an aneurysm of the ascending aorta.

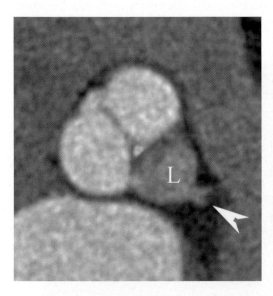
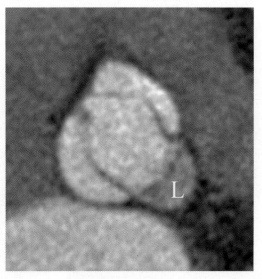

Fig. 10.12 Rare aortic valve anomaly resulting in a functionally bicuspid valve with an associated aneurysm of the ascending aorta. **(A)** Short-axis view of the aortic valve in diastole demonstrates a lack of contrast opacification in the left sinus of Valsalva (L), associated with lack of contrast in the origin of the left coronary artery (*arrowhead*). A small central regurgitant orifice is present. **(B)** Systolic view demonstrates that two of the aortic cusps open normally. The triangular appearance of the open aortic valve clearly demonstrates the presence of three aortic leaflets. However, the left coronary cusp remains unchanged in position, fixed over the left sinus of Valsalva. (*Continued on page 238*)

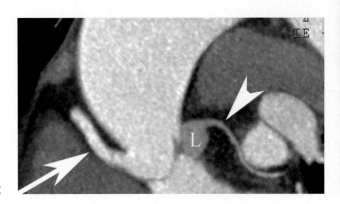

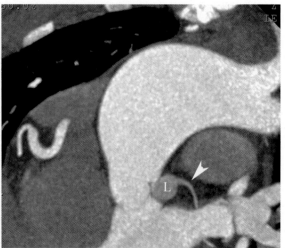

C

D

Fig. 10.12 (*Continued*) Rare aortic valve anomaly resulting in a functionally bicuspid valve with an associated aneurysm of the ascending aorta. **(C)** Coronal view of the aortic root during diastole. There is a lack of opacification of the left sinus of Valsalva (L) and the left coronary artery (*arrowhead*). A large right coronary artery (*arrow*) supplies the

left system via collaterals. **(D)** Oblique view of the ascending aorta demonstrates the presence of an aneurysm that measured greater than 4 cm. Again noted is the lack of opacification of the left sinus of Valsalva (L) and the left coronary artery (*arrowhead*).

◆ Aortic Regurgitation

The diagnosis and grading of aortic regurgitation are usually performed by echocardiography. Diameter of the regurgitant jet, vena contracta measurement, pressure half-time measurement, and hemodynamic calculations may be used for echocardiographic grading of the severity of aortic regurgitation. Cardiac CTA can demonstrate incomplete coaptation of the aortic valve in diastole and can be used to measure the regurgitant orifice (**Fig. 10.13**) but cannot provide hemodynamic data to assess the severity of aortic insufficiency. Although CT is sensitive for the presence of

moderate to severe aortic insufficiency, CT is relatively less sensitive for the presence of mild aortic insufficiency, especially in the setting of a calcified or bicuspid valve.[22] Enlargement of left ventricular chamber size accompanies chronic severe aortic regurgitation and suggests that the regurgitant lesion is hemodynamically significant. Measurements of left ventricular volume in systole and diastole are useful when deciding on surgical intervention for aortic regurgitation.

Common causes for aortic regurgitation include primary abnormalities of the aortic valve (bicuspid valve, myxomatous degeneration) or dilatation of the aortic root (hypertension,

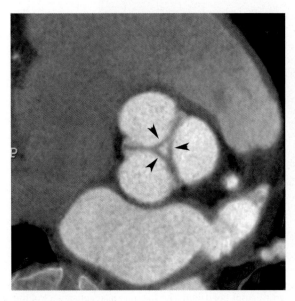

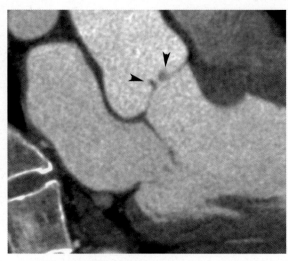

A

B

Fig. 10.13 Two cases of mild aortic insufficiency. **(A)** Short-axis view through the aortic valve in diastole demonstrates mildly thickened commissures, with incomplete coaptation at the center of the valve (*arrowheads*). **(B)** Three-chamber view through the aortic valve again

demonstrates thickened aortic leaflets with incomplete coaptation (*arrowheads*). Incomplete coaptation is associated with a central regurgitant jet through the aortic valve.

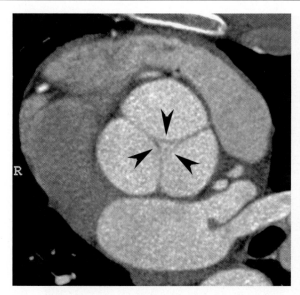

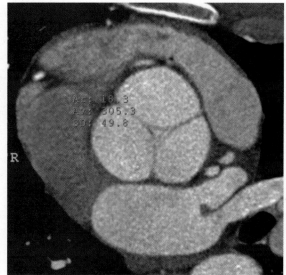

C

D

Fig. 10.13 (*Continued*) **(C)** Short-axis view through the aortic valve in another patient demonstrates incomplete coaptation at the center of an otherwise normal valve (*arrowheads*). **(D)** Planimetry demonstrates a regurgitant orifice of 0.18 cm², compatible with the history of mild aortic insufficiency.

connective tissue disorders). Hypertension is the most common cause of aortic dilatation, followed by congenital abnormalities of collagen synthesis. Dilatation of the aortic root leads to displacement of the commissural attachments of the valve leaflets with resultant malcoaptation. Less common causes of aortic regurgitation include endocarditis and aortic dissection (see discussion later in this chapter).

Incomplete coaptation of the aortic valve may be demonstrated in both short axis and long axis during diastole (**Figs. 10.12 and 10.13**). Aortic insufficiency may be associated with abnormalities of the adjacent cardiac structures, such as the membranous ventricular septum (**Fig. 10.14**). Finally, aortic insufficiency may be present concomitantly with aortic

stenosis when thickening of the valve leaflets restricts opening and also prevents adequate coaptation (**Fig. 10.15**).

◆ Aortic Tumors, Vegetations, and Dissection

Aortic valve leaflets are sharply defined on cardiac CT as three discrete structures. Small, soft tissue tags along the aortic leaflets, ranging in length from 0.3 to 0.6 mm, are described on pathologic studies. These Lambl's excrescences have been reported in 70 to 90% of valves during autopsy, but they are not

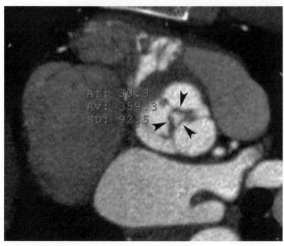

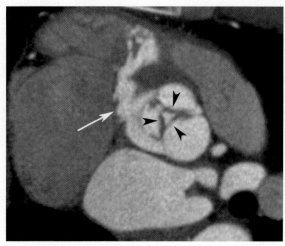

A

B

Fig. 10.14 Thickened aortic valve with mild aortic insufficiency and an associated ventral septal defect (VSD) in the aortic outflow tract. **(A)** Short-axis image through the aortic valve in diastole demonstrates thickened commissures with incomplete coaptation (*arrowheads*). The regurgitant valve orifice is measured at 0.3 cm². **(B)** Short-axis image with a slightly modified angulation demonstrates a VSD that is immediately below the aortic valve (*arrow*). The VSD may contribute to abnormal flow patterns around the aortic valve and lead to early degeneration of the valve leaflets. (*Continued on page 240*)

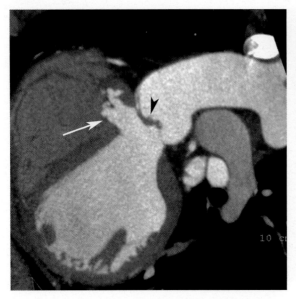

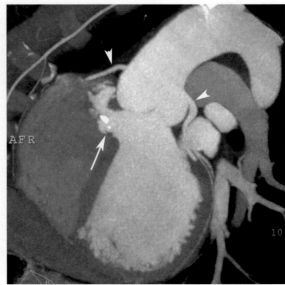

C

D

Fig. 10.14 (*Continued*) Thickened aortic valve with mild aortic insufficiency and an associated ventral septal defect (VSD) in the aortic outflow tract. **(C)** Coronal view of the aortic root demonstrates the thickened aortic valve (*arrowhead*), with a high VSD present immediately below the valve. **(D)** Left anterior oblique view demonstrates the relationship of the coronary arteries (*arrowheads*), to the aortic valve and the VSD (*arrow*).

visible with current cardiac CT technology. Another normal pathology finding, the nodules of Arantius, is small collections of fibrous tissue located near the free edges of the aortic cusps. These anatomic variations are not visible on CT, although in theory they could mimic the presence of a small tumor.

Cardiac CTA may be used to demonstrate a variety of valvular abnormalities.[23] The most common primary tumor of the aortic valve is the fibroelastoma, which generally appears as a small ball on a stalk, with frond-like protrusions. These can occur on either side of the valve, but are more commonly found on the aortic surface or affixed to the commissural attachments of the valve (**Fig. 10.16**). Despite the benign histologic appearance, aortic fibroelastomas may embolize and result in stroke. They are most commonly diagnosed by transesophageal echocardiography.

Noninfectious vegetations of the heart valves in a setting of systemic lupus erythematosus were first described by Libman and Sacks in 1924.[24] These verrucous projections usually occur on the ventricular surface of the valve, along the valve ring or commissures (**Fig. 10.17**). In

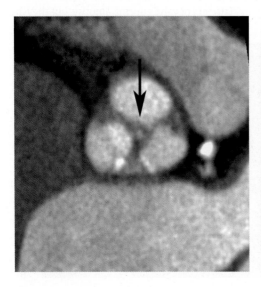

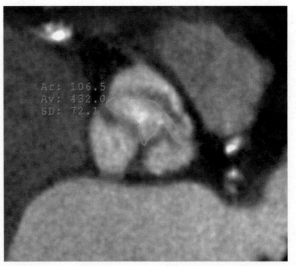

A

B

Fig. 10.15 Thickened aortic valve with mild regurgitation and moderate to severe stenosis. **(A)** Short-axis image of the aortic valve in diastole demonstrates thickened commissures as well as incomplete coaptation at the center of the valve (*arrow*). **(B)** Short-axis image through the aortic valve in systole again demonstrates the thickened valve leaflets. There is a triangular opening with restriction of leaflet motion. Planimetric measurement of 1.06 cm² is compatible with moderate to severe aortic stenosis.

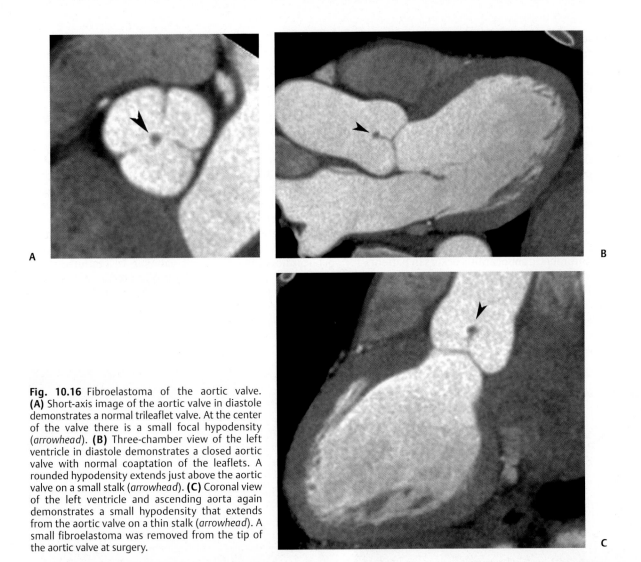

Fig. 10.16 Fibroelastoma of the aortic valve. **(A)** Short-axis image of the aortic valve in diastole demonstrates a normal trileaflet valve. At the center of the valve there is a small focal hypodensity (*arrowhead*). **(B)** Three-chamber view of the left ventricle in diastole demonstrates a closed aortic valve with normal coaptation of the leaflets. A rounded hypodensity extends just above the aortic valve on a small stalk (*arrowhead*). **(C)** Coronal view of the left ventricle and ascending aorta again demonstrates a small hypodensity that extends from the aortic valve on a thin stalk (*arrowhead*). A small fibroelastoma was removed from the tip of the aortic valve at surgery.

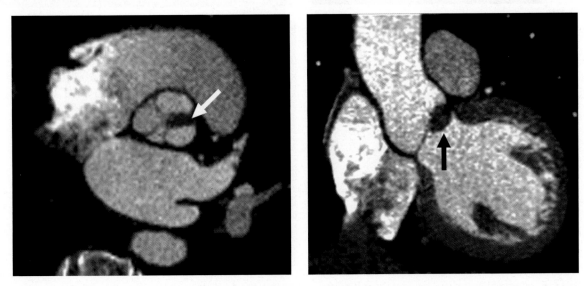

Fig. 10.17 Libman–Sacks endocarditis in a patient with systemic lupus erythematosus and peripheral arterial emboli. **(A)** Short-axis through the aortic valve demonstrates a soft tissue mass along the commissure between the left and right coronary cusps. **(B)** Coronal image through the aortic valve confirms this well-defined soft tissue vegetation. At surgery the vegetation was consistent with Libman–Sacks endocarditis. (Reprinted with permission from Gilkeson RC, Markowitz AH, Balude A, Sachs PB. MDCT evaluation of aortic valvular disease. AJR Am J Roentgenol. 2006;186(2):350–360.)

autopsy studies of lupus patients, the prevalence of Lib-man–Sacks vegetations ranges from 13 to 74%.[25] Similar lesions are described in the anti-phospholipid antibody syndromes.[26] These noninfectious vegetations have been shown to frequently change over time on serial echocardiograms.[27] There is debate whether the incidence of these lesions has decreased in the era of increased steroid use. There is no clear association with other markers of disease activity, but these are thought to represent valvulitis. Diffuse valvular thickening commonly occurs in systemic lupus erythematosus, and extensive valvular thickening is associated with progressive valvular deterioration requiring valve replacement.[25]

Nonbacterial thrombotic endocarditis occurs in patients with malignancy and consists of acellular thrombus deposition on the ventricular surface of the aortic and pulmonic valves and the atrial surface of the mitral and tricuspid valves. These lesions are rarely diagnosed before death but

are seen in 0.3 to 9.3% of autopsies in patients with malignancy. There is an association with metastatic adenocarcinomas and disseminated intravascular coagulation.[26]

Bacterial endocarditis may present with valvular vegetations, which distort the normal morphology and function of the aortic valve (**Fig. 10.18**). Patients with congenitally abnormal or diseased valves are more prone to infection of the valves (**Fig. 10.19**). Native valve vegetations predominantly occur on the ventricular surface of the valve and can appear as small, adherent masses or large, pedunculated lesions. Variable degrees of leaflet destruction may occur, and involvement of the annulus can lead to abscess formation. Because of the relative insensitivity of transthoracic echocardiography for small valvular vegetations, transesophageal echocardiography is often recommended. The true sensitivity of cardiac CT for the diagnosis of endocarditis has not been studied, although CT may be useful in preoperative planning for bacterial endocarditis.[28]

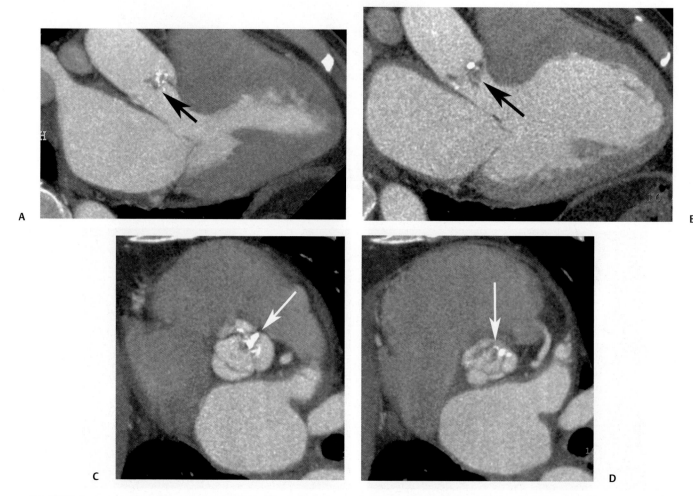

Fig. 10.18 Bacterial endocarditis with a vegetation of the aortic valve. **(A)** Three-chamber view during systole demonstrates calcification of the aortic valve with focal thickening of the anterior leaflet (*arrow*). **(B)** Three-chamber view during diastole demonstrates incomplete coaptation of the aortic valve with prolapse of a large vegetation attached to the anterior leaflet (*arrow*). **(C)** Short-axis view during systole demonstrates calcification of the aortic valve along the commissure between the left and right coronary cusps (*arrow*). A soft tissue density is present within the open valve, adjacent to the calfication. **(D)** Short-axis view during diastole demonstrates imcomplete coaptation of the valve leaflets. The vegetation is identified as it prolapses through this regurgitant orifice (*arrow*).

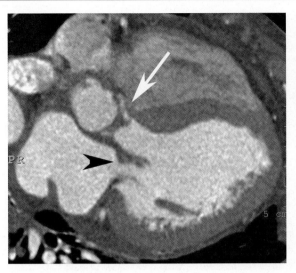

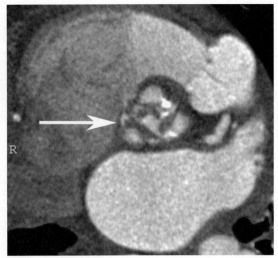

Fig. 10.19 Bacterial endocarditis of a bicuspid aortic valve. The presence of a congenitally deformed valve predisposes to the development of endocarditis. **(A)** Three-chamber view demonstrates markedly thickened and deformed aortic valve leaflets with prolapse of a large vegetation into the left ventricular outflow tract (*arrow*). The anterior mitral leaflet was also involved by endocarditis and appears thickened (*arrowhead*). **(B)** Short-axis image demonstrates a markedly thickened and deformed aortic valve with scattered calcification. The valvular calcification is likely related to premature degeneration of the bicuspid aortic valve.

Atherosclerotic disease tends to involve the abdominal aorta to a greater extent than it involves the thoracic aorta. Atherosclerotic plaque with ulceration in the thoracic aorta may be identified during CTA and is infrequently associated with thrombosis or embolization (**Fig. 10.20**).[29] Atherosclerotic involvement of the thoracic aorta may result in narrowing at the origins of the great vessels, aneurysm or pseudoaneurysm formation, and dissection. Aortic dissection may extend into the aortic root and may involve the aortic valve (**Fig. 10.21**), with complications including obstruction of the coronary arteries, loss of normal aortic valve function, and hemorrhage into the pericardial space. In an unusual complication of aortic dissection, the intimal flap may prolapse through the aortic valve (**Fig. 10.22**), resulting in severe aortic insufficiency.

◆ Prosthetic Aortic Valves

Cardiac CT is useful for both pre-operative planning and postoperative evaluation of aortic valve replacement surgery. In pre-operative planning, cardiac CT may be used to measure

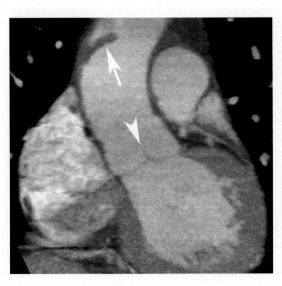

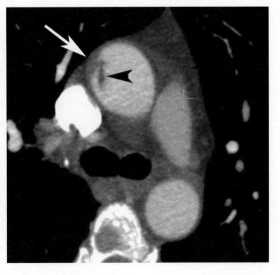

Fig. 10.20 Patient with initial transient ischemic attack (TIA) and subsequent stroke: atherosclerotic plaque with associated clot in the ascending aorta and fibroelastoma of the aortic valve. **(A)** Coronal image through the left ventricle and ascending aorta in diastole. There is a normal appearance of the closed aortic valve (*arrowhead*). No tumor is identified. Approximately 5 cm above the level of the valve, there is thickening of the aortic wall with an associated thrombus that extends into the lumen (*arrow*). **(B)** Axial image through the aorta 5 cm above the valve demonstrates thickening of the right side of the aortic wall (*arrow*), as well as thrombus within the lumen (*arrowhead*). (Continued on page 244)

Fig. 10.20 (*Continued*) Patient with initial transient ischemic attack (TIA) and subsequent stroke: atherosclerotic plaque with associated clot in the ascending aorta and fibroelastoma of the aortic valve. **(C)** Repeat study after a stroke again demonstrates a normal aortic valve (*arrowhead*) with thickening along the right side of the ascending aorta (*arrow*), but the intraluminal thrombus is no longer present. This thrombus has presumably embolized and was the cause of the stroke. A fibroelastoma was removed from the aortic valve but was not apparent on either the first or second CT scan.

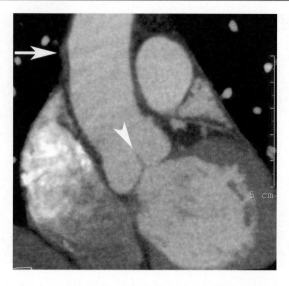

C

the diameter of the LVOT and the aortic annulus for appropriate sizing of the prosthetic valve, as well as for evaluation of the coronary circulation.[30] The echocardiographic literature suggests that end diastolic measurements bear the greatest similarity to intraoperative measurement[31] and should be obtained in a plane that is parallel to the aortic annulus (see **Fig. 9.2D,E**). Following surgery, cardiac CT can be used to document the size and position of the prosthesis, the apposition of the prosthesis to the annulus, and normal motion of the prosthetic leaflets.[32] In the setting of an elevated postoperative gradient in the aortic outflow tract, planimetric measurements with CT can help to distinguish whether the obstruction is related to the valve or the outflow tract.

Bioprosthetic aortic valves may be identified by radiopaque struts, by a radiopaque annulus around the valve leaflets, or by a thick appearance of a prosthetic valve annulus. Although the valve material is often fixed to metallic struts, some newer bioprosthetic "stentless" valves may be more difficult to identify as they are directly sewn into the aortic wall (**Fig. 10.23**).

Mechanical valves are often difficult to evaluate by echocardiography because of artifact from the valve material. Older style caged-ball valves have been supplanted by tilting disk prostheses and bileaflet valves. Two commonly placed mechanical valves in the aortic position are the St. Jude and CarboMedics valves. Each of these valves has

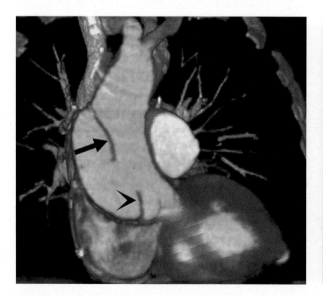

A

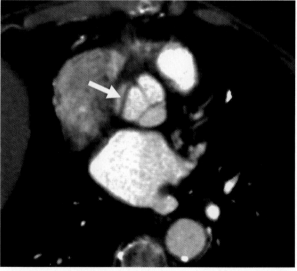

B

Fig. 10.21 Dissection of the ascending aorta involving the aortic valve. **(A)** Coronal image demonstrates a dissection flap in the ascending aorta (*arrow* and *arrowhead*). The inferior portion of the dissection extends to the aortic root (*arrowhead*). **(B)** Short-axis image through the aortic valve demonstrates that the dissection extends to the noncoronary cusp (*arrow*). Extension into the aortic valve with sudden onset of severe insufficiency is a potentially lethal complication of aortic dissection. (Reprinted with permission from Gilkeson RC, Markowitz AH, Balgude A, Sachs PB. MDCT evaluation of aortic valvular disease. AJR Am J Roentgenol. 2006;186(2):350–360.)

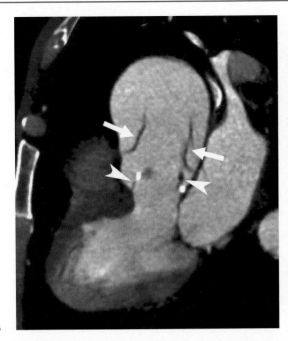

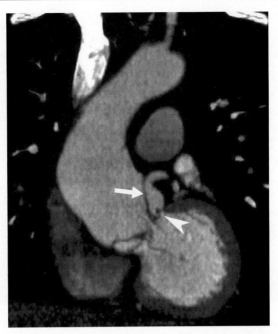

Fig. 10.22 Dissection of the proximal ascending aorta with prolapse through the aortic valve. **(A)** Three-chamber view through the left ventricle and proximal ascending aorta in systole. There is a dissection flap in the proximal ascending aorta (*arrows*), which is just above the aortic valve (*arrowheads*). **(B)** Coronal image during diastole. The dissection flap (*arrow*) is now prolapsed through the aortic valve (*arrowhead*). The dissection flap overlies the orifice of the left coronary artery during diastole. The appearance suggests that there will be associated aortic insufficiency. (Reprinted with permission from Gilkeson RC, Markowitz AH, Balgude A, Sachs PB. MDCT evaluation of aortic valvular disease. AJR Am J Roentgenol. 2006;186(2):350–360.)

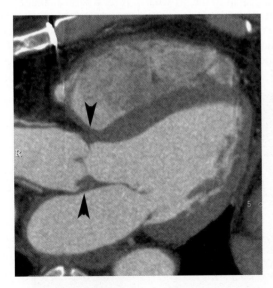

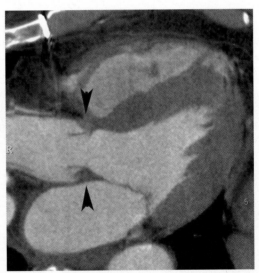

Fig. 10.23 Normally functioning bioprosthetic aortic valve. **(A)** Three-chamber view during diastole demonstrates a normal closed position of the aortic valve. The struts are seen as areas of thickening along the margins of the valve (*arrowheads*). **(B)** Three-chamber view during systole demonstrates a normal open position of the valve leaflets. (*Continued on page 246*)

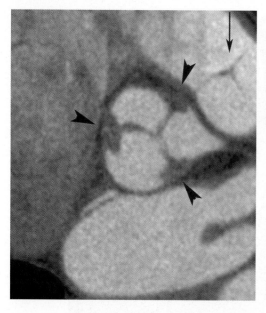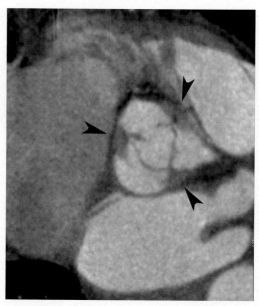

C

D

Fig. 10.23 (*Continued*) Normally functioning bioprosthetic **(C)** Short-axis image during diastole demonstrates the three struts (*arrowheads*) of the bioprosthetic. Although the commissures appear mildly thick on this short-axis view, they appeared normal in all other views. **(D)** Short-axis image during systole demonstrates a normal triangular opening of the aortic valve.

two metallic leaflets in the shape of a half-circle. The valve ring and leaflets are well defined by CT in both the closed and open positions to document normal valve function (**Fig. 10.24**). Pannus or thrombus around a prosthetic valve may present with loss of normal valve motion, which can be identified by CT.[33]

Prosthetic cardiac valves predispose patients to a higher risk for endocarditis compared with native valves. In the setting of a bioprosthetic valve, endocarditis may present as a focal vegetation or as diffuse valvular thickening on CT

(**Fig. 10.25**). Additional complications of aortic valve replacement are often related to infection and include paravalvular abscess formation, pseudoaneurysms, and dehiscence of the prosthetic valve from the valve annulus. Paravalvular abscess should appear as a low-density collection adjacent to the prosthesis. After a paravalvular abscess has ruptured into the adjacent chamber, a pseudoaneurysm is diagnosed by enhancement with contrast material. Cardiac CT is useful to demonstrate the valvular abnormality along with the location and extent of paravalvular

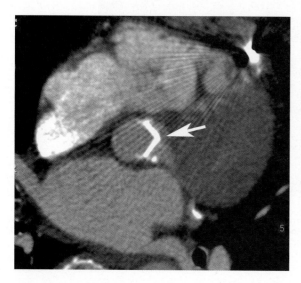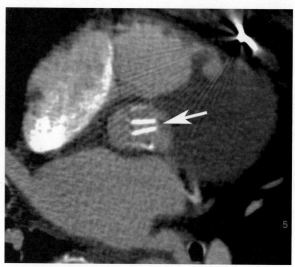

A

B

Fig. 10.24 Normally functioning St. Jude's prostatic aortic valve. **(A)** Axial image through the aortic root in diastole demonstrates the normal closed position (*arrow*) of the mechanical St Jude's valve. **(B)** Axial image through the aortic root in systole demonstrates a normal open position (*arrow*) of the St. Jude's valve.

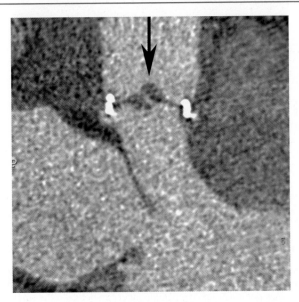

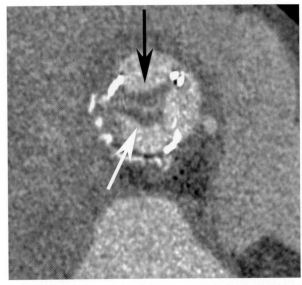

Fig. 10.25 Bacterial endocarditis of a bioprosthetic aortic valve. **(A)** Three-chamber view demonstrates thickened leaflets of a prosthetic aortic valve in the closed diastolic position (*arrow*). Metallic struts are visible at bases of the valve leaflets. **(B)** Short-axis image demonstrates thickening of the anterior right coronary leaflet (*black arrow*), as well as the noncoronary leaflet (*white arrow*) related to endocarditis.

pseudoaneurysms (**Figs. 10.26, 10.27,** and **10.28**). Systolic and diastolic phase images may be used to demonstrate dynamic changes in the size of a pseudoaneurysm during the cardiac cycle (**Fig. 10.29**). The location and extent of valvular dehiscence may also be evaluated for pre-operative planning (**Figs. 10.30** and **10.31**). Replacement of the aortic valve is often performed in combination with replacement of the ascending aorta. Pseudoaneurysms or leaks in the ascending aorta may be discovered at the anastomosis site or at the site of the aortic cannulation during surgery (**Fig. 10.32**).

◆ Mitral Valve Anatomy

The mitral valve has two leaflets, the anterior and the posterior leaflets. Normal mitral leaflets are thin, open widely during diastole, and demonstrate complete coaptation with

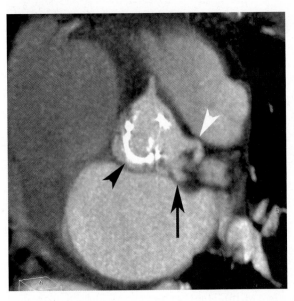

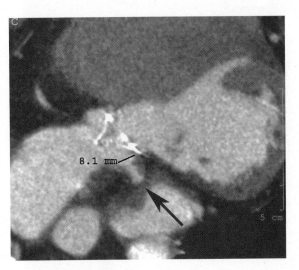

Fig. 10.26 Pseudoaneurysm of the aortic root following aortic valve replacement. **(A)** Short-axis image through the aortic root demonstrates the ring of an aortic bioprosthesis (*black arrowhead*), with a pseudoaneurysm of the left sinus of Valsalva (*black arrow*) just below the left main coronary artery (*white arrowhead*). **(B)** Three-chamber view demonstrates a focal pseudoaneurysm just above the level of the aortic valve replacement (*black arrow*).

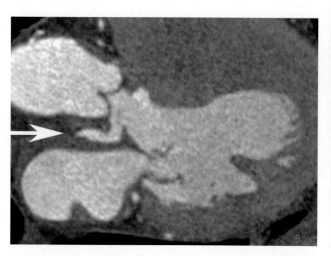

A

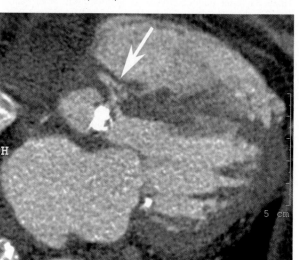

B

Fig. 10.27 Aortic valve bioprosthesis with pseudoaneurysm extending into the intervalvular fibrosa. **(A)** Three-chamber view demonstrates a focal pseudoaneurysm extending from the left ventricular outflow tract into the intervalvular fibrosa between the aortic valve and left atrium (*arrow*). There is increased distance between the aortic and mitral valves secondary to disruption of the intervalvular fibrosa. **(B)** Short-axis view demonstrates the pseudoaneurysm between the aortic root and the left atrium (*arrow*).

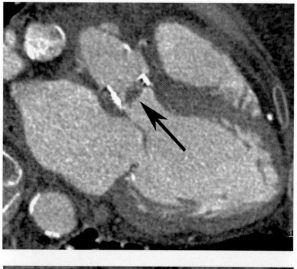

A

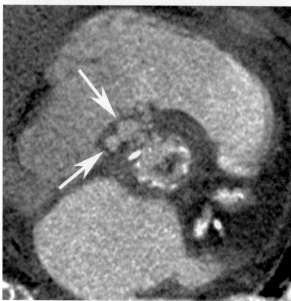

B

C

Fig. 10.28 Aortic valve bioprosthesis with pseudoaneurysm extending between the aortic root and the right ventricular outflow tract secondary to endocarditis. **(A)** Three-chamber view demonstrates thickening of the leaflets of the bioprosthetic aortic valve (*arrow*). **(B)** Three-chamber view shifted slightly to the right side demonstrates a focal pseudoaneurysm extending from the left ventricular outflow tract into the space between the aortic root and the right ventricular outflow tract (*arrow*). **(C)** Short-axis view confirms the location of the pseudoaneurysm between the aortic root and the right ventricular outflow tract (*arrows*).

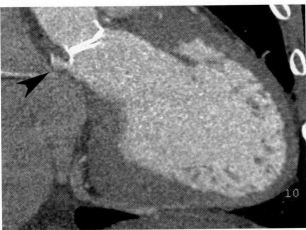
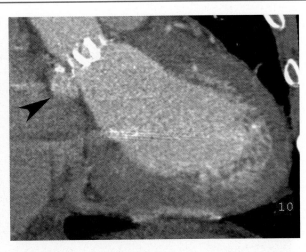

Fig. 10.29 St. Jude's mechanical aortic valve with pseudoaneurysm extending inferiorly from the left ventricular outflow tract. **(A)** Aortic outflow view demonstrates a mechanical aortic valve in a normal closed position during diastole. A pseudoaneurysm is identified just below the prosthesis (*arrowhead*). **(B)** Systolic image demonstrates the normal open position of the mechanical prosthesis. The pseudoaneurysm appears to enlarge during systole (*arrowhead*).

overlap during systole (**Fig. 10.33**). The posterior leaflet is divided into three scallops, called P1, P2, and P3, and the corresponding parts of the anterior leaflet are named A1, A2, and A3. The subvalvular apparatus of the mitral valve consists of two papillary muscles, an anterolateral muscle and a posteromedial muscle, along with the chordal structures that attach each of these muscles to both of the mitral valve leaflets. Considerable variation in the number of muscle bundles within each papillary muscle can be visualized on CT.[34] Multiple heads of the papillary muscles may be demonstrated as they insert into the left ventricular wall (**Fig. 10.33C,D**).

Short-axis images through the mitral valve during diastole demonstrate a bean-shaped opening. In a patient with normal sinus rhythm, the mitral valve opens rapidly during early diastolic filling. However, unlike the aortic valve leaflets, the mitral valve leaflets do not remain open in a fixed position for an extended portion of the cardiac cycle. Rather, these leaflets begin to float toward a closed position in mid-diastole, and then open again during atrial

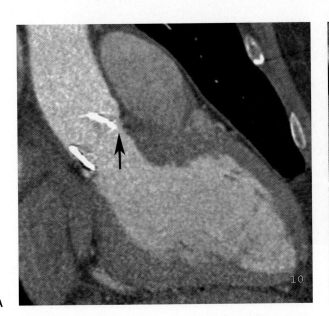
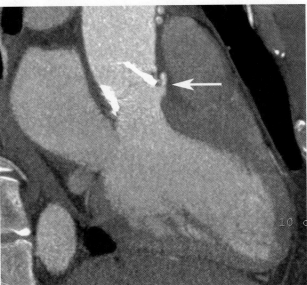

Fig. 10.30 Bioprosthetic aortic valve with anterior dehiscence and pseudoaneurysm secondary to infection. **(A)** Aortic outflow view demonstrates tilting of the bioprosthesis secondary to disruption of the anterior attachment, which is superiorly displaced. Contrast material passes around the bioprosthesis anteriorly at the site of dehiscence (*arrow*). **(B)** Three-chamber view demonstrates a small pseudoaneurysm extending anteriorly from the left ventricular outflow tract into the space between the aortic root and the right ventricular outflow tract (*arrow*).

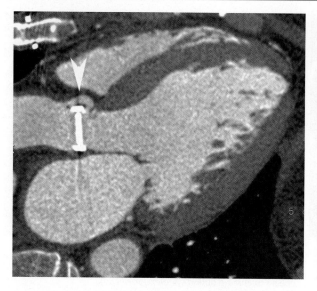

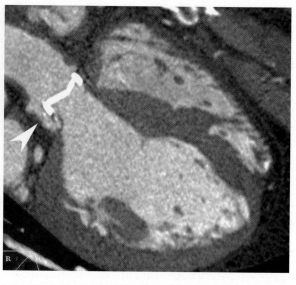

Fig. 10.31 St. Jude's mechanical aortic valve with dehiscence along the anterior and lateral portions of the valve ring. **(A)** Three-chamber view during diastole demonstrates that the anterior attachment of the mechanical aortic valve is disrupted with superior displacement and tilting of the valve relative to the aortic annulus. Contrast material passes anterior to the prosthetic valve (*arrowhead*). **(B)** A modified five-chamber view demonstrates that the lateral attachment of the mechanical aortic valve is also disrupted with contrast material passing lateral to the prosthesis (*arrowhead*).

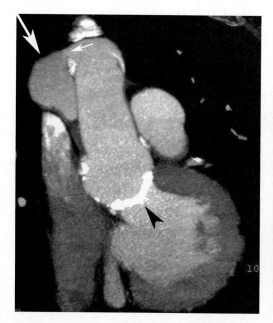

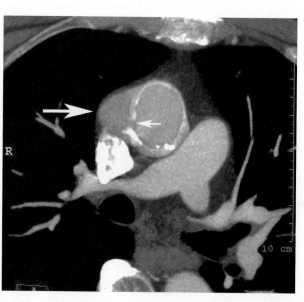

Fig. 10.32 Pseudoaneurysm of the ascending aorta following aortic valve replacement. **(A)** Coronal view through the ascending aorta demonstrates a mechanical aortic valve replacement in a normal closed position during diastole (*arrowhead*). The proximal ascending aorta has been replaced by a tube graft. There is a large pseudo-aneurysm at the site of the anastomosis of the tube graft with the native aortic arch (*arrow*). The site of leak at the upper suture line is identified (*small arrow*). **(B)** Axial image at the level of the aortic leak. A small area of discontinuity is identified along the suture line within the ascending aorta (*small arrow*). The associated pseudoaneurysm is clearly defined (*large arrow*).

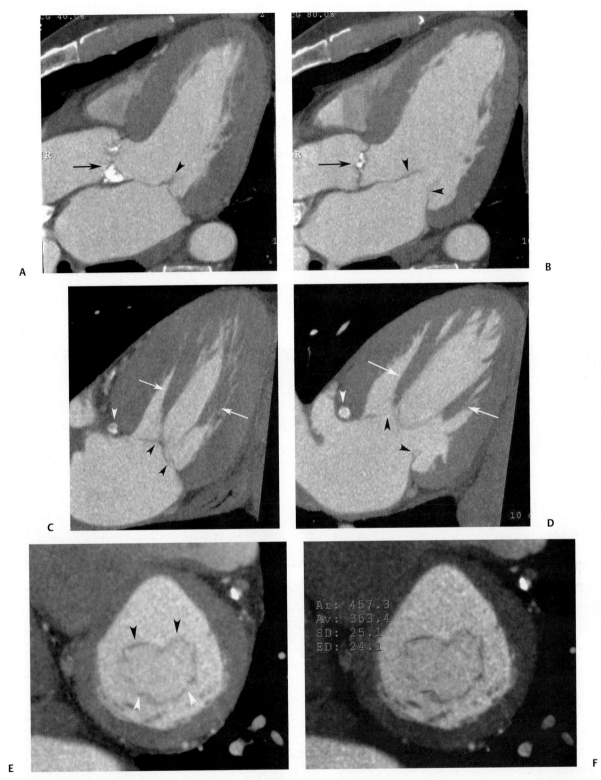

Fig. 10.33 Normal mitral valve. **(A)** Three-chamber view of the left ventricle during systole demonstrates a calcified aortic valve (*arrow*) with normal closure of the mitral valve (*arrowhead*). There is complete coaptation of the mitral leaflets. The mitral valve leaflets close up to the plane of the mitral annulus but do not extend beyond that plane into the left atrium. **(B)** Diastolic image demonstrates normal opening of the mitral valve (*arrowheads*). Papillary muscles are not generally visible on the three-chamber view through the left ventricle and mitral valve. **(C)** Two-chamber view in this same patient during systole demonstrates the papillary muscles (*arrows*), as well as the chordal attachments to the mitral valve (*arrowheads*). Once again, the mitral valve closes to the annulus but does not extend above the plane of the mitral annulus. **(D)** Diastolic view demonstrates the papillary muscles (*arrows*), as well as the open mitral leaflets (*arrowheads*). The chordal attachments are not well visualized in this view. A patent stent is present in the circumflex artery (*white arrowhead*). **(E)** Short-axis image through the mitral valve demonstrates normal thickness of the open mitral valve. The anterior leaflet (*black arrowheads*) and the posterior leaflet (*white arrowheads*) demonstrate a thin undulating contour. **(F)** A normal mitral valve area is demonstrated by planimetry with an area of 4.6 cm².

systole. This complex motion pattern of the mitral leaflets complicates CT imaging of the mitral valve and is further complicated in non–sinus rhythm. In general, mitral valve excursion is greatest at about 50 to 60% of the RR interval and again at 80% of the RR interval.

A normal mitral valve area (**Fig. 10.33F**) is in the range of 4.0 to 6.0 cm². A thickened mitral valve may appear to be restricted (**Fig. 10.34**), although symptoms of mitral stenosis do not typically develop unless the valve area is reduced to less than 2.5 cm².[35] The mean pressure gradient across the normal mitral valve is less than 5 mm. In a small series of normal subjects reviewed at Thomas Jefferson University, planimetry of the mitral valve on cardiac CT demonstrated a mean valve area of 5.5 cm². However, interobserver variation of this mitral measurement (up to 1.8 cm²) is much greater than interobserver variation in the measurement of aortic valve area (<1 cm²). Mitral planimetry is complicated by continuous motion of the

mitral valve, redundancy of the valve leaflets, and poor demarcation between the edges of the mitral leaflets and the attached chordal structures.

◆ Mitral Stenosis

Although the normal area of the mitral valve is about 4.0 to 6.0 cm², the diagnosis of mitral stenosis is not generally suggested until the valve area is reduced to below 2.5 cm², or a mean valve pressure gradient greater than 5 mm Hg is identified. ACC/AHA values for grading of mitral stenosis are summarized in **Table 10.1**. Mild mitral stenosis is generally diagnosed with a valve area greater than 1.5 cm² (**Fig. 10.35**). Moderate mitral stenosis is suggested by a valve area between 1.0 and 1.5 cm² (**Fig. 10.36**). Severe mitral stenosis is diagnosed with a valve area less than 1 cm² or a valve gradient greater than 10 mm Hg. Severe mitral stenosis is

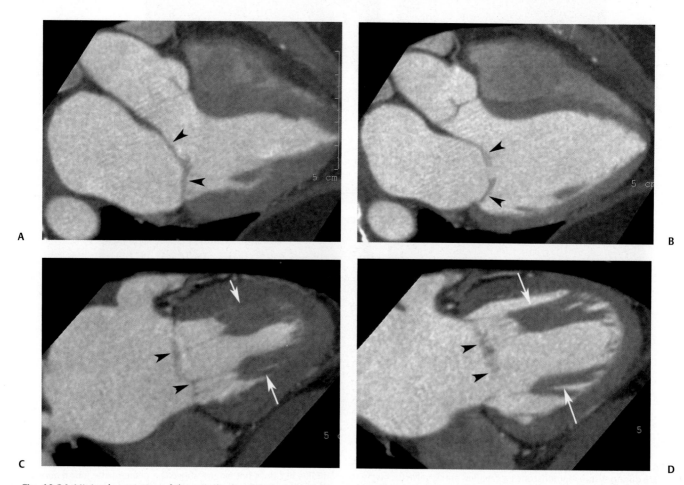

Fig. 10.34 Minimal restriction of the mitral valve. **(A)** Three-chamber view through the left ventricle during systole demonstrates a closed mitral valve (*arrowheads*). The aortic valve is faintly visualized in the open position just above the mitral valve. **(B)** Three-chamber view during diastole demonstrates the mitral valve in open position (*arrowheads*). The mitral valve leaflets are mildly thickened and appear domed, suggesting mild restriction of motion. A similar appearance of doming with no significant gradient was confirmed by echocardiogra-phy. The aortic valve is visualized above the mitral valve in a closed diastolic position. **(C)** Systolic frame demonstrating the anterolateral and posteromedial papillary muscles (*arrows*) as well as the chordae tendinea, which attach these muscles to the mitral valve (*arrowheads*). **(D)** Diastolic frame demonstrating better definition of the papillary muscles, which are now separated from the left ventricular wall. Chordal attachments are identified to a mildly thick mitral valve leaflet (*arrowheads*).

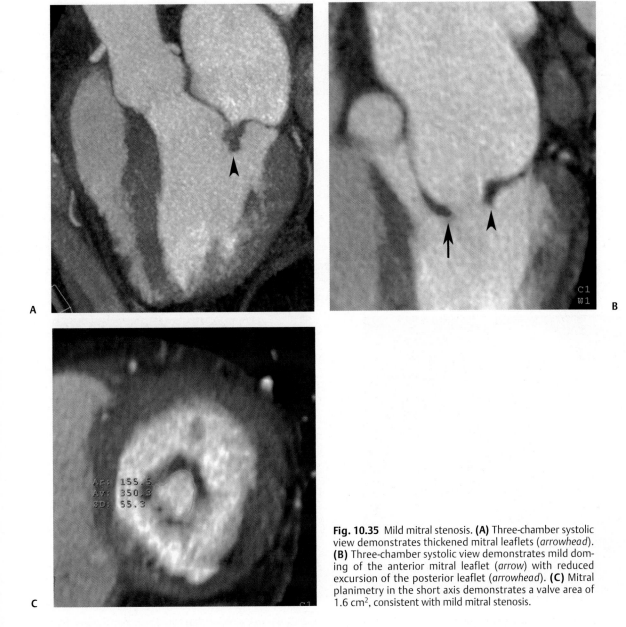

Fig. 10.35 Mild mitral stenosis. **(A)** Three-chamber systolic view demonstrates thickened mitral leaflets (*arrowhead*). **(B)** Three-chamber systolic view demonstrates mild doming of the anterior mitral leaflet (*arrow*) with reduced excursion of the posterior leaflet (*arrowhead*). **(C)** Mitral planimetry in the short axis demonstrates a valve area of 1.6 cm², consistent with mild mitral stenosis.

often associated with dilatation of the left atrium (**Fig. 10.37**) and elevated pulmonary pressures.

Rheumatic fever is by far the most common cause of mitral stenosis, resulting in thickening and calcification of the leaflets with commisural and chordal fusion.[36] With the decline of rheumatic fever, mitral stenosis has become distinctly less common.

Calcification of the mitral annulus is a relatively common entity (**Fig. 10.38**). The posterior annulus is involved more frequently and to a greater extent than the anterior annulus. Annular calcification does not generally interfere with valve function. However, mitral annular calcification (MAC) may extend to the valve leaflets and may cause some restriction of leaflet motion, most commonly at the base of the posterior leaflet. Caseous calcification of the mitral annulus is an

uncommon variation of MAC (frequency is less than 1% of all MACs)[37] that may present as a heterogeneous or echogenic mass on echocardiography and is sometimes referred to CT for further evaluation.[38] The characteristic CT appearance of caseous calcification of the mitral annulus is related to the presence of a thick slurry of calcium within the annulus (**Fig. 10.39**). The calcification may appear denser in the dependent portion of the mass and should not enhance between baseline and post-contrast imaging. Although caseous calcification is not a neoplasm, the process can appear to extend into the overlying myocardium as well as to infiltrate the posterior mitral leaflet (**Fig. 10.40**). Cardiac CT provides complementary information to echocardiography and may be useful for serial follow-up to document progression of caseous calcification in the mitral annulus or into the mitral valve.[39] As

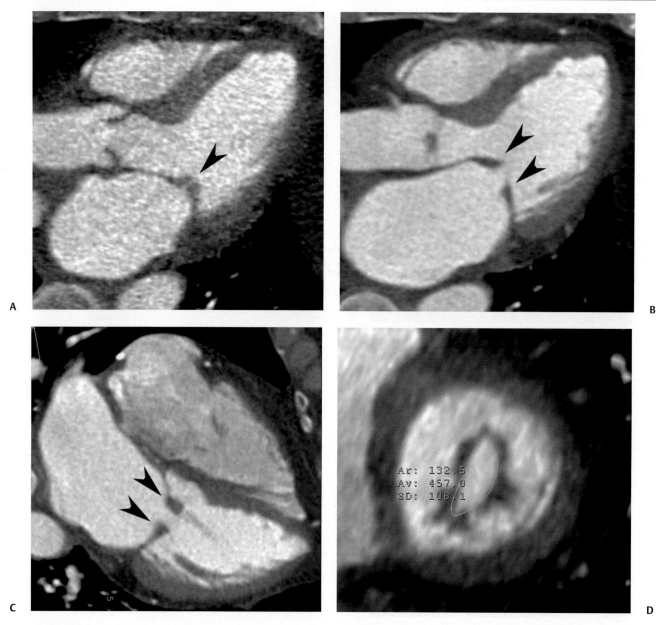

Fig. 10.36 Moderate mitral stenosis. **(A)** Three-chamber systolic view demonstrates thickened mitral leaflets (*arrowhead*). **(B)** Three-chamber systolic view demonstrates doming of the mitral leaflets (*arrowheads*). **(C)** Four-chamber systolic view also demonstrates reduced opening of the mitral leaflets (*arrowheads*). **(D)** Mitral planimetry in the short axis demonstrates a valve area of 1.3 cm², consistent with moderate mitral stenosis.

an unusual presentation, extensive mitral annular calcification may actually progress to mitral stenosis (**Fig. 10.41**).[40] MAC has been associated with calcific atherosclerosis in the aorta and the carotid arteries, but not in the coronary vasculature.[41]

◆ Mitral Regurgitation

Mitral regurgitation is now the most commonly encountered clinically significant cardiac valve lesion.[42] Echocardiography and ventriculography generally serve as the standard to judge the severity of mitral regurgitation for clinical management of patients. A recent study has demonstrated that quantification of the regurgitant mitral orifice by cardiac CT is highly correlated with the degree of mitral regurgitation documented by transesophageal echocardiography and ventriculograhy.[43]

Mitral valve prolapse, an entity present in 1 to 2.5% of the population, is commonly associated with mitral insufficiency.[44] Mitral valve prolapse was first described by Barlow and Bosman, who recognized the association of late systolic murmurs and clicks with the mitral valve.[45] With the widespread use of echocardiography in the early 1980s, mitral valve prolapse was diagnosed with a prevalence as high as

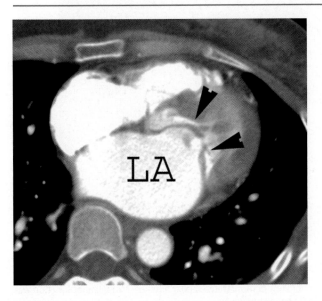

Fig. 10.37 Mitral stenosis with dilated left atrium. Four-chamber view demonstrates thickened mitral leaflets (*arrowheads*) with doming of the mitral valve and a markedly enlarged left atrium (LA). The dilated LA is related to longstanding mitral stenosis.

mitral valve prolapse include prolapse of the leaflets by 2 mm or more above the mitral annulus in the three-chamber view of the heart.[48] Prolapse is observed more frequently in the posterior mitral leaflet (**Figs. 10.43** and **10.44**). Although the cause of mitral valve prolapse is generally related to proliferation of myxomatous connective tissue within the leaflets, mitral valve prolapse may be seen with or without overt thickening of the mitral leaflets. In a minority of patients, prolapse may be related to an underlying connective tissue disorder such as Marfan disease or Ehlers-Danlos syndrome. Prolapse associated with thickening of the valve leaflets to greater than 5 mm is termed *classic* prolapse.[49] Myxomatous infiltration of the papillary muscles may result in papillary muscle dysfunction. Thickening of the mitral leaflets in patients with mitral valve prolapse is a major predictor of poor prognosis with a higher risk of mitral regurgitation, endocarditis, and sudden death.

Mitral regurgitation often results from a combination of factors. Mitral regurgitation may result from focal regions of malcoaptation resulting from myxomatous thickening of the mitral valve, with or without evidence of prolapse. In the setting of mitral valve prolapse, the billowing of the leaflet is accentuated as systole progresses, further displacing the leaflet tip and increasing the regurgitant orifice area. Dilatation of the mitral annulus with enlargement of the left atrium in atrial fibrillation or diastolic dysfunction may result in incomplete coaptation of the valve leaflets and associated mitral regurgitation. A dilated annulus is often observed in a setting of ischemic heart disease along with ventricular enlargement and myocardial dysfunction (**Fig. 10.45**). Papillary muscle displacement due to ventricular enlargement or dysfunction of the myocardium beneath the papillary muscle may lead to valve tethering and malcoaptation of leaflets. Dysfunction of

38%.[46] However, work by Levine and colleagues demonstrated that the mitral annulus is saddle-shaped, with the anterior and posterior portions of the annulus tilted away from the cardiac apex. The annular portions of the mitral valve visible on a four chamber view are closer to the cardiac apex. As a result of this geometry, the mitral leaflets can appear to break the plane of the annulus in the four chamber view in the absence of true prolapse (**Fig. 10.42**).[47] Current echocardiographic criteria for the diagnosis of

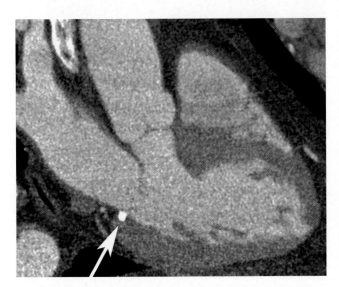

A

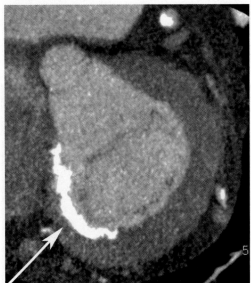

B

Fig. 10.38 Mitral annular calcification. **(A)** Three-chamber view of the left ventricle during diastole demonstrates calcification along the posterior mitral annulus (*arrow*). Annular calcification is most common along the posterior mitral annulus and is rarely of clinical significance.

(B) Short-axis view through the base of the left ventricle. The annular calcification extends along the medial aspect of the mitral valve (*arrow*). Annular calcification does not usually interfere with mitral valve function.

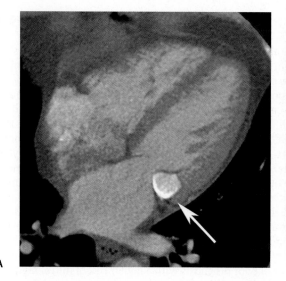

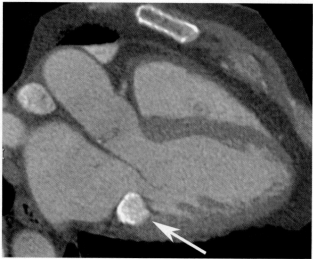

Fig. 10.39 Caseous calcification of the mitral annulus. **(A)** Four-chamber view demonstrates a large calcified mass in the posterior mitral annulus (*arrow*) with layering of calcium in the more dependent portion of the mass. The graded shading within the mass is related to varying density of the toothpaste-like milk of calcium within the annulus. The mass extends into the base of the posterior mitral leaflet. **(B)** Three-chamber view demonstrates similar findings. Mitral leaflet function was normal on cine images.

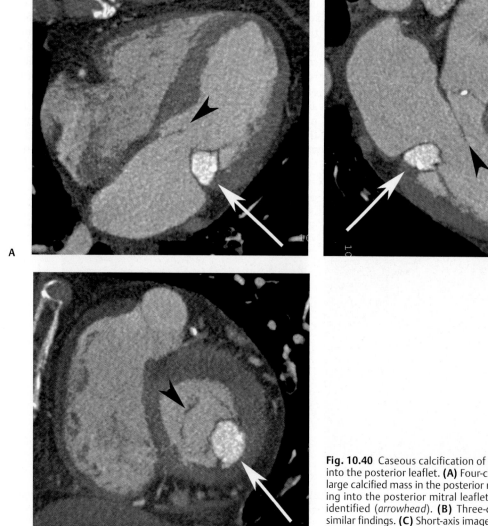

Fig. 10.40 Caseous calcification of the mitral annulus extending into the posterior leaflet. **(A)** Four-chamber view demonstrates a large calcified mass in the posterior mitral annulus (*arrow*) extending into the posterior mitral leaflet. A normal anterior leaflet is identified (*arrowhead*). **(B)** Three-chamber view demonstrates similar findings. **(C)** Short-axis image demonstrates that the annular calcification extends into the posterior mitral leaflet but that the valve area is preserved.

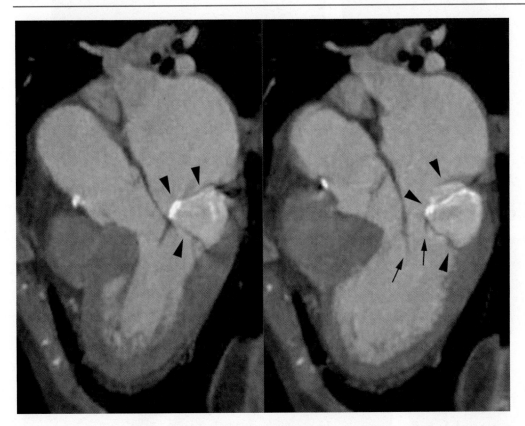

Fig. 10.41 Caseous calcification of the mitral annulus resulting in mitral stenosis. Three-chamber views in systole (on the left) and diastole (on the right) demonstrate a peripherally calcified mass (*arrowheads*) in the posterior mitral annulus. The mitral leaflets (*arrows*) are normal in thickness. However, the large calcified mass in the posterior annulus restricts the opening of the posterior leaflet. (Reprinted from Alkadhi H, Leschka S, Prêtre R, Perren A, Marincek B, Wildermuch S. Caseous calcification of the mitral annulus. J Thorac Cardiovasc Surg. 2005; 129(6):1438–1440, with permission from the American Association for Thoracic Surgery.)

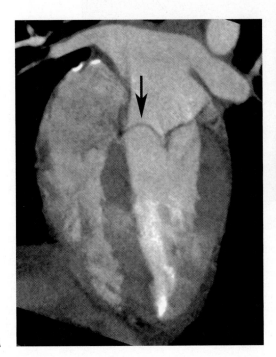

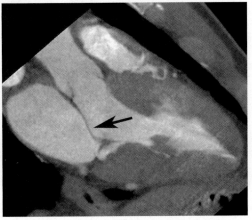

Fig. 10.42 Mitral valve pseudoprolapse. **(A)** Four-chamber view during systole demonstrates apparent prolapse of the anterior mitral leaflet (*arrow*). **(B)** Three-chamber view during systole demonstrates normal coaptation of the mitral leaflets with no prolapse.

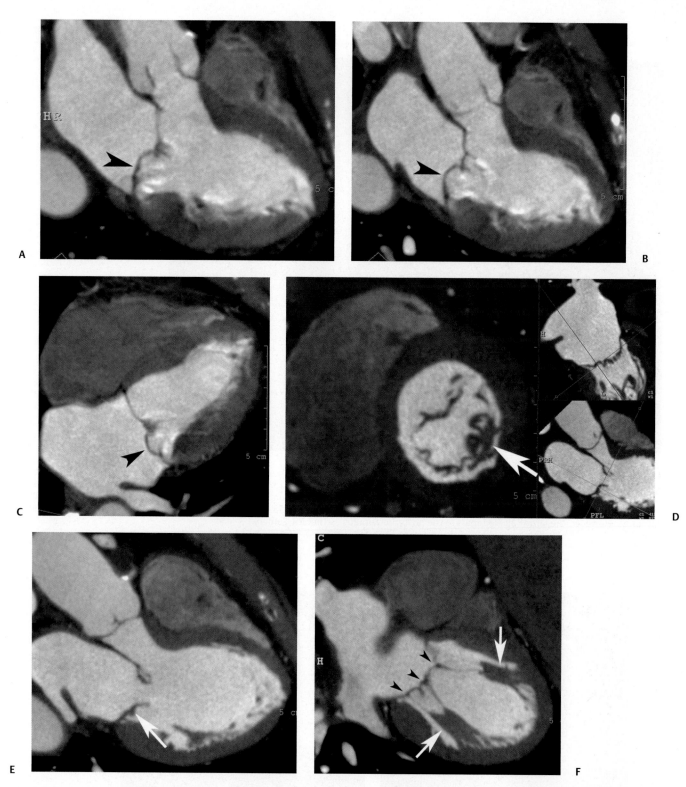

Fig. 10.43 Mitral valve prolapse. **(A)** Three-chamber view through the left ventricle during systole demonstrates a thickened posterior leaflet (*arrowhead*). Extension of the posterior leaflet above the plane of the mitral annulus into the left atrium is diagnostic of mitral prolapse. **(B)** A slightly off-axis view more clearly demonstrates prolapse of the posterior leaflet (*arrowhead*). **(C)** Four-chamber view again demonstrates prolapse of the mitral valve leaflet (*arrowhead*). Prolapse should not be diagnosed in the four-chamber view alone because extension of the mitral valve above the mitral annulus may provide a false-positive diagnosis in this projection. In this case, however, the three-chamber view clearly demonstrates prolapse of the posterior mitral leaflet. The four-chamber view demonstrates left atrial enlargement related to mitral insufficiency. **(D)** Short-axis image through the mitral valve demonstrates thickening of the mitral leaflets, particularly the posterior mitral leaflet (*arrow*). This leaflet appears thickened and redundant, compatible with myxomatous degeneration associated with mitral prolapse (*arrow*). **(E)** Three-chamber view in diastole again demonstrates the thickened posterior mitral leaflet (*arrow*), with normal diastolic opening of the mitral valve. **(F)** Diastolic image through the papillary muscles demonstrates a normal appearance of both papillary muscles (*arrows*), as well as a normal appearance of the chordal attachments to the mitral valve (*arrowheads*).

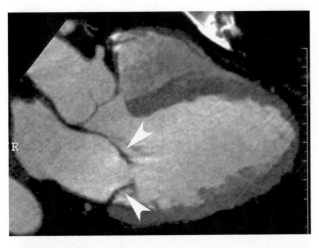

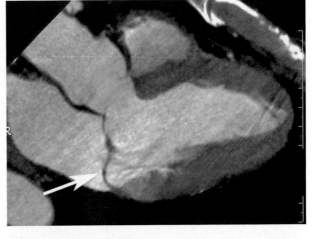

Fig. 10.44 Mitral valve prolapse. **(A)** Three-chamber view of the left ventricle during diastole demonstrates mildly thickened mitral leaflets (*arrowheads*). **(B)** Three-chamber view during systole demonstrates mild prolapse of the posterior leaflet (*arrow*) above the plane of the mitral annulus. The anterior leaflet closes to the plane of the annulus, but it does not prolapse through the annulus.

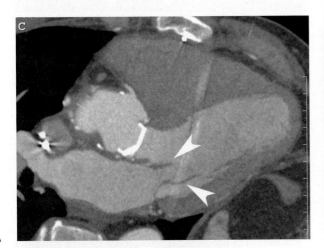

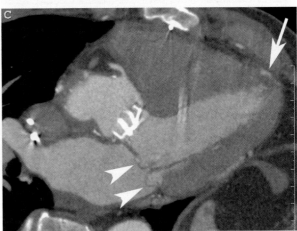

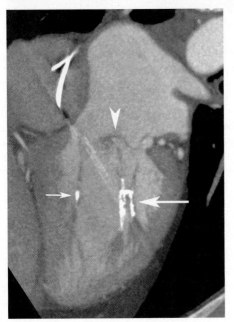

Fig. 10.45 Mitral valve prolapse with thinned or calcified chordal structures and mitral insufficiency in the setting of ischemic heart disease. **(A)** Three-chamber view of the left ventricle during diastole demonstrates mildly thickened mitral leaflets (*arrowheads*). The mitral valve is in the open position; the St. Jude's prosthetic aortic valve is in the closed position. **(B)** Three-chamber view during systole demonstrates prolapse of both mitral leaflets (*arrowheads*) above the plane of the mitral annulus with incomplete coaptation of the mitral leaflets. The St. Jude's valve is now in the open position. Calcification in the left ventricular apex is related to a previous infarct (*arrow*). **(C)** Coronal view through the papillary muscles again demonstrates a thickened mitral valve (*arrowhead*). The anterolateral chordal apparatus is heavily calcified (*large arrow*); the posteromedial chordal apparatus is mildly calcified (*small arrow*). Both sets of chordal structures appear atrophic. The chordal changes in this patient are related to the prior infarct and likely contribute to the mitral prolapse.

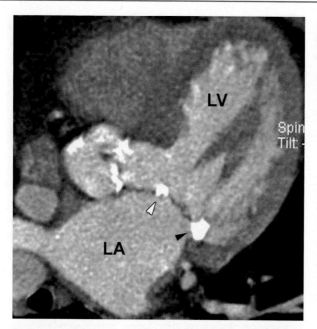

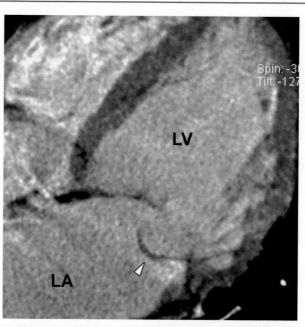

A

B

Fig. 10.46 Flail posterior mitral valve leaflet. **(A)** Three-chamber view in early systole demonstrates a closed mitral valve. There is calcification of the anterior mitral leaflet (*white arrowhead*). There is also extensive calcification of the posterior mitral annulus (*black arrowhead*). Prolapse is not appreciated in this view. **(B)** Oblique four-chamber view demonstrates clear prolapse of a portion of the posterior mitral leaflet (*white*

arrowhead). This finding was confirmed on transesophageal echocardiogram. Chordal rupture was demonstrated on the transesophageal echocardiogram but is not demonstrated on CT. LA, left atrium; LV, left ventricle. (Reprinted with permission from Alkadhi H, Wildermuth S, Bettex DA, et al. Mitral regurgitation: quantification with 16-detector row CT—initial experience. Radiology 2006;238(2):454–463.)

the papillary muscles themselves is a less common cause of mitral regurgitation. In a setting of papillary muscle or chordal disruption, a flail mitral leaflet may result in acute severe mitral regurgitation. (**Fig. 10.46**). Leaflet destruction from endocarditis results in mitral regurgitation, sometimes from a leaflet perforation rather than a coaptation point. Distortion and calcification in the setting of rheumatic disease also lead to mitral regurgitation and can be the primary lesion of rheumatic disease, usually in male patients. Systolic anterior motion of the mitral leaflets, as seen in hypertrophic obstructive cardiomyopathy, can also result in late systolic mitral regurgitation. As the anterior leaflet is pulled into the LVOT by the Venturi forces, it moves away from the posterior leaflet, disrupting their normal coaptation (see **Fig. 9.49**).[50]

As with aortic regurgitation, the diagnosis of mitral regurgitation by CT depends entirely on visualization of the regurgitant mitral orifice (**Fig. 10.47**). Hemodynamic measurements and visualization of the regurgitant jet are not possible with CT. A short-axis CT image of the incompletely coapted leaflets may be obtained for measurement of a regurgitant orifice, but planimetry of the regurgitant mitral orifice is often complicated by the unusual geometry of the orifice related to overlapping, redundant mitral leaflets.

◆ **Mitral Prostheses**

Dilatation of the mitral annulus is often associated with mitral insufficiency. Dilatation of the mitral annulus may be a cause of incomplete coaptation of the mitral leaflets. Alternatively, mitral insufficiency may result in dilatation of

the left atrium and enlargement of the mitral annulus. Thus, enlargement of the mitral annulus may be both a cause and a consequence of mitral insufficiency, with a vicious cycle resulting in increasing mitral regurgitation. Surgical treatment of an enlarged annulus may be accomplished by placing an annular ring to restrict dilatation of the mitral annulus to allow proper coaptation of the mitral leaflets (**Fig. 10.48**). CTA may be useful in pre-operative evaluation of the annulus to evaluate for size and calcification, as well as in the post-operative evaluation of the mitral annulus and mitral valve coaptation (**Fig. 10.49**). Rarely, annular rings may be placed into both the mitral and tricuspid positions (**Fig. 10.50**). Extensive mitral annular calcification may adversely affect the ability of the surgeon to sew into the annulus and also may significantly increase surgical morbidity and mortality.[51]

A prosthetic valve in the mitral position is easily visualized on CTA. As with the aortic valve, the mitral prosthesis can be evaluated for position within the annulus and for function of the valve leaflets (**Fig. 10.51**). As with aortic valve prostheses, complications of mitral prostheses include infection and dehiscence of the valve from the annulus (**Fig. 10.52**).

◆ **Right-Sided Valves**

The right-sided heart valves are often not visualized on coronary CTA because a saline flush is used to remove high-density contrast material from the right side of the heart. Even when contrast material is present, the mixing of saline, unopacified blood from the inferior vena cava (IVC) and

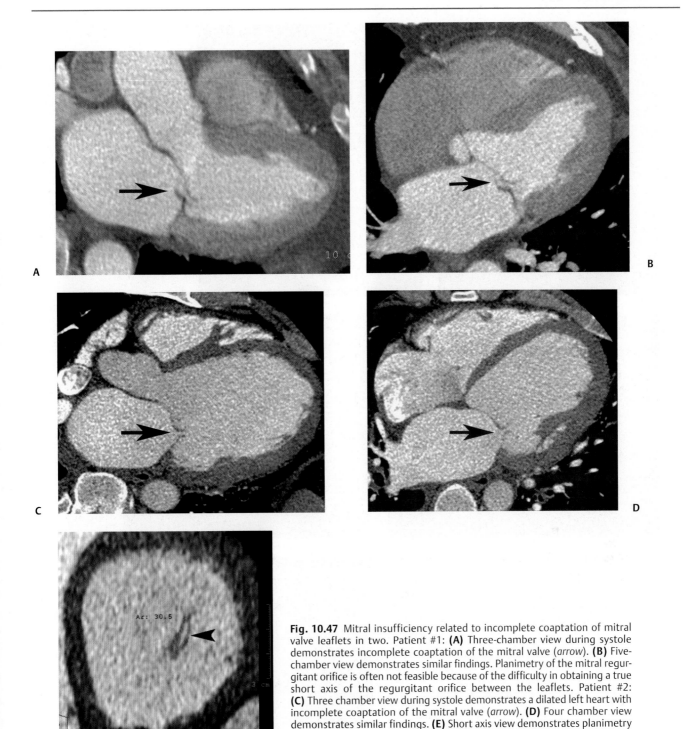

Fig. 10.47 Mitral insufficiency related to incomplete coaptation of mitral valve leaflets in two. Patient #1: **(A)** Three-chamber view during systole demonstrates incomplete coaptation of the mitral valve (*arrow*). **(B)** Five-chamber view demonstrates similar findings. Planimetry of the mitral regurgitant orifice is often not feasible because of the difficulty in obtaining a true short axis of the regurgitant orifice between the leaflets. Patient #2: **(C)** Three chamber view during systole demonstrates a dilated left heart with incomplete coaptation of the mitral valve (*arrow*). **(D)** Four chamber view demonstrates similar findings. **(E)** Short axis view demonstrates planimetry of the mitral regurgitant orifice (*arrowhead*) with an area of 0.3 cm², corresponding to moderate mitral insufficiency.

high-density contrast often creates a confusing picture that obscures visualization of the tricuspid valve (**Fig. 10.53**). Furthermore, the tricuspid valve, like the mitral valve, has a complex motion pattern throughout the cardiac cycle and a redundant complex structure that is difficult to evaluate. This mixing artifact is less a problem for evaluation of the pulmonic valve when sufficient contrast is present in the right side of the heart (**Fig. 10.53A**).

When cardiac CT is performed as a "triple rule-out" (for coronary disease, aortic dissection, and pulmonary embolism), dilute contrast is used in the second phase of the injection in place of a saline flush. The tricuspid and

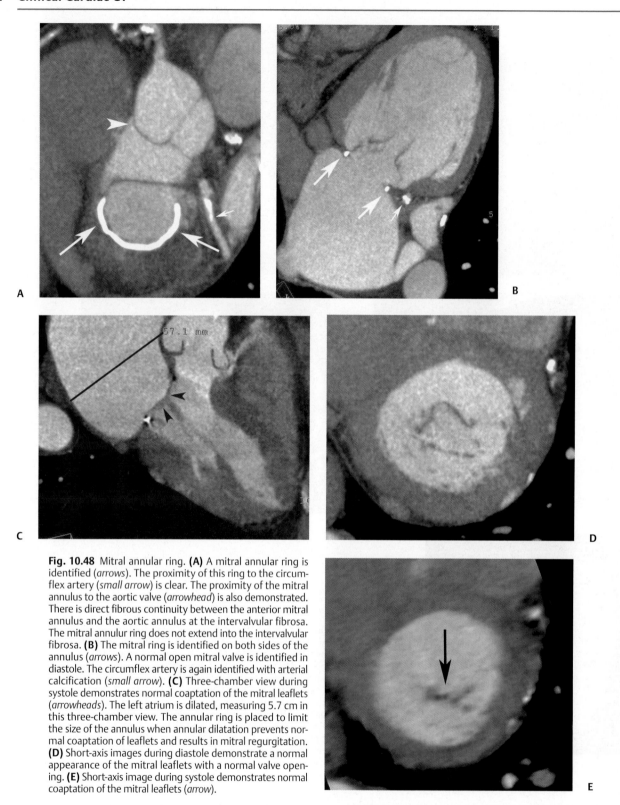

Fig. 10.48 Mitral annular ring. **(A)** A mitral annular ring is identified (*arrows*). The proximity of this ring to the circumflex artery (*small arrow*) is clear. The proximity of the mitral annulus to the aortic valve (*arrowhead*) is also demonstrated. There is direct fibrous continuity between the anterior mitral annulus and the aortic annulus at the intervalvular fibrosa. The mitral annulur ring does not extend into the intervalvular fibrosa. **(B)** The mitral ring is identified on both sides of the annulus (*arrows*). A normal open mitral valve is identified in diastole. The circumflex artery is again identified with arterial calcification (*small arrow*). **(C)** Three-chamber view during systole demonstrates normal coaptation of the mitral leaflets (*arrowheads*). The left atrium is dilated, measuring 5.7 cm in this three-chamber view. The annular ring is placed to limit the size of the annulus when annular dilatation prevents normal coaptation of leaflets and results in mitral regurgitation. **(D)** Short-axis images during diastole demonstrate a normal appearance of the mitral leaflets with a normal valve opening. **(E)** Short-axis image during systole demonstrates normal coaptation of the mitral leaflets (*arrow*).

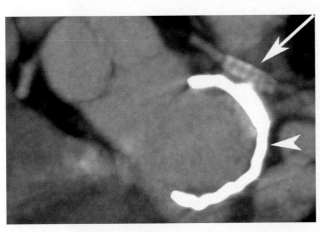

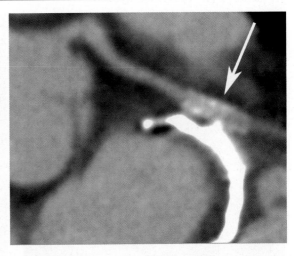

Fig. 10.49 Injury to the circumflex artery during placement of a mitral annular ring. The circumflex artery was stented to occlude a small pseudoaneurysm that was created by a stitch placed to stabilize the annular ring. **(A)** The aortic root is identified at the top of the image. A stent is present in the circumflex artery (*arrow*), immediately adjacent to the mitral annular ring (*arrowhead*). **(B)** Different obliquity demonstrates the course of the proximal circumflex artery from the aorta. Note the proximity of the annular ring to the stented portion of the circumflex artery (*arrow*).

pulmonic valves are more frequently visualized on these studies because of better opacification in the right-sided cardiac chambers (**Fig. 10.54**). Nonetheless, evaluation of the tricuspid valve is often limited by heterogeneous enhancement related to unopacified blood return from the IVC.

As with the aortic and mitral valves, evaluation of the tricuspid and pulmonic valves is dependent on adequate

contrast material, temporal resolution, and electrocardiographic gating. Compared with aortic and mitral disease, disease processes involving the tricuspid and pulmonic valves are less common causes of clinically significant cardiac disease in adults and usually result from pulmonary hypertension or right ventricular enlargement and dysfunction. It is important to realize that mild regurgitation of the

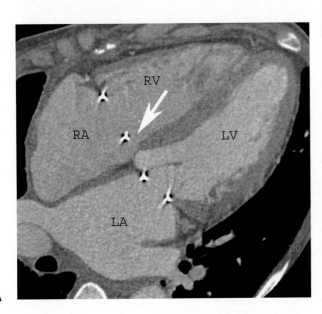

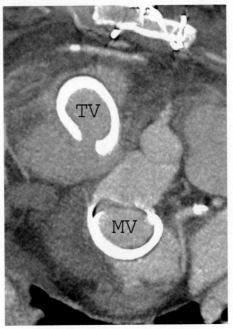

Fig. 10.50 Annular rings in the mitral and tricuspid positions with a paravalvular leak along the septal side of the tricuspid annulus. **(A)** Four-chamber view demonstrates annuluar rings in both the mitral and tricuspid positions. The mitral ring demonstrates contiguity with the annulus on both its septal and lateral sides. A discontinuity is identified between the tricuspid ring and the septum (*arrow*) with a paravalvular leak along the septal side of the tricuspid annulus. **(B)** Short-axis image demonstrates the position of both the mitral and tricuspid rings. MV, mitral valve; TV, tricuspid valve.

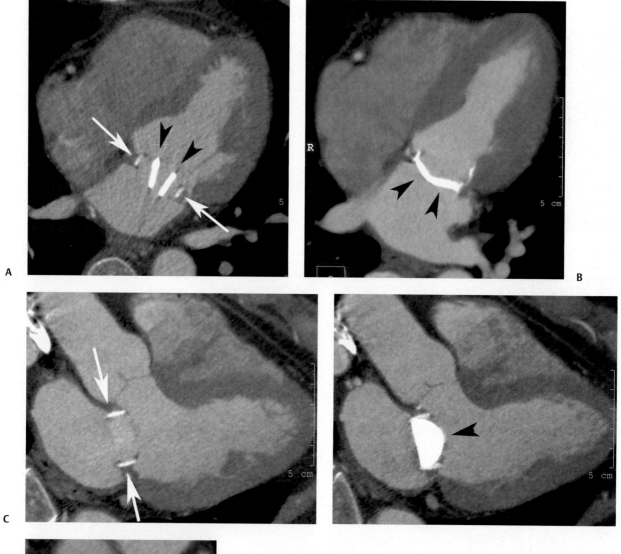

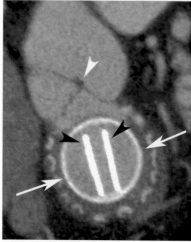

Fig. 10.51 Normal appearance of a St. Jude's mechanical mitral valve replacement. **(A)** Four-chamber view during diastole demonstrates the annulus of the prosthesis (*arrows*) and the two leaflets in open position (*arrowheads*). **(B)** Four-chamber view during systole demonstrates normal function of the prosthesis with coaptation of the leaflets (*arrowheads*). **(C)** Three-chamber view through the center of the prosthetic valve during diastole demonstrates only the annulus (*arrows*). The leaflets are open and out of the plane of the image. **(D)** Three-chamber view obtained slightly off axis demonstrates the "half-circle" shape of an individual leaflet in the mitral prosthesis (*arrowhead*). **(E)** Short-axis view through the mitral prosthesis during diastole demonstrates the annular ring (*arrows*) as well as the valve leaflets (*black arrowheads*). Note the proximity of the aortic valve (*white arrowhead*) to the mitral valve.

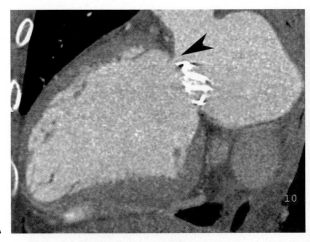
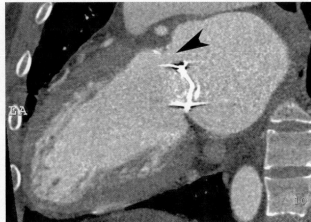

A   B

Fig. 10.52 St. Jude's mechanical mitral valve with anterior dehiscence. **(A)** Two-chamber view during diastole demonstrates the leaflets of the prosthesis in the open position. Contrast is seen to extend across the mitral annulus just anterior to the valve ring (*arrowhead*). **(B)** Two-chamber view during systole demonstrates the leaflets of the prosthesis in the closed position. The paravalvular leak (*arrowhead*) is more obvious during systole because the mitral annulus appears to be pulled further from the anterior aspect of the prosthetic valve.

tricuspid and pulmonic valves is a common, normal variation. However, more severe insufficiency is often associated with elevated right-sided heart pressure and a dilated IVC. In the setting of intravenous drug abuse, vegetations on the tricuspid valve are likely related to infective endocarditis. Rheumatic heart disease may also affect the tricuspid valve, leading to thickened, shortened leaflets with doming. Carcinoid heart disease is present in 50 to 70% of patients with carcinoid syndrome, characterized by the formation of endocardial plaques, which primarily affect the right-sided valves and endocardium. CT imaging reveals thickening of the tricuspid and pulmonic leaflets without calcification. The subvalvular apparatus is involved as well, leading to leaflet shortening and central malcoaptation.[52]

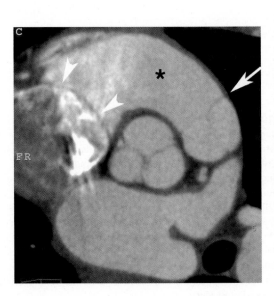
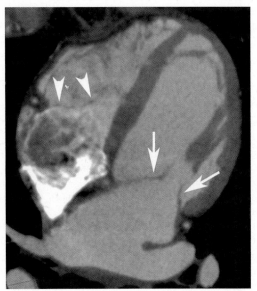

A   B

Fig. 10.53 Evaluation of the right-sided cardiac valves. **(A)** Short-axis image through the aortic valve demonstrates the right ventricular outflow tract as it crosses anterior to the aorta (*). The tricuspid valve is at the 10 o'clock location (*arrowheads*); the pulmonic valve is at the 2 o'clock position (*arrow*). The right-sided valves are of normal thickness. A combination of a dense contrast material, streak artifact, and unopacified saline in the right atrium combine to obscure visualization of the adjacent tricuspid valve (*arrowheads*). **(B)** Four-chamber view during diastole demonstrates normal opening of the mitral (*arrows*) and tricuspid (*arrowheads*) valves. The tricuspid valve is poorly visualized secondary to the presence of a mixture of dense contrast from the superior vena cava and unopacified flow from the inferior vena cava into the right atrium. Normal trabeculations in the right ventricle further limit visualization of the tricuspid valve.

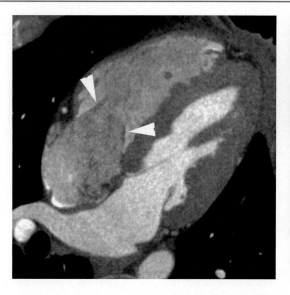
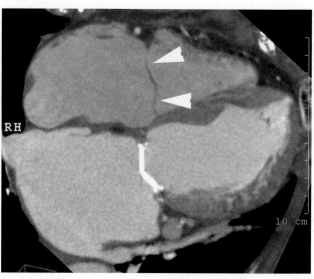

A   B

Fig. 10.54 Normal tricuspid anatomy. **(A)** Four-chamber view demonstrates low-level heterogeneous opacification of the right side of the heart with suboptimal visualization of the normal tricuspid valve (*arrowheads*). **(B)** Four-chamber view in a different patient with homogeneous enhancement of the right side of the heart and excellent visualization of the tricuspid valve (*arrowheads*). This patient has a St. Jude's mitral valve with a dilated left atrium.

◆ Conclusion

Assessment of cardiac valves is an integral part of comprehensive imaging assessment of the heart. Both the aortic and mitral valves are visualized during coronary CTA without the need for additional contrast or imaging time. Pathologic processes that affect these valves may be related to congenital or acquired disease and can adversely impact cardiac morphology and function.

Coronary CTA is useful before valve replacement for surgical planning and to assess the coronary vessels in patients at risk for coronary artery disease. In the patient scheduled for aortic valve surgery, CT is helpful in evaluating the ascending aorta, measuring the size of the LVOT, and demonstrating the relationship between the coronary arteries and the aortic valve or aortic annulus.

Normal Aortic Valve

Cine 10.1   Normal trileaflet aortic valve. Thin leaflets open into a triangular valve orifice.
Cine 10.2   Normal aortic valve. Leaflet motion is assessed most easily on the long axis views while the area of the valve opening is assessed most easily by planimetry in the short axis view.
Cine 10.3   Normal aortic valve. The relationship of the right and left coronary arteries to the associated aortic sinuses and valve cusps is demonstrated in the short axis view. There is no coronary artery associated with the posterior non-coronary cusp.
Cine 10.4   Incomplete opening of a trileaflet aortic valve secondary to poor LV function. The cannula of a left ventricular assist device is present anterior to the right ventricle.

Aortic Insufficiency

Cine 10.5   Myxomatous aortic valve. Thickening of the aortic valve by myxomatous infiltration is a cause of aortic insufficiency. This aortic valve appears to prolapse into the outflow tract during diastole, and a small regurgitant orifice is identified on the short axis views.

Cine 10.6   Trileaflet aortic valve with incomplete coaptation, resulting in moderate to severe aortic insufficiency. Incomplete coaptation is identified on both the short axis and long axis views.
Cine 10.7   Trileaflet aortic valve with incomplete coaptation, resulting in mild aortic insufficiency. Incomplete coaptation is identified on both the short axis and long axis views.
Cine 10.8   Trileaflet aortic valve with dilated aortic root and incomplete coaptation, resulting in aortic insufficiency. Dilatation of the aortic root secondary to hypertension is a common cause of aortic insufficiency.
Cine 10.9   Trileaflet aortic valve with dilated aortic root, effacement of the sinotubular junction and incomplete coaptation, resulting in aortic insufficiency.
Cine 10.10   Calcified trileaflet aortic valve with mild insufficiency along with minimal restriction of leaflet motion.
Cine 10.11   Calcified trileaflet aortic valve with moderate insufficiency and mild stenosis. There is mildly restricted motion of the non-coronary cusp with central lack of coaptation during diastole.

Aortic Stenosis

Cine 10.12 Calcified aortic valve without significant stenosis. Although the valve and the annulus both demonstrate mild calcification, there is no significant restriction to aortic valve opening.

Cine 10.13 Calcified aortic valve without significant stenosis. The aortic valve opens to a full equilateral triangle in the short axis view.

Cine 10.14 Calcified aortic valve with mild to moderate stenosis. The severity of stenosis is assessed most easily by planimetry of the open aortic valve in the short axis view.

Cine 10.15 Calcified aortic valve with mild to moderate stenosis. Calcification crosses the right and left coronary cusps which are functionally fused. Aortic valve area measures 1.4 to 1.5 cm^2 by planimetry.

Cine 10.16 Calcified aortic valve with moderate stenosis. There is little motion of the calcified leaflet associated with the non-coronary sinus of Valsalva.

Cine 10.17 Calcified aortic valve with moderate stenosis. The eccentric coaptation point of the valve on the three chamber view, and lack of opening between the left and right coronary cusps suggest that this may be a bicuspid valve.

Cine 10.18 Calcified aortic valve with moderate stenosis and mild insufficiency. A small regurgitant orifice is visible during diastole.

Cine 10.19 Calcified aortic valve with severe stenosis (see Figure 10.7).

Cine 10.20 Calcified and thickened aortic valve with a measured valve area of 0.9 cm^2 by planimetry.

Cine 10.21 Critical aortic stenosis. Three leaflets are identified, but there is marked restriction of opening during systole. Planimetry of this valve is demonstrated in Figure 10.8 in the text.

Cine 10.22 Porcelain aortic root with aortic stenosis and mild insufficiency. Heavily calcified aortic root with mildly restricted aortic leaflets. A central regurgitant orifice is present during diastole. Although the cine appearance suggests only mild aortic stenosis, the aortic valve area was only 0.7 cm^2 by planimetry (the calcified root measures only 2.1 cm in diameter). Mild restriction of this small valve resulted in a Doppler gradient of 80 mmHg and a clinical presentation of severe aortic stenosis.

Bicuspid Aortic Valve

Cine 10.23 Bicuspid aortic valve with fusion of the commissure between the right and left coronary cusps. A pseudoraphe at the site of a fused commissure can mimic a normal trileaflet valve during diastole. However, the systolic short axis view demonstrates a classic "fishmouth" opening.

Cine 10.24 Bicuspid aortic valve with fusion of the commissure between the right and left coronary cusps. Once again, this pseudoraphae suggests a normal trileaflet valve during diastole.

Cine 10.25 Bicuspid aortic valve with fusion of the commissure between the right and left coronary cusps. A pseudoraphae is demonstrated.

Cine 10.26 Bicuspid aortic valve with fusion of the commissure between the right and left coronary cusps. A pseudoraphae is demonstrated. There is mild valvular calcification without restriction of motion.

Cine 10.27 Bicuspid aortic valve with only one visible commissure– no pseudoraphe.

Cine 10.28 Bicuspid aortic valve with dilated ascending aorta.

Cine 10.29 Trileaflet valve presenting as a functionally bicuspid valve secondary to fusion of the left aortic cusp to the left sinus of Valsalva (see Figure 10.12).

Bicuspid Aortic Valve with Stenosis

Cine 10.30 Bicuspid aortic valve with aneurysm of the ascending aorta. Note the eccentric opening aortic valve with a single leaflet extending across the right and non coronary sinuses of Valsalva. There is mild calcification of the left coronary cusp with restriction of motion on the three chamber view (top left). However, the larger right-sided cusp moves freely so that there is no hemodynamically significant stenosis.

Cine 10.31 Bicuspid aortic valve. There is no visible commissure between the right and left coronary cusps. There is mild valvular calcification with minimal restriction of motion. However, the aortic valve area was normal by planimetry.

Cine 10.32 Bicuspid aortic valve with heavy valvular calcification and mild to moderate aortic stenosis.

Cine 10.33 Bicuspid aortic valve with moderate aortic stenosis and ascending aortic aneurysm. Bicuspid aortic valves are associated with connective tissue disease that may predispose patients to aortic aneurysms and aortic rupture.

Cine 10.34 Bicuspid aortic valve with fusion of the right and non-coronary cusps, and moderate to severe aortic stenosis. The presence of heavy valvular calcification does not compromise measurement of aortic valve area on the short axis projection in this case.

Cine 10.35 Bicuspid aortic valve with fusion of right and non-coronary cusps, and moderate to severe aortic stenosis. The presence of heavy valvular calcification creates artifact which may limit the accuracy of measurement of the aortic valve area.

Cine 10.36 Bicuspid aortic valve with severe stenosis. The calcified leaflets demonstrate a straight commissure across the valve in short axis with only minimal motion.

Aortic Valve Masses / Vegetation

Cine 10.37 Fibroelastoma of the aortic valve. A small round fibroelastoma is present at the tip of the aortic valve, and is visible in the closed diastolic position. The diagnosis of fibrolastoma is usually made by transesophageal echocardiography. These lesions are often not visible on CT because of their small size and their characteristic vibratory motion.

Cine 10.38 (A,B) Bacterial endocarditis with a vegetation on the aortic valve and severe aortic insufficiency. A diseased valve is more susceptible to endocarditis. The presence of calcification in this patient suggests that this valve had pre-existing disease. The vegetation extends from the calcified leaflet/commissure and prolapses into the left ventricular outflow tract during diastole.

Prosthetic Aortic Valves

Cine 10.39 Normally functioning bioprosthetic aortic valve with metallic struts. A trileaflet valve is identified with normal opening of the cusps on the short axis view. Imaging of the cusps is limited by artifact from the metallic struts.

(Continued on page 268)

Cine 10.40   Normally functioning bioprosthetic aortic valve with metallic struts. The leaflets are normal in thickness, and normal motion is identified on long and short axis views. Once again, imaging of the cusps is limited by artifact from the metallic struts.

Cine 10.41   Normally functioning bioprosthetic aortic valve without metallic struts. The valve cusps are more clearly identified in this prosthesis with no metallic artifact.

Cine 10.42   Normally functioning Carbomedics prosthetic aortic valve. Both leaflets of this bileaflet mechanical valve are identified and demonstrate a normal motion pattern.

Cine 10.43   Normally functioning St. Judes prosthetic aortic valve. The valve is normally seated in the aortic annulus. Both leaflets of this bileaflet mechanical valve demonstrate a normal motion pattern.

Cine 10.44   Normally functioning St. Judes prosthetic aortic valve. The valve is seated in the aortic annulus. The larger diameter of the aortic root is appreciated just above the valve plane. The sinuses of Valsalva project around the valve on the short axis view.

Cine 10.45   Normally function Medtronic-Hall prosthetic aortic valve. A single disc serves as the valve leaflet. The valve hinge is visible, extending to the center of the disc.

Normal Mitral Valve

Cine 10.46   Normally functioning mitral valve. Valve motion is best appreciated on long axis images, and specifically, in the five chamber view in this case. Note the biphasic opening of the mitral valve during diastole, corresponding to the diastolic filling phases of rapid early diastolic filling and atrial systole in late diastole.

Cine 10.47   Normally functioning mitral valve with short axis imaging. Although the long axis views are best to demonstrate leaflet motion, the short axis view is best for planimetry to demonstrate mitral valve area.

Mitral Valve Prolapse

Cine 10.48   Myxomatous mitral valve with prolapse of the posterior mitral leaflet. The mitral leaflets appear thick. The diagnosis of prolapse is made on the three chamber view. In this case, the posterior mitral leaflet prolapses above the plane of the mitral annulus in the three chamber view.

Cine 10.49   Myxomatous mitral valve with prolapse of both the anterior and posterior mitral leaflets. The mitral leaflets appear thick. The diagnosis of prolapse is made on the three chamber view. Both mitral leaflets prolapse approximately 4–5mm above the plane of the mitral annulus in the three chamber view. The image appears grainy during systole because of tube current modulation.

Cine 10.50   Prolapse of the posterior mitral leaflet. Prolapse is identified in both the four chamber and three chamber views. However, the diagnosis of prolapse should be based upon the three chamber view. Visualization of mitral prolapse in the four chamber view may lead to false positive diagnosis when prolapse is not present in the three chamber view.

Cine 10.51   Prolapse of both the anterior and posterior mitral leaflets. Both leaflets are demonstrated to prolapse above the mitral annulus in the three chamber view.

Cine 10.52   Redundant posterior mitral leaflet. A focal bulge of the posterior mitral leaflet toward the atrium is identified during systole in the four chamber and five chamber views. This bulge does not break the plane of the annulus, and was not visualized on the three chamber view. This bulge does not meet the criteria for prolapse of the mitral valve.

Cine 10.53   Pseudoprolapse of the anterior mitral leaflet on the four chamber view. The anterior mitral leaflet extends above the plane of the mitral annulus in the four chamber view during systole. The three chamber view demonstrates normal mitral valve coaptation with no prolapse.

Mitral Annular Calcification

Cine 10.54   Mitral annuluar calcification without restriction of mitral leaflet motion. Calcification is present at the base of the anterior mitral leaflet on the four chamber, five chamber and two chamber views. There is no restriction of mitral leaflet motion. Mitral annular calcification is generally a benign finding, common in the posterior annulus, and more common with increasing age.

Cine 10.55   **(A,B)** Caseous calcification of the mitral annulus. The annular calcification is seen best in the three chamber and five chamber views where it is visualized to extend into the posterior mitral leaflet.

Cine 10.56   Caseous calcification of the mitral annulus. The annular calcification is visible along the posterior annulus on the three chamber and two chamber views.

Mitral Stenosis

Cine 10.57   **(A,B)** Mild mitral stenosis with thickened mitral leaflets and mild restriction of the posterior leaflet on the four chamber and three chamber views.

Cine 10.58   Mild to moderate mitral stenosis with a valve area of 1.6 cm^2. The leaflets are thickened with a "hockey stick" bowed configuration of the anterior leaflet and an immobile posterior leaflet.

Mitral Insufficiency

Cine 10.59   Mitral insufficiency with marked dilatation of the left ventricle, a stretched anterior leaflet, a posterior leaflet that appears short/restricted, and failure of mitral coaptation in the two chamber view.

Cine 10.60   **(A,B)** Mitral insufficiency secondary to lack of coaptation of the mitral valve.

Cine 10.61   Myxomatous anterior mitral leaflet with inadequate mitral coaptation (two chamber view) and subtle prolapse of the anterior leaflet (three chamber view).

Endocarditis of Native Aortic and Mitral Valves

Cine 10.62   **(A–D)** Aortic and mitral valve endocarditis with marked valve thickening. (A & B): Thickened and calcified aortic valve with a flail leaflet/vegetation. (C & D): Thickened mitral valve, particularly the anterior leaflet, with inadequate coaptation.

Mitral Annular Ring / Prosthetic Mitral Valve

Cine 10.63   Annular rings in the mitral and tricuspid positions.

Cine 10.64   Normally functioning St. Judes prosthesis in the mitral position.

Cine 10.65 **(A,B)** Normal functioning St. Judes valves in the aortic and mitral positions.

Cine 10.66 Normally functioning ball in cage (Star Edwards) valve in the mitral position.

Infection / Complications of Valve Prostheses

Cine 10.67 Aortic bioprosthesis in a patient with persistent bacteremia. The prosthetic leaflets appear mildly thickened, but no definite vegetation was identified.

Cine 10.68 Aortic bioprosthesis with endocarditis and pseudoaneurysm. The bioprosthetic valve is markedly thickened secondary to vegetations. A small pseudoaneurysm is present just below the anterior attachment of the bioprosthesis, visible on the three chamber and short axis views.

Cine 10.69 St. Judes prosthetic aortic valve with anterior paravalvular leak related to dehiscence along the anterior attachment on the three chamber view (top left).

Cine 10.70 St. Judes prosthetic aortic valve with posterior dehiscence visible along the posterior attachment of the prosthesis on the three chamber view (top right).

Cine 10.71 **(A,B)** Pseudoaneurysm of the LVOT status post replacement of the aortic and mitral valves with St. Judes prostheses.

Cine 10.71 **(C,D)** Six-month follow-up demonstrates no significant change in the bilobed pseudoaneurysm between the aorta and the right ventricular outflow tract.

Cine 10.72 **(A,B)** St. Judes aortic valve with posterior dehiscence and pseudoaneurysm between the aorta and left atrium.

Cine 10.73 **(A,B)** Aortic valve bioprosthesis with pseudoaneurysm of the left ventricular outflow tract as a complication of endocarditis with abscess formation and rupture. A. The bioprosthetic valve demonstrates normal function in long axis (left-sided images) and short axis (top right). A kink is appreciated at the upper anastomosis of the short tube graft. A small, pulsatile pseudoaneurysm is present within the intervalvular fibrosa, between the bioprosthesis and the left atrium. Mild systolic anterior motion of the mitral valve is present (top left image). B. Three chamber view obtained slightly off axis demonstrates the origin of the pseudoaneurysm from the posterior aspect of the left ventricular outflow tract with extension into the intervalvular fibrosa. The reimplanted right coronary artery is visible anterior to the aortic root, with a high grade stenosis at the site of reimplantation into the tube graft.

Cine 10.74 Status post Bentall procedure with a mechanical aortic valve and tube graft of the ascending aorta. The coronary arteries have been reimplanted into the tube graft (top left image). Although the mechanical valve appears to function normally and does not "rock" excessively, there is complete dehiscence of the proximal anastamosis to the LVOT with a pseudoaneurysm around the proximal tube graft contained by the surgical scar tissue. Note that the tube graft is compressed by the enlarging pseudoaneurysm during systole (bottom left image).

Cine 10.75 Bioprosthetic aortic valve with post-infectious pseudoaneurysm extending from the LVOT into the intervalvular fibrosa.

Cine 10.76 Bioprosthetic mitral valve with paravalvular leak related to dehiscence along the lateral aspect of the valve annulus, best appreciated on the four chamber view (top left).

Tricuspid Valve

Cine 10.77 Normal tricuspid valve. The tricuspid valve is visualized on the four chamber and short axis views. Heterogeneous opacification of the right atrium is a common limiting factor in evaluation of the tricuspid valve.

Cine 10.78 Normal tricuspid valve. Both the mitral and tricuspid valve demonstrate a normal appearance on the four chamber and short axis views. The tricuspid valve attachment to the septum is slightly more apical as compared to the mitral valve. The left ventricle demonstrates a large infarct involving the inferior and inferolateral walls with a patch repair.

Cine 10.79 **(A)** Ebstein anomaly. Markedly enlarged right heart with redundant tricuspid valve demonstrating inferior displacement of the septal leaflet on the four chamber view (top left).

Cine 10.79 **(B)** Ebstein anomaly. Thickened tricuspid valve is demonstrated on the right ventricular inflow view (top left). Three redundant tricuspid leaflets are demonstrated on the short axis view (bottom left).

References

1. Chen JJ, Manning MA, Frazier AA, Jeudy J, White CS. CT angiography of the cardiac valves: normal, diseased, and postoperative appearances. Radiographics. 2009;29(5):1393–1412

2. Al-Attar N, Himbert D, Descoutures F, et al. Transcatheter aortic valve implantation: selection strategy is crucial for outcome. Ann Thorac Surg. 2009;87(6):1757–1762, discussion 1762–1763

3. Himbert D, Descoutures F, Al-Attar N, et al. Results of transfemoral or transapical aortic valve implantation following a uniform assessment in high-risk patients with aortic stenosis. J Am Coll Cardiol. 2009; 54(4):303–311

4. Zoghbi WA, Farmer KL, Soto JG, Nelson JG, Quinones MA. Accurate noninvasive quantification of stenotic aortic valve area by Doppler echocardiography. Circulation. 1986;73(3):452–459

5. Rahimtoola SH. Severe aortic stenosis with low systolic gradient: the good and bad news. Circulation. 2000;101(16):1892–1894

6. Alkadhi H, Wildermuth S, Plass A, et al. Aortic stenosis: comparative evaluation of 16-detector row CT and echocardiography. Radiology. 2006;240(1):47–55

7. LaBounty TM, Sundaram B, Agarwal P, Armstrong WA, Kazerooni EA, Yamada E. Aortic valve area on 64-MDCT correlates with transesophageal echocardiography in aortic stenosis. AJR Am J Roentgenol. 2008;191(6):1652–1658

8. Shah RG, Novaro GM, Blandon RJ, Whiteman MS, Asher CR, Kirsch J. Aortic valve area: meta-analysis of diagnostic performance of multidetector computed tomography for aortic valve area measurements as compared to transthoracic echocardiography. Int J Cardiovasc Imaging. 2009;25(6):601–609

9. Halpern EJ, Mallya R, Sewell M, Shulman M, Zwas DR. Differences in aortic valve area measured with CT planimetry and echocardiography (continuity equation) are related to divergent estimates of left ventricular outflow tract area. AJR Am J Roentgenol. 2009;192(6):1668–1673

10. Rajamannan NM, Gersh B, Bonow RO. Calcific aortic stenosis: from bench to the bedside—emerging clinical and cellular concepts. Heart. 2003;89(7):801–805

11. Stewart BF, Siscovick D, Lind BK, et al. Clinical factors associated with calcific aortic valve disease. Cardiovascular Health Study. J Am Coll Cardiol. 1997;29(3):630–634

12. Otto CM, Lind BK, Kitzman DW, Gersh BJ, Siscovick DS. Association of aortic-valve sclerosis with cardiovascular mortality and morbidity in the elderly. N Engl J Med. 1999;341(3):142–147

13. LaBounty TM, Sundaram B, Agarwal P, Armstrong WA, Kazerooni EA, Yamada E. Aortic valve area on 64-MDCT correlates with transesophageal echocardiography in aortic stenosis. AJR Am J Roentgenol. 2008;191(6):1652–1658

14. Halpern EJ, Zhang S, Wansaicheong GK. Assessment of the aortic valve area and morphology during cardiac CT angiography. Proceedings of the 92nd annual meeting of the Radiological Society of North America. Chicago, Ill, December 2006. Abstract #SSQ08–06, p. 533

15. Bonow RO, Carabello BA, Kanu C, et al; American College of Cardiology/American Heart Association Task Force on Practice Guidelines; Society of Cardiovascular Anesthesiologists; Society for Cardiovascular Angiography and Interventions; Society of Thoracic Surgeons. ACC/AHA 2006 guidelines for the management of patients with valvular heart disease: a report of the American College of Cardiology/American Heart Association Task Force on Practice Guidelines (writing committee to revise the 1998 Guidelines for the Management of Patients With Valvular Heart Disease): developed in collaboration with the Society of Cardiovascular Anesthesiologists: endorsed by the Society for Cardiovascular Angiography and Interventions and the Society of Thoracic Surgeons. Circulation. 2006; 114(5):e84–e231

16. Otto CM, Burwash IG, Legget ME, et al. Prospective study of asymptomatic valvular aortic stenosis. Clinical, echocardiographic, and exercise predictors of outcome. Circulation. 1997;95(9):2262–2270

17. Nataatmadja M, West M, West J, et al. Abnormal extracellular matrix protein transport associated with increased apoptosis of vascular smooth muscle cells in marfan syndrome and bicuspid aortic valve thoracic aortic aneurysm. Circulation. 2003;108(Suppl 1): II329–II334

18. Hahn RT, Roman MJ, Mogtader AH, Devereux RB. Association of aortic dilation with regurgitant, stenotic and functionally normal bicuspid aortic valves. J Am Coll Cardiol. 1992;19(2):283–288

19. Nistri S, Sorbo MD, Marin M, Palisi M, Scognamiglio R, Thiene G. Aortic root dilatation in young men with normally functioning bicuspid aortic valves. Heart. 1999;82(1):19–22

20. Borger MA, Preston M, Ivanov J, et al. Should the ascending aorta be replaced more frequently in patients with bicuspid aortic valve disease? J Thorac Cardiovasc Surg. 2004;128(5):677–683

21. Mussa S, Miller P, Barron DJ, Brawn WJ. Occlusion of the left coronary ostium by an aortic valve leaflet. J Thorac Cardiovasc Surg. 2007; 134(6):1586–1587

22. Feuchtner GM, Dichtl W, Müller S, et al. 64-MDCT for diagnosis of aortic regurgitation in patients referred to CT coronary angiography. AJR Am J Roentgenol. 2008;191(1):W1–7

23. Gilkeson RC, Markowitz AH, Balgude A, Sachs PB. MDCT evaluation of aortic valvular disease. AJR Am J Roentgenol. 2006;186(2):350–360

24. Libman E, Sacks B. A hitherto undescribed form of valvular and mural endocarditis. Arch Intern Med. 1924;33:701–737

25. Moder KG, Miller TD, Tazelaar HD. Cardiac involvement in systemic lupus erythematosus. Mayo Clin Proc. 1999;74(3):275–284

26. Joffe II, Jacobs LE, Owen AN, Ioli A, Kotler MN. Noninfective valvular masses: review of the literature with emphasis on imaging techniques and management. Am Heart J. 1996;131(6):1175–1183

27. Roldan CA, Shively BK, Crawford MH. An echocardiographic study of valvular heart disease associated with systemic lupus erythematosus. N Engl J Med. 1996;335(19):1424–1430

28. Lentini S, Monaco F, Tancredi F, Savasta M, Gaeta R. Aortic valve infective endocarditis: could multi-detector CT scan be proposed for routine screening of concomitant coronary artery disease before surgery? Ann Thorac Surg. 2009;87(5):1585–1587

29. Hoey ET, Mansoubi H, Gopalan D, Tasker AD, Screaton NJ. MDCT features of cardiothoracic sources of stroke. Clin Radiol. 2009;64(5):550–559

30. Bettencourt N, Rocha J, Carvalho M, et al. Multislice computed tomography in the exclusion of coronary artery disease in patients with presurgical valve disease. Circ Cardiovasc Imaging. 2009;2(4): 306–313

31. Harpaz D, Shah P, Bezante G, et al. Transthoracic and transesophageal echocardiographic sizing of the aortic annulus to determine prosthesis size. Am J Cardiol. 1993;72(18):1411–1417

32. LaBounty TM, Agarwal PP, Chughtai A, Bach DS, Wizauer E, Kazerooni EA. Evaluation of mechanical heart valve size and function with ECG-gated 64-MDCT. AJR Am J Roentgenol. 2009;193(5):W389–96

33. Chan J, Marwan M, Schepis T, Ropers D, Du L, Achenbach S. Images in cardiovascular medicine. Cardiac CT assessment of prosthetic aortic valve dysfunction secondary to acute thrombosis and response to thrombolysis. Circulation. 2009;120(19):1933–1934

34. Berdajs D, Lajos P, Turina MI. A new classification of the mitral papillary muscle. Med Sci Monit. 2005;11(1):BR18–BR21

35. Gorlin R, Gorlin SG. Hydraulic formula for calculation of the area of the stenotic mitral valve, other cardiac valves, and central circulatory shunts. I. Am Heart J. 1951;41(1):1–29

36. Roberts WC, Perloff JK. Mitral valvular disease. A clinicopathologic survey of the conditions causing the mitral valve to function abnormally. Ann Intern Med. 1972;77(6):939–975

37. Harpaz D, Auerbach I, Vered Z, Motro M, Tobar A, Rosenblatt S. Caseous calcification of the mitral annulus: a neglected, unrecognized diagnosis. J Am Soc Echocardiogr. 2001;14(8):825–831

38. Biteker M, Duran NE, Ozkan M. Caseous calcification of the mitral annulus imaged with 64-slice multidetector CT. Echocardiography. 2009;26(6):744–745

39. Blankstein R, Durst R, Picard MH, Cury RC. Progression of mitral annulus calcification to caseous necrosis of the mitral valve: complementary role of multi-modality imaging. Eur Heart J. 2009;30(3):304

40. Alkadhi H, Leschka S, Prêtre R, Perren A, Marincek B, Wildermuth S. Caseous calcification of the mitral annulus. J Thorac Cardiovasc Surg. 2005;129(6):1438–1440

41. Jeon DS, Atar S, Brasch AV, et al. Association of mitral annulus calcification, aortic valve sclerosis and aortic root calcification with abnormal myocardial perfusion single photon emission tomography in subjects age < or =65 years old. J Am Coll Cardiol. 2001;38(7):1988–1993

42. Jones EC, Devereux RB, Roman MJ, et al. Prevalence and correlates of mitral regurgitation in a population-based sample (the Strong Heart Study). Am J Cardiol. 2001;87(3):298–304

43. Alkadhi H, Wildermuth S, Bettex DA, et al. Mitral regurgitation: quantification with 16-detector row CT—initial experience. Radiology. 2006;238(2):454–463

44. Freed LA, Levy D, Levine RA, et al. Prevalence and clinical outcome of mitral-valve prolapse. N Engl J Med. 1999;341(1):1–7

45. Barlow JB, Bosman CK. Aneurysmal protrusion of the posterior leaflet of the mitral valve. An auscultatory-electrocardiographic syndrome. Am Heart J. 1966;71(2):166–178

46. Warth DC, King ME, Cohen JM, Tesoriero VL, Marcus E, Weyman AE. Prevalence of mitral valve prolapse in normal children. J Am Coll Cardiol. 1985;5(5):1173–1177

47. Levine RA, Triulzi MO, Harrigan P, Weyman AE. The relationship of mitral annular shape to the diagnosis of mitral valve prolapse. Circulation. 1987;75(4):756–767

48. Freed LA, Benjamin EJ, Levy D, et al. Mitral valve prolapse in the general population: the benign nature of echocardiographic features in the Framingham Heart Study. J Am Coll Cardiol. 2002;40(7): 1298–1304

49. Hayek E, Gring CN, Griffin BP. Mitral valve prolapse. Lancet. 2005; 365(9458):507–518

50. Schwammenthal E, Nakatani S, He S, et al. Mechanism of mitral regurgitation in hypertrophic cardiomyopathy: mismatch of posterior to anterior leaflet length and mobility. Circulation. 1998;98(9):856–865

51. Cammack PL, Edie RN, Edmunds LH Jr. Bar calcification of the mitral anulus. A risk factor in mitral valve operations. J Thorac Cardiovasc Surg. 1987;94(3):399–404

52. Veitch AM, Morgan-Hughes GJ, Roobottom CA. Carcinoid heart disease as shown by 64-slice CT coronary angiography. Eur Heart J. 2006; 27(19):2271

11

Ablation in the Left Atrium

Behzad B. Pavri and Ethan J. Halpern

◆ Pathophysiology of Atrial Fibrillation

Atrial fibrillation (AF) is the most common cardiac rhythm disturbance in humans, with an incidence that increases with age and doubles through many decades of life.[1] Because pharmacologic therapy for this arrhythmia is only modestly successful, treatment of AF remains a challenging problem. In the last decade, since the seminal recognition that rapid firing from within the pulmonary veins (PVs) is a common triggering mechanism for AF,[2] ablation in the left atrium (LA) has become increasingly common as a treatment strategy. It is now well recognized that the LA musculature extends to variable degrees into the pulmonary veins.[3] These extensions of atrial myocardium are the most common sites for rapidly firing triggers that initiate AF. Electrical recordings obtained from circular multipolar ("lasso") catheters positioned at the mouth of the PVs reveal sharp electrograms, termed *PV potentials*. PV potentials are recorded during sinus rhythm and during repetitive firing at the initiation of AF. Although AF may sometimes be provoked by electrical depolarizations from non-PV locations[4] (such as the coronary sinus, the ligament of Marshall, the superior vena cava, the crista terminalis, the fossa ovalis), it is clear that most paroxysmal and persistent AF is related to the PVs. Electrical isolation of the PVs has become a central tenet in ablation strategies for AF.

◆ Ablation Strategies to "Cure" Atrial Fibrillation

Various ablation strategies have been developed to attempt a "cure" for AF. Most of these approaches rely on ablation around the junction of the PVs and the body of the LA, the so-called pulmonary antrum, to achieve electrical disconnection of the PVs from the atrial myocardium. Ablation is most often accomplished with radiofrequency (RF) energy, although alternate energy sources, such as cryoablation, focused ultrasound, and microwave ablation have been investigated. RF energy is delivered around the pulmonary antrum until PV potentials are abolished and electrical disconnection of the PV from the body of the atrium is achieved. Additional RF energy is often delivered in linear patterns ("lines") to electrically compartmentalize the LA or to create lines of block. Such strategies are anatomically guided and are dependent on a clear understanding of LA anatomy. Not unexpectedly, such extensive ablation strategies in the relatively thin-walled LA are associated with a low, but not insignificant, complication rate.

◆ "Normal" (Conventional) Left Atrial Anatomy

The LA is the most superior and posterior chamber in the heart. The posterior wall of the LA abuts the esophagus. The LA cavity is not amenable to comparison with any standard geometric figure but may be thought of as approximating an oblate spheroid. The mitral annulus is located at the anterior–inferior aspect of the LA chamber. The right and left superior PVs enter the posterior aspect of the "roof" of the LA, whereas the right and left inferior PVs enter at the inferoposterior aspect of the LA, close to the posterior aspect of the mitral annulus (**Figs. 11.1 and 11.2**). In saggital section, the superior PVs are often more anterior than the inferior PVs, yet the superior PVs are farther from the mitral annulus because of the anteroinferior orientation of the mitral annulus (**Fig. 11.3**). This anatomic relationship is of clinical importance because ablation strategies often involve creation of a "line of block" by placing contiguous RF lesions from the inferolateral mitral annulus to the left inferior PV to prevent LA flutter.[5] On average, the left-sided PVs tend to be slightly larger than the right-sided PVs, and the superior PVs tend to be slightly larger than the inferior PVs. PVs in patients with AF tend to be larger compared with those in control groups without AF. Often the PV ostia are oval rather than circular.[6]

The LA appendage is a highly trabeculated, "cauliflower-like" protuberance from the upper left side of the LA, extending anteriorly along the left superolateral margin of the LA (**Fig. 11.4**). The orifice of the LA appendage is

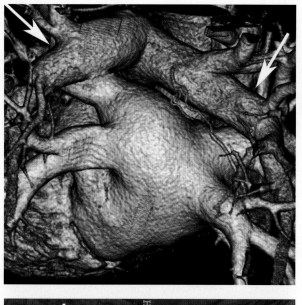

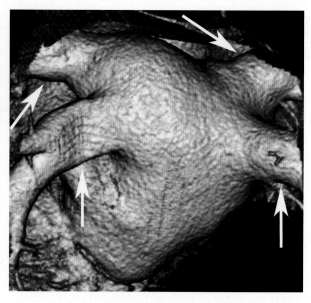

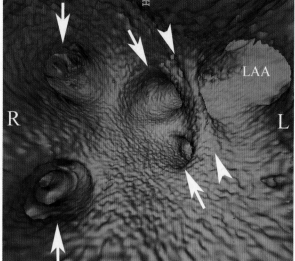

Fig. 11.1 Conventional left atrial anatomy (LAA). **(A)** Surface image demonstrates the posterior wall of the left atrium with associated pulmonary veins. The pulmonary arteries have not been removed (*arrows*) and do obscure the pulmonary veins. **(B)** The pulmonary arteries have now been removed, and the four pulmonary veins are clearly identified (*arrows*). **(C)** Endoluminal view demonstrates four pulmonary veins (*arrows*). The ridge that separates the two left-sided pulmonary veins from the left atrial appendage is clearly defined (*arrowheads*).

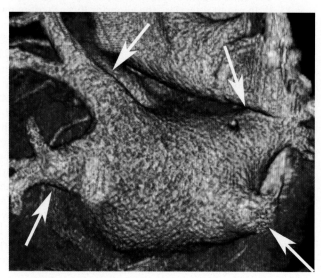

Fig. 11.2 Conventional left atrial anatomy. **(A)** Surface image demonstrates four pulmonary veins (*arrows*). There is a superior and an inferior pulmonary vein on each side.

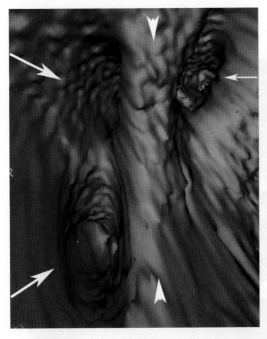

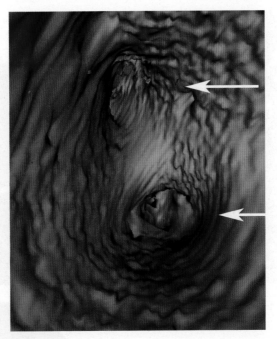

B

C

Fig. 11.2 (*Continued*) **(B)** Endoluminal view of the left side of the left atrium demonstrates the left pulmonary veins (*large arrows*), separated from the left atrial appendage (*small arrow*) by a ridge (*arrowheads*).

(C) Endoluminal evaluation of the right side of the atrium clearly demonstrates two separate right pulmonary veins (*arrows*).

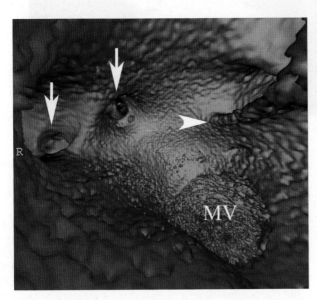

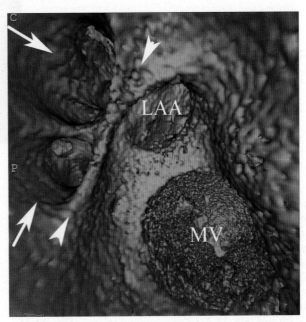

A

B

Fig. 11.3 Relationship of pulmonary veins to mitral annulus. **(A)** Endoluminal view looking posteriorly–inferiorly from the anterior–superior aspect of the left atrium demonstrates the right-sided pulmonary veins (*arrows*). The left pulmonary veins are blocked from view by the ridge (*arrowhead*) that separates these veins from the left atrial appendage.

The mitral valve (MV) is located anterior–inferior to this ridge. **(B)** Endoluminal view of the left side of the left atrium demonstrates the left pulmonary veins (*arrows*), separated from the left atrial appendage (LAA) by a ridge (*arrowheads*). The MV is anterior–inferior to the pulmonary veins and closer to the inferior pulmonary veins.

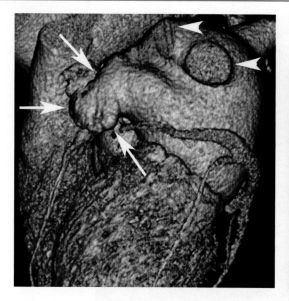

A

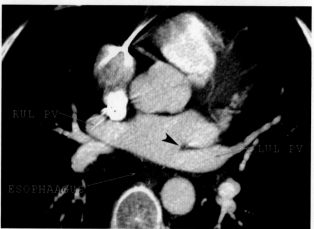

B

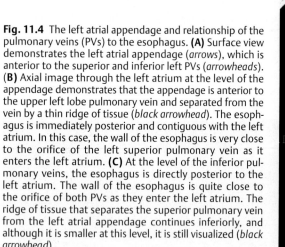

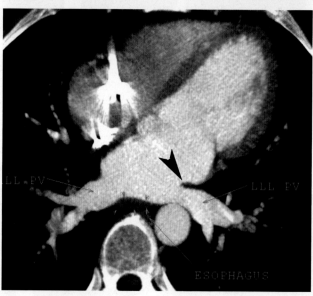

C

Fig. 11.4 The left atrial appendage and relationship of the pulmonary veins (PVs) to the esophagus. **(A)** Surface view demonstrates the left atrial appendage (*arrows*), which is anterior to the superior and inferior left PVs (*arrowheads*). **(B)** Axial image through the left atrium at the level of the appendage demonstrates that the appendage is anterior to the upper left lobe pulmonary vein and separated from the vein by a thin ridge of tissue (*black arrowhead*). The esophagus is immediately posterior and contiguous with the left atrium. In this case, the wall of the esophagus is very close to the orifice of the left superior pulmonary vein as it enters the left atrium. **(C)** At the level of the inferior pulmonary veins, the esophagus is directly posterior to the left atrium. The wall of the esophagus is quite close to the orifice of both PVs as they enter the left atrium. The ridge of tissue that separates the superior pulmonary vein from the left atrial appendage continues inferiorly, and although it is smaller at this level, it is still visualized (*black arrowhead*).

generally anterior to the insertion of the superior left PVs, but it may be positioned slightly superior to or slightly inferior to the left superior PV.[7] The mouth of the LA appendage is oval and tends to be larger in patients with AF compared with normal hearts. The posterior wall of the LA appendage abuts the anterior walls of the left-sided PVs. The posterior walls of the left-sided PVs often abut the esophagus and descending aorta. The ridge or crest of tissue separating the left PVs from the appendage may be visualized on axial images (**Fig. 11.4**) or endoluminal images (**Figs. 11.1C, 11.2B,** and **11.3B**). This ridge is sometimes called the "warfarin ridge" because it can be mistaken for a LA clot during echocardiography. The thickness and orientation of this ridge are of great importance to the electrophysiologist during ablation to achieve PV isolation. It is generally not possible to position the ablation catheter on this ridge. Hence ablation is often attempted on the posterior aspect of

this structure (ie, the anterior wall of the left PV antrum). Recent studies have demonstrated that pre-procedural CT reconstruction is useful to classify a wide range of variations in morphology of the left atrial appendage.[8]

Although most patients have the standard pulmonary venous anatomy described above, a substantial minority of the population demonstrates variation in the number, size, and orientation of PVs (**Figs. 11.5, 11.6, 11.7, 11.8, 11.9, 11.10, 11.11** and **11.12**). This variability is of clinical importance to the electrophysiologist performing LA ablation because the procedure is anatomically driven. A single antrum for the left-sided pulmonary veins is probably the most commonly encountered variation (**Fig. 11.5**). In addition, we and others have recently reported additional appendage-like diverticula at varying locations in a significant minority of patients.[9] Ablation within these "ectopic" or "supernumary" appendages may be required but may also result in complications

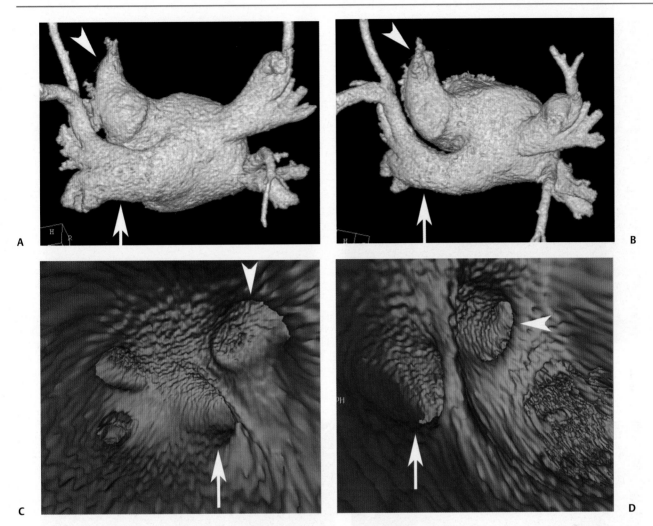

Fig. 11.5 Single antrum of the left-sided pulmonary veins. **(A)** Surface image from the back of the left atrium demonstrates the left atrial appendage (*arrowhead*) is superior to the single pulmonary vein that enters the left side of the left atrium (*arrow*). **(B)** Surface image from a cranial position demonstrates the roof of the left atrium with the left atrial appendage anteriorly (*arrowhead*) and the solitary left pulmonary vein more posteriorly (*arrow*). **(C)** Endoluminal view of the posterior wall of the left atrium demonstrates the orifice of the left atrial appendage (*arrowhead*) superior and anterior to the orifice of the single left pulmonary vein (*arrow*). These two structures are separated by the warfarin ridge. The two right-sided pulmonary vein orifices are also visible. **(D)** Close-up endoluminal view again demonstrates the orifices of the left atrial appendage (*arrowhead*) and left pulmonary vein (*arrow*) separated by the warfarin ridge. The mitral valve annulus is visible on the bottom right of the image.

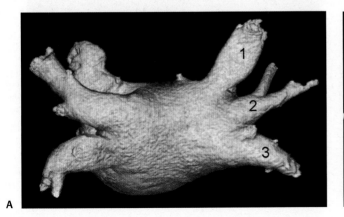

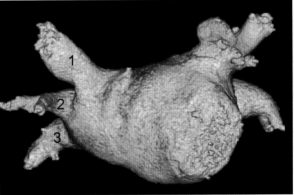

Fig. 11.6 Accessory right pulmonary vein. **(A)** Surface image of the back of the left atrium demonstrates three right-sided pulmonary veins (*numbered*). **(B)** Surface image in an anteroposterior projection again demonstrates three numbered right-sided pulmonary veins. The left-sided pulmonary veins are obscured by the left atrial appendage.

(Continued on page 276)

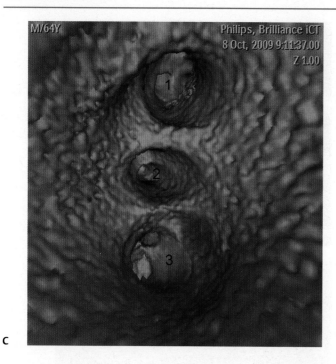

C

Fig. 11.6 (*Continued*) Accessory right pulmonary vein. **(C)** Endoluminal view along the right side of the left atrium demonstrates the three pulmonary veins (*numbered*).

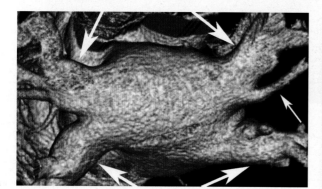

A

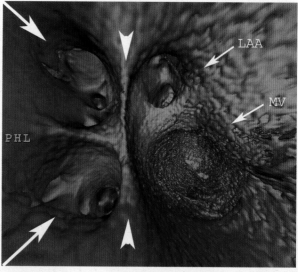

B

Fig. 11.7 Small accessory right pulmonary vein. **(A)** Surface image of the posterior left atrium demonstrates four large pulmonary veins (*arrows*), as well as a small accessory right middle pulmonary vein (*small arrow*). **(B)** Endoluminal view of left side of the left atrium demonstrates the left pulmonary veins (*arrows*), which are separated from the left atrial appendage (LAA) and mitral valve (MV) annulus by a thin ridge of tissue (*arrowheads*). Evaluation of the thickness of this ridge is important because it may dictate how the ablation is performed in this area.

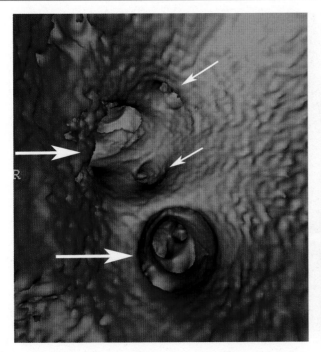

C

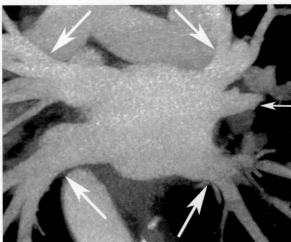

D

Fig. 11.7 (*Continued*) **(C)** Endoluminal view on the right side demonstrates two large pulmonary veins emptying into the left atrium (*arrows*). Although the surface image suggested only one accessory vein, the endoluminal image demonstrates two accessory veins (*small arrows*), emptying into the left atrium near the insertion of the superior right pulmonary vein. **(D)** Maximum intensity projection image through the left atrium again demonstrates the four larger pulmonary veins emptying into the left atrium as well as one of the accessory pulmonary veins (*small arrow*).

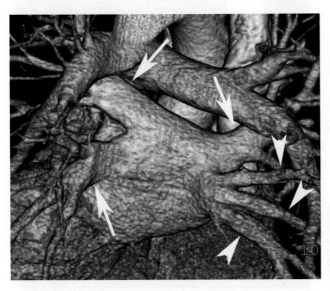

A

Fig. 11.8 Compound inferior right pulmonary vein. **(A)** Surface image of the posterior left atrial wall demonstrates three large pulmonary veins (*arrows*), representing the left superior and inferior pulmonary veins, as well as the right superior pulmonary vein. The right inferior pulmonary vein is composed of three smaller vessels that empty into a common orifice (*arrowheads*). (*Continued on page 278*)

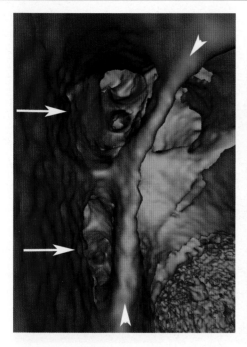

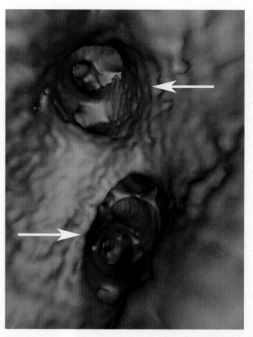

Fig. 11.8 (*Continued*) Compound inferior right pulmonary vein. **(B)** Endoluminal view along the left side of the left atrium demonstrates the two left pulmonary veins (*arrows*) separated from the atrial appendage by a thin ridge (*arrowheads*). **(C)** Endoluminal view of the right pulmonary veins demonstrates two orifices with immediate branching of the inferior right pulmonary vein. The branching pattern into the inferior orifice should be evaluated with both the surface and endoluminal views before attempted ablation around these vessels.

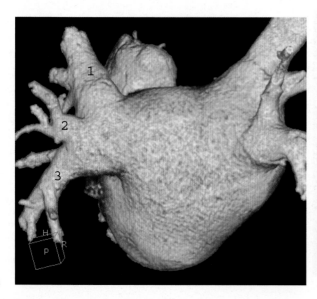

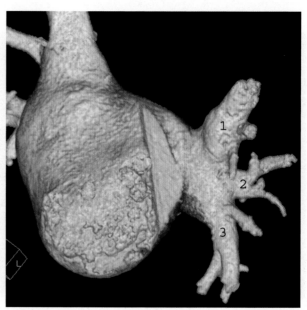

Fig. 11.9 Accessory left pulmonary vein. **(A)** Surface image of the back of the left atrium demonstrates three left-sided pulmonary veins (*numbered*) with a common ostium into the left atrium. **(B)** Surface image in an anteroposterior projection following removal of the left atrial appendage again demonstrates three numbered left-sided pulmonary veins.

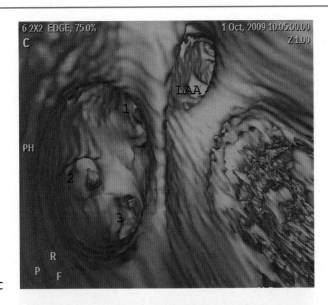

Fig. 11.9 (*Continued*) **(C)** Endoluminal view along the left side of the left atrium demonstrates the three pulmonary veins (*numbered*) with a common ostium separated from the left atrial appendage (LAA) by a ridge of tissue.

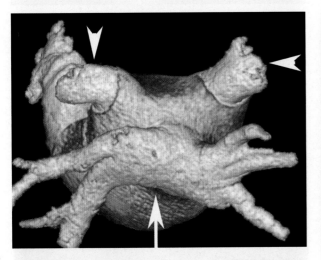

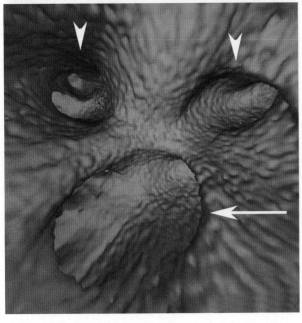

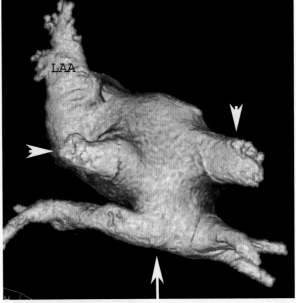

Fig. 11.10 Common ostium of the right and left inferior pulmonary veins. **(A)** Surface image of the back of the left atrium demonstrates two superior pulmonary veins (*arrowheads*) as well as a common truck of the inferior pulmonary veins (*arrow*). **(B)** Surface image from above again demonstrates two superior pulmonary veins (*arrowheads*) with the anteriorly located left atrial appendage (LAA). The common trunk of the inferior pulmonary veins enters the left atrium posteriorly (*arrow*). **(C)** Endoluminal view of the posterior wall of the left atrium demonstrates the independent ostia of the two superior pulmonary veins (*arrowheads*), as well as the common ostium of the inferior pulmonary veins (*arrow*).

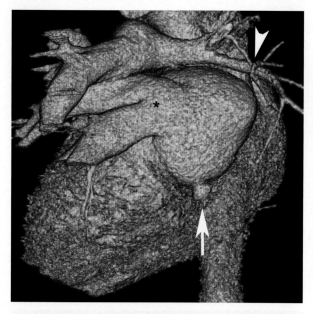

A

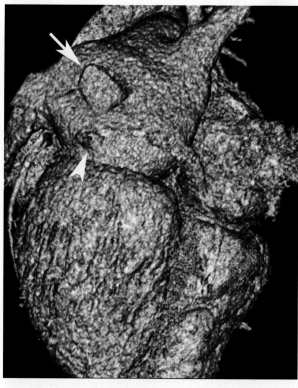

B

Fig. 11.11 Unilateral absence of the right pulmonary veins, common trunk of the left pulmonary veins, hypoplasia of the right pulmonary artery, and a left atrial diverticulum. **(A,B)** Surface renderings of the left atrium from a posterior projection demonstrate two large left pulmonary veins that join into a common trunk (*) before entering the

left atrium. The right pulmonary artery (*arrowhead*) is hypoplastic, and there are no right-sided pulmonary veins. A solitary diverticulum is present along the inferior margin of the left atrium (*arrow*). Cine images of this case are provided on the accompanying CD.

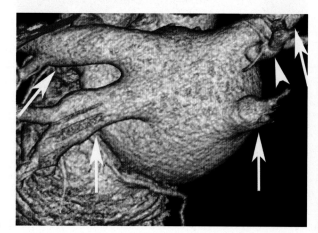

A

Fig. 11.12 Accessory right pulmonary vein and left atrial diverticula. **(A)** Surface view of the left posterior atrium demonstrates the four expected pulmonary veins (*arrows*), as well as a small upper lobe accessory right-sided pulmonary vein (*arrowhead*). **(B)** A different obliquity of the surface view with the pulmonary veins removed from view demonstrates two diverticula of the left atrium, a larger one more superiorly (*arrow*), and a smaller one more inferiorly (*arrowhead*).

B

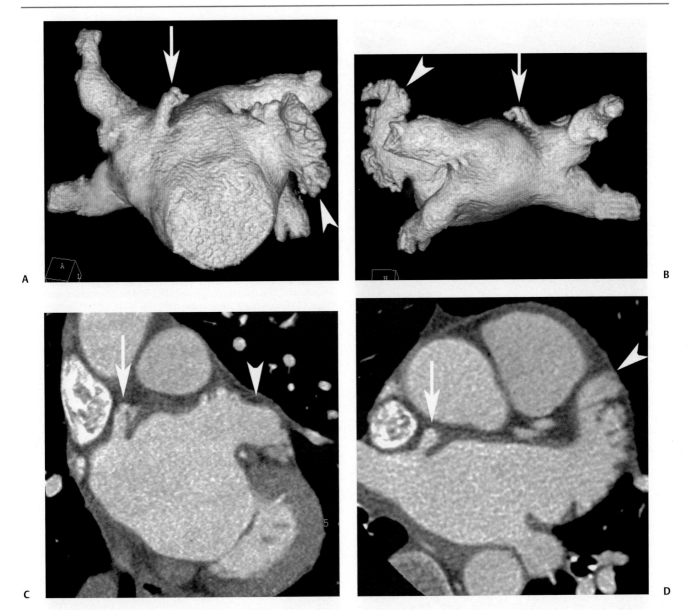

Fig. 11.13 Diverticulum in the roof of the left atrium, anterior to the right superior pulmonary vein. **(A)** Surface view of the left atrium from the anterior projection demonstrates a trabeculated diverticulum (*arrow*) and the trabeculated left atrial appendage (*arrowhead*). **(B)** Surface view from a posterior projection again demonstrates a trabeculated diverticulum (*arrow*) and the trabeculated left atrial appendage (*arrowhead*). **(C)** Coronal maximum intensity projection (MIP) demonstrates the trabeculation within the diverticulum to better advantage (*arrow*) as well as the left atrial appendage (*arrowhead*). **(D)** Axial MIP demonstrates similar findings.

(**Figs. 11.11, 11.12, 11.13, 11.14, 11.15,** and **11.16** and following discussion). To achieve adequate electrical isolation of the PVs and to avoid complications, the electrophysiologist must have precise prior knowledge of these anatomic details in the LA chamber and PVs.[10]

The interatrial septum separates the right from the left atrium. A thinned portion in the center of the interatrial septum is termed the *fossa ovalis* (**Fig. 11.17**). A patent foramen ovale allows the electrophysiologist to cross the interatrial septum easily without having to create a transseptal puncture. CT angiography (CTA) may identify patency of the fossa ovalis by extension of a jet of contrast material into the right atrium (**Figs. 11.18** and **11.19**). When the fossa ovalis is closed (and not "probe-patent"), the electrophysiologist performs a transseptal puncture(s) at this site to allow catheter access into the LA cavity from the right atrium. Normally, the interatrial septum bows slightly toward the right side but can be aneurysmal or undulating (**Fig. 11.17**). Aneurysmal fossae may harbor foci capable of rapid firing that may initiate AF.

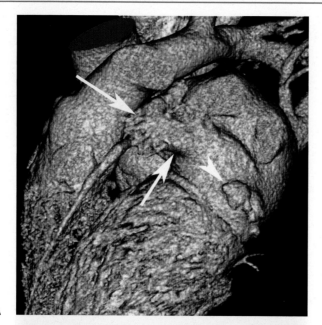

A

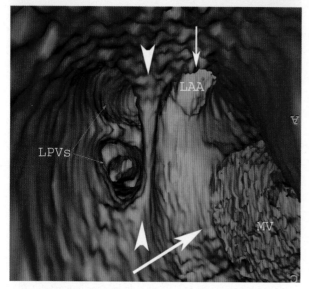

B

Fig. 11.14 Diverticulum at the base of the left atrial appendage. **(A)** Surface-rendered image of the left atrium demonstrates the atrial appendage (*arrows*). At the base of the left atrial appendage, there is a diverticulum (*arrowhead*). **(B)** Endoluminal view of the left side of the atrium demonstrates the left atrial appendage (LAA) (*small arrow*) above the mitral valve (MV) (*large arrow*) and separated from the left-sided pulmonary veins (LPVs) by a ridge of tissue (*arrowheads*). The diverticulum is not identified on this endoluminal image. **(C)** Endoluminal view on the right side of the atrium demonstrates two right-sided pulmonary veins (*arrows*).

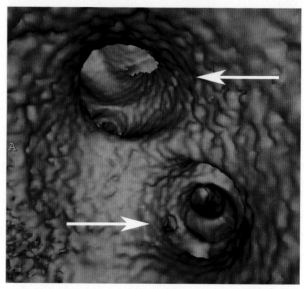

C

◆ Ablation Strategies as Related to Left Atrial Anatomy

The left-sided PVs usually enter the LA directly behind the LA appendage. The anterior wall of the left PV antrum is separated from the posterior wall of the LA appendage by a ridge of tissue (**Figs. 11.1C, 11.2B,** and **11.3B**). In some patients, the LA appendage may be situated at a slightly higher plane than the antrum of the left-sided PVs. To achieve electrical isolation of the left sided PVs, it is critical to ablate along this ridge of tissue, yet avoid ablation within the thin-walled appendage. In practice, it is often impossible to position the ablation catheter along this ridge, so most electrophysiologists will deliver RF energy along the PV side of the ridge (ie, the anterior wall of the

antrum). Appreciation of individual anatomic variations of this region is key to planning and achieving successful left PV isolation, especially when additional PVs or proximal branches are present.

It is now well recognized that a significant proportion of patients will have anatomic variations in the number of PVs, their entrance into the LA, and proximal branching patterns. Not uncommonly, the left superior and left inferior PVs enter the body of the LA as a common trunk or a common antrum (**Fig. 11.5**). It is important to measure the size of this trunk to select an appropriately sized mapping catheter. There is a well-recognized right middle PV (**Fig. 11.6**), which is often of smaller diameter (**Fig. 11.7**), or a right "top" PV. Less frequently, multiple PVs may enter the LA in a compound orifice (**Fig. 11.8**). The presence of an

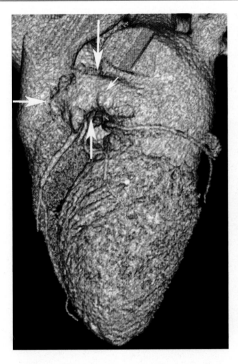

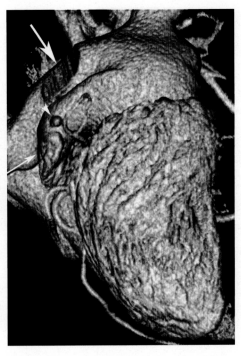

A

B

Fig. 11.15 Diverticulum of the left atrial appendage. **(A)** Surface view demonstrates the left atrial appendage (*arrows*), as well as a small diverticulum near the base of the left atrial appendage (*small arrow*). **(B)** Second, similar case with a small diverticulum (*arrowhead*) at the base of the left atrial appendage (*small arrow*). The pulmonary veins were removed from this image so that the appendage was visible (*larger arrow*).

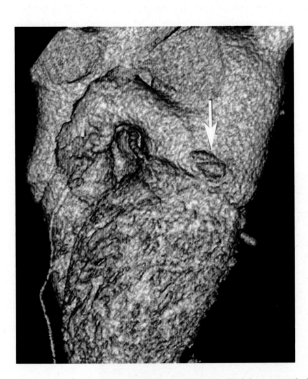

Fig. 11.16 Diverticulum along the posterior wall of the atrium behind the left atrial appendage. A diverticulum of the left atrium (*arrow*) is identified in the left atrial wall just posterior to the base of the left atrial appendage. Just as the atrial appendage has a thin wall, a diverticulum in the atrium will also have a thin wall, which should be avoided during the ablation process.

accessory left-sided pulmonary vein is somewhat less common (**Fig. 11.9**). A common ostium of left pulmonary veins is found in 17%; accessory pulmonary veins are found in 29%.[11] We recently encountered an unusual variation of pulmonary venous anatomy where the inferior PVs from both sides empty into a common chamber that communicates with the body of the left atrium (**Fig. 11.10**). The common trunk must be carefully measured to ensure that an appropriately sized mapping catheter is available for the ablation procedure. In an extremely rare variation, PVs may be unilaterally absent in the setting of a hypoplastic lung (**Fig. 11.11**). Many patients will thus have either three or five (sometimes six) PVs.

A priori knowledge of anatomic variations in pulmonary venous anatomy is vital in planning the optimal ablation strategy. For example, the presence of three (often with a small diameter) right-sided PVs would prompt RF delivery as an all-encompassing "oval" around the PVs rather than attempting to isolate each vein individually. Small-diameter PVs are unlikely to harbor triggering myocardial fascicles and are more likely to develop stenosis or occlusion after ablation; small-diameter PVs should be avoided as ablation targets. Recognition of a large-diameter PV identifies a likely culprit vein that deserves careful attention to attain complete electrical isolation. It is important to recognize that cardiac CTA is generally performed with gating of image acquisition to the QRS complex. CT acquisition may be performed in atrial systole or diastole, but PV ostial dimensions decrease by about 32% during atrial systole.[12] The reported size of the

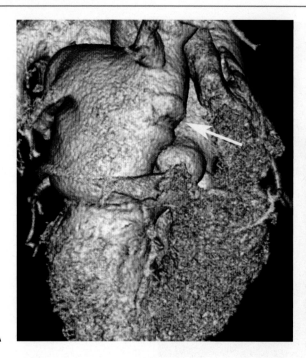

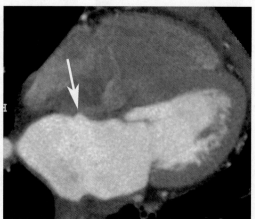

Fig. 11.17 Fossa ovalis. **(A)** Surface-rendered image demonstrates the interatrial septum with an undulating margin at the level of the fossa ovalis (*arrow*). **(B)** Axial image through the same heart demonstrates the thin undulating contour of the left atrium at the level of the fossa ovalis (*arrow*).

PV ostia should be interpreted in light of the phase in the cardiac cycle when selecting ostial ablation sites.

A clear picture of LA anatomy and the relationship of the LA to adjacent mediastinal structures is vital to achieve a successful and safe outcome during LA ablation. Complications of ablation, both cardiac-related and involving adjacent structures, may be minimized by detailed pre-procedural knowledge of LA and PV anatomy. The possibility of death as a complication of catheter ablation in the LA is reported in 0.1% of patients.[13] It should be noted that magnetic

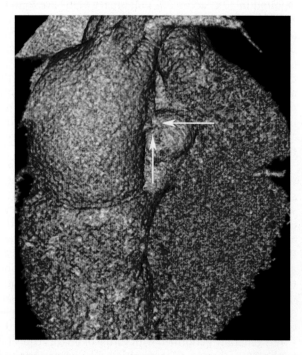

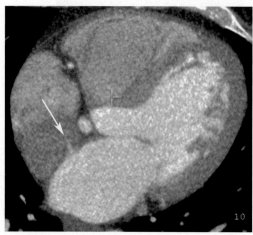

Fig. 11.18 Patent foramen ovale. **(A)** Surface image demonstrates the left atrium with a small out pouching corresponding to a small jet of contrast extending through the patent foramen ovale (*arrows*). **(B)** Axial image through the heart at the same level demonstrates a small jet of contrast extending from the left atrium toward the right atrium (*arrow*).

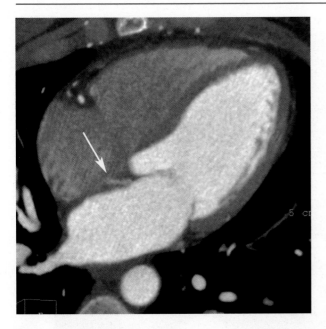

Fig. 11.19 Patent foramen ovale. Axial image in a different patient demonstrates a small jet of contrast extending from the left atrium toward the right atrium (*arrow*). A patent foramen ovale is not an uncommon finding and is of little clinical significance unless there is evidence of embolic disease or a hemodynamically significant shunt.

resonance imaging (MRI) and magnetic resonance angiography (MRA) can provide similar anatomic information as that provided by CTA.[14,15] An understanding of the individual patient's anatomy and clinical factors must be considered to minimize the complications described below.

◆ Left Atrial Perforation and Tamponade

The LA myocardium varies from 1 to 4 mm in thickness. The left atrial appendage is a trabeculated pouch, highly variable in its dimensions. Muscular trabeculations within the LA appendage may be separated by intervening tissue that is less than 1 mm thick, making inadvertent ablation at such locations potentially dangerous. Based on this anatomic observation, ablation is generally avoided within the LA appendage. Our group has shown that a small number of patients will have diverticula or "supernumary"/"ectopic" appendages,[15] often at unexpected locations (**Figs. 11.11, 11.12, 11.13, 11.14, 11.15,** and **11.16**); such information would allow the electrophysiologist to avoid inadvertent ablation within small diverticula/pouches, and thus avoid potentially catastrophic perforations. Tamponade remains the most common complication of ablation within the LA, with an occurrence rate of just over 1%;[17] recent medicare data suggest that the risk may be higher.[18] It must be noted that ablation within the LA for AF is performed with systemic anticoagulation with heparin (target-activated clotting time of ~300 seconds), thus greatly increasing the probability of serious bleeding and tamponade with any perforation.

◆ Esophageal Damage and Creation of Atrio-Esophageal Fistula

The esophagus runs behind the LA, most often in direct contact with the posterior wall of the LA (**Fig. 11.4**).[19,20] In a series of 80 patients reported from our institution, all 80 patients demonstrated a portion of the posterior LA wall in direct contact with the esophagus. The distance between the esophagus and the antrum of each PV was measured on axial images (**Fig. 11.20**). The average distance of the esophagus was 19.5 mm from the right superior PV antrum, 10.1 mm from the right inferior PV antrum, 4.1 mm from the left superior PV antrum, and 5.4 mm from the left inferior PV antrum.[21] In a substantial minority of patients, the antrum of a left-sided PV may be located immediately anterior to and contiguous with the esophagus. One of the rare but almost always fatal complications of AF ablation is the development of a fistula between the LA and the esophagus as a result of thermal injury. Knowledge of the atrio-esophageal relationship is vital to preventing this type of lethal complication,[22] which has become increasingly infrequent since it was first reported because of the use of such imaging.[23]

◆ Pulmonary Vein Stenosis

Earlier approaches to PV isolation involved ablation within or at the ostium of the PVs, resulting in a high rate of PV stenosis.[24] With recognition of this complication, ablation strategies have changed. In place of ablation within the ostium, antral ablation away from the mouth of the PV is performed. As a result of this change in technique, PV stenosis is now a rare event. Nonetheless, in evaluation of patients with dyspnea following AF ablation, CTA provides an excellent tool to evaluate for PV stenosis.[25]

◆ Newer Applications of CT Imaging: Real-Time "Fusion Imaging"

Although three-dimensional (3-D) electroanatomic reconstruction of the LA is routinely performed during the ablation procedure, this anatomic "shell" of the LA is, at best, a rough approximation of true atrial and PV anatomy. Numerous systems are commercially available that will "register" anatomic landmarks in real time with the same structures on previously acquired 3-D CTA images.[26] Computer software can merge real-time electroanatomic imaging with the 3-D CTA image and allow mapping and ablation to be performed with anatomically accurate 3-D images. "Fusion images," when accurately merged, provide superior anatomic detail, more precise accuracy of lesion placement, and potentially improved safety with reduced radiation exposure.[27] Fusion imaging during ablation has become the standard of care, making preablation CTA an essential step. Competing imaging technologies, such as real-time intracardiac ultrasound

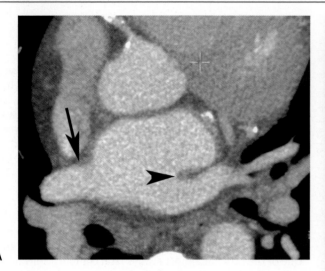

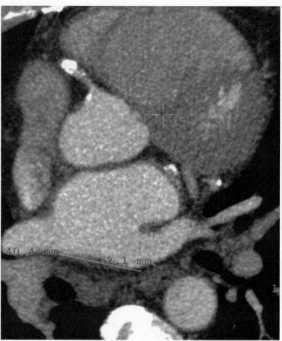

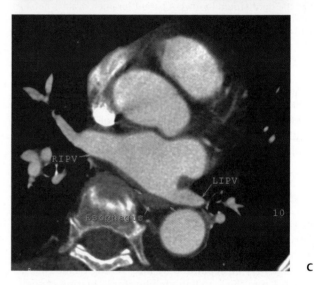

Fig. 11.20 Relationship of the esophagus to the left atrium. **(A)** Superior pulmonary veins are identified on a single axial image. The right superior pulmonary vein (*arrow*) and left superior pulmonary vein enter the atrium at the same level. The left-sided vein enters just posterior to a thin ridge of tissue (*arrowhead*), which separates it from the atrial appendage. Note that the esophagus is immediately posterior to the left superior pulmonary vein in this image. **(B)** The distance between the esophagus and the orifice of the superior pulmonary veins is measured. There is a 2-mm distance between the esophagus and the orifice of the left superior pulmonary vein. The esophagus is much farther from the orifice of the right superior pulmonary vein. In this situation, the electrophysiologist should be aware that while ablating around the left superior pulmonary vein, the esophagus is in close proximity. **(C)** Axial image at the level of the inferior pulmonary veins. The esophagus is shifted farther to the left side and is immediately contiguous with the left inferior pulmonary vein (LIPV) as it enters the left atrium. RIPV, right inferior pulmonary vein.

with 3-D reconstruction, are proving to be a viable alternative to CT imaging and have the advantage of providing real-time anatomic information. It has been recommended that ultrasound imaging should be merged with previously acquired CT images for optimal outcomes because CT and ultrasound may provide complementary information,[28] and real-time ultrasound may improve accuracy of lesion placement.[29]

◆ Coronary Sinus

The venous drainage of the heart is returned to the right atrium by the coronary sinus. The proximal third of the coronary sinus is a muscular structure with myocardium that is contiguous with that of the LA.[30] It is now recognized

that, in a minority of patients, the coronary sinus may provide the electrical triggers that initiate AF.[31] Ablation strategies often involve electrical "disconnection" of the coronary sinus by ablation at the ostium, ablation inside the proximal third of the coronary sinus, and inside the LA along the posterior mitral annulus. The size, angulation, and branching of the coronary sinus can be readily appreciated by CTA before any ablation procedure (**Fig. 11.21**).

◆ Conclusion

Valuable anatomic and relational information is readily obtained by preablation CTA. There is increasing consensus that preablation imaging of the LA and PVs, whether by CTA

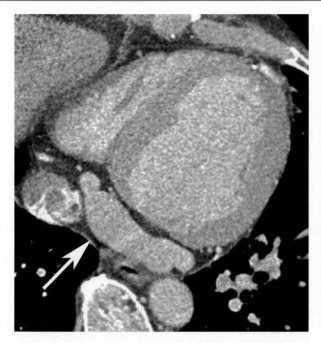
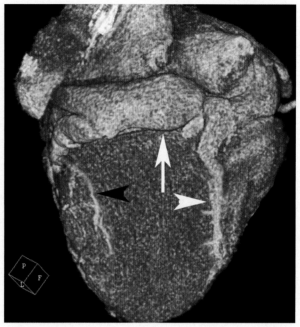

Fig. 11.21 Coronary sinus anatomy in a patient with markedly dilated coronary veins. **(A)** Axial image demonstrates a markedly dilated coronary sinus in the left posterior atrioventricular groove (*arrow*). **(B)** Surface-rendered image again demonstrates the dilated coronary sinus (*arrow*) as well as a dilated middle coronary vein in the posterior interventricular groove (*white arrowhead*). Another dilated vein is present along the surface of the left ventricle (*black arrowhead*).

or MRI/MRA, helps in planning ablation strategies, guides catheter manipulation, and helps avoid complications. This anatomic information, acquired noninvasively and with little risk to the patient, is crucial in the management of patients with AF who are selected for ablation therapy.

Finally, although real-time imaging technologies such as intracardiac ultrasound are becoming more commonplace, integration of CTA image data during ablation in the LA is often useful to shorten procedure times and improve patient outcome.[32]

Cine 11.1 Unilateral absence of the right pulmonary veins, common trunk of the left pulmonary veins, hypoplasia of the right pulmonary artery, and left atrial diverticulum (see Fig. 11.11). Cine surface rendering of the left atrium begins with a view from the left side, demonstrating the left pulmonary veins, and then rotates to demonstrate the posterior wall of the left atrium with an inferior diverticulum. As the heart is rotated to demonstrate the right side of the left atrium, a hypoplastic right pulmonary artery is identified with no right-sided pulmonary veins.

References

1. Kannel WB, Wolf PA, Benjamin EJ, Levy D. Prevalence, incidence, prognosis, and predisposing conditions for atrial fibrillation: population-based estimates. Am J Cardiol. 1998;82(8A, 8A):2N–9N

2. Haïssaguerre M, Jaïs P, Shah DC, et al. Spontaneous initiation of atrial fibrillation by ectopic beats originating in the pulmonary veins. N Engl J Med. 1998;339(10):659–666

3. Nathan H, Eliakim M. The junction between the left atrium and the pulmonary veins: an anatomic study of human hearts. Circulation. 1966;34(3):412–422

4. Lin WS, Tai CT, Hsieh MH, et al. Catheter ablation of paroxysmal atrial fibrillation initiated by non-pulmonary vein ectopy. Circulation. 2003;107(25):3176–3183

5. Jaïs P, Hocini M, Hsu LF, et al. Technique and results of linear ablation at the mitral isthmus. Circulation. 2004;110(19):2996–3002

6. Wittkampf FH, Vonken EJ, Derksen R, et al. Pulmonary vein ostium geometry: analysis by magnetic resonance angiography. Circulation. 2003;107(1):21–23

7. Wongcharoen W, Tsao HM, Wu MH, et al. Morphologic characteristics of the left atrial appendage, roof, and septum: implications for the ablation of atrial fibrillation. J Cardiovasc Electrophysiol. 2006;17(9):951–956

8. Wang Y, di Base L, Horton RP, Nguyen T, Mohanty P, Natale A. Left atrial appendage studied by computer tomography to help planning for appendage closure device placement. J Cardiovase Electrophysiol 2010;21:973–982

9. Killeen RP, O'Connor SA, Keane D, Dodd JD. Ectopic focus in an accessory left atrial appendage: radiofrequency ablation of refractory atrial fibrillation. Circulation. 2009;120(8):e60–e62

10. Mansour M, Holmvang G, Ruskin J. Role of imaging techniques in preparation for catheter ablation of atrial fibrillation. J Cardiovasc Electrophysiol. 2004;15(9):1107–1108

11. Joshi SB, Blum AR, Mansour M, Abbara S. CT applications in electrophysiology. Cardiol Clin. 2009;27(4):619–631

12. Lickfett L, Dickfeld T, Kato R, et al. Changes of pulmonary vein orifice size and location throughout the cardiac cycle: dynamic analysis using magnetic resonance cine imaging. J Cardiovasc Electrophysiol.2005; 16(6):582–588

13. Cappato R, Calkins H, Chen SA, et al. Prevalence and causes of fatal outcome in catheter ablation of atrial fibrillation. J Am Coll Cardiol. 2009;53(19):1798–1803

14. Kato R, Lickfett L, Meininger G, et al. Pulmonary vein anatomy in patients undergoing catheter ablation of atrial fibrillation: lessons learned by use of magnetic resonance imaging. Circulation. 2003;107(15):2004–2010

15. Mansour M, Holmvang G, Sosnovik D, et al. Assessment of pulmonary vein anatomic variability by magnetic resonance imaging: implications for catheter ablation techniques for atrial fibrillation. J Cardiovasc Electrophysiol. 2004;15(4):387–393

16. Dheer S, Pavri BB, Halpern EJ. Variant anatomy of the left atrial appendage: potential impact on planning for electrophysiologic ablation procedures. Proceedings of the Radiological Society of North America. Chicago, Ill. Nov 2006; Abstract #LL-CA4118–R04, p. 673

17. Dagres N, Hindricks G, Kottkamp H, et al. Complications of atrial fibrillation ablation in a high-volume center in 1,000 procedures: still cause for concern? J Cardiovasc Electrophysiol. 2009;20(9):1014–1019

18. Ellis ER, Culler SD, Simon AW, Reynolds MR. Trends in utilization and complications of catheter ablation for atrial fibrillation in Medicare beneficiaries. Heart Rhytm 2009;6(9):1267–1273

19. Cury RC, Abbara S, Schmidt S, et al. Relationship of the esophagus and aorta to the left atrium and pulmonary veins: implications for catheter ablation of atrial fibrillation. Heart Rhythm. 2005;2(12):1317–1323

20. Lemola K, Sneider M, Desjardins B, et al. Computed tomographic analysis of the anatomy of the left atrium and the esophagus: implications for left atrial catheter ablation. Circulation. 2004;110(24):3655–3660

21. Halpern EJ, Pavri BB. Assessment of pulmonary venous anatomy during coronary CT angiography. Proceedings of the Radiological Society of North America. Chicago, Ill. Nov 2005; Abstract #SSC05–04, p. 244

22. Sánchez-Quintana D, Cabrera JA, Climent V, Farré J, Mendonça MC, Ho SY. Anatomic relations between the esophagus and left atrium and relevance for ablation of atrial fibrillation. Circulation. 2005;112(10): 1400–1405

23. Vijayaraman P, Netrebko P, Geyfman V, Dandamudi G, Casey K, Ellenbogen KA. Esophageal fistula formation despite esophageal monitoring and low-power radiofrequency catheter ablation for atrial fibrillation. Circ Arrhythm Electrophysiol. 2009;2(5):e31–e33

24. Robbins IM, Colvin EV, Doyle TP, et al. Pulmonary vein stenosis after catheter ablation of atrial fibrillation. Circulation. 1998;98(17): 1769–1775

25. Scharf C, Sneider M, Case I, et al. Anatomy of the pulmonary veins in patients with atrial fibrillation and effects of segmental ostial ablation analyzed by computed tomography. J Cardiovasc Electrophysiol. 2003; 14(2):150–155

26. Reddy VY, Malchano ZJ, Neuzil P, Brem E, Ruskin JN. Early clinical experience with CARTO-Merge for integration of 3D-CT imaging with real-time mapping to guide catheter ablation of atrial fibrillation. Heart Rhythm. 2005;2(Suppl):S160

27. Caponi D, Corleto A, Scaglione M, Blandino A, Biasco L, Cristoforetti Y, Cerrato N, Toso E, Morello M, Gaita F. Ablation of atrial fibrillation: does the addition of three-dimensional magnetic resonance imaging of the left atrium

28. Burke SJ, Aggarwala G, Stanford W, Mullan B, Thompson B, van Beek EJ. Preablation assessment for the left atrium: comparison of ECG-gated cardiac CT with echocardiography. Acad Radiol. 2008;15(7): 835–843

29. Daccarett M, Segerson NM, Günther J, et al. Blinded correlation study of three-dimensional electro-anatomical image integration and phased array intra-cardiac echocardiography for left atrial mapping. Europace. 2007;9(10):923–926

30. Ho SY, Sanchez-Quintana D, Cabrera JA, Anderson RH. Anatomy of the left atrium: implications for radiofrequency ablation of atrial fibrillation. J Cardiovasc Electrophysiol. 1999;10(11):1525–1533

31. Jaïs P, Haïssaguerre M, Shah DC, et al. A focal source of atrial fibrillation treated by discrete radiofrequency ablation. Circulation. 1997; 95(3): 572–576

32. Tops LF, Schalij MJ. Multislice CT: is it essential before atrial fibrillation ablation? Heart. 2008;94(8):973–975

12

Cardiac Interventions

Panayotis Fasseas and Daniel J. McCormick

◆ Multislice–Multidetector CT and Planning of Cardiac Interventions

The rapid evolution of interventional techniques for the heart, the introduction of new devices, and improvements in adjunctive pharmacotherapy have led to explosive growth in the field of interventional cardiology. Meticulous attention to patient selection, risk stratification, choice of appropriate equipment, and procedural skills is essential for the successful outcome of a percutaneous coronary intervention (PCI). In addition, attention to specific angiographic characteristics is critical for planning of PCIs (**Table 12.1**). Multislice–multidetector computed tomography (MDCT) can accurately provide anatomic information in a noninvasive manner to improve the planning and outcome of PCI.

Estimation of periprocedural risk identifies those patients who are at higher risk for PCI-related complications and allows the implementation of measures aimed at reducing that risk (eg, hemodynamic support, optimizing volume status, surgical standby). Demographic and clinical characteristics (eg, age, gender, diabetes mellitus, renal failure) play an important role in determining risk. MDCT can further refine the risk stratification by providing information on the presence of significant left main disease, multivessel coronary artery disease, and determination of left ventricular (LV) systolic function.[1]

The purpose of this chapter is to review the role of coronary MDCT imaging in the planning and follow-up of percutaneous and surgical coronary interventions.

◆ Vascular Access

Patients with severe diffuse peripheral vascular disease, especially those with prior revascularization procedures, require careful assessment of vascular anatomy and access sites. Appropriate selection of percutaneous access is essential in complex interventions requiring the use of large-diameter guiding catheters and high-risk interventions where the use of an intra-aortic balloon pump may be necessary. In such patients, CT angiography (CTA) provides a noninvasive roadmap that can assist the interventionalist in selecting the most appropriate access sites. An appropriate access route should avoid significant obstructive disease in the aortoileofemoral system, as well as excessively tortuous vessels and calcifications that may preclude advancement of interventional equipment. In patients with prior surgical revascularization, such as aortobifemoral bypass surgery, CTA angiography can determine whether the grafts represent appropriate vascular access sites.

When upper extremity access (brachial or radial artery) is contemplated, CTA allows evaluation of the aortic arch branches for atherosclerosis and tortuosity. Manipulation of catheters and interventional wires in severely atherosclerotic aortic arch branches may result in cerebral embolization.

◆ Calcified Lesions

Calcified coronary artery stenoses pose significant technical challenges to the interventional cardiologist. PCI of calcified lesions is associated with a higher rate of procedural failure and increased risk of periprocedural and long-term major adverse clinical events (eg, death, myocardial infarction, need for repeat target-vessel revascularization).[2,3] The presence of coronary calcium makes the stenotic vessel rigid and may affect the ability to deliver interventional devices to the target lesion. Furthermore, calcification of the vessel wall may render the vessel resistant to dilatation by conventional balloon angioplasty (PTCA).[4] This occurs more commonly in vessels with circumferential (360-degree) calcification and with intimal–medial (as opposed to adventitial) calcification.[3,5,6] In such cases, the use of atheroablative devices such as rotational atherectomy is indicated.[4] However, unnecessary atheroablation of long-calcified coronary segments may result in significant embolization of the distal microvasculature, resulting in periprocedural myocardial infarction.[6] MDCT can accurately identify characteristics of a complex calcified lesion. Specifically, MDCT can demonstrate the presence, location, severity, and length of calcification. In addition, it can display the distribution of calcium in the vessel wall (circumferential versus focal, intimal

Table 12.1 Angiographic Characteristics

Aortic root size
Selection of guiding catheters
Vessel characteristics in native coronaries
Presence of coronary anomalies
Location of the coronary ostia
Spatial orientation of the proximal segment of the vessel
Vessel diameter
Vessel tortuosity
Vessel calcification
Amount of myocardium supplied by vessel
Vessel characteristics in bypass grafts
Proximal anastomosis site
Vessel course (anterior to the aorta versus retroaortic)
Type of graft (single, sequential, Y-graft)
Degenerated saphenous vein graft
Graft size
Amount of myocardium supplied by grafted vessel
Lesion characteristics
Location
Length
Vessel diameter
Bifurcation
Severity of stenosis
Calcification (severity, pattern of vessel involvement)
Vessel angulation at the stenosis
Plaque characterization
High-risk lesions
Left main
Ostial stenosis
Bifurcation lesions
Left ventricular systolic function
Congenital heart disease
Atrial and ventricular septal defects
Coronary fistulae

versus adventitial) (**Fig. 12.1**). This information is critical in deciding whether to use atheroablative devices and in estimating the risk and likely success of the planned PCI.

◆ Vessel Tortuosity and Angulated Lesions

Target-vessel tortuosity is a known complicating angiographic variable for PCI.[7] Tortuosity complicates the delivery of interventional devices and can result in incomplete stent apposition in an angulated segment.[8] Incomplete stent apposition is associated with increased risk of stent thrombosis and with drug-eluting stents, with incomplete elution of drug to the vessel wall, and a potentially increased rate of restenosis.[9]

Adequate PCI outcomes in tortuous vessels frequently require the use of more "aggressive" devices, such as larger-caliber guides and stiffer guidewires. The use of such devices may result in vascular injury, such as dissection, acute closure, or perforation.[10] MDCT can accurately define the severity of tortuosity, demonstrate the presence of angulation at the target lesion, and guide the interventional cardiologist in the choice of appropriate equipment (**Fig. 12.2**).

◆ Chronic Total Occlusions

PCI of chronic total occlusions (CTO) is associated with lower success (recanalization) rates, mainly related to the difficulty of crossing the occlusion with a guidewire.[11] PCI of a CTO may be a relatively lengthy procedure, resulting in increased radiation exposure and use of contrast. Several angiographic characteristics may be identified by MDCT to assist in predicting the recanalization success rate. Chronic total occlusions with a tapered vessel stump, the absence of side branches at the site of the occlusion, and the lack of significant bridging collateral circulation are favorable angiographic predictors.[12] MDCT may also serve as a roadmap for recanalization of occluded vessels, as it provides information on vessel tortuosity, length of occlusion, and the presence and pattern of calcification (**Fig. 12.3**). Yokayama et al reviewed the utility of MDCT imaging for lesion and plaque characterization before attempting PCI of a CTO in 22 patients. They report that the use of MDCT resulted in procedural success in 21 CTOs (91.3%). The ability to identify the various components of the atherosclerotic plaque and obtain three-dimensional renderings of the occluded segment plays a significant role in the ability to recanalize the stenosis. They also suggest that presence of calcified plaque in the proximal and distal portions of the CTO may reduce the success rate of the procedure.[13]

◆ Bifurcation Lesions

The success rate of PCI of bifurcation lesions has improved significantly over the past decade. The development of drug-eluting stents and improved stent designs have led to the development of effective bifurcation stenting techniques.[14]

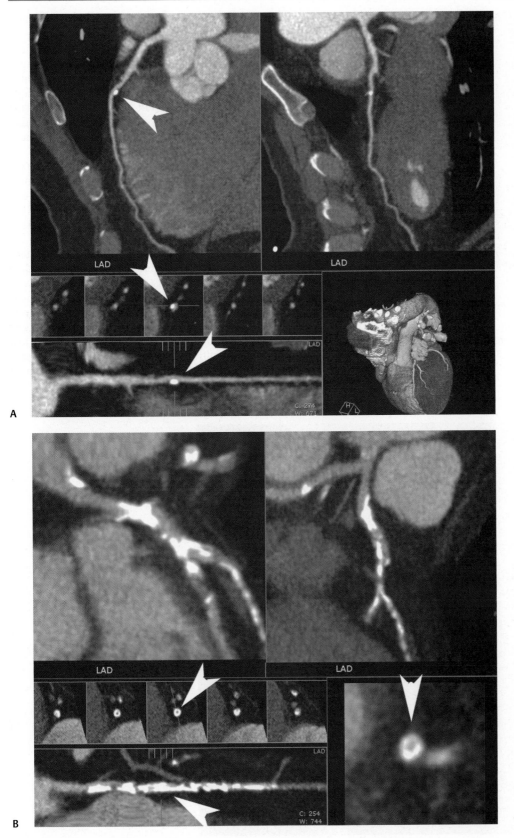

Fig. 12.1 Coronary calcification. **(A)** Curved maximum intensity projection (MIP) images demonstrate focal calcification of the left anterior descending artery (LAD) with positive remodeling. The calcium involves the adventitia of the vessel (*arrowhead*) without involvement of the intima. **(B)** Curved MIP images in a different patient demonstrate diffuse calcification of the left anterior descending artery. Straightened lumen and orthogonal views confirm luminal narrowing with involvement of all layers of the vessel wall (*arrowhead*).

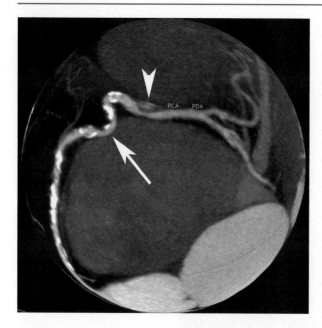

Fig. 12.2 Globe maximum intensity projection of the right coronary artery (RCA). There is eccentric stenosis of the distal RCA with associated ulceration (*arrowhead*). A segment with severe tortuosity and calcification is identified just proximal to the eccentric stenosis (*arrow*).

The pattern of atheromatous involvement and the morphology of bifurcation lesions can be extremely variable. In bifurcation lesions with a small side branch or without significant ostial disease, initial stenting of the main branch with provisional stenting of the side branch may represent a reasonable approach. For lesions with extensive plaque burden involving both the parent vessel and a larger side branch, stenting of both branches will decrease the possibility of plaque shifting with potential side branch loss or suboptimal angiographic result.

For bifurcation lesions, the interventional cardiologist will decide which bifurcation stenting technique is most appropriate based on the diameter of the parent vessel and side branch and the angle between the two vessels. If the diameters of the two vessels are similar and the angle is acute, "culotte" stenting will provide good coverage of the bifurcation without overexpansion of the side-branch stent in the parent vessel. If the side-branch stent is smaller than the main vessel and the angle is acute, "crush" stenting will allow adequate coverage of the lesion without overexpansion of the sidebranch stent. The "kissing" stent technique is ideal for lesions with mild angulation in which the bulk of the plaque involves the parent and side-branch vessels just distal to the bifurcation, especially if the parent vessel proximal to the bifurcation is larger. In situations where

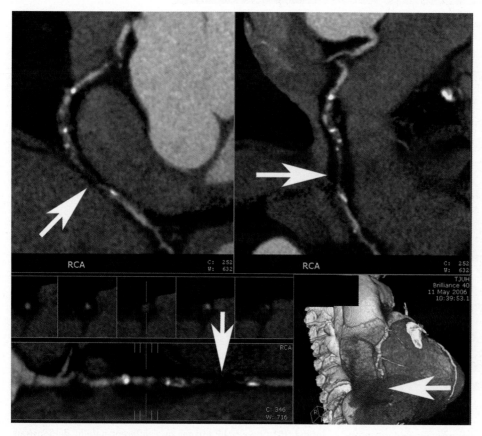

Fig. 12.3 Orthogonal curved maximum intensity projection images demonstrate chronic total occlusion of the mid right coronary artery (RCA) (*arrow*), with moderate proximal calcification and tortuosity.

continuous control of both branches of the bifurcation is required, such as left main PCI, the crush stent and kissing stent techniques allow bifurcation stenting without leaving one of the two branches temporarily unprotected. If the angle between the parent vessel and the side branch is obtuse or at a right angle, T-stenting will provide adequate coverage of the bifurcation. An important limitation of this technique is the potential for incomplete coverage of the side-branch ostium, which may result in ostial restenosis.[15]

An important decision faced by the interventional cardiologist when treating bifurcation lesions is to determine whether side-branch protection is necessary. This is an important issue because side branch protection with stenting results in increased PCI complexity, thrombosis, and restenosis. Leaving the side branch unprotected may be a reasonable approach if the vessel is small in diameter and supplies a small amount of myocardium (**Fig. 12.4**). Side-branch protection is advisable when the side-branch diameter is greater than 2.0 mm, when the side branch originates from a diseased segment of the parent vessel, and when there is greater than 50% ostial stenosis (**Fig. 12.5**).

Assessment of the presence and severity of calcification in bifurcation lesions is essential because calcified vessels are less compliant. Calcification may interfere with the delivery and deployment of interventional devices (**Fig. 12.1**). In such cases lesion modification with rotational atherectomy will result in improved lesion compliance. MDCT can provide the interventional cardiologist with all the necessary angiographic information (eg, vessel size, angulation, plaque distribution pattern, calcification) to select the appropriate stenting technique and assess the need for debulking.

◆ Aorto-Ostial Lesions

The performance of PCI in aorto-ostial lesions is associated with unique challenges that are not encountered in other coronary segments.[16] These lesions are frequently calcified, less compliant, and more difficult to dilate. In addition, because of the ostial location of the stenosis, the ability to engage selectively the vessel in a coaxial manner and maintain a stable guiding catheter position is limited.[17] The presence of an anomalous origin of the vessel ostium may further increase the complexity of the PCI and require the use of guiding catheters with a special tip shape. Because of the large amount of myocardium in jeopardy with aorto-ostial lesions, complications resulting in dissection or acute closure can lead to significant myocardial injury and hemodynamic instability.

MDCT allows accurate assessment of aorto-ostial lesion severity, the angle of vessel take-off from the aorta, length of stenosis, anomalous origin of the vessel, presence of calcification, and need for plaque debulking. All these angiographic variables are very important in the selection of guiding catheters of appropriate type and size.

◆ Left Main Disease

With the improvement in interventional equipment, advent of stents, introduction of drug-eluting stents, potent antiplatelet agents, and improved operator technical skills, unprotected left main PCI is being performed with increasing frequency.[18] This is a high-risk interventional procedure, the success of which relies on optimal visualization of the vessel and meticulous planning. MDCT can identify all the

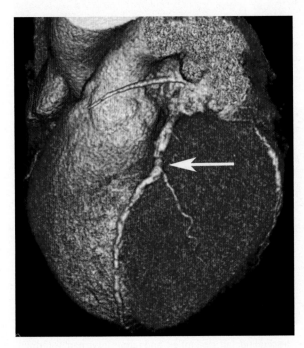

Fig. 12.4 Surface volumetric rendering in the left anterior oblique projection. A bifurcation lesion involves the left anterior descending artery and a small diagonal branch (*arrow*).

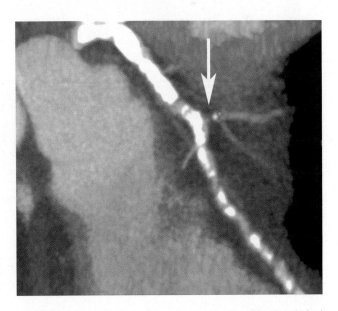

Fig. 12.5 Slab maximum intensity projection of a diffusely calcified left anterior descending artery (LAD). A high-grade ostial stenosis is present in a medium-size diagonal branch originating at a right angle from the LAD (*arrow*).

functional and angiographic characteristics that will allow the interventional cardiologist to assess the level of risk, to determine the feasibility of the procedure, and to select the appropriate equipment. Patients with impaired LV systolic function and severe atherosclerosis of the remaining vessels are at increased risk for periprocedural complications.[19] Other important characteristics include vessel size and length, presence and severity of calcification, and the location of stenosis (ostial, mid or, distal) (**Fig. 12.6**). The complexity and risk of left main PCI are greater for distal left main bifurcation lesions involving the left anterior descending, left circumflex, and ramus intermedius branches.

In the era before stents, left main PCI was performed with balloon angioplasty and was associated with inferior angiographic and clinical outcomes. The application of stents to left main PCI improves procedural success by decreasing the risk of dissection, acute closure, spasm, and elastic recoil.[20] Unfortunately, in-stent restenosis (ISR) remains a potential problem, even with the use of drug-eluting stents. ISR is the

result of neointimal hyperplasia within the stent that results in reduction of the vessel lumen. ISR in the left main places a large amount of myocardium at risk and may lead to adverse clinical events. Routine angiographic follow-up is currently recommended for patients treated with left main PCI.[20] As the ability of MDCT to image stented segments improves, MDCT may become an alternative to invasive angiography in these patients.

◆ **In-Stent Restenosis and Stent Thrombosis**

The advent of coronary stents has led to excellent acute angiographic results and significantly lower rates of angiographic and clinical restenosis compared with balloon angioplasty. However, the use of stents is associated with the potential risk for development of ISR and stent thrombosis.

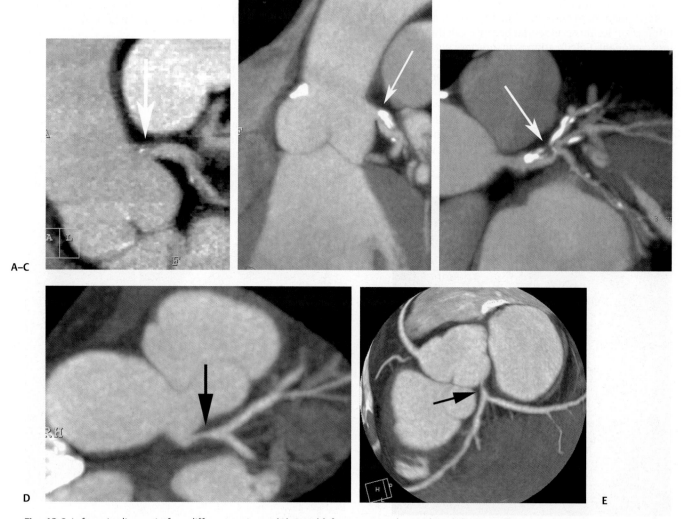

A–C

D

E

Fig. 12.6 Left main disease in four different patients. **(A)** Ostial left main stenosis with mild eccentric calcification (*arrow*). **(B)** Ostial left main stenosis with severe eccentric calcification (*arrow*). **(C)** Severe eccentric distal left main calcified stenosis with ostial involvement of the left anterior descending, left circumflex, and ramus intermedius (*arrow*). **(D)** Moderate stenosis of the left main coronary artery with low-density plaque (*opposite the arrow*). **(E)** Globe maximum intensity projection in the same patient as part (D).

ISR is caused by neointimal hyperplasia and, in most patients, presents with symptoms of recurrent ischemia. ISR is seldom associated with an acute coronary syndrome. Conversely, stent thrombosis commonly results in an ST-elevation myocardial infarction and is associated with poor short- and long-term outcomes. The development of drug eluting stents has led to a significant reduction in the incidence of ISR. However, drug-eluting stents are associated with delayed endotheliazation, which may account for a reported increased incidence of stent thrombosis.[21]

The utility of MDCT for assessment of stent patency is discussed in detail in Chapter 7. MDCT imaging of stented segments can detect the presence of ISR but is not commonly used for evaluation of stent thrombosis because these patients usually present acutely and are taken to the catheter laboratory. Occasionally, patients with stent thrombosis and adequate collateral coronary circulation may present with minimal or no symptoms and are evaluated by CT (**Fig. 12.7**). In these patients, MDCT may be useful in

diagnosis and can assist the interventional cardiologist in the choice of the appropriate treatment strategy based on the angiographic characteristics of the lesion. Unfortunately, the ability of MDCT to differentiate severe ISR with subtotal occlusion of the stented segment from stent thrombosis is limited by the fact that both processes result in lack of vessel lumen contrast enhancement.

◆ Coronary Artery Bypass Grafts

MDCT imaging can play an important role in the evaluation of patients with prior coronary artery bypass graft (CABG). The utility of MDCT for assessment of graft patency is discussed in Chapter 8. In addition to assessment of graft patency, MDCT provides angiographic information for the planning of PCI in and around grafts. Locating the proximal anastomotic site of the graft can occasionally be challenging, especially if radiopaque graft locator markers were not

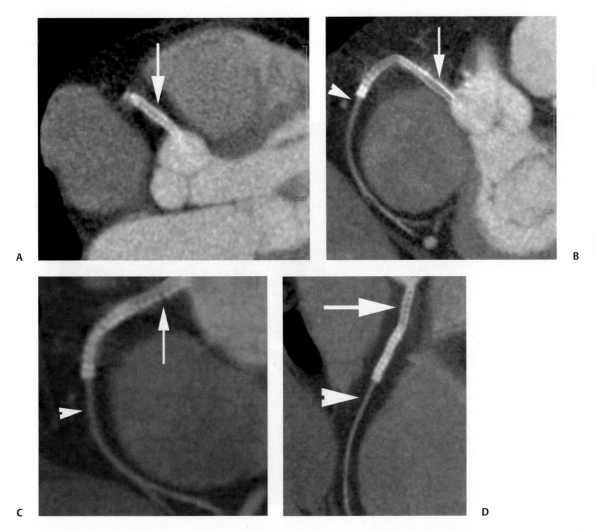

Fig. 12.7 Segmental thrombosis of a right coronary artery (RCA) stent. **(A)** Axial image of the proximal RCA demonstrates a stent with thrombus (*arrow*). **(B)** Slab maximum intensity projection (MIP) demonstrates thrombosis of the proximal stent (*arrow*) with reconstitution of the distal RCA (*arrowhead*). **(C,D)** Tracked, curved MIP images in two orthogonal views demonstrate the full extent of the RCA with in-stent thrombus (*arrow*) and distal reconstitution (*arrowhead*).   (*Continued on page 296*)

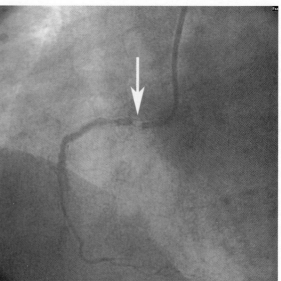

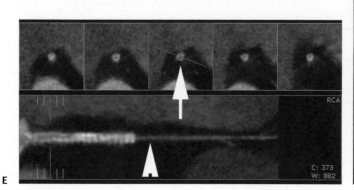

Fig. 12.7 (*Continued*) Segmental thrombosis of a right coronary artery (RCA) stent. **(E)** The straightened lumen view provides perpendicular images to the stent, clearly demonstrating the thrombus within the proximal stent lumen (*arrow*). **(F)** Conventional arteriogram with RCA injection demonstrates subtotal occlusion of the stented segment in the proximal RCA (*arrow*) with filling of the more distal portions of the vessel.

placed on the aorta at the time of surgery. Knowing the exact location of the proximal anastomosis, the course (anterior to the aorta versus retroaortic), and the angle between the graft and the aorta facilitates the selection of appropriate guiding catheters and may reduce the amount of radiation and contrast used during angiography (**Fig. 12.8**).

Saphenous vein graft (SVG) atherosclerosis usually begins after 3 years post-operatively and is characterized by development of atheromatous debris that is friable, soft, bulky, and frequently associated with thrombus. Graft manipulation during PCI may cause dislodgement of this debris, distal embolization of the microvasculature of the grafted vessel, and periprocedural myocardial infarction resulting in high adverse cardiac event rates.[22] Embolic protection devices (EPDs) are placed in the SVG distal to the target lesion in an attempt to capture and retrieve embolic material. The routine use of EPDs during SVG interventions has resulted in significant reduction in the adverse cardiac event rate.[23] MDCT can identify the SVG characteristics that may preclude the use of specific types of EPDs, including graft diameter (>7 mm, <3 mm), extreme graft tortuosity and angulation, and location of stenosis in the ostium or in close proximity to the distal anastomosis (<3 cm). Similarly, angiographic information on the grafted vessel, such as size, extent of atherosclerosis, and myocardial territory supplied, is essential. The interventional cardiologist might elect not to intervene in a graft supplying a vessel that is small, diffusely diseased, or that supplies only a small myocardial territory.

Another important application of MDCT angiography is the detection of subclavian disease in patients with internal mammary artery (IMA) grafts. Hemodynamically significant stenosis of the proximal subclavian artery can compromise

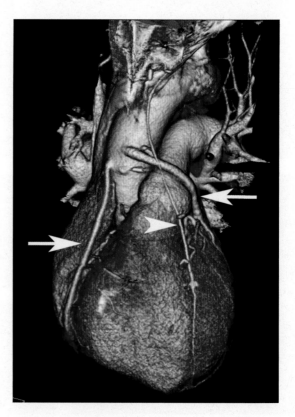

Fig. 12.8 Surface volumetric rendering demonstrates patent coronary artery bypass grafts. The left internal mammary artery graft to the left anterior descending (*arrowhead*) is smaller in caliber compared with the saphenous vein grafts to the right coronary artery and obtuse marginal artery (*arrows*).

blood flow to the IMA and result in ischemia in the grafted vessel territory.

Advanced knowledge about the presence of a significant stenosis, the location of the diseased segment, and disease involving important branches of the subclavian artery (IMA, vertebral), is essential in planning PCI of the subclavian artery. Routine evaluation of the aortic arch vessels should be performed in all patients with IMA grafts.

◆ Coronary Artery Fistulae

A coronary artery fistula is an abnormal communication between a coronary artery and either a cardiac chamber or any segment of the pulmonary, cardiac, or systemic circulation. Coronary artery fistulae (CAF) account for 0.2 to 0.4% of congenital cardiac anomalies. CAF frequently arise from the right coronary artery (50–60%) or the left coronary artery (30–40%). The vast majority of CAF (>90%) empty into the right side of the heart, most frequently into the right ventricle. Although Most CAF are congenital in origin, iatrogenic causes have been described. Small, asymptomatic CAF can be managed conservatively because they do not typically cause hemodynamic compromise and may close spontaneously.[24] Larger fistulae may enlarge with time and become symptomatic secondary to coronary steal with resultant ischemia or shunting with resultant volume overload and congestive heart failure. Potential complications include aneurysm formation, mural thrombosis with distal embolization, arrhythmias, infectious endocarditis, and, rarely, rupture.[24,25]

Although coronary angiography is considered the gold standard in the evaluation of CAF, MDCT imaging allows three-dimensional reconstruction of the fistula (see **Figs. 4.22** and **4.23**) with accurate sizing of the native vessel and the CAF, evaluation of the vessel wall, and detection of aneurysmal dilatation that can be missed by conventional angiography in the presence of mural thrombus.[26,27] All the aforementioned angiographic characteristics are essential in planning for percutaneous embolization. Patients with large tortuous fistulae, with multiple fistulous communications, with aneurysmal dilatation, and with fistulae providing important branches to the myocardium might not be amenable to percutaneous closure.[28,29]

Percutaneous occlusion can be performed using a variety of materials, including coils, umbrella devices, vascular occluders, detachable balloons, and others. The choice of the closure device is based on the anatomic characteristics of the fistula. When coil embolization is performed, the coil diameter should be 20 to 25% larger than the fistula to obtain a stable position and to achieve thrombosis with the least amount of coils possible. MDCT can play an important role in planning the appropriate embolization technique and can provide a noninvasive angiographic follow-up of these patients. Although MDCT does assess chamber size, a limitation of MDCT is the inability to assess hemodynamic flow parameters within a CAF.

◆ Multivessel Coronary Artery Disease

Optimal management of patients with multivessel coronary artery disease (percutaneous versus surgical) is a matter of controversy that is beyond the scope of this chapter. Over the last decade, several randomized trials have compared CABG with percutaneous revascularization. Overall, these studies revealed no significant difference in survival benefit between the two treatment modalities. However, the subset of patients with diabetes and multivessel CAD did derive a mortality benefit from surgical revascularization, particularly those with impaired LV function. Furthermore, CABG was shown to provide more effective relief from angina, and PCI was associated with the need for repeat revascularization.[30]

MDCT coronary imaging may provide a useful adjunct for management of multivessel CAD. Specifically, MDCT may optimize the selection of a specific revascularization modality by identifying lesion subtypes that are associated with a higher or lower PCI success rate. For example, patients with chronic total occlusions, long lesions, left main disease, severe vessel tortuosity, ostial disease, calcification, and complex bifurcation lesions might be better candidates for surgical management.

A unique advantage of MDCT over conventional coronary angiography is the ability to image the vessel wall and provide important information on the composition of the atherosclerotic plaque, with the potential to distinguish lipid-rich from fibrotic and calcified plaques.[31] Diffuse coronary artery wall involvement with predominantly calcified or lipid-rich plaque may favor CABG, whereas focal wall involvement with fibrotic plaque might identify patients who are better candidates for percutaneous revascularization.

◆ Congenital Heart Disease

Percutaneous repair of congenital cardiac anomalies such as atrial septal defects (ASD), ventricular septal defects (VSD), patent ductus arteriosus (PDA), and aorctic coarctation has become a common occurrence in the cardiac catheterization laboratory. Planning a percutaneous repair of such congenital anomalies requires detailed anatomic information to determine the patient's candidacy for the procedure and to select the appropriate device for the specific defect.

There are several subtypes of ASDs and VSDs; these are classified on the basis of their anatomic location (see **Figs. 9.14, 9.15,** and **9.16**), and not all defects are amenable to catheter-based closure. MDCT provides three-dimensional images of the defect and surrounding anatomic structures that are very useful for planning percutaneous closure of ASDs (**Figs. 12.9, 12.10**), VSDs (**Figs. 12.11** and **12.12**), and PDAs (**Fig. 12.13**). Specifically, MDCT provides accurate assessment of the defect diameter, the presence of a tissue rim to support a closure device, location, spatial orientation, length (tunneled defects), and the presence of multiple fenestrations. Accuracy of these anatomic details is critical because a measurement error can result in the choice of an incorrect device type or device size, with resultant complications such as device embolization or incomplete sealing of

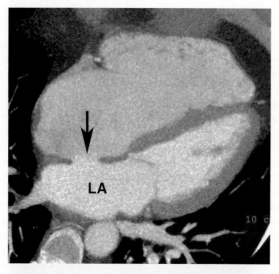

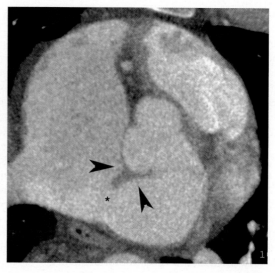

A

B

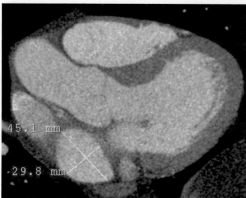

C

Fig. 12.9 Large ostium secundum atrial septal defect (ASD). **(A)** Four-chamber view demonstrates a normal size left atrium (LA) with an ostium secundum atrial septal defect (*arrow*). The right side of the heart is enlarged secondary to this shunt. **(B)** Short-axis maximum intensity projection image demonstrates the relationship of the defect to the aortic root. A closure device will overlap the atrial septum adjacent to the aortic root (*arrowheads*). **(C)** Long-axis image demonstrates the ASD en face and allows perpendicular measurements of its size. **(D,E)** Endoluminal views demonstrate the relationship of the ASD to the mitral annulus and to the pulmonary veins. Structures adjacent to the ASD, including the aortic root, the mitral annulus, and the pulmonary veins, must be identified so that they are not injured during placement of a closure device. MV, mitral valve.

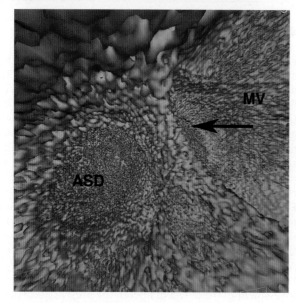

D

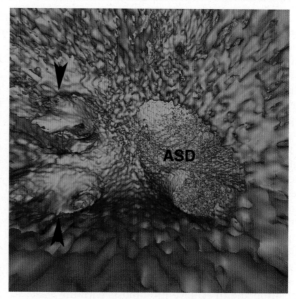

E

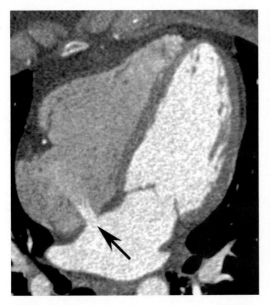 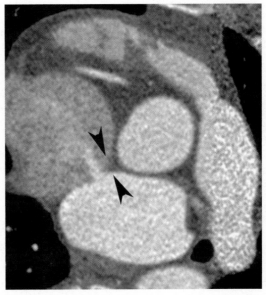

Fig. 12.10 Ostium secundum atrial septal defect adjacent to the aortic root. **(A)** Four-chamber view demonstrates an atrial septal defect (ASD) measuring about 5 mm in diameter at the level of the foramen ovale (*arrow*) with left-to-right shunting of contrast material. **(B)** Short-axis maximum intensity projection demonstrates the relationship of the ASD to the aortic root. Only a short segment of septum is available between the ASD and the aortic root (*arrowheads*) for fixation of a closure device.

the defect with continuous shunting. It is essential to measure the proximity of the defect to important cardiac structures, such as the aorta, atrial and ventricular free walls, and the valvular structures, because repetitive injury from an oversized device can result in delayed perforation.[32] In addition

to assessment of the defect and adjacent anatomic structures, MDCT can exclude the presence of thrombus in the cardiac chambers (especially the left atrium) before the closure procedure. Unnoticed thombus may lead to thromboembolic complications during catheter manipulation.

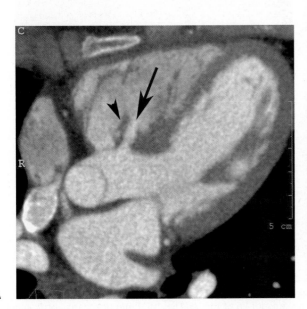 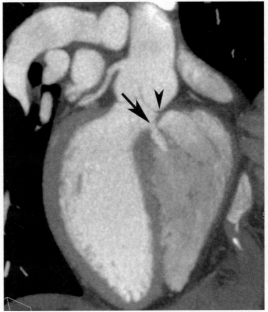

Fig. 12.11 Membranous ventricular septal defect (VSD). **(A)** Slab maximum intensity projection (MIP) three-chamber view demonstrates a communication across the upper portion of the ventricular septum (*arrow*). The VSD tunnel is elongated by the presence of a windsock of tissue that extends into the right ventricle (*arrowhead*). **(B)** Slab MIP long-axis projection demonstrates that there is only a very short lip of tissue between the VSD (*arrow*) and the aortic annulus (*arrowhead*). The presence of the windsock and the short lip above the VSD are complicating factors for percutaneous closure. (*Continued on page 300*)

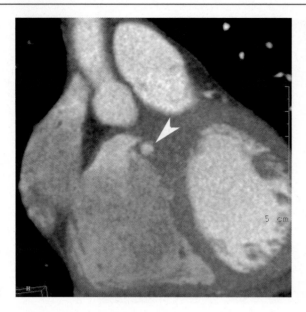

C

Fig. 12.11 (*Continued*) Membranous ventricular septal defect (VSD). **(C)** Slab MIP in a perpendicular plane demonstrates the round contour of the defect (*arrowhead*) and allows measurement of its diameter.

PDA closure can be achieved with either surgical or catheter-based techniques. Several clinical and anatomic parameters are essential to the planning of optimal treatment. Although percutaneous closure has become the procedure of choice in adults, surgical repair is more appropriate in patients with infection (endarteritis), thrombus, and other cardiac conditions that require surgical correction.[33]

Conversely, surgical repair of PDA is not technically feasible in the presence of moderate to severe duct calcification or aneurysmal dilatation.[33] MDCT can play an important role in selecting the optimal treatment modality by providing detailed images and measurements of the PDA. These include diameter, length, shape (eg, conic, tubular, with constrictions, dilated aortic ampulla), angulation, calcification,

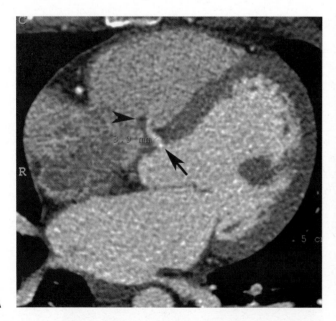

A

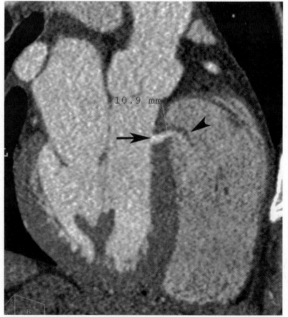

B

Fig. 12.12 Perimembranous ventricular septal defect (VSD). **(A)** Four-chamber view demonstrates a 3.9-mm communication across the upper portion of the ventricular septum (*arrow*) with a small windsock of tissue extending into the right ventricle (*arrowhead*). The windsock was located immediately adjacent to the chordal structures of the tricuspid valve. The presence of this tissue extending into the right ventricle complicated the placement of a closure device. **(B)** Three-chamber view again demonstrates the VSD (*arrow*) and windsock (*arrowhead*). The superior lip of the VSD lies 10.9 mm below the aortic annulus, allowing just enough tissue for placement of a closure device. Successful percutaneous closure was performed. The closure device had to be passed across the defect from the left ventricular side because of the windsock.

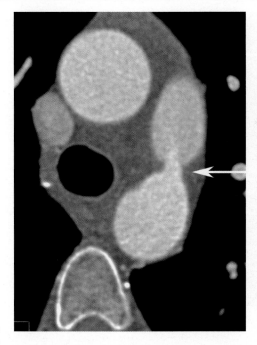

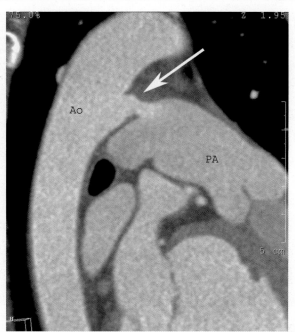

A

B

Fig. 12.13 Patent ductus arteriosus. **(A)** Axial image demonstrates a communication between the distal main pulmonary artery (PA) and the descending aorta (Ao) (*arrow*). **(B)** Sagittal maximum intensity projection again demonstrates a communication between the distal main PA and the descending aorta (*arrow*). The aortic side of the communication demonstrates a wide neck that must be considered when placing a closure device.

aneurysmal dilatation, and presence of thrombus.[34] Size and shape are essential in the selection of the correct closure device. Furthermore, three-dimensional images of the PDA and the spatial relations with adjacent structures can be very useful when surgical repair is contemplated.

Endovascular balloon dilatation and stent implantation are now increasingly used for both native aortic coarctation and recoarctation in older children and adults.[35] Percutaneous treatment of coarctation poses unique difficulties in view of the size of the aorta, the vicinity to the arch branches, and the presence of associated conditions such as transverse aortic arch hypoplasia and sequela of prior surgical or balloon dilatation, such as aneurysms.[36] MDCT imaging can provide detailed information on the diameter of the aorta proximal and distal to the coarctation (site of post-stenotic dilation), detect the presence of aneurysms (potential need for covered stents or coiling), detect the presence of aortic arch hypoplasia, determine proximity to the arch branches, and ascertain the length of the coarctation (discrete versus tubular). CTA of the aorta and iliac arteries is valuable in older adults to evaluate presence of peripheral arterial disease at the ileofemoral level, given the large profile of the balloons and stents used in these procedures. Follow-up imaging is essential following repair to detect recurrence of coarctation (after balloon dilatation) and aneurysm formation. MDCT may be superior to magnetic resonance imaging (MRI) in patients who underwent stent implantation because of artifacts produced by the stent and the limited accuracy of MRI in detecting small aneurysms.[35]

Following placement of a percutaneous closure device, MDCT can demonstrate the position of the device, the presence of any residual shunt, and the relationship of the device to adjacent anatomic structures (**Fig. 12.14**).

◆ Cardiovascular Surgery Applications

MDCT imaging can be useful to the cardiothoracic surgeon by providing essential anatomic information. In addition to basic angiographic and functional data, such as the presence of congenital coronary anomalies, the location of the stenoses, the size of the vessels to be grafted, and LV size and function, MDCT can detect additional important characteristics that are not easily identifiable by conventional angiography. CT imaging can demonstrate the presence of atherosclerosis and calcification in the ascending aorta and guide the surgeon to select an appropriate site for the proximal anastomosis of aortocoronary bypass grafts. Furthermore, MDCT can distinguish an epicardial coronary segment that can be used as a target site for a bypass graft from a bridged segment with an intramyocardial course. These graft issues are discussed in more detail in Chapter 8.

Repeat open heart surgery is associated with increased risk because of the potential for injury to pre-existing grafts and cardiac structures. MDCT with three-dimensional image reconstruction can accurately identify these important structures (**Fig. 12.15**). Gasparovic et al reported a series of 33 patients who underwent preoperative MDCT imaging before reoperative cardiac surgery. Their study showed that MDCT imaging was superior to conventional coronary angiography and chest radiography in defining the position

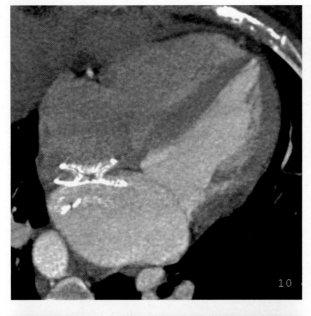

A

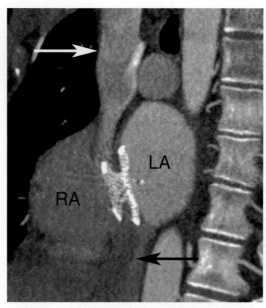

B

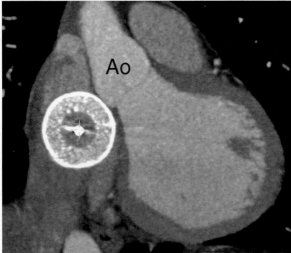

C

Ao

Fig. 12.14 Percutaneously placed 24-mm Amplatzer ASD occluder (AGA Medical Corp; Golden Valley, MN) in an ostium secundum atrial septal defect (ASD). **(A)** Four-chamber view demonstrates the closure device extending along both sides of the interatrial septum with no evidence of residual interatrial shunting. **(B)** Coronal maximum intensity projection (MIP) demonstrates the closure device between the two atria, with the superior vena cava (*white arrow*) and the inferior vena cava (*black arrow*) entering the right atrium (RA) adjacent to the device. The device is appropriately sized to close the ASD but does not block the inflow of blood into the RA. **(C)** Sagittal MIP demonstrates the proximity of the closure device to the aortic root. Once again, the device is appropriately sized and positioned so that it does not injure the aortic root. Ao, aorta; LA, left atrium.

of the bypass grafts and cardiac structures in relation to the sternum.[37]

MDCT can be useful in the pre-operative evaluation of patients undergoing surgical resection of LV pseudo-aneurysms. It is vital to distinguish a pseudoaneurysm from a true LV aneurysm because the latter could be managed medically (see **Figs. 9.23, 9.24,** and **9.25**). The key identifying characteristic is the lack of myocardial tissue in the wall of the pseudoaneurysm. Additional information can be obtained on the pseudoaneurysm's location, shape, size, presence of mural thrombus or calcification, LV geometry and function, and the potential need for mitral valve or papillary muscle repair (**Fig. 12.16**).[38,39]

MDCT can identify the subgroup of patients with ventricular pseudoaneurysms who may be candidates for percutaneous closure. Anatomic characteristics that do not favor

percutaneous device closure include the presence of a large pseudoaneurysm neck with irregular margins that could result in incomplete sealing of the defect and inadequate tissue rim to retain the device in place. The need for mitral valve or papillary muscle repair, and the possible interference of the device with these cardiac structures, may preclude percutaneous treatment.

In patients with LV systolic dysfunction, especially those with ischemic etiology, surgical ventricular restoration (SVR) is becoming a promising treatment modality. SVR corrects LV geometry by resection of scarred segments of myocardium, reduction of LV volume, and restoration of the LV elliptical shape. MDCT can provide the necessary anatomic information for patient selection, operative planning, and post-operative follow-up (**Fig. 12.17**). The following anatomic characteristics are essential for the identification

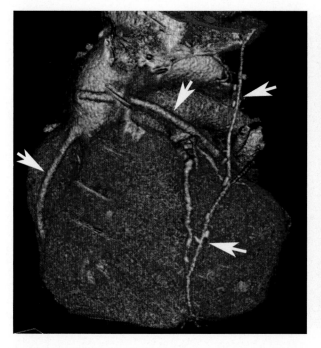

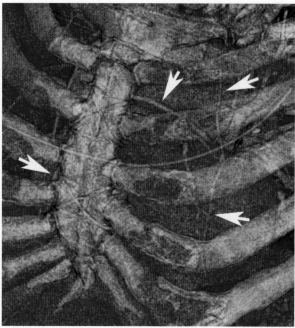

Fig. 12.15 Relationship of coronary anatomy to the chest wall. **(A)** Surface-rendered volumetric image of the heart demonstrates multiple bypass grafts (*arrows*). **(B)** Surface-rendered volumetric image in the identical orientation with visible translucent rib cage. The relationship of the bypass grafts (*arrows*) to the bony structures is demonstrated.

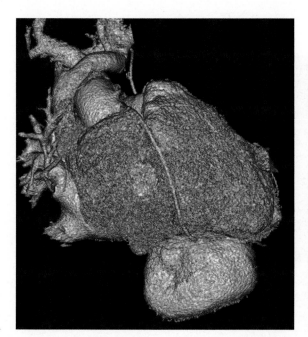

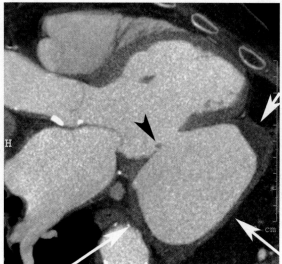

Fig. 12.16 Left ventricular (LV) pseudoaneurysm involving the inferior wall. **(A)** Surface-rendered image demonstrates the size of the pseudoaneurysm and the relationship of the pseudoaneurysm to the LV but does not demonstrate details of the aneurysm neck. **(B,C)** Orthogonal slab maximum intensity projection (MIP) images demonstrate the pseudoaneurysm (*arrows*) with a wide neck (*white arrowheads*) and with a chordal structure/papillary muscle crossing the neck (*black arrowhead*). (*Continued on page 304*)

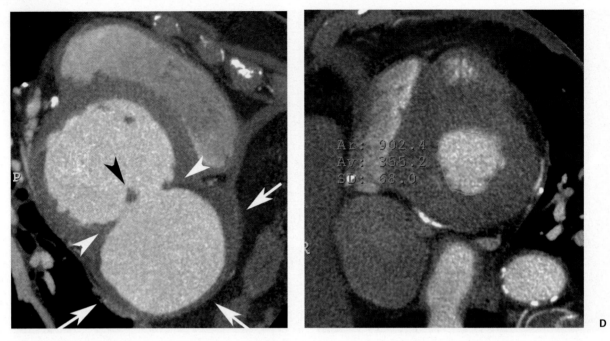

Fig. 12.16 (*Continued*) Left ventricular (LV) pseudoaneurysm involving the inferior wall. **(D)** Slab MIP image of the neck of the pseudoaneurysm en face provides an assessment of the size and contour of the defect for selection of a closure device. Unfortunately, the presence of chordal structures across the neck of the pseudoaneurysm precluded a percutaneous closure procedure. Cine images of the pseudoaneurysm are provided on the accompanying CD.

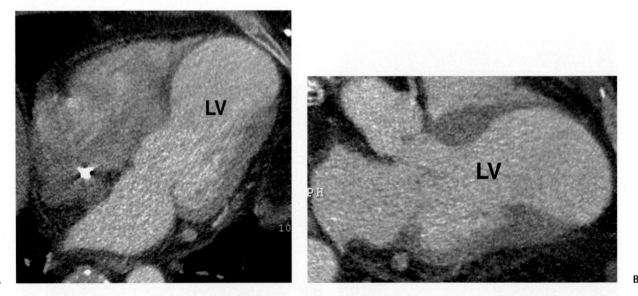

Fig. 12.17 Ventricular remodeling surgery. **(A,B)** Four-chamber and long-axis views of the left ventricle (LV) demonstrate a large apical aneurysm. Cine images demonstrate akinesis of the apex with hypokinesis of the proximal walls.

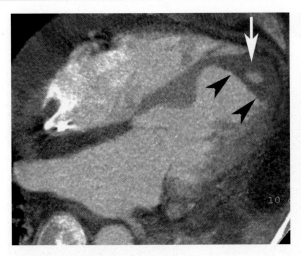

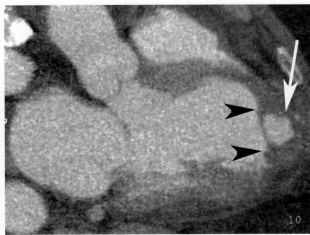

C   D

Fig. 12.17 (*Continued*) **(C,D)** Post-operative four-chamber and long-axis views of the LV demonstrate a patch across the apex (*black arrowheads*) intended to exclude the akinetic segment. Unfortunately, there is a leak with contrast extending beyond the patch into the apex (*white arrow*). Cine images of the apical aneurysm and postoperative repair are provided on the accompanying CD.

of those patients who may benefit from the procedure: mitral annular size, extent of scarred and akinetic myocardium, interpapillary muscle distance, LV systolic volume, and LV systolic volume index. Myocardial viability is an additional parameter necessary for the pre-operative evaluation of these patients. The data on evaluation of myocardial viability by cardiac CT are limited and experimental at this time.[40,41]

MDCT can play an important role in the planning of aortic or mitral valve replacement. As illustrated in Chapter 10, the ability to examine the valve in multiple planes provides valuable information on the morphology of the valve and surrounding cardiac structures. Specifically, MDCT provides excellent evaluation of the valve annulus size, annular calcification, valve leaflet calcification, valve motion, valve area, LV outflow tract dimensions, and mitral subvalvular apparatus (**Fig. 12.18**).[42] Aortic valve disease may be associated with enlargement of the aortic root and ascending aorta, requiring surgical repair at the time of valve surgery.[42] Imaging of the aorta is imperative in patients

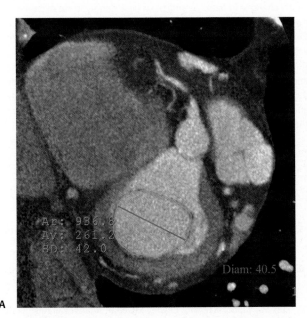

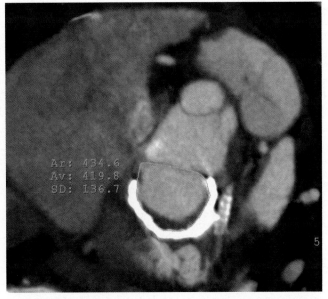

A   B

Fig. 12.18 Measurement of the mitral and aortic valve annulus. **(A)** Short axis through the mitral annulus demonstrates planimetry of the annulus area (9.4 cm²) and measurement of the annulus diameter (4.1 cm). **(B)** Short-axis through the mitral annulus after placement of an annular ring demonstrates planimetry of the annulus area (4.4 cm²). (*Continued on page 306*)

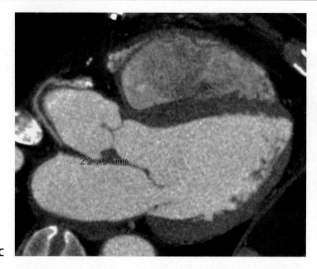

C

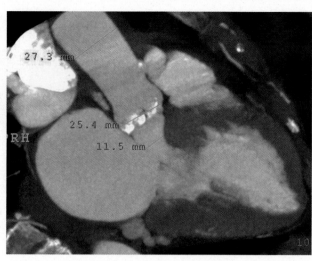

D

Fig. 12.18 (*Continued*) Measurement of the mitral and aortic valve annulus. **(C)** Long-axis image demonstrates measurement of a normal left ventricular outflow tract in a patient with a bioprosthetic aortic valve. **(D)** Long-axis image in a patient with calcific aortic stenosis demonstrates measurement of the outflow tract (1.2 cm), the annulus (2.5 cm), and the ascending aorta (2.7 cm). The outflow tract is narrowed by hypertrophy of the upper ventricular septum.

with aortic valve disease (**Fig. 12.18D**). In patients with mitral valve disease and atrial fibrillation, cardiac CT can detect the presence of left atrial thrombus. MDCT also allows determination of the LV function and cardiac chamber sizes. It is important to identify patients with impaired LV function because the risk of perioperative complications is increased in this subgroup.

◆ Conclusion

The rapid evolution of interventional cardiology techniques over the past decade has provided a wealth of new percutaneous and surgical procedures. MDCT evaluation provides an excellent method for patient selection, technical planning, and follow-up for many of these new procedures.

Cine 12.1 Large pseudoaneurysm of the proximal inferior–inferolateral left ventricle (LV) wall (see Fig. 12.16). **(A)** Surface display demonstrates a large pseudoaneurysm under the LV. The cine begins in the right anterior oblique projection and demonstrates the proximity of the pseudoaneurysm to a right coronary artery–posterior descending artery bypass graft. The cine then rotates to the left side of the heart and demonstrates the relationship between the pseudoaneurysm and the right internal mammary graft to the circumflex territory. **(B)** Functional cine demonstrates poor LV contractility with akinesis of the inferior–inferolateral walls and a large pseudoaneurysm. While

the LV contracts during systole, the pseudoaneurysm is not significantly changed in size. The short-axis view demonstrates a papillary muscle crossing over the neck of the pseudoaneurysm.

Cine 12.2 Ventricular remodeling surgery. Apical aneurysm treated with a patch across the left ventricular apex (see Fig. 12.17). **(A)** Functional cine in the five-chamber view demonstrates a large akinetic apical aneurysm of the left ventricle (LV). **(B)** Postoperative study demonstrates a patch placed across the distal LV to exclude the aneurysm. There is a leak in the patch with contrast extending into the apical aneurysm.

References

1. Wu C, Hannan EL, Walford G, et al. A risk score to predict in-hospital mortality for percutaneous coronary interventions. J Am Coll Cardiol. 2006;47(3):654–660

2. Iliadis EA, Zaacks SM, Calvin JE, Allen J, Parrillo JE, Klein LW. The relative influence of lesion length and other stenosis morphologies on procedural success of coronary intervention. Angiology. 2000;51(1):39–52

3. Holmes DR Jr. Long and calcified lesions. In: Ellis SG, Holmes DR, eds. Strategic approaches in coronary intervention. 3rd ed. Philadelphia, PA: Lippincott Williams & Wilkins; 2006:295–298

4. Rosenblum J, Stertzer SH, Shaw RE, et al. Rotational ablation of balloon angioplasty failures. J Invasive Cardiol. 1992;4(6):312–318

5. Mintz GS, Douek P, Pichard AD, et al. Target lesion calcification in coronary artery disease: an intravascular ultrasound study. J Am Coll Cardiol. 1992;20(5):1149–1155

6. Freed MS. Calcified lesions. In: Safian RD, Freed MS, eds. The manual of interventional cardiology. 3rd ed. Royal Oak, MI: Physicians' Press; 2001:245–54

7. Ellis SG, Vandormael MG, Cowley MJ, et al; Multivessel Angioplasty Prognosis Study Group. Coronary morphologic and clinical determinants of procedural outcome with angioplasty for multivessel coronary disease. Implications for patient selection. Circulation. 1990; 82(4):1193–1202

8. Abhyankar AD, Luyue G, Bailey BP. Stent implantation in severely angulated lesions: safety, efficacy, and morphological remodelling. Cathet Cardiovasc Diagn. 1997;40(3):261–264

9. Joner M, Finn AV, Farb A, et al. Pathology of drug-eluting stents in humans: delayed healing and late thrombotic risk. J Am Coll Cardiol. 2006;48(1):193–202

10. Flood RD, Popma JJ, Chuang YC, et al. Incidence, angiographic predictors, and clinical significance of coronary perforation occurring after new device angioplasty. J Am Coll Cardiol. 1994;23(Suppl 1):301A

11. Ivanhoe RJ, Weintraub WS, Douglas JS Jr, et al. Percutaneous transluminal coronary angioplasty of chronic total occlusions: primary success, restenosis, and long-term clinical follow-up. Circulation. 1992;85(1):106–115

12. Freed MS. Chronic total occlusion. In: Safian RD, Freed MS, eds. The manual of interventional cardiology. 3rd ed. Royal Oak, MI: Physicians' Press; 2001:287–315

13. Yokoyama N, Yamamoto Y, Suzuki S, et al. Impact of 16-slice computed tomography in percutaneous coronary intervention of chronic total occlusions. Catheter Cardiovasc Interv 2006;68(1):1–7

14. Colombo A, Stankovic G, Reimers B. Bifurcation lesions—the role of stents. In: Ellis SG, Holmes DR, eds. Strategic approaches in coronary intervention. 3rd ed. Philadelphia, PA: Lippincott Williams & Wilkins; 2006:304–319

15. Safian RD. Bifurcation lesions. In: Safian RD, Freed MS, eds. The manual of interventional cardiology. 3rd ed. Royal Oak, MI: Physicians' Press; 2001:221–254

16. Stewart JT, Ward DE, Davies MJ, Pepper JR. Isolated coronary ostial stenosis: observations on the pathology. Eur Heart J. 1987;8(8):917–920

17. Freed MS. Ostial lesions. In: Safian RD, Freed MS, eds. The manual of interventional cardiology. 3rd ed. Royal Oak, MI: Physicians' Press, 2001:261–272

18. Park SJ, Park SW, Lee CW, Hong MK, Kim JJ. Stenting of unprotected left main stenosis: acute and long term results of the first 100 cases: elective intervention of left main coronary artery stenosis. J Am Coll Cardiol. 2000;35(Suppl 1):61

19. Fajadet J, Black A, Hayeruzadeh B, et al. Unprotected left main stenting. In: Fajadet J, ed. Syllabus for EuroPCR 2001.

20. Fasseas P, Holmes DR Jr. Unprotected left main percutaneous coronary intervention. Rev Cardiovasc Med. 2002;3(3):157–160

21. Iakovou I, Schmidt T, Bonizzoni E, et al. Incidence, predictors, and outcome of thrombosis after successful implantation of drug-eluting stents. JAMA. 2005;293(17):2126–2130

22. Douglas JS Jr, Savage MP. Saphenous vein graft disease. In: Ellis SG, Holmes DR, eds. Strategic approaches in coronary intervention. 3rd ed. Philadelphia, PA: Lippincott Williams & Wilkins, 2006:386–393

23. Fasseas P, Orford JL, Denktas AE, Berger PB. Distal protection devices during percutaneous coronary and carotid interventions. Curr Control Trials Cardiovasc Med. 2001;2(6):286–291

24. Angelini P. Normal and anomalous coronary arteries in humans. In: Coronary artery anomalies. Philadelphia, PA: Lippincott Williams & Wilkins; 1999:60–63

25. Carrel T, Tkebuchava T, Jenni R, Arbenz U, Turina M. Congenital coronary fistulas in children and adults: diagnosis, surgical technique and results. Cardiology. 1996;87(4):325–330

26. Morra A, Romano S, Del Borrello M, Ramondo A, Greco P. Noninvasive evaluation of a fistula between a giant coronary aneurysm and coronary sinus performed via multidetector row computed tomography. Clin Imaging. 2006;30(4):275–277

27. Hara H, Moroi M, Araki T, et al. Coronary artery fistula with an associated aneurysm detected by 16-slice multidetector row computed tomographic angiography. Heart Vessels. 2005;20(4):184–185

28. Mavroudis C, Backer CL, Rocchini AP, Muster AJ, Gevitz M. Coronary artery fistulas in infants and children: a surgical review and discussion of coil embolization. Ann Thorac Surg. 1997;63(5):1235–1242

29. Perry SB, Rome J, Keane JF, Baim DS, Lock JE. Transcatheter closure of coronary artery fistulas. J Am Coll Cardiol. 1992;20(1):205–209

30. Casserly IP. The optimal revascularization strategy for multivessel coronary artery disease: the debate continues. Cleve Clin J Med. 2006;73(4):317–318, 320–322, 324 passim

31. Leber AW, Knez A, White CW, et al. Composition of coronary atherosclerotic plaques in patients with acute myocardial infarction and stable angina pectoris determined by contrast-enhanced multislice computed tomography. Am J Cardiol. 2003;91(6):714–718

32. Chessa M, Carminati M, Butera G, et al. Early and late complications associated with transcatheter occlusion of secundum atrial septal defect. J Am Coll Cardiol. 2002;39(6):1061–1065

33. Warnes CA, Williams RG, Bashore TM, et al; American College of Cardiology; American Heart Association Task Force on Practice Guidelines (Writing Committee to Develop Guidelines on the Management of Adults with Congenital Heart Disease); American Society of Echocardiography; Heart Rhythm Society; International Society for Adult Congenital Heart Disease; Society for Cardiovascular Angiography and Interventions; Society of Thoracic Surgeons. ACC/AHA 2008 guidelines for the management of adults with congenital heart disease: a report of the American College of Cardiology/American Heart Association Task Force on Practice Guidelines (Writing Committee to Develop Guidelines on the Management of Adults with Congenital Heart Disease). Developed in Collaboration with the American Society of Echocardiography, Heart Rhythm Society, International Society for Adult Congenital Heart Disease, Society for Cardiovascular Angiography and Interventions, and Society of Thoracic Surgeons. J Am Coll Cardiol. 2008;52(23):e1–e121

34. Morgan-Hughes GJ, Marshall AJ, Roobottom C. Morphologic assessment of patent ductus arteriosus in adults using retrospectively ECG-gated multidetector CT. AJR Am J Roentgenol. 2003;181(3):749–754

35. Rosenthal E. Stent implantation for aortic coarctation: the treatment of choice in adults? J Am Coll Cardiol. 2001;38(5):1524–1527

36. Hamdan MA, Maheshwari S, Fahey JT, Hellenbrand WE. Endovascular stents for coarctation of the aorta: initial results and intermediate-term follow-up. J Am Coll Cardiol. 2001;38(5):1518–1523

37. Gasparovic H, Rybicki FJ, Millstine J, et al. Three dimensional computed tomographic imaging in planning the surgical approach for redo cardiac surgery after coronary revascularization. Eur J Cardiothorac Surg. 2005;28(2):244–249

38. Baks T, Cademartiri F, Spierenburg HA, de Feyter PJ. Chronic pseudoaneurysm of the left ventricle. Int J Cardiovasc Imaging. 2006;22(3-4):497–499

39. Frances C, Romero A, Grady D. Left ventricular pseudoaneurysm. J Am Coll Cardiol. 1998;32(3):557–561

40. Baks T, Cademartiri F, Moelker AD, et al. Multislice computed tomography and magnetic resonance imaging for the assessment of reperfused avute myocardial infarction. J Am Coll Cardiol. 2006;48:144–152

41. Mahnken AH, Koos R, Katoh M, et al. Assessment of myocardial viability in reperfused acute myocardial infarction using 16-slice computed tomography in comparison to magnetic resonance imaging. J Am Coll Cardiol. 2005;45(12):2042–2047

42. Boxt LM. CT of valvular heart disease. Int J Cardiovasc Imaging. 2005;21(1):105–113

13

Thoracic Aorta

Scott C. Silvestry, James T. Diehl, and Ethan J. Halpern

Assessment of the thoracic aorta is integral to evaluation of the cardiovascular system during cardiac CT. Changes in the structure and function of the thoracic aorta may significantly impact left ventricular function, coronary blood flow, and cerebral and peripheral circulation. Although dedicated coronary CT angiography (CTA) will not image the aortic arch, a complete interpretation of every cardiac CT should comment on the presence of thoracic aortic disease in visualized portions of the aorta. For patients in whom more complete evaluation of the aorta is desired, the electrocardiogrphic (ECG)-gated examination is easily extended from the aortic arch down through the diaphragm. Aortic anomalies, variants, aneurysmal disease, dissection, intramural hematoma, and penetrating atherosclerotic ulcers are clearly defined by ECG-gated CTA. This information allows the clinician to evaluate thoroughly aortic disease, stratify risk and prognosis, target medical therapy, plan endovascular and surgical interventions, and assess follow-up. Changes on serial assessment of the thoracic aorta can identify patients at increased risk for adverse outcome. Patients with rapid progression of disease over time may warrant more aggressive risk factor modification; blood pressure control; or early, timely surgical intervention. Finally, follow-up imaging after surgical intervention on the heart and thoracic aorta is essential for the early detection and treatment of complications and progression of disease.

◆ Normal Anatomy of the Aorta

The thoracic aorta is divided into five segments: aortic root, ascending aorta, proximal aortic arch, distal aortic arch, and descending thoracic aorta (**Fig. 13.1A**).

The aortic root is the cylindrical segment of aorta from the ventriculoaortic junction to the sinotubular junction, which contains the aortic valve, the aortic annulus, and the sinuses of Valsalva (see **Fig. 3.1**). The three aortic root sinuses or sinuses of Valsalva are functionally identical. The left and right coronary arteries normally arise from ostia in the left and right sinuses, respectively. The third, posterior, sinus is normally without a coronary origin and is termed the *noncoronary sinus*.

The semilunar attachments of the aortic valve cusps form the hemodynamic junction between the left ventricle and the aorta. Structures distal to this boundary are exposed to arterial pressure; structures proximal to this boundary are subject to ventricular pressure. This relationship becomes more important in interpreting anatomic and physiologic changes in diseases affecting the aortic root. The attachments of the aortic valve cusps to the aortic wall are not planar, but rather crown-like, from the top of the commissures at the level of the sinotubular junction to the nadir of the cusps in the left ventricular outflow tract.[1] Because of this anatomy, significant dilation of the aorta at the sinotubular junction leads to loss of valvular support with aortic valve incompetence.[1,2] Understanding this mechanism of aortic insufficiency is essential to understanding changes in the aortic valve from diseases such as aortic dissection and annuloaortic ectasia.

Aortic root size measurements are made at the annulus (nadir of the aortic leaflets), at the midpoint of the sinuses of Valsalva, and at the sinotubular junction (**Figs. 13.1C,D**). Assessing these dimensions allows accurate serial comparison of changes in aortic root size and defines the root morphology to allow disease classification and to plan surgical intervention.[1,3,4]

The size of the normal aortic root is related to body size, height, and sex. Aortic root size changes with age and with hypertension.[4–6] Enlargement of the aortic root may lead to significant aortic valvular regurgitation in patients with hypertension, collagen vascular diseases (such as Marfan syndrome or Ehler-Danlos syndrome), and aortic dissection through loss of valve support and central aortic insufficiency. The normal diameter of the adult aorta just above the sinotubular junction averages 3.6 cm (range, 2.4–4.7 cm).[7,8]

The ascending aorta extends from the sinotubular junction to the origin of the innominate artery. The average diameter of the adult ascending aorta is 3.5 cm (range, 2.2–4.7 cm).[8] A diameter greater than 4.0 cm is generally classified as aneurysmal (**Figs. 13.1D,E**). The aortic arch begins at the origin of the right innominate artery and ends at the attachment of the ligamentum arteriosum. The proximal arch extends from the origin of the right innominate artery to the origin of the left subclavian artery and includes the origin of the left common carotid artery. The distal arch, called the *aortic isthmus*, includes the aorta from the origin of the left subclavian artery to the ligamentum arteriosum. The distal aortic arch may be slightly narrower than the proximal descending thoracic aorta, particularly in infants and children.

The descending thoracic aorta begins distal to the ligamentum arteriosum and extends to the aortic hiatus of the diaphragm. Its proximal portion may appear slightly dilated and is thus termed the *aortic spindle*. The mid-descending thoracic aorta has an average diameter of 2.5 cm (range, 1.6–3.7 cm). The distal descending thoracic aorta

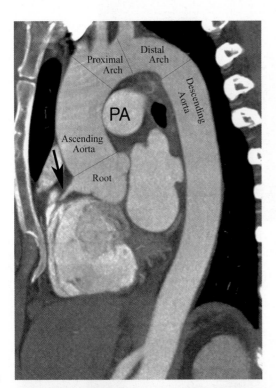

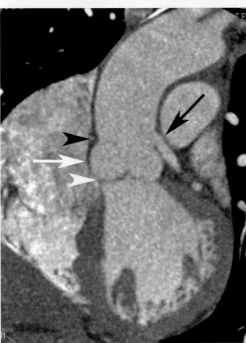

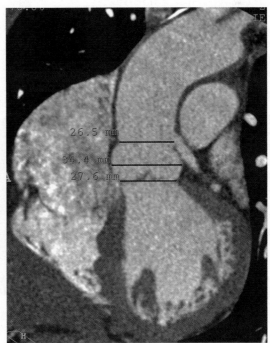

Fig. 13.1 Segments of the thoracic aorta. **(A)** The aortic root is visualized with three sinuses of Valsalva and the origin of the right coronary artery from the anterior sinus (*arrow*). The ascending aorta extends from the sinotubular junction to the origin of the innominate artery. The arch is divided into a proximal segment that extends to the origin of the left subclavian artery and a distal segment that extends to the ligamentum arteriosum. The mild dilatation of the descending aorta beyond the aortic isthmus is known as the aortic spindle. PA, pulmonary artery. **(B)** The normal proximal aorta demonstrates a tapered waist at the sinotubular junction (*black arrowhead*). Measurements of the proximal aorta include the diameter of the annulus at the level of the aortic valve (*white arrowhead*), the diameter of the root at the sinuses of Valsalva (*white arrow*), and the diameter of the aorta at the sinotubular junction (*black arrowhead*). Although the coronary arteries normally originate just below the sinotubular junction, the origin of the left coronary artery in this patient (*black arrow*) is just superior to the sinotubular junction. **(C)** Measurements of the aortic root are demonstrated at the aortic annulus (27.6 mm), the aortic root (34.4 mm), and the sinotubular junction (26.5 mm). (*Continued on page 310*)

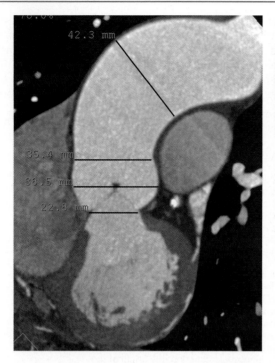

D

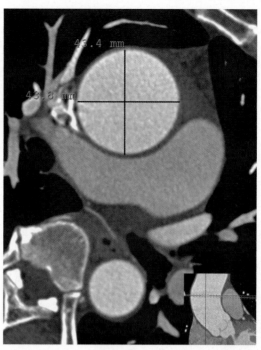

E

Fig. 13.1 (*Continued*) Segments of the thoracic aorta. **(D)** Measurements of the aortic root and ascending aorta in a different patient demonstrate a top normal-size root (38.5 mm) and a mildly dilated ascending aorta (42.3 mm). A tapered diameter is measured at the sinotubular junction (35.4 mm). **(E)** Short-axis measurement of the ascending aorta in the same patient as (D) demonstrates aneurismal dilatation to 4.3 × 4.4 cm. Inset in the bottom right corner demonstrates angulation used to obtain short-axis measurement.

above the diaphragm has an average diameter of 2.4 cm (range, 1.4– 3.3 cm).[7,8]

◆ **Thoracic Aorta: Normal Variants**

The unique properties and anatomic relationships of the ligamentum arteriosum may create radiographic appearances that mimic thoracic aortic disease states. The ductus diverticulum is a focal, convex bulge on the undersurface of the isthmic region of the aortic arch (**Fig. 13.2**). This bulge is commonly thought to arise from the remnant of the ductus arteriosus, although some have theorized its presence as a vestige of the embryonic right dorsal aortic root.[9] The importance of this structure is differentiating its appearance from the presence of a post-traumatic or atherosclerotic pseudoaneurysm in this location (**Figs. 13.19** and **13.20**). The ductus diverticulum may be differentiated from an aortic pseudoaneurysm by its smooth margins and symmetric appearance. Pseudocoarctation of the aorta may occur when the aorta elongates and kinks in this location resulting from tethering of the aorta at the ligamentum arteriosum. The appearance of the aorta in pseudocoarctation is similar to true coarctation, but the absence of collateral circulation readily differentiates the two states.

Three sequential arterial branches arise from the aortic arch. The right innominate (brachiocephalic) artery arises first and is the largest, giving rise to the right subclavian and right common carotid arteries. The left common carotid

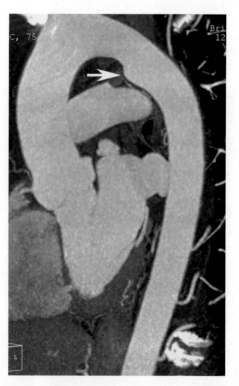

A

Fig. 13.2 Ductus diverticulum in two patients. **(A)** Ductus diverticulum presents as a focal, convex bulge on the anterior undersurface of the isthmic region of the aortic arch (*arrow*). The smooth contour of the ductus diverticulum distinguishes this structure from a pseudoaneurysm.

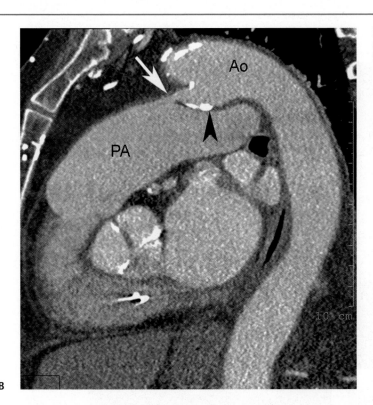

B

Fig. 13.2 (*Continued*) **(B)** Ductus diverticulum (*arrowhead*) associated with a patent ductus arteriosus (*arrow*) between the aorta (Ao) and pulmonary artery (PA).

artery arises next and is typically the smallest artery of the great vessels. The left subclavian artery branches next, arising from the distal arch posteriorly. The standard branching pattern is seen overall in about 70% of individuals.[10] The most common variation is a combined origin of the innominate and left common carotid arteries in about 10 to 13% of individuals, often termed a bovine aortic arch. The term *bovine aortic arch* is actually a misnomer because the branching pattern in cattle has a single trunk that splits into all the great vessels. In about 5% of the population, the left vertebral artery arises as a separate branch directly from the aorta, between the left common carotid artery and the left subclavian artery.[10]

◆ Congenital Anomalies of the Aorta and the Great Vessels

Congenital anomalies of the aorta and branching pattern of the great vessels may present as isolated anomalies or in association with other congenital cardiac malformations. Definition of the aortic malformation is based on the position and caliber of the aortic arch and its branches, the descending aorta, and the ductus or ligamentum arteriosum. Vascular rings are unusual congenital abnormalities in which the anomalous configuration of the arch or associated vessels forms a complete ring surrounding the trachea and esophagus and may result in symptoms related to compression. Vascular rings result from malformations of the primarily paired aortic arch or branching pulmonary arteries during embryogenesis.

The two most common types of complete vascular rings are double aortic arch (**Fig. 13.3**) and right aortic arch with an aberrant left subclavian artery (**Fig. 13.4**), comprising 85 to 95% of vascular rings. Double aortic arch results from a persistence of the embryologic double aortic arch with right and left arches arising from the ascending aorta and rejoining posteriorly after giving rise to their respective carotid and subclavian arteries. In the right aortic arch with an aberrant left subclavian artery, a left ligamentum arteriosum may connect the aberrant subclavian artery to the left pulmonary artery to complete the ring. Two other complete vascular rings that are extremely rare (<1%) include the right aortic arch with mirror-image branching and a left ligamentum arteriosum (**Fig. 13.5**) and left aortic arch with an aberrant retroesophageal right subclavian artery (**Fig. 13.6**), right-sided descending aorta, and right ligamentum arteriosum.[11] In infants and children, compression of the trachea and esophagus from vascular rings frequently cause symptoms of respiratory distress, recurrent pneumonia, bronchitis, stridor, and poor intake.[12]

Related vascular anomalies involving arch vessels that do not form a complete ring may produce similar symptoms from compression of the trachea or esophagus or may remain asymptomatic.[12] A right aortic arch crosses the mediastinum to the right of the trachea and esophagus and occurs in 0.1% of adults.[13,14] Right aortic arch anomalies include right aortic arch with an aberrant left subclavian artery; right aortic arch with mirror image branching; and right aortic arch with isolated left subclavian artery arising from the left pulmonary artery. Of these, only the right aortic arch with aberrant left subclavian artery is likely to be a source of symptomatic

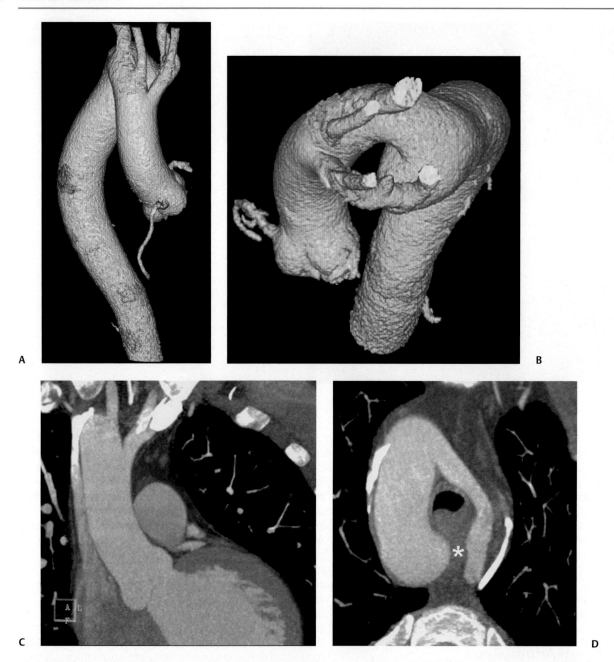

Fig. 13.3 Double aortic arch forms a vascular ring around the trachea and esophagus. **(A)** Anterior view demonstrates a larger right arch and a smaller left arch, each giving rise to an ipsilateral carotid and subclavian artery. **(B)** View from above clearly demonstrates the ring created by the two arches. **(C)** Coronal maximum intensity projection image demonstrates the ascending aorta as it divides into a larger right arch and a smaller left arch. **(D)** Axial view demonstrates that the trachea and esophagus are encircled by the vascular ring. The esophagus (*) is compressed from both sides.

tracheal–esophageal compression. Right aortic arch with mirror-image branching has a high likelihood of association with other forms of complex congenital heart disease but is not usually itself a cause of symptoms.[14] Isolated left subclavian artery is a rare cause of upper extremity ischemia.

Vascular rings are rare in adults. In one series of vascular rings first diagnosed in adults, the most common anomaly was double aortic arch (46%) (**Fig. 13.3**), followed by right

aortic arch with aberrant left subclavian artery and ligamentum arteriosum (30%) (**Fig. 13.4**). Only two thirds of adults in this report were symptomatic at diagnosis. Dysphagia and respiratory symptoms were the predominant presenting symptom in adults.[15–17] Exercise-induced dilatation of the aortic arch and age-dependent changes in thoracic compliance have been proposed as potential mechanisms of new-onset symptoms in the adult-diagnosed

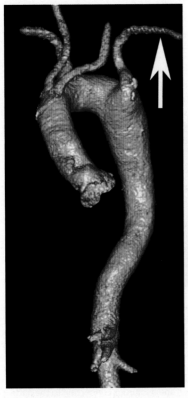

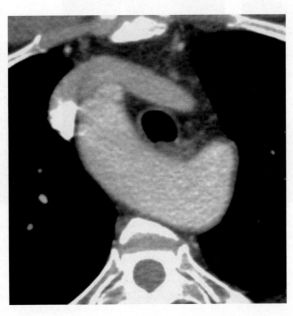

A

B

Fig. 13.4 Right-sided aortic arch with aberrant left subclavian artery. **(A)** Left anterior oblique view demonstrates four vessels arising from the right-sided arch. In the order of their origins from the arch, these vessels are the left common carotid artery, the right common carotid artery, the right subclavian artery, and the left subclavian artery (*arrow*). Note that the left subclavian artery originates with a broad-based origin—the diverticulum of Kommerell—from the distal aortic arch. **(B)** Axial image demonstrates the right-sided arch with the diverticulum of Kommerell passing behind the trachea and esophagus and giving rise to the aberrant left subclavian artery. A vascular ring may be completed by a left-sided ductus arteriosus (or its remnant, the ligamentum arteriosum) passing from the aberrant left subclavian artery to the proximal left pulmonary artery.

vascular ring patient.[15,16] Symptomatic vascular rings require operative intervention.

CTA is the ideal imaging modality to assess vascular rings. Three-dimensional reconstruction with and without volume rendering defines the morphology of the great vessels and their topography in relation to the adjacent soft tissue structures and allows pre-operative planning for surgical intervention. CT offers significant advantage over echocardiography in the delineation of the great vessels to the adjacent esophagus, trachea, and bronchi for surgical planning as well.[11]

◆ Aneurysmal Disease of the Ascending Aorta

Aneurysms of the thoracic aorta are most common in the ascending portion (**Fig. 13.7**). Whereas atherosclerosis is a common cause of all thoracic aortic aneurysms, this cause is rare for isolated ascending aortic aneurysms. The mechanism for isolated ascending aortic aneurysms is likely based on a genetic or acquired weakness in the aortic wall that renders these patients susceptible to hemodynamic-induced enlargement with time. Cystic medial degeneration is the most common cause of isolated ascending aortic aneurysm disease. In many patients, cystic medial degeneration may be the result of susceptibilities from genetic disorders such as Marfan syndrome, Ehler-Danlos syndrome, familial aneurysm disease, bicuspid aortic valve disease, or the inflammatory processes of infectious or noninfectious aortitis, including syphilis and Takayasu arteritis. Up to one third of cases are idiopathic with acceleration of the normal aging processes of elastic fiber fragmentation and smooth cell necrosis for unknown reasons.[18] Idiopathic cystic medial degeneration may represent an undefined susceptibility for accelerated degeneration in response to risk factors such as smoking and hypertension.

Marfan syndrome, a common inherited connective tissue disease caused by deficiency of the matrix protein fibrillin-1, affects the ocular, skeletal, and cardiovascular system.[19,20] Patients with Marfan syndrome demonstrate accelerated aneurysm growth and tend to dissect and rupture at smaller sizes, especially in patients with a family history of early complications and death. The average age of death for untreated patients with Marfan syndrome is 32 years, with aortic root complications implicated in

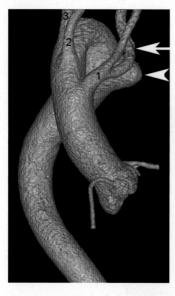
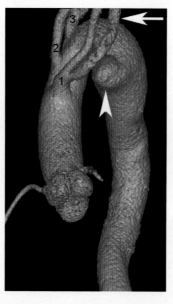
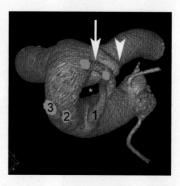

A–C

Fig. 13.5 Right-sided aortic arch with mirror image branching in an adult patient with dysphagia lusoria presenting as chest pain. **(A)** AP view demonstrates a right sided aortic arch with three great vessels. The first branch is a left innominate artery (1), followed by a right common carotid artery (2), and finally a right subclavian artery (3). The descending aorta is on the right side. A remnant of the distal portion of the left aortic arch presents as a diverticulum of the descending aorta (*arrowhead*), just posterior to the left subclavian artery (*arrow*). **(B)** Steep left anterior oblique projection demonstrates the proximity of the left subclavian artery (*arrow*) to the aortic diverticulum (*arrowhead*). In this highly unusual case, a fibrous connection between these two structures results in a vascular ring with associated esophageal compression. More commonly, a vascular ring may be present in a right-sided arch when a left-sided ductus arteriosus or ligamentum arteriosum passes between the left-sided descending aorta and the proximal left pulmonary artery. **(C)** View from above demonstrates the ring formed by the right arch, the left subclavian artery (*arrow*) and its fibrous connection to the aortic diverticulum (*arrowhead*). The trachea and esophagus pass within the ring (*).

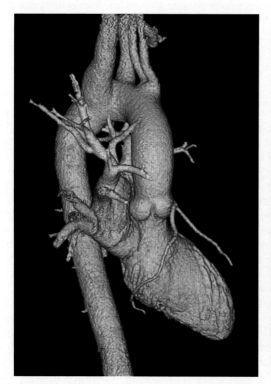
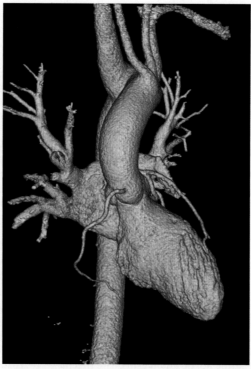

A

B

Fig. 13.6 Left-sided aortic arch with aberrant right subclavian artery. **(A)** Anterior view demonstrates the left-sided arch and left-sided heart structures, including the pulmonary veins. An aberrant subclavian artery originates from a broad-based diverticulum of Kommerell in the distal aortic arch. **(B)** Left anterior oblique view demonstrates the right coronary artery originating from the anterior sinus of Valsalva. The large aberrant subclavian artery is the fourth and final branch of the arch.

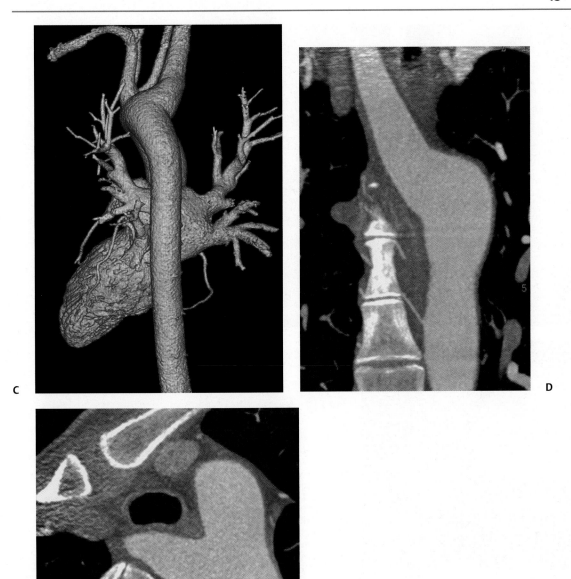

Fig. 13.6 (*Continued*) **(C)** Posterior view and **(D)** coronal maximum intensity projection demonstrate the aberrant origin of the right subclavian artery with a broad base from the distal aortic arch. The descending aorta remains on the left side. **(E)** Oblique axial view demonstrates the aortic arch to the left of the trachea and the origin of the aberrant right subclavian artery posterior to the trachea. A vascular ring is present when a right-sided ductus arteriosus or ligamentum arteriosum passes from the aberrant subclavian artery to the right pulmonary artery.

60 to 80% of deaths from acute heart failure, acute aortic dissection, and aortic rupture.[21] The classic aneurysm features in Marfan syndrome include a pear-shaped aneurysmal ascending aorta with smooth tapering to a normal aortic arch and has been termed *annuloaortic ectasia*. This condition is characterized by dilated sinuses of Valsalva with effacement of the sinotubular junction (**Fig. 13.8**).

Bicuspid aortic valve disease is the most common cardiac congenital anomaly, occurring in up to 2.0% of the population in the United States. Bicuspid aortic valve patients have an intrinsic smooth muscle abnormality that predisposes them to higher rates of cystic medial degeneration and ascending aortic enlargement and dissection.[22] These patients have an increased incidence of both aortic root enlargement and ascending aortic aneurysms independent of the function

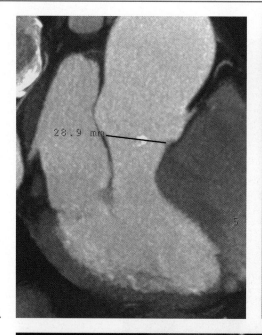

A

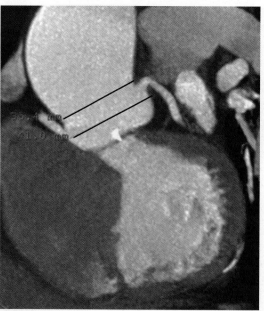

B

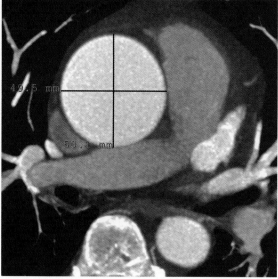

C

Fig. 13.7 Aneurysm of the aortic root and ascending aorta with preservation of the sinotubular junction. **(A)** Three-chamber view demonstrates measurement of the aortic annulus (2.9 cm) at the level of a mildly calcified aortic valve. **(B)** Left anterior oblique view demonstrates measurement of the aortic root at the level of the sinuses of Valsalva (4.1 cm) and at the sinotubular junction (3.5 cm). Although the root is dilated, a normal tapered appearance is present at the sinotubular junction. **(C)** Axial image through the ascending aorta demonstrates an aneurysm measuring 5 cm in diameter.

of their bicuspid valves, age, body size, and hypertension.[6,22] Patients with bicuspid aortic valve disease and aneurysmal dilation of the ascending aorta should be considered for earlier surgery because of the intrinsic weakness of the aorta (**Fig. 13.9**).

Syphilitic aortitis causes destruction of the aortic media with loss of elastic and smooth muscle fibers and subintimal scarring. These changes lead to aortic dilatation and aneurysms. The most common site of a syphilitic thoracic aneurysm is the ascending thoracic aorta, followed by the aortic arch, proximal descending thoracic aorta, and distal descending thoracic aorta. Sinus of Valsalva involvement is rare and usually asymmetric. Despite infrequent sinus involvement, syphilitic aortitis may be associated with narrowing of the coronary ostia due to subintimal scarring with myocardial ischemia.[23]

Aneurysm Size

The goal of surgical intervention on asymptomatic patients with aortic dilatation is to prevent rupture (**Fig. 13.10**) and aortic dissection (**Figs. 13.11** and **13.12**). In persons younger than 60 years, an ascending aortic diameter greater than 4 cm and a descending aortic diameter greater than 3 cm indicates dilatation; a diameter

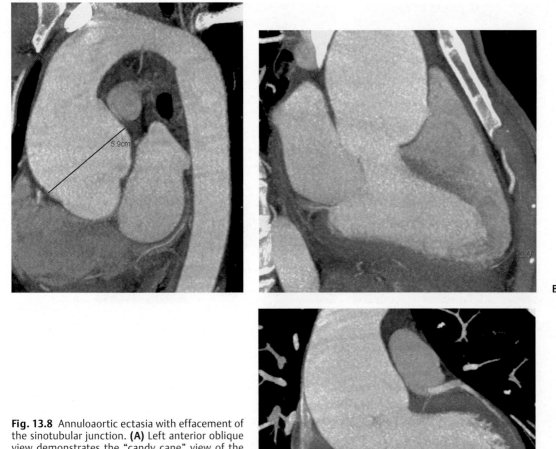

Fig. 13.8 Annuloaortic ectasia with effacement of the sinotubular junction. **(A)** Left anterior oblique view demonstrates the "candy cane" view of the thoracic aorta with dilatation of the aortic root and proximal ascending aorta to 5.9 cm. **(B)** Three-chamber view is approximately perpendicular to the view in (A) and again demonstrates dilatation of the proximal aorta with effacement of the sinotubular junction. **(C)** Coronal view demonstrates a dilated aorta above the aortic valve with no hint of a sinotubular junction.

greater than 1.5 times the expected normal diameter is defined as a thoracic aortic aneurysm.[24] The diameter of an aneurysm strongly correlates with the risk of rupture or dissection, but there is not a clear consensus of an absolute size indication for elective surgical repair in ascending aortic aneurysms.[20]

The Yale group reported rupture or dissection at a median size of 5.9 cm in the ascending aorta and 7.2 cm in the descending aorta with yearly rates of rupture or dissection about 7% and death 12% at or above these sizes.[19,20] On the basis of these data, the traditional threshold for elective surgical therapy in good-risk candidates has been 5.5 cm for ascending aortic aneurysms. To improve risk stratification, some centers have advocated using cross-sectional area with indexing to body size. Although volume measurements have been advanced by some as the best estimate of the risk of rupture, there are no adequate

natural history data for this approach.[24] Others have suggested the use of ratios of measured to expected size based on the body surface area and age, adjusted according to the underlying etiology.[25]

Growth

The rate of expansion is also an important consideration in thoracic aneurysm disease. In a large longitudinal study, the average rate of growth for all thoracic aneurysms was found to be 0.12 cm per year.[19] Longitudinal studies of the rate of expansion have reported greater rates of expansion in the descending aorta with Marfan syndrome, chronic dissection, and bicuspid valve disease.[26] Growth at a rate of greater than 1.0 cm per year is a widely accepted indication for surgical intervention.[25]

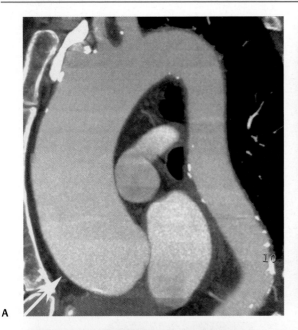

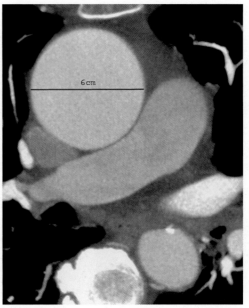

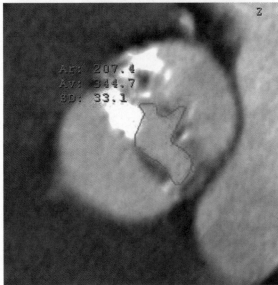

Fig. 13.9 Aortic aneurysm with bicuspid aortic valve. **(A)** Left anterior oblique view demonstrates a diffusely dilated ascending aorta (*arrow*) with no evidence of normal tapering at the sinotubular junction. **(B)** Axial image demonstrates a maximum diameter of 6 cm in the ascending aorta. **(C)** Systolic phase image through the aortic valve demonstrates a calcified bicuspid aortic valve with mild stenosis (valve area = 2.1 cm²). A bicuspid aortic valve is associated with abnormal properties of the ascending aorta that predispose to aortic aneurysm, dissection, and rupture at smaller diameters than the general population.

The Influence of Etiology

The individual benefit–risk assessment for intervention is based on the patient's composite risk of rupture and dissection as a function of size, rate of growth, etiology, associated disease, and surgical risk. Size thresholds for intervention in individual patients are adjusted for underlying etiology, recent rate of growth, and family history of complications. Patients with Marfan syndrome, Ehler-Danlos syndrome, familial aneurysms, and chronic dissection all likely benefit from earlier intervention. Patients with bicuspid aortic valves may be at increased risk and may warrant early surgical treatment.[6,27]

Surgical Planning

Preoperative CTA of the aorta is essential for surgical planning. Accurate assessment of aortic root size, rate of change, morphology of the aortic valve leaflets, and distal extent of the ascending aortic aneurysm is critical to plan the appropriate operation. Further presurgical assessment includes the presence of concomitant coronary disease, aortic valvular stenosis, and regurgitation and the status of the mitral valve. In patients with large aneurysms and effacement of the sinotubular junction, measurements of the aortic root diameter may be misleading. In these cases, assessing the cephalad displacement of the coronary ostia provides a

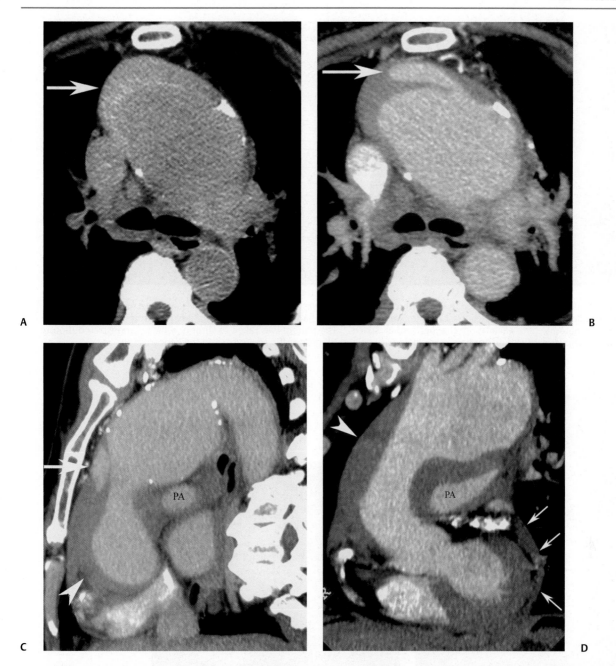

Fig. 13.10 Ascending aortic aneurysm with contained rupture into the pericardial space. **(A)** Axial view without intravenous contrast demonstrates a dense rim of hematoma (*arrow*) around the ascending aorta. **(B)** Post-contrast view at the same level demonstrates an aneurismal ascending aorta with contrast extending beyond the aorta anteriorly (*arrow*) into the hematoma. **(C)** Sagittal view again demonstrates contrast (*arrow*) anterior to the true lumen of the ascending aorta with hematoma extending down to the aortic root (*arrowhead*) and surrounding the pulmonary artery (PA). **(D)** Oblique view demonstrates hematoma anterior to the ascending aorta (*arrowhead*), surrounding the PA, and extending caudally inside the pericardium. (*Continued on page 320*)

measure of the integrity of the sinuses of Valsalva and the aortic root (**Fig. 13.13**). Assessing whether aortic regurgitation is related to the valve itself or to loss of sinotubular support (as seen in annuloaortic ectasia) is important when considering root preservation and valve-sparing techniques.

Ascending aortic aneurysms with normal sinuses and a normal aortic annulus may be treated with replacement of the ascending aorta from the sinotubular ridge to the origin of the innominate artery using a simple tube graft. If the aortic valve is diseased, a standard aortic valve replacement

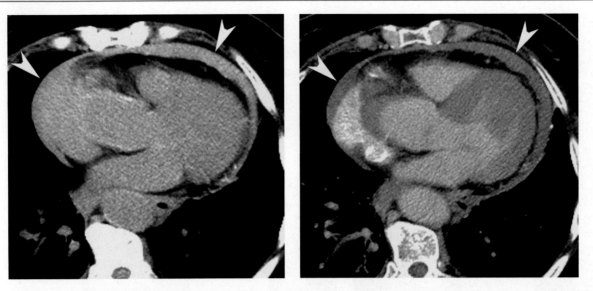

E   F

Fig. 13.10 (*Continued*) Ascending aortic aneurysm with contained rupture into the pericardial space. **(E)** Pre-contrast axial image demonstrates dense hematoma (*arrowheads*) in the pericardial space around the heart. **(F)** Pericardial fluid appears lower in density on a contrast-enhanced image at the same level (*arrowheads*). These findings had progressed from a study performed earlier the same day. The patient was taken to surgery, which demonstrated rupture of a thoracic aortic aneurysm into the pericardial space.

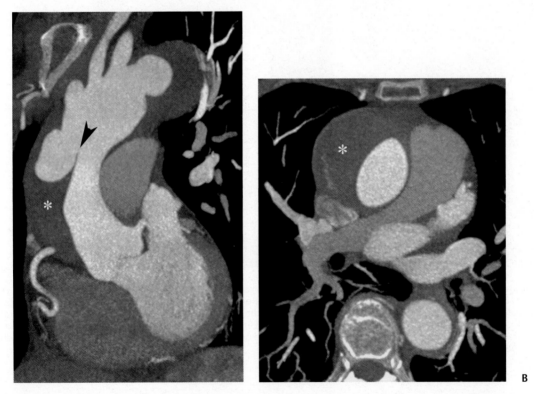

A   B

Fig. 13.11 Type A dissection with aneurysm of the ascending aorta (DeBakey type I). **(A)** Left anterior oblique projection of the ascending aorta demonstrates a dissection flap just proximal to the arch vessels (*arrowhead*). Extensive thrombus is present in the false lumen (***), extending down to the aortic root. **(B)** Axial view through the ascending aorta demonstrates aneurismal dilatation of the aorta with compression of the true lumen of the aorta by a thrombus-filled false lumen (***).

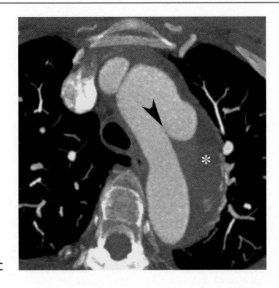

C

Fig. 13.11 (*Continued*) **(C)** Axial image through the arch demonstrates a more distal dissection flap (*arrowhead*) with thrombus in the false lumen along the arch (*). Any extension of this dissection may threaten the integrity of the aortic root, the coronary arteries, or the great vessels.

may be performed. In patients with marked effacement of the sinotubular junction and cephalad displacement of the coronary ostia, the aortic root should be replaced as a part of the index procedure. Patients with Marfan syndrome with significant dilatation of the aortic root and ascending aortic aneurysm should undergo replacement of both the aorta and root because of the high frequency of subsequent root-related complications and death. This approach involves replacing the ascending aorta and root with a valve

conduit, and reimplantation of the coronary arteries into the neosinuses.

Involvement of the sinuses of Valsalva in non-Marfan syndrome patients may be treated with valve-sparing aortic root reconstruction techniques or replacement of the aortic valve and reimplantation of the coronary arteries. In patients with extensive disease involving the arch or descending thoracic aorta, additional procedures such as arch replacement and "elephant trunk" procedures may be

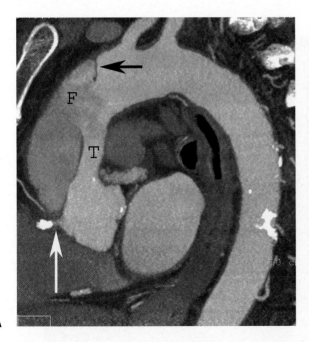

A

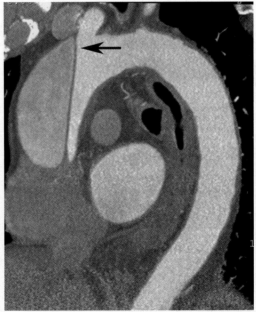

B

Fig. 13.12 Type A dissection of an aneurysmal ascending aorta (DeBakey Type II). **(A)** Left anterior oblique view demonstrates that the proximal extent of the dissection flap is at the ostium of the stented right coronary artery (*white arrow*). The distal extent of the flap is in the proximal arch (*black arrow*). There is bidirectional flow of blood between the true lumen (T) and false lumen (F) though a rent in the intimal flap. **(B)** Slightly different obliquity demonstrates that the distal extent of the dissection flap ends at the origin of the innominate artery (*arrow*). Dissection into a coronary artery or into a great vessel is an important source of morbidity and mortality with type A dissection. (*Continued on page 322*)

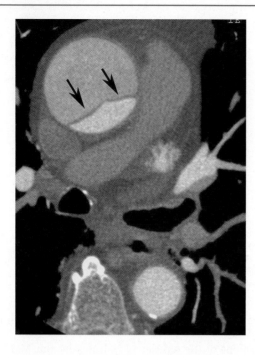

C

Fig. 13.12 (*Continued*) Type A dissection of an aneurysmal ascending aorta (DeBakey Type II). **(C)** Axial image demonstrates the intimal flap (*arrows*) with a brightly enhanced true lumen and a larger false lumen. The diameter of the ascending aorta at the level of the dissection (5.6 cm) measures approximately twice the diameter of the descending aorta.

performed under the same deep hypothermic circulatory arrest to treat all diseased aortic tissue and plan for additional future procedures. Novel approaches to treating aortic arch and descending thoracic aortic disease simultaneously through combined open surgery and endovascular stent graft deployment are currently under development.[28]

Follow-up

All patients who have undergone thoracic aortic surgery should have long-term follow-up with repeat imaging. Because complete resection of aortic tissue is not feasible and residual aortic tissue is often not normal, patients are at risk

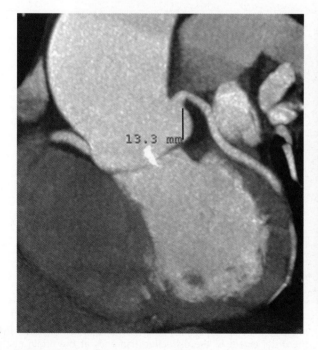

A

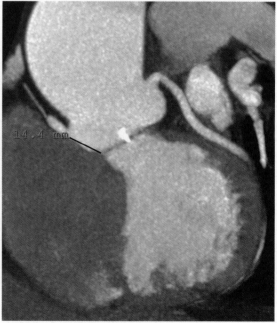

B

Fig. 13.13 Evaluation of the aortic root with measurement of the cephalad displacement of the coronary ostia from the aortic annulus. **(A)** Measurement of the superior displacement of the ostium of the left main coronary artery (in the same patient as figure 13.7). **(B)** Measurement of the superior displacement of the ostium of the right coronary artery. The coronary ostia are located just below the sinotubular junction (in the same patient as Fig. 13.7).

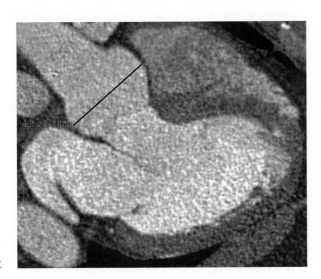

C

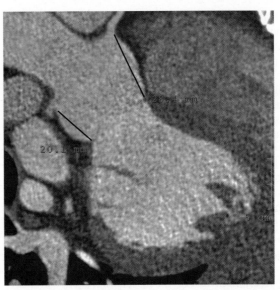

D

Fig. 13.13 (*Continued*) **(C)** Three chamber view in a different patient demonstrates dilatation of the aortic root to 4.3cm. **(D)** Measurements of the superior displacement of the coronary ostia in this second patient demonstrate that most of the dilatation is related to the right sinus of Valsalva. The RCA origin is 2.8cm above the aortic annulus, while the LCA origin is 2.0cm above the aortic annulus. The superior displacement of the coronary ostia provides the surgeon with a measurement of expansion and deformation of the aortic root.

for the subsequent aortic dissection, aneurysmal degeneration, and pseudoaneurysm formation. Routine scheduled surveillance CT or magnetic resonance imaging (MRI) is ideal for monitoring disease progression and for early detection of complications to avoid the increased morbidity and mortality of emergency reoperation. Patients at increased risk of reoperation, such as those with Marfan syndrome, familial aneurysms, or dissections, require more frequent follow-up.

◆ Sinus of Valsalva Aneurysm

Coronary sinus aneurysms are rare congenital anomalies more commonly reported in non-Western countries. These defects are thought to be congenital in origin, but up to half of the reported cases are defined as "acquired."[29] Sinus of Valsalva aneurysms may be associated with cystic medial necrosis, representing an anatomically localized aortic sinus defect of muscular and elastic tissue; however, these defects are rarely reported to be associated with ascending aortic aneurysm on presentation or follow-up. Sinus of Valsalva aneurysms most commonly involve a single sinus; the right aortic root sinus is involved in 70% of patients, the noncoronary sinus is involved in 29%, and the left coronary sinus is involved in only 1%.[30,31]

Sinus of Valsalva aneurysms commonly present with chest pain, cardiac arrest, or heart failure after rupture and development of an aortocardiac fistula.[30,31] Sinus of Valsalva aneurysms have been reported to rupture into all cardiac chambers, with fistulous communication seen most commonly into the right atrium and right ventricle. Intact sinus of Valsalva aneurysms should be treated when diagnosed because of the risk of rupture as well as the risk of enlargement with potential right ventricular outflow tract

obstruction, coronary artery occlusion, aortic regurgitation, complete heart block, and ventricular tachycardia.[29]

◆ Acute Aortic Diseases

Aortic dissection, intramural hematoma, and penetrating atherosclerotic ulcer represent a spectrum of pathologic processes in which the integrity of the aortic wall is breached. These entities are typically diagnosed in patients with acute chest pain who undergo imaging on an emergent basis. With increasing utilization of the "triple rule-out" scan in the emergency department (see Chapter 15), the detection of acute aortic disease is likely to increase.[32] In addition, these diagnoses may be found in the subacute or chronic phase in patients undergoing multislice–multidetector CT (MDCT) imaging for other indications. Establishing the precise disease entity and stage is essential for the timely treatment of acute aortic disease.

◆ Aortic Dissection

Aortic dissection is the most common acute aortic disorder, occurring in up to 0.8% of reported populations.[33] Prompt diagnosis is critical bcause mortality associated with this condition increases based on the time until detection and treatment. Aortic dissection is caused by blood entering the wall through an intimal tear with propagation in the media proximally or distally. Propagation of blood displaces the intima inward, resulting in a dissection flap that defines two lumina: a false lumen and true lumen. Aortic dissection may extend centrally to the aortic root, coronary ostia, and aortic valve or distally to the arch vessels, descending thoracic aorta, and mesenteric vessels.

The original DeBakey classification of aortic dissection categorized aortic dissection by the site of origin and the extent of dissection. Type 1 and 2 dissections originate in the ascending aorta. Type 1 extends to involve the arch and may extend beyond the arch (**Fig. 13.11**); type 2 is limited to the ascending aorta (**Fig. 13.12**). Type 3 dissection originates and involves the descending thoracic aorta. The Stanford system divides aortic dissection into type A and type B. Stanford type A dissection involves the ascending aorta (regardless of the site of origin), with or without involvement of descending aorta. Stanford type B involves the descending aorta with or without distal propagation. The Stanford classification has superseded the Debakey system because it reflects the dichotomy of treatment of aortic dissection: surgical intervention for type A dissection and medical treatment for type B dissection.

Ascending Aortic Dissection

When dissection involving the ascending aorta extends toward the aortic root (**Fig. 13.14**), potential complications include aortic valve regurgitation, occlusion of coronary artery ostia, and dissection or rupture into the pericardial cavity. Extension of the aortic dissection into the pericardium is associated with a high risk of cardiac tamponade. Extension of a dissection into the arch may result in involvement of the great vessels (**Fig. 13.15**). Death from aortic dissection is usually caused by acute aortic regurgitation, major branch-vessel obstruction, pericardial tamponade, aortic rupture, or stroke.

Conventional treatment of dissection involving the ascending aorta is surgical. Pre-operative imaging is used to demonstrate the extent of dissection, aortic root and arch vessel involvement, and the presence of re-entry tears. Additional imaging considerations include identifying sites for peripheral cardiopulmonary bypass (typically the right axillary or femoral arteries) and the status of cerebral, visceral, and extremity perfusion. The presence of aortic aneurysmal disease as well as underlying conditions that may predispose to dissection and rupture should be evaluated on pre-operative imaging. Whereas most patients with type A aortic dissection are effectively treated by grafting from the sinotubular ridge to the arch, patients with Marfan syndrome, extensive aortic aneurysmal disease, or bicuspid aortic valve may be treated with root, valve, and "elephant trunk" procedures as appropriate.[34-36] In addition to its application to pre-operative planning, CTA can be useful for post-operative evaluation following ascending aorta and aortic root surgery (**Fig. 13.16**).

Descending Thoracic Aortic Dissection

Type B dissection tends to affect an older population with a higher prevalence of hypertension compared with type A dissection. Medical treatment of type B aortic dissection is aimed at effective blood pressure control and monitoring for complications of dissection, including poor end-organ perfusion, retrograde extension, and signs of impending rupture. Ischemic complications to the kidneys, spinal cord,

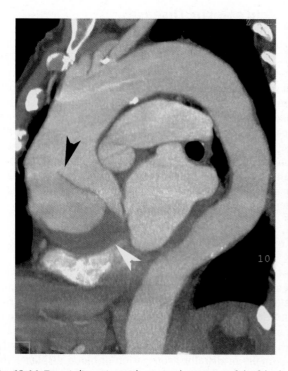 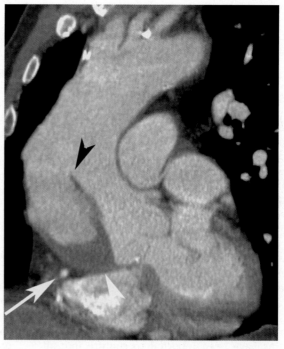

A   **B**

Fig. 13.14 Type A dissection with proximal extension of the false lumen alongside the aortic root, extending down to the level of the aortic valve. **(A)** Left anterior oblique view demonstrates a dissection flap in the ascending aorta (*black arrowhead*) with thrombus within the false lumen (*white arrowhead*). **(B)** Coronal view demonstrates a dissection flap in the ascending aorta (*black arrowhead*) with a false lumen extending down along the right side of the aortic root, between the aortic root and the right coronary artery (*arrow*). Thrombus is present at the inferior extent of the false lumen (*white arrowhead*), which is at the level of the aortic annulus. There is no evidence of pericardial effusion at this time.

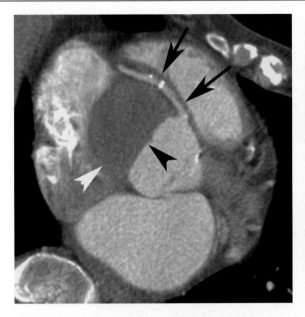

C

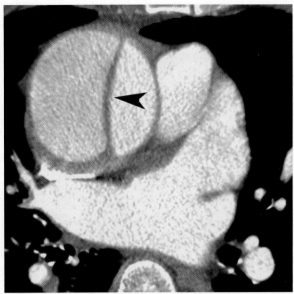

D

Fig. 13.14 (*Continued*) **(C)** Short-axis image through the aortic root demonstrates the thrombosed false lumen (*white arrowhead*) with mass effect on the aortic root (*black arrowhead*). The right coronary artery (*arrows*) is draped around the thrombosed false lumen. **(D)** Axial image demonstrates the dissection flap in the dilated ascending aorta (*arrowhead*). The smaller true lumen on the left side demonstrates a greater level of contrast enhancement compared with the larger false lumen on the right side. The dissection flap is often convex away from the true lumen.

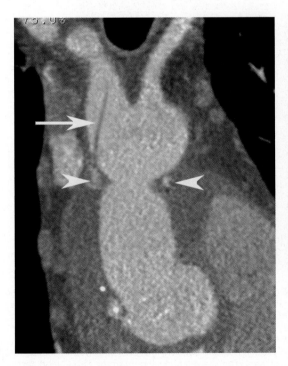

A

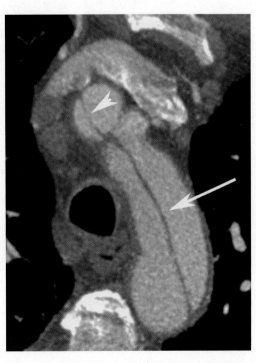

B

Fig. 13.15 Two patients with type A dissection, status-post repair with graft in the ascending aorta. A residual dissection flap is present in the native ascending aorta just beyond the graft anastomosis, extending into the innominate artery and down the descending thoracic aorta. Patient 1: **(A)** Coronal view of the ascending aorta demonstrates mild narrowing at the level of an anastomosis between a tube graft and the proximal aortic arch (*arrowheads*), with a dissection flap extending from the anastomosis into the innominate artery (*arrow*). **(B)** Axial view of the aortic arch demonstrates a dissection flap within the arch (*arrow*) and also extending into the innominate artery (*arrowhead*). (*Continued on page 326*)

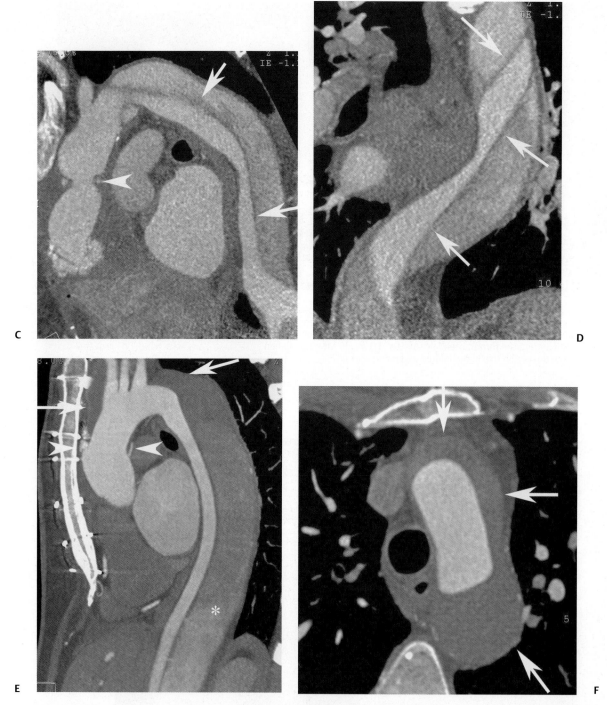

C

D

E

F

Fig. 13.15 (*Continued*) Two patients with type A dissection, status-post repair with graft in the ascending aorta. A residual dissection flap is present in the native ascending aorta just beyond the graft anastomosis, extending into the innominate artery and down the descending thoracic aorta. **(C)** Left anterior oblique view of the thoracic aorta demonstrates narrowing at the distal anastomosis of the ascending aortic graft (*arrowhead*) with a dissection flap extending through the arch and descending thoracic aorta (*arrows*). **(D)** Coronal view of the descending thoracic aorta demonstrates the spiral course of the dissection flap, extending into the abdomen. The presence of a persistent false lumen is associated with a poorer long-term prognosis. Patient 2: **(E)** Left anterior oblique view of the thoracic aorta demonstrates suture at the upper end of the ascending aortic graft (*arrowheads*) with an unopacified false lumen anterior to the native ascending aorta and surrounding the arch (*arrows*). The false lumen demonstrates progressive enhancement in the descending aorta (*). **(F)** Axial slice through the arch demonstrates the opacified true lumen surrounded by an unopacified false lumen (*arrows*).

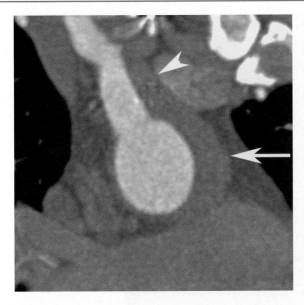
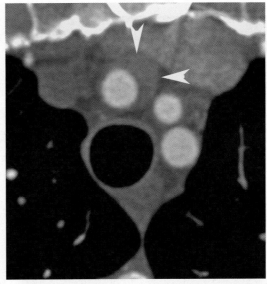

Fig. 13.15 (*Continued*) **(G)** Oblique coronal view through the aortic arch again demonstrates the false lumen around the left side of the arch (*arrow*) and extending along the innominate artery (*arrowhead*). **(H)** Axial slice through the great vessels demonstrates the false lumen extending around the innominate artery. The false lumen in this patient presents as unopacified tissue surrounding the innominate artery rather than an obvious flap within the vessel.

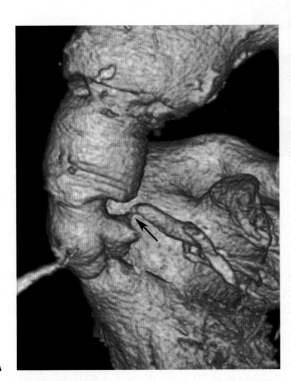
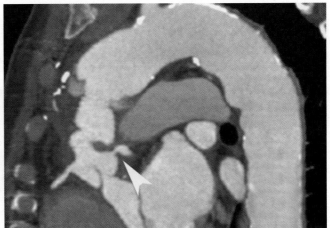
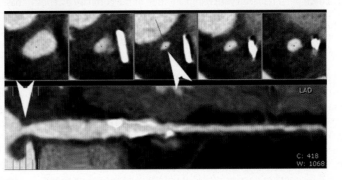

Fig. 13.16 Evaluation of the proximal aorta after a Bentall procedure in two patients. The aortic valve, aortic root, and ascending aorta have been replaced with reimplantation of the coronary arteries into the graft. First patient: **(A)** Volumetric rendering demonstrates the origins of both coronary arteries from the prosthetic aortic root with narrowing of the left coronary artery (*arrow*). **(B)** Slab MIP of the aortic arch again demonstrates the graft in the ascending aorta with a small amount of fluid anteriorly and narrowing at the origin of the left coronary artery (*arrowhead*). **(C)** Straightened lumen view of the left coronary artery based upon a tracked reconstruction confirms the stenosis at the origin of the left coronary artery (*arrowhead*) with flattening of the vessel origin on short axis (*arrowhead*). (Images courtesy of Robert Quaife, MD; University of Colorado–Denver). (*Continued on page 328*)

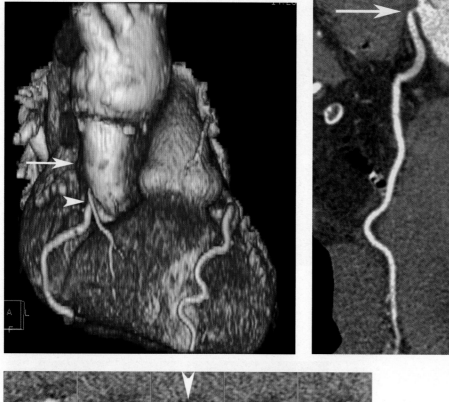

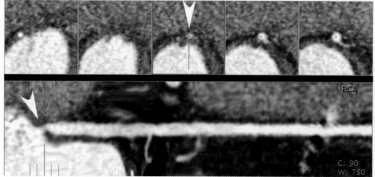

Fig. 13.16 (*Continued*) Evaluation of the proximal aorta after a Bentall procedure in two patients. The aortic valve, aortic root, and ascending aorta have been replaced with reimplantation of the coronary arteries into the graft. Second patient: **(D)** Volumetric rendering demonstrates a graft which replaces the aortic root and proximal ascending aorta (*arrow*). The right coronary artery originates from the graft (*arrowhead*).

(E) Slab MIP demonstrates an anastomatic stricture at the origin of the RCA (*arrow*). **(F)** Straightened lumen view of the right coronary artery based upon a tracked reconstruction confirms a high grade anastomatic stricture at the origin of the RCA (*arrowheads*), with no other evidence of coronary disease.

viscera, or extremities may prompt classic open surgery, endovascular fenestration, or thoracic endovascular aortic repair.[37–39] Data from the International Registry of Aortic Dissection (IRAD) report that the survival rate with the medical management of uncomplicated type B dissection approaches 90%, with most deaths occurring during the first week of hospitalization.[33] Open surgery for complications of type B dissection carries a risk of spinal cord injury or mortality of up to 67%.[40]

CTA is the method of choice for diagnostic imaging and follow-up of type B dissection. The radiologic evaluation of the type B dissection should assess the origin of the tear, aortic size, retrograde propagation, extent of dissection, and perfusion of the abdominal viscera and extremities. The aorta is evaluated for evidence of rupture, which may be suggested by loss of definition of the aortic wall, adjacent hematoma, or high-density pleural fluid.

Descending Thoracic Aortic Dissection with Retrograde Extension to the Ascending Aorta

The management of patients with an intimal tear in the descending aorta and retrograde extension into the arch and ascending aorta is controversial. This subset was identified in up to 20% of patients in several series of acute ascending aortic dissection.[41,42] Data from IRAD on patients treated with medical management did not show a difference in survival between patients with an intimal tear in the descending aorta and retrograde extension into the arch and standard type B dissection patients.[43] Indications for early surgery in this patient subset include continued patency of the false lumen, enlargement of the ascending aorta and arch, moderate to severe aortic regurgitation, and rupture of the aorta.[44]

Progression of Aortic Dissection

Long-term follow-up is necessary for all patients after acute aortic dissection, along with medical therapy to control underlying hypertension and modification of cardiovascular risk factors. The disrupted layers of the aorta are less resistant to the pulsatile force of arterial blood and are at risk for subsequent diameter expansion and rupture. Aortic size at the time of initial type B dissection is an important predictor of future need for descending aortic replacement. Other prognostic factors include patency of the false lumen after repair of type A aortic dissection and rate of growth of the descending thoracic aorta during the first post-operative year.[45,46] Timing of surgery to replace a dissecting thoracic aneurysm is based on aneurysm size, rate of growth, extent of dissection, and underlying etiology.[47,48] The role of emerging endovascular techniques in chronic dissection is undefined at present because of a lack of proven benefit and complication rates.[49]

The role of endovascular therapy in acute and subacute type B dissection is currently under investigation in randomized trials. If re-establishing aortic continuity with endovascular repair can alter the natural history of the dissected aorta, dissecting aneurysm may be preventable.[37,50] However, current reports of endovascular repair for acute type B dissection do not show improvement in short- or medium-term survival despite significantly increased rates of aortic remodeling compared with medical therapy.[50] The lack of survival benefit in initial randomized clinical trials brings into question the benefit of intervening in the acutely injured aorta.

◆ Intramural Hematoma

Intramural hematoma (IMH) is defined as hemorrhage within the media without evidence of an intimal tear. IMH results from spontaneous hemorrhage of the vasa vasorum of the medial layer. This hematoma weakens the medial layer but does not displace the intima inward as in classic aortic dissection. IMH has been viewed as a precursor of aortic dissection, representing either an early stage or a variant of dissection. Localized intramural hematoma, diffuse hemorrhage into the aortic media, and penetrating aortic ulcers are now considered abnormalities on the continuum of aortic wall injury, with possible outcomes leading to acute aortic dissection, aortic rupture, and aortic aneurysm formation.[51] Intramural hematoma comprises

about 8% of all acute aortic syndromes,[52] with an age distribution very similar to type B aortic dissection.[20]

Mortality risk is highest with a proximal site of IMH (**Fig. 13.17**) and progressively lower with a more distal site (**Fig. 13.18**). Mortality is 60% from IMH in the aortic root, 50% in the proximal ascending aorta, 33% in the distal ascending aorta, and 10% in the descending thoracic aorta.[33] The nonclassic aortic dissection entities have been classified by Svensson et al as types I through V according to the extent of aortic injury[53] and by Eggebrecht and colleagues into communicating, noncommunicating, antegrade, and retrograde dissection types.[51] These descriptive classifications provide insight into the natural history and prognosis for IMH beyond the risk of rupture and death in the IRAD registry.

CT evidence for IMH includes hyperattenuating cresentic hematoma eccentrically within the aortic wall (best defined on noncontrast CT) (**Fig. 13.17A**), absence of a dissection membrane, and circular or crescentic thickening of the aortic wall with central displacement of intimal calcification. Characteristic clinical symptoms are often required to differentiate IMH from the radiographically similar entities of subacute noncommunicating dissection with a thrombosed false channel, aortitis, tumor, and soft plaque. MRI criteria for acute IMH include high signal on T2-weighted images with isointense signal on T1-weighted images and no enhancement after injection of contrast media.[54] In some instances, depending on the initial imaging study, IMH may be difficult to differentiate from mural thrombus related to penetrating ulcer of the aorta. Transesophageal echocardiography may offer advantages for the diagnosis of IMH by showing the intact aortic intima, excluding a Doppler flow communication with the aortic lumen, and demonstrating the "echo-free space" seen in 60% of IMH cases.[55]

Aortic wall configuration in IMH has been observed to change rapidly.[55] Hemorrhage into the aortic media may be self-limiting, but this event triggers a dynamic process that may progress to circumferential and longitudinal extension of medial hemorrhage, classic dissection, aortic rupture, or rapid aneurysmal dilatation of the aorta. Temporal information about progression of IMH can sometimes be inferred from MRI. T1-weighted spin-echo images show intermediate signal intensity caused by the presence of oxyhemoglobin in the acute stage and hyperintensity with the formation of methemoglobin within the evolving hematoma.[54] The temporal discrimination of MRI in IMH may be helpful in estimating acuity at the time of presentation to guide medical versus surgical therapy.

Given the dynamic nature of IMH and mortality risk of acute type A dissection, emergent surgical therapy is traditionally recommended for type A IMH (**Fig. 13.17**). However, older patients treated by medical therapy alone may have a favorable outcome, with mortality approaching 10%.[56] Studies observing complete resolution of IMH on short-term imaging reassessment have supported a noninterventional approach to IMH.[57] With selective operation, Kang and colleagues reported progression rates

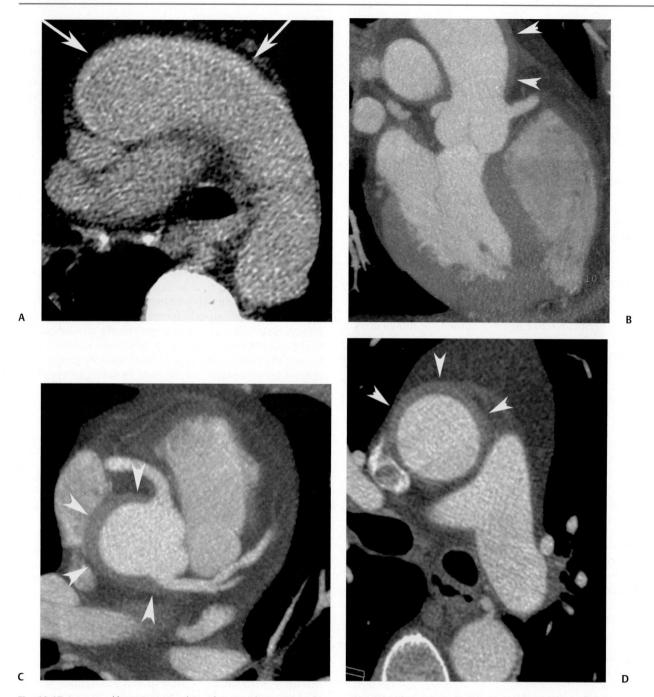

Fig. 13.17 Intramural hematoma involving the ascending aorta and extending from the aortic root into the aortic arch. **(A)** Pre-constrast image through the arch demonstrates intramural density corresponding to hematoma within the wall of the ascending aorta and proximal arch (*arrows*). **(B)** CT angiography (CTA) confirms mural thickening and demon-strates extension of the thickening down to the aortic root (*arrowheads*). **(C)** Axial image from CTA confirms that the intramural hematoma extends into the aortic root (*arrowheads*) up to the origins of the coronary arteries. **(D)** Axial image in the ascending aorta demonstrates the circumferential nature of the intramural hematoma in the ascending aorta.

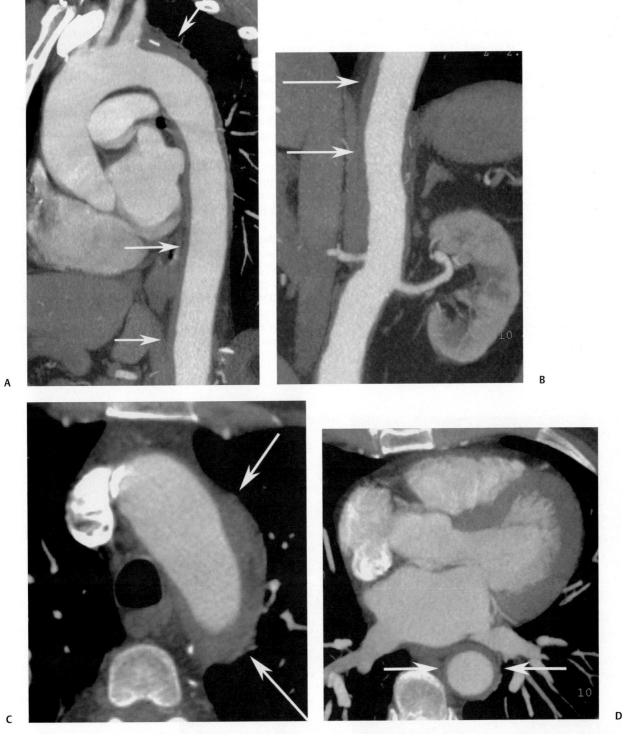

Fig. 13.18 Intramural hematoma extending from the distal aortic arch into the descending thoracic and upper abdominal aorta. **(A)** Left anterior oblique view of the aortic arch demonstrates diffuse thickening of the distal arch and descending aorta beyond the subclavian artery (*arrows*). **(B)** Coronal view of the lower thoracic and upper abdominal aorta demonstrates that the thickening persists (*arrows*) down to the level of the renal arteries (*arrowheads*). **(C)** Axial image of the aortic arch demonstrates mural thickening along the distal half of the aortic arch. **(D)** Axial image of the descending aorta confirms the circumferential mural thickening of the descending aorta (*arrows*). This patient appeared stable but progressed to a frank symptomatic dissection the day after this scan.

of only 15% and acceptable survival of medically treated type A IMH patients despite initial presentation with pericardial or mediastinal effusions.[58] Factors predictive of IMH progression include recurrent or persisting pain, the presence of penetrating aortic ulcer, and an ascending aortic diameter greater than 5 cm at the first examination.[59] Predictors of an overall favorable prognosis and regression of IMH include an aortic diameter less than 5 cm, regression of the hematoma during medical therapy, younger age, and hematoma thickness less than 1.0 cm.[59,60]

Treatment strategies for IMH should be individualized under close monitoring conditions.[61] Symptomatic patients, patients with progression on repeat imaging, and patients with an ascending aorta size larger than 5 cm should undergo emergent/urgent surgery. Patients who can be stabilized with antihypertensive therapy and medical management as well as patients with a high surgical risk may be treated medically with acceptable results. To date, no prospective randomized clinical trial has explored advanced imaging to direct therapy. However, the dynamic nature of IMH with propensity for regression and progression to classic dissection necessitates that all patients, regardless of outcome from the acute event, have long-term follow-up by aortic specialists.[62]

◆ Penetrating Atherosclerotic Ulcer

Penetrating atherosclerotic ulcer (PAU) is defined as an ulceration of atheromatous plaque that has eroded the inner, elastic layer of the aortic wall, reached the medial layer, and produced a hematoma in the media (**Fig. 13.19**). This pathologic condition is distinct from classic aortic dissection and aortic rupture but may represent a midpoint (or an alternative pathway) in the evolution of this process. The evolution of a penetrating atherosclerotic ulcer begins with aortic atheroma and progresses to plaque ulceration. Penetrating ulcers are initially contained in the intima, then extend into the media, then to hematoma formation with adventitial false aneurysm, and finally to transmural rupture (**Fig. 13.20**). Penetrating atherosclerotic ulcer is typically seen in older hypertensive individuals in a similar distribution to type B aortic dissection.

The natural history of PAU is variable, with both progression and resolution reported in the literature. Some clinicians suggest that PAU may have a poorer prognosis than classic aortic dissection based on observational studies.[63,64] Most reports document slow rates of disease progression and low rates of acute rupture in asymptomatic patients. Symptomatic patients with back or chest pain demonstrate higher rates of progression and complications.[63,65] Pain may

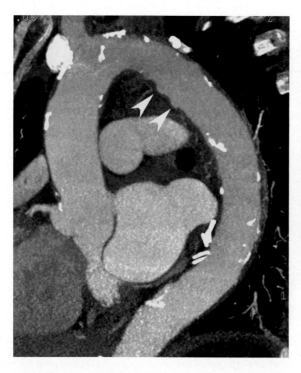
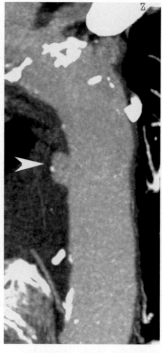

A

B

Fig. 13.19 Atherosclerotic disease of the aorta with penetrating atherosclerotic ulcers on the undersurface of the aortic arch. **(A)** Slab maximum intensity projection (MIP) view of the aortic arch in the left anterior oblique projection demonstrates diffuse atherosclerotic calcifications as well as intimal irregularity. In addition, two small penetrating ulcers are identified on the undersurface of the arch (*arrowheads*). **(B)** MIP view of the proximal descending aorta in a slightly different obliquity demonstrates one of the two penetrating ulcers to better advantage, clearly demonstrating projection of the contrast material beyond the expected location of the aortic intima. Based on the level of penetration, this ulcer would be classified as a pseudoaneurysm. Although a ductus diverticulum (Fig 13.2) might be seen at this location, the presence of two outpouchings extending from an atherosclerotic aorta at acute angles suggests that these represent ulcerations.

be one of the most important prognostic variables for progression and to identify patients who may benefit from surgical intervention.[66,67]

Accepted indications for considering surgical intervention with grafting of the affected area include persistent or recurrent pain, hemodynamic instability, rapidly expanding aortic diameter, contained hematoma, or impending aortic rupture. Many of these lesions are amenable to endovascular treatment.[51,58,61,63] Current clinical investigations seek to identify patients at increased risk for disease progression to define an emerging role for endovascular treatment of PAU.[51] An increasing role of endovascular therapy may shift the benefit–risk profile for treatment of patients with penetrating atherosclerotic ulcers of the aorta.

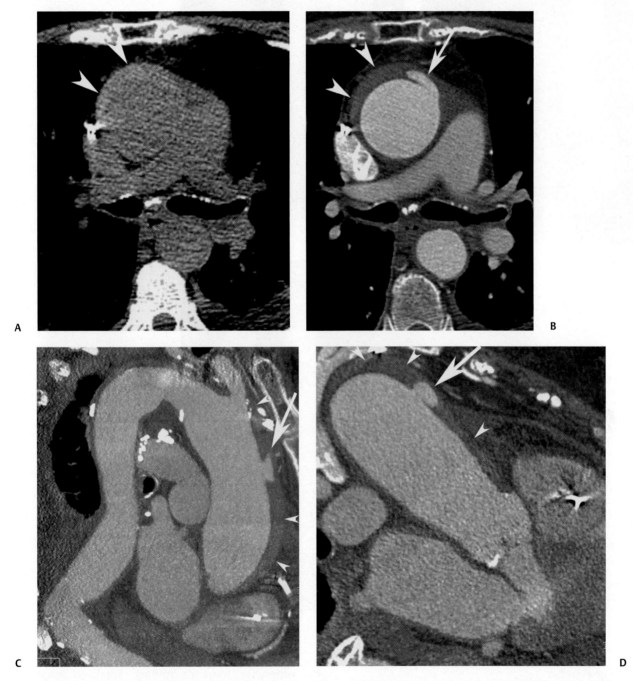

Fig. 13.20 Penetrating atherosclerotic ulcer with rupture into the subadventitial space of the ascending aorta. **(A)** Pre-contrast axial image demonstrates a subtle rim of high-density hematoma around the anterior aspect of the ascending aorta (*arrowheads*). **(B)** CT angiogram with axial image at the same level demonstrates a penetrating ulcer from the left anterior aspect of the ascending aorta (*arrow*) within the hematoma (*arrowheads*). **(C)** Right anterior oblique projection again demonstrates the penetrating ulcer (*arrow*) as well as the hematoma that extends from the aortic root to the origin of the innominate artery (*arrowheads*). **(D)** Three-chamber view demonstrates the penetrating ulcer (*arrow*) as well as the surrounding hematoma (*arrowheads*). (Continued on page 334)

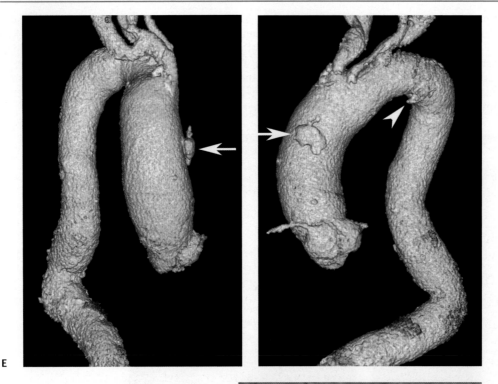

E   F

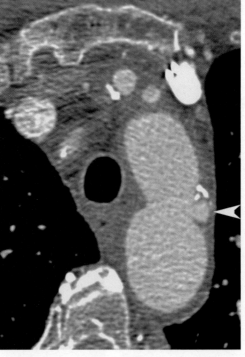

Fig. 13.20 (*Continued*) Penetrating athero-sclerotic ulcer with rupture into the sub-adventitial space of the ascending aorta. **(E)** Volumetric rendering in a right anterior oblique projection demonstrates the penetrating ulcer (*arrow*) projecting off the left anterior aspect of the ascending aorta. **(F)** Volumetric rendering in a left anterior oblique projection again demonstrates the penetrating ulcer on the anterior aspect of the ascending aorta (*arrow*), along with a second penetrating ulcer along the left side of the aortic arch (*arrowhead*). **(G)** Axial image through the aortic arch demonstrates the second penetrating ulcer (*arrowhead*) with no evidence of surrounding hematoma. Note that this ulcer extends laterally from the arch and has a narrow neck, in contrast to a ductus diverticulum that would extend inferiorly with a smooth, wide neck.

G

◆ Post-Operative Appearance of the Aorta

The post-surgical appearance after thoracic aortic surgery depends on the surgical technique and changes with time. Small pockets of air in the perigraft space may dissipate in the immediate post-operative period; however, the use of surgical hemostatic adjuvants and fibrin glue may prolong this otherwise transient finding. Small to moderate amounts of low-attenuation perigraft material within the first several months following graft replacement are common (**Fig. 13.21**). This material probably represents a combination of seroma, resolving hematoma, inflammatory fluid, and granulation tissue. Such collections tend to

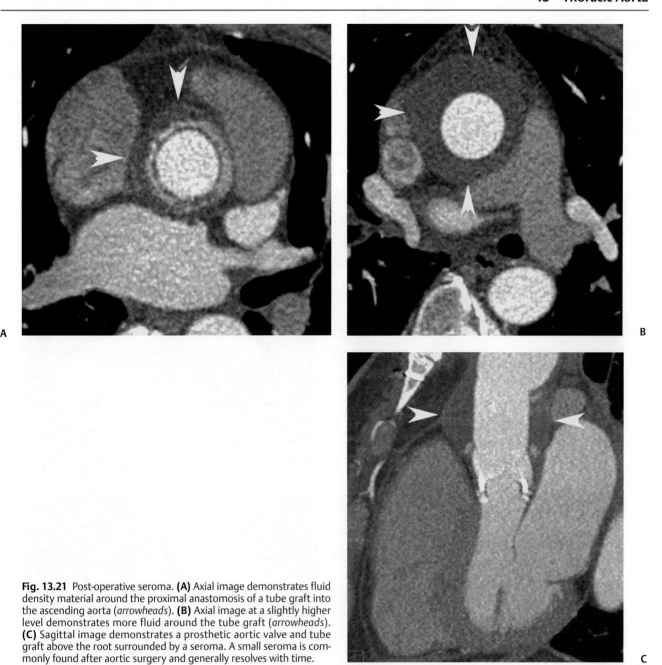

Fig. 13.21 Post-operative seroma. **(A)** Axial image demonstrates fluid density material around the proximal anastomosis of a tube graft into the ascending aorta (*arrowheads*). **(B)** Axial image at a slightly higher level demonstrates more fluid around the tube graft (*arrowheads*). **(C)** Sagittal image demonstrates a prosthetic aortic valve and tube graft above the root surrounded by a seroma. A small seroma is commonly found after aortic surgery and generally resolves with time.

resolve slowly over time, although some remain stable for months (**Fig. 13.22**).[69] Familiarity with these aspects of the radiographic appearances of the post-surgical aorta is essential to identify normal post-operative findings and to recognize potentially life-threatening complications.[69–71]

The anatomic appearance of the reconstructed aorta and graft may be confounding. In the setting of excess graft length and kinking, axial imaging assessment alone may suggest the appearance of a residual dissection flap.[70,71] Multiplanar reconstructions can be helpful in confirming the integrity of graft–aorta anastomosis and assessing the length and alignment (**Figs. 13.22** and **13.23**). Three-dimensional reconstructed images may also assist in

differentiating post-operative pseudoaneurysms from ligated graft branches, and in defining extra-anatomic reconstruction such as arch reconstruction techniques and hybrid debranching procedures.[28,72]

The CT finding of perigraft flow in the early or intermediate post-surgical periods may be normal, depending on timing and subsequent evolution. Small wisps of contrast extravasation in the immediate post-surgical period are often benign and resolve without intervention. Patients with requirements for anticoagulation may have persistent small jets of perigraft flow communicating into perigraft clot. If the size of perigraft clot increases significantly over time, infection and graft dehiscence should be considered. A further increase in low-attenuation perigraft fluid suggests concomitant infection.[70,73]

Following thoracic aorta surgery, surveillance imaging should be obtained at suitable intervals for life because the time of onset of complications is highly variable. Dehiscence may be seen at any time following surgery, even many years afterward. New or significantly enlarged contrast extravasation usually represents an urgent finding on any follow-up imaging study. Whereas small amounts of contrast material may pool between the graft and the surrounding native aorta in patients with residual aortic tissue, an increase in the amount of material in this space suggests graft dehiscence and may be an indication for closer radiographic follow-up or surgical intervention.[69,70,73,74] Lastly, lifetime follow-up for endovascular intervention of the thoracic aorta is also necessary to monitor aneurysm progression, the presence or progression of endoleaks, and the stability of the aortic prosthesis.

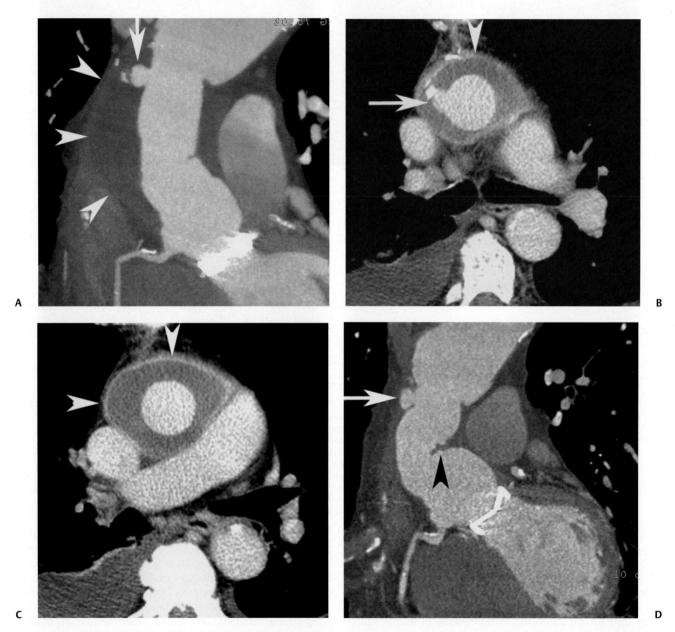

Fig. 13.22 Post-operative seroma with pseudoaneurysm. **(A)** Maximum intensity projection (MIP) view in the left anterior oblique projection after replacement of the aortic root and ascending aorta demonstrates the presence of a moderate size perigraft seroma (*arrowheads*) anterior to the graft, along with a pseudoaneurysm in the upper portion of the graft (*top arrow*). Axial images through the graft **(B)** at the level of the pseudoaneurysm (*arrow*) and **(C)** in the more proximal ascending aorta demonstrate the moderate size perigraft seroma (*arrowheads*) with enhancing tissue around the seroma. **(D)** MIP view in the left anterior oblique projection 2 years later demonstrates resolution of the perigraft seroma with a residual pseudoaneurysm in the upper portion of the graft (*top arrow*). Note that the components of the graft have changed in position with a resulting kink in the ascending aorta (*arrowhead*).

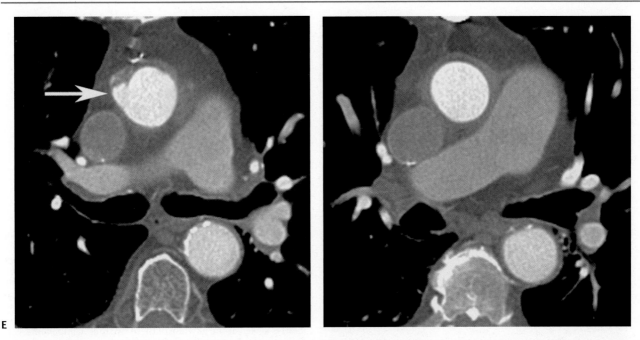

E   F

Fig. 13.22 (*Continued*) Axial images **(E)** at the level of the pseudoaneurysm (*arrow*) and **(F)** in the more proximal ascending aorta confirm the small persistent pseudoaneurysm with complete resolution of the perigraft seroma.

◆ Pseudoaneurysms of the Aorta

Pseudoaneurysm, or false aneurysm formation, of the thoracic aorta results from transmural disruption of the aorta, with the leak contained by the surrounding mediastinal structures preventing frank rupture. Pseudoaneurysms related to penetrating atherosclerotic aortic ulcers were discussed in a preceding section. Additional causes include previous cardiac surgery, infection, or trauma. Previous cardiac surgery is the most frequent cause of thoracic

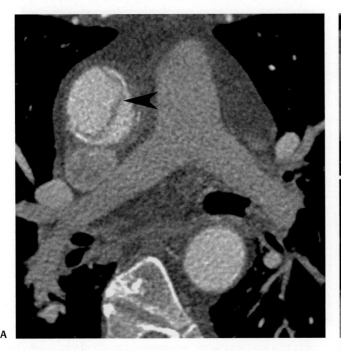

A

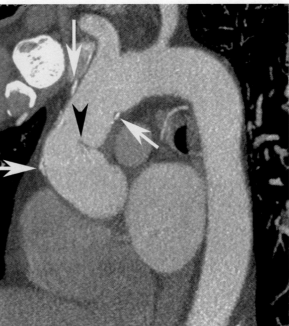

B

Fig. 13.23 Kinked graft in the ascending aorta mimicking the presence of a dissection flap on axial imaging. **(A)** Axial scan through the ascending and descending aorta demonstrates an apparent flap within the lumen of the ascending aorta (*arrowhead*), suggesting the presence of a dissection. **(B)** Slab maximum intensity projection view of the thoracic aorta in the left anterior oblique projection demonstrates suture lines along the graft (*arrows*) as well as a linear projection extending into the lumen of the aorta (*black arrowhead*).   (*Continued on page 338*)

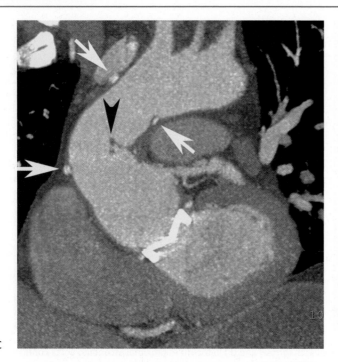

C

Fig. 13.23 (*Continued*) Kinked graft in the ascending aorta mimicking the presence of a dissection flap on axial imaging. **(C)** In a slightly different obliquity, the mechanical aortic prosthesis is seen along with the suture lines in the ascending aorta (*arrows*). The linear projection extending into the lumen (*black arrowhead*) corresponds to the suture line between two components of the graft. The more central component extends from the mechanical valve, while the more distal component ends just proximal to the arch vessels. The graft is kinked at the junction of these two graft components, with the suture line projecting into the lumen of the grafts.

aortic pseudoaneurysms, with an estimated incidence of less than 0.5% of all cardiac surgical cases.[75] Sites of previous aortotomy, graft anastomosis (**Fig. 13.24**), cannulation (**Fig. 13.25**), vent needles (**Fig. 13.26**), and proximal vein graft anastomosis have all been reported as sites of pseudoaneurysm formation.[76] Infection, poor anastomotic technique, and intrinsic aortic wall disease have been implicated as predisposing risk factors for pseudoaneurysm

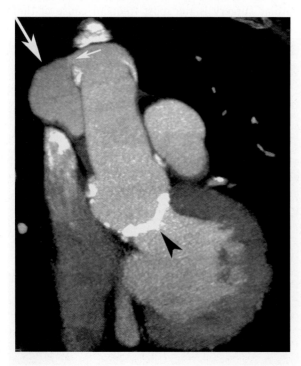

A

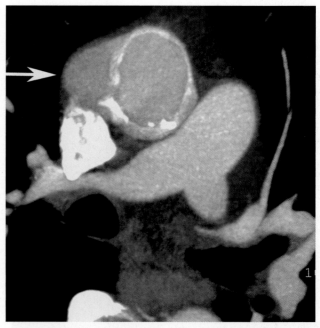

B

Fig. 13.24 Pseudoaneurysm of the ascending aorta following aortic valve and proximal ascending aortic replacement. **(A)** Coronal view through the ascending aorta demonstrates a mechanical aortic valve replacement in a normal closed position during diastole (*arrowhead*). The proximal ascending aorta has been replaced by a tube graft. There is a large pseudoaneurysm at the site of the anastomosis of the tube graft with the native aortic arch (*arrow*). The site of leak at the upper suture line is identified (*small arrow*). **(B)** Axial image at the level of the aortic leak. A small area of discontinuity is identified along the suture line within the ascending aorta. The associated pseudoaneurysm is clearly defined (*large arrow*).

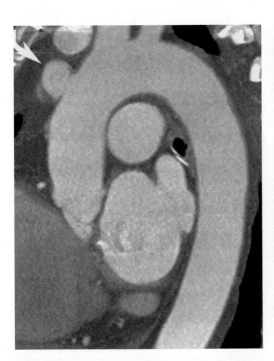

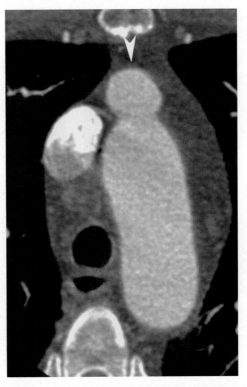

Fig. 13.25 Pseudoaneurysm of the ascending aorta at a cannula site. **(A)** Left anterior oblique projection of the aortic arch demonstrates a round pseudoaneurysm of the ascending aorta at the site of a cannula placed while the patient was on a bypass pump (*arrow*). **(B)** Axial image demonstrates the same pseudoaneurysm (*arrowhead*).

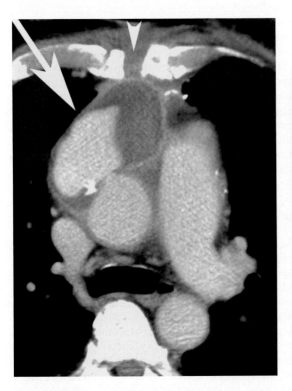

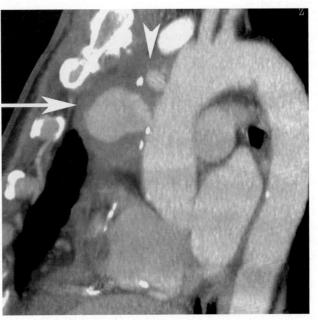

Fig. 13.26 Retrosternal infection with pseudoaneurysms of the ascending aorta at the previous sites of a cardioplegia needle and a cannula. **(A)** Axial image at the level of the carina demonstrates a large pseudoaneurysm extending from the ascending aorta into the retrosternal space (*arrow*) with associated dehiscence of the sternotomy site (*arrowhead*). Infected fluid was leaking from the sternotomy site. **(B)** Oblique maximum intensity projection (MIP) again demonstrates the large pseudoaneurysm (*arrow*) as well as a smaller pseudoaneurysm at a slightly superior location (*arrowhead*). (*Continued on page 340*)

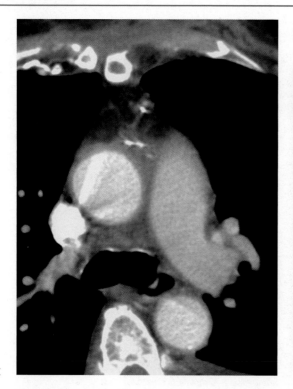

C

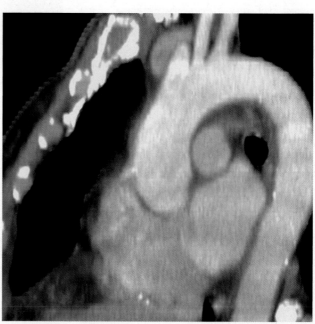

D

Fig. 13.26 (*Continued*) Retrosternal infection with pseudoaneurysms of the ascending aorta at the previous sites of a cardioplegia needle and a cannula. (**C**) Follow-up axial image 10 months after surgical debridement and repair demonstrates interval resolution of the large pseudoaneurysm. (**D**) Resolution of both pseudoaneurysms is confirmed on the oblique MIP.

formation after cardiac surgery (**Fig. 13.27**).[77] Although previous cardiac surgery and graft infection are the most common causes for pseudoaneurysm in the ascending aorta, trauma may be more common in the descending aorta (**Fig. 13.28**).[75]

Most patients requiring surgery for thoracic aortic pseudoaneurysm have been reported to present within 2 years of the original surgery.[75,77] Timing of presentation for the remaining patients is almost equally distributed up to 15 years after initial cardiac surgery, with nonmycotic pseudoaneurysms reported as long as 25 years later.[78] Presenting symptoms commonly arise from the mass effect of an enlarging pseudoaneurysm or distortion of the aortic valve with valvular regurgitation and resultant heart failure. These symptoms may include chest pain or fullness, shortness of breath, hoarseness, and dysphagia. Patients who present with a sentinel bleed or new pulsatile chest mass along the previous incision may harbor an eroding pseudoaneurysm and should be treated emergently.

In general, the presence of an aortic pseudoaneurysm is an indication for repair, with patient symptoms and pseudoaneurysm size guiding the timing of surgical intervention. Most patients in reported series undergo operation within 3 weeks of presentation with about 10% undergoing emergency surgery for heart failure, compression, and hemodynamic or radiographic instability. The presence of infection should be assumed for operative planning using cardiac CT or chest CTA as a guide (**Fig. 13.26**). The presence of a saccular aneurysm of the ascending aorta in a patient with previous cardiac surgery is an infected pseudoaneurysm until proven otherwise. Three-dimensional reconstructions allow surgical planning for proximal and distal control, access for cardiopulmonary bypass, and myocardial protection.[79]

Small pseudoaneurysms at sites of previous instrumentation that are noted as an incidental finding on follow-up imaging in asymptomatic patients are not likely to need surgical repair but require subsequent imaging to assess continued stability. Small pseudoaneurysms may be safely followed by serial CTA if they have been stable with no sign of infection, and the cause is linked to anticoagulation or other factors.[75,77]

Surgical Treatment

The treatment of post-operative ascending aortic graft pseudoaneurysm is surgical. The presence of pseudoaneurysm suggests occult infection and requires an operative plan that incorporates wide debridement of infected tissue and removal of any compromised graft. Small pseudoaneurysms may be surgically treated by resection of the pseudoaneurysm, debridement of the infected vascular structure, and reconstruction with autologous or prosthetic graft material. Most are treated with resection and interposition grafting when possible. Some investigators have suggested the finding of a narrow neck in post-surgical pseudoaneurysms indicates a noninfectious etiology and have advocated a less aggressive approach in these circumstances.

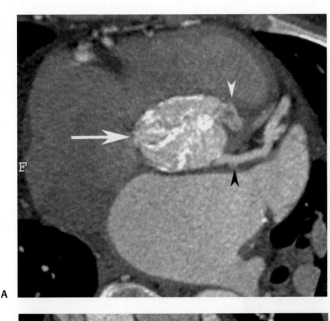

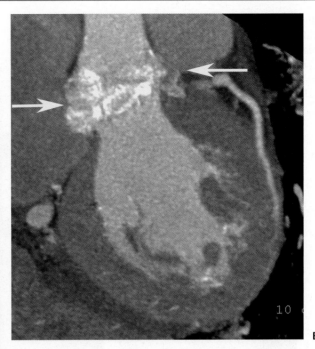

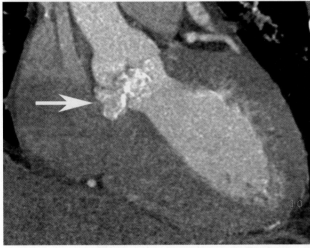

Fig. 13.27 Calcification with pseudoaneurysm of the aortic root after replacement of the ascending aorta with a graft. **(A)** Axial image demonstrates extensive calcification of the aortic valve and root (*arrow*) with a pseudoaneurysm on the left side of the root (*white arrowhead*) anterior to the origin of the left coronary artery (*black arrowhead*). **(B,C)** Long-axis views of the left ventricle and aorta demonstrate extensive calcification of the aortic root with bilateral pseudoaneurysms involving the aortic root and left ventricular outflow tract (*arrows*) on both sides of the aortic valve.

The surgical treatment of post-cardiac surgical pseudoaneurysms is complex and technically challenging. Successful surgical treatment often relies on establishing control of the aorta by using peripheral cannulation, systemic cooling, early ventricular decompression, and deep hypothermic circulatory arrest.[77,80] Inadvertent entry into the pseudoaneurysm before cannulation for cardiopulmonary bypass and control of the aorta may be catastrophic. CTA is essential to planning cardiopulmonary bypass and successful surgical treatment of aortic pseudoaneursyms.[79]

Although the traditional treatment of post-traumatic pseudoaneurysms has been surgical, these aneurysms are ideally suited to treatment with endovascular approaches. Descending thoracic pseudoaneurysms are anatomically amenable to endovascular grafting (**Fig. 13.28**), but enthusiasm for this approach is tempered by caution in placing new prosthetic material into a potentially infected vascular field. Endovascular repairs in this setting have reported good short-term outcomes, but the long-term results are unknown.[74]

◆ Aortitis

Acute aortitis is an uncommon clinical entity. The presentation of aortitis in the setting of acute chest pain may overlap with other, more prevalent sources of chest pain such as acute myocardial infarction, acute aortic dissection, and pulmonary embolism. CTA may demonstrate a thickened thoracic aorta that is normal or enlarged, mimicking the appearance of intramural hematoma (**Fig. 13.29**), with a variable finding of associated pleural effusion.[81]

Patients have undergone surgical exploration with and without replacement of the aorta in this setting based on the clinical presentation and radiographic abnormalities. Subsequent pathologic evaluation of the resected aorta may reveal the underlying inflammatory cause. Additional pre-surgical evaluation by magnetic resonance angiography or transesophageal echocardiography may be helpful in ruling out an aortic dissection.

◆ Assessment of Aortic Atheroma

Evaluation of the thoracic aorta should include a thorough assessment of aortic atheroma. The normal aorta has a smooth intimal surface. Atherosclerotic plaque within the aorta generally appears as low-density material with an

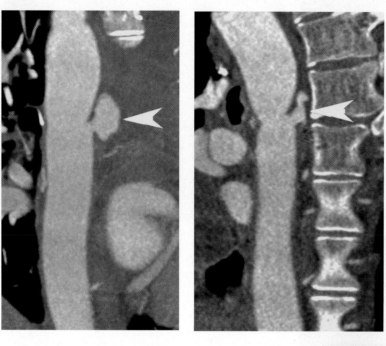

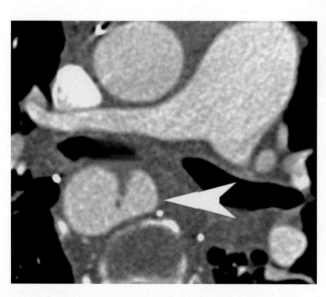

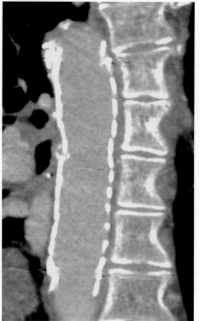

Fig. 13.28 Post-traumatic pseudoaneurysm of the descending thoracic aorta with endovascular repair. **(A)** Anteroposterior view of the descending thoracic aorta demonstrates a pseudoaneurysm extending to the left side (*arrowhead*). **(B)** Left anterior oblique view again demonstrates the pseudoaneurysm (*arrowhead*) with an abrupt change in caliber of the aorta just above the pseudoaneurysm corresponding to the site of traumatic injury. **(C)** Axial view again demonstrates the pseudoaneurysm (*arrowhead*) with minimal surrounding hematoma in the posterior mediastinum. **(D)** Left anterior oblique view in the same projection as in (B) following placement of a covered stent. The pseudoaneurysm is no longer present.

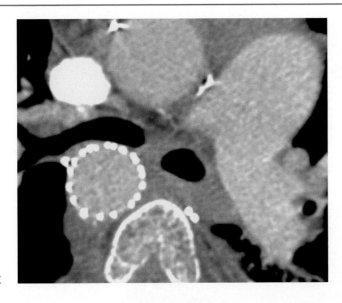

E

Fig. 13.28 (Continued) (E) Axial view at the same level as (C) confirms that the pseudoaneurysm has been successfully excluded.

irregular contour along the intimal lining and may be difficult to distinguish from thrombus in an aneurysmal aorta (**Fig. 13.30**). The detection of focal plaque projecting into the lumen of the aorta (**Fig. 13.31**) or mobile atheroma (**Figs. 13.32** and **13.33**; see associated cine clips) of the ascending aorta and arch has significant prognostic value for predicting stroke and peripheral embolism.[82] Although the causality is unclear, the risk of stroke and peripheral embolism is increased fourfold by the presence of severe atheroma (>4 mm) in the aortic arch and 12-fold by the presence of mobile atheroma.[83] This increased risk has been corroborated in multiple studies and suggests an important role of aortic atheroma in the pathogenesis of stroke.[84,85] A five-grade ranking system has been proposed for atherosclerotic plaque within the thoracic aorta: 1 = normal, 2 = flat thickening, 3 = protruding atheroma less than 5 mm, 4 = protruding atheroma 5 mm or greater, and 5 = mobile thrombus.[82,86]

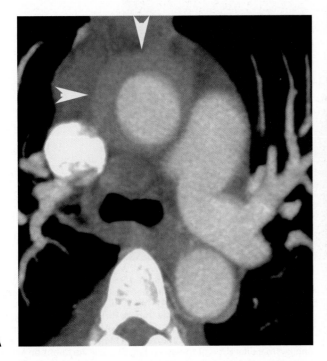

A

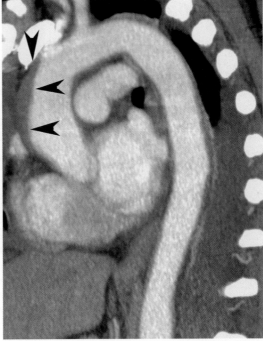

B

Fig. 13.29 Aortitis with mediastinal fibrosis. **(A)** Axial image demonstrates circumferential thickening around the proximal ascending aorta (*arrowheads*). In the setting of acute chest pain, this finding was believed to be suspicious for an intramural hematoma. **(B)** Maximum intensity projection of the aortic arch again demonstrates thickening along the anterior wall of the aorta (*arrowheads*). The patient was taken for median sternotomy. Biopsy of the tissue around the ascending aorta demonstrated aortitis associated with mediastinal fibrosis.

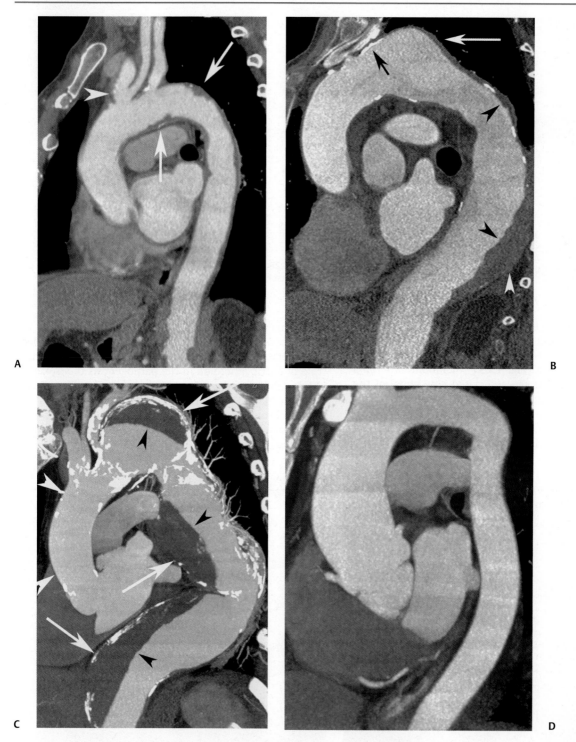

Fig. 13.30 Atherosclerotic disease of the aorta in three patients. **(A)** Normal-caliber aorta with a common origin of the innominate and left common carotid arteries (*arrowhead*). Atherosclerotic plaque is identified as irregular, low-density material along the lumen of the aortic arch (*arrows*). Additional focal areas of atherosclerosis are present in the upper abdominal aorta in the lower portion of the image. **(B)** Aneurysmal aorta with dilatation in the arch (*white arrow*) and descending aorta (*white arrowhead*) and areas of calcified plaque (*black arrow*) as well as low-density plaque or thrombus (*black arrowheads*). It is difficult to distinguish noncalcified plaque from thombus, especially in the nonaneurysmal segments of the aorta. **(C)** Diffusely aneurismal aorta (*arrows*) with a tube graft in the ascending aorta (*arrowheads*). Large areas of low-density material within the aneurismal segments of the aorta demonstrate a relatively smooth surface and likely represent thrombus that has formed within the aneurismal portions of the aorta. **(D)** Comparison view of the thoracic aorta in a fourth patient with aneurysmal dilatation of the ascending thoracic aorta but no significant atherosclerotic disease. Note that the wall thickness is barely perceptible in the absence of atherosclerotic disease or thrombus.

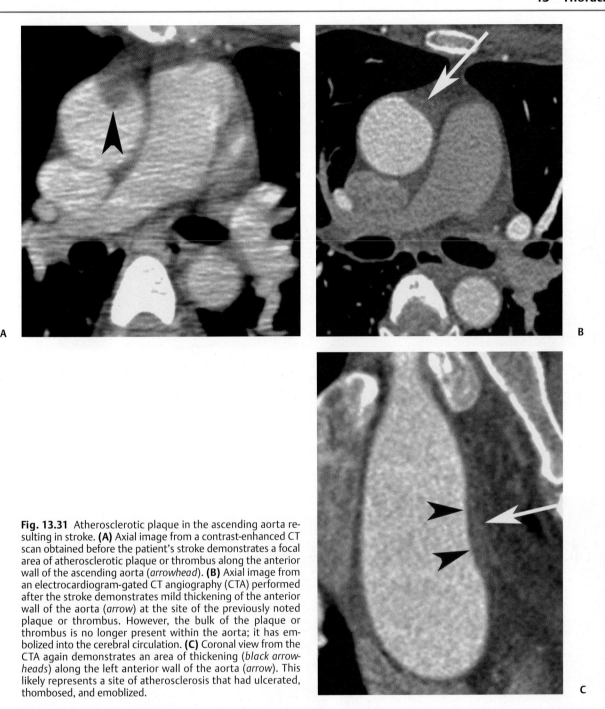

Fig. 13.31 Atherosclerotic plaque in the ascending aorta resulting in stroke. **(A)** Axial image from a contrast-enhanced CT scan obtained before the patient's stroke demonstrates a focal area of atherosclerotic plaque or thrombus along the anterior wall of the ascending aorta (*arrowhead*). **(B)** Axial image from an electrocardiogram-gated CT angiography (CTA) performed after the stroke demonstrates mild thickening of the anterior wall of the aorta (*arrow*) at the site of the previously noted plaque or thrombus. However, the bulk of the plaque or thrombus is no longer present within the aorta; it has embolized into the cerebral circulation. **(C)** Coronal view from the CTA again demonstrates an area of thickening (*black arrowheads*) along the left anterior wall of the aorta (*arrow*). This likely represents a site of atherosclerosis that had ulcerated, thombosed, and emoblized.

Although there is agreement regarding the prognostic significance of these findings, there is no consensus statement or accepted evidence-based algorithm guiding clinical management. Acute treatment options include thrombolysis and surgery. However, these invasive therapies are rarely used except in limited clinical scenarios.[87] Secondary preventative measures include the use of antiplatelet agents, anticoagulants, and statins. In general, combination antiplatelet therapy with aspirin and clopidogrel is favored as an alternative to warfarin.[87] Ongoing clinical trials are being conducted to determine which therapies are more effective in minimizing ischemic stroke, intracranial hemorrhage, myocardial infarction, peripheral embolism, and death. Additional management strategies include aggressive risk factor control with blood pressure and lipid-lowering therapies and diabetic control when indicated.

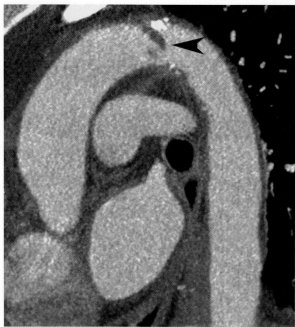

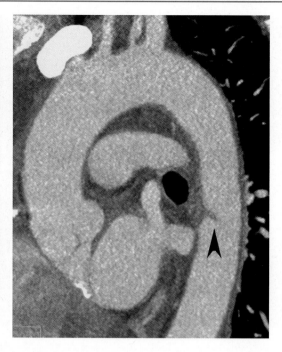

A

B

Fig. 13.32 Mobile atherosclerotic plaque/thombus in the aortic arch. **(A)** Maximum intensity projection view of the arch demonstrates the presence of calcified atherosclerotic disease at the top of the arch with a focal extension of low-density material into the arch (*arrowhead*). This material was visualized to move in real time (see cine on DVD). **(B)** Slightly different obliquity of the aortic arch demonstrates a second focus of plaque or thrombus extending from the wall of the descending thoracic aorta (*arrowhead*).

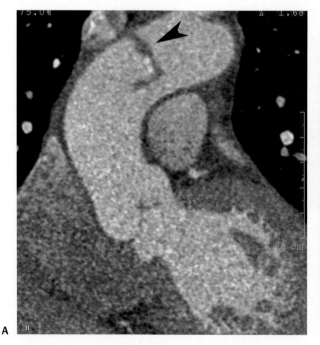

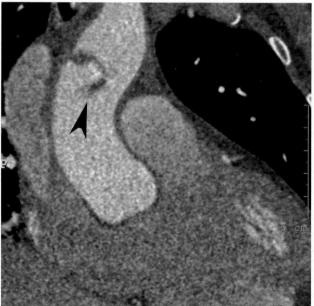

A

B

Fig. 13.33 Mobile atherosclerotic plaque or thrombus in the aortic arch of a patient with history of a transient ischemic event. Two views of the proximal aorta demonstrate a focal comma-shaped linear structure attached to the wall of the aortic arch (*arrowhead*). This material was visualized to move in real time (see cine on DVD).

◆ Conclusion

Assessment of the thoracic aorta is an essential component of the comprehensive imaging assessment of the heart and vascular system. The presence, extent, and type of disease in the thoracic aorta may mandate or alter intervention in the context of cardiac disease. Assessment of pathologic findings of the heart and thoracic aorta on cardiac CT must be evaluated together to allow optimal management. Longitudinal assessment of the thoracic aorta with CTA allows estimation of the impact of risk factor modification, stratification of apparently similar aortic aneurysmal disease, monitoring of post-intervention complications, and surveillance of the post-dissection aorta to plan timely surgical intervention.

Cine 13.1 Mobile atherosclerotic plaque–thrombus in the aortic arch (see Fig. 13.32). **(A)** Oblique sagittal cine of the aortic valve and proximal arch demonstrates a linear, low-density plaque–thrombus that is fixed to the ascending aorta just proximal to the innominate artery origin but is freely mobile within the aortic lumen. **(B)** Axial cine again demonstrates the mobile linear structure that is fixed to the right side of the ascending aorta and extends across to the left. **(C)** Coronal cine again demonstrates the mobile plaque–thrombus as it flips proximally and distally with each cardiac cycle.

Cine 13.2 **(A,B)** Mobile atherosclerotic plaque–thrombus in the distal ascending aorta in a patient with recent stroke. Low-density plaque–thrombus is fixed to the right side of the distal ascending aorta but is freely mobile within the lumen.

References

1. Anderson RH. The surgical anatomy of the aortic root. Multimedia manual of cardiothoracic surgery. MMCTS. European Association for Cardio-thoracic Surgery, 2007. pp. 1–8

2. Brewer RJ, Deck JD, Capati B, Nolan SP. The dynamic aortic root. Its role in aortic valve function. J Thorac Cardiovasc Surg. 1976;72(3):413–417

3. Burman ED, Keegan J, Kilner PJ. Aortic root measurement by cardiovascular magnetic resonance: specification of planes and lines of measurement and corresponding normal values. Circ Cardiovasc Imaging. 2008;1(2):104–113

4. Anderson RH, Ho SY, Brecker SJ. Anatomic basis of cross-sectional echocardiography. Heart. 2001;85(6):716–720

5. Vasan RS, Larson MG, Levy D. Determinants of echocardiographic aortic root size. The Framingham Heart Study. Circulation. 1995;91(3):734–740

6. Nistri S, Sorbo MD, Marin M, Palisi M, Scognamiglio R, Thiene G. Aortic root dilatation in young men with normally functioning bicuspid aortic valves. Heart. 1999;82(1):19–22

7. Bickerstaff LK, Pairolero PC, Hollier LH, et al. Thoracic aortic aneurysms: a population-based study. Surgery. 1982;92(6):1103–1108

8. Aronberg DJ, Glazer HS, Madsen K, Sagel SS. Normal thoracic aortic diameters by computed tomography. J Comput Assist Tomogr. 1984;8(2):247–250

9. Grollman JH. The aortic diverticulum: a remnant of the partially involuted dorsal aortic root. Cardiovasc Intervent Radiol. 1989;12(1):14–17

10. Layton KF, Kallmes DF, Cloft HJ, Lindell EP, Cox VS. Bovine aortic arch variant in humans: clarification of a common misnomer. AJNR Am J Neuroradiol. 2006;27(7):1541–1542

11. Eichhorn J, Fink C, Delorme S, Ulmer H. Rings, slings and other vascular abnormalities. Ultrafast computed tomography and magnetic resonance angiography in pediatric cardiology. Z Kardiol. 2004;93(3):201–208

12. Berdon WE. Rings, slings, and other things: vascular compression of the infant trachea updated from the midcentury to the millennium—the legacy of Robert E. Gross, MD, and Edward B. D. Neuhauser, MD. Radiology. 2000;216(3):624–632

13. Gomes AS, Lois JF, George B, Alpan G, Williams RG. Congenital abnormalities of the aortic arch: MR imaging. Radiology. 1987;165(3):691–695

14. Soler R, Rodríguez E, Requejo I, Fernández R, Raposo I. Magnetic resonance imaging of congenital abnormalities of the thoracic aorta. Eur Radiol. 1998;8(4):540–546

15. Grathwohl KW, Afifi AY, Dillard TA, Olson JP, Heric BR. Vascular rings of the thoracic aorta in adults. Am Surg. 1999;65(11):1077–1083

16. Stoica SC, Lockowandt U, Coulden R, Ward R, Bilton D, Dunning J. Double aortic arch masquerading as asthma for thirty years. Respiration. 2002;69(1):92–95

17. Adkins RB Jr, Maples MD, Graham BS, Witt TT, Davies J. Dysphagia associated with an aortic arch anomaly in adults. Am Surg. 1986;52(5):238–245

18. Pearce WH, Slaughter MS, LeMaire S, et al. Aortic diameter as a function of age, gender, and body surface area. Surgery. 1993;114(4):691–697

19. Davies RR, Goldstein LJ, Coady MA, et al. Yearly rupture or dissection rates for thoracic aortic aneurysms: simple prediction based on size. Ann Thorac Surg. 2002;73(1):17–27, discussion 27–28

20. Coady MA, Rizzo JA, Elefteriades JA. Developing surgical intervention criteria for thoracic aortic aneurysms. Cardiol Clin. 1999;17(4):827–839

21. Judge DP, Dietz HC. Therapy of Marfan syndrome. Annu Rev Med. 2008;59:43–59

22. Tadros TM, Klein MD, Shapira OM. Ascending aortic dilatation associated with bicuspid aortic valve: pathophysiology, molecular biology, and clinical implications. Circulation. 2009;119(6):880–890

23. Homme JL, Aubry MC, Edwards WD, et al. Surgical pathology of the ascending aorta: a clinicopathologic study of 513 cases. Am J Surg Pathol. 2006;30(9):1159–1168

24. Litmanovich D, Bankier AA, Cantin L, Raptopoulos V, Boiselle PM. CT and MRI in diseases of the aorta. AJR Am J Roentgenol. 2009;193(4):928–940

25. Ergin MA, Spielvogel D, Apaydin A, et al. Surgical treatment of the dilated ascending aorta: when and how? Ann Thorac Surg. 1999;67(6):1834–1839, discussion 1853–1856

26. Borger MA, Preston M, Ivanov J, et al. Should the ascending aorta be replaced more frequently in patients with bicuspid aortic valve disease? J Thorac Cardiovasc Surg. 2004;128(5):677–683

27. Fedak PW, Verma S, David TE, Leask RL, Weisel RD, Butany J. Clinical and pathophysiological implications of a bicuspid aortic valve. Circulation. 2002;106(8):900–904

28. Brinkman WT, Szeto WY, Bavaria JE. Stent graft treatment for transverse arch and descending thoracic aorta aneurysms. Curr Opin Cardiol. 2007;22(6):510–516

29. Akashi H, Tayama E, Tayama K, Kosuga T, Takagi K, Aoyagi S. Remodeling operation for unruptured aneurysms of three sinuses of Valsalva. J Thorac Cardiovasc. Surg 2005;129(4):951–952

30. Golzari M, Riebman JB. The four seasons of ruptured sinus of valsalva aneurysms: case presentations and review. Heart Surg Forum. 2004;7(6):E577–E583

31. Goldberg N, Krasnow N. Sinus of Valsalva aneurysms. Clin Cardiol. 1990;13(12):831–836

32. Johnson TR, Nikolaou K, Wintersperger BJ, et al. ECG-gated 64-MDCT angiography in the differential diagnosis of acute chest pain. AJR Am J Roentgenol. 2007;188(1):76–82

33. Tsai TT, Trimarchi S, Nienaber CA. Acute aortic dissection: perspectives from the International Registry of Acute Aortic Dissection (IRAD). Eur J Vasc Endovasc Surg. 2009;37(2):149–159

34. David TE. Surgery of the aortic valve. Curr Probl Surg. 1999;36(6):426–501

35. David TE. Remodeling of aortic root and preservation of the native aortic valve. Op Tech Card Thorac Surg. 1996;1:44–56

36. Estrera AL, Miller CC III, Villa MA, et al. Proximal reoperations after repaired acute type A aortic dissection. Ann Thorac Surg. 2007; 83(5): 1603–1608, discussion 1608–1609

37. Verhoye JP, Miller DC, Sze D, Dake MD, Mitchell RS. Complicated acute type B aortic dissection: midterm results of emergency endovascular stent-grafting. J Thorac Cardiovasc Surg. 2008;136(2):424–430

38. Elefteriades JA, Hammond GL, Gusberg RJ, Kopf GS, Baldwin JC. Fenestration revisited: a safe and effective procedure for descending aortic dissection. Arch Surg. 1990;125(6):786–790

39. Elefteriades JA, Hartleroad J, Gusberg RJ, et al. Long-term experience with descending aortic dissection: the complication-specific approach. Ann Thorac Surg. 1992;53(1):11–20, discussion 20–21

40. Tsai TT, Fattori R, Trimarchi S, et al; International Registry of Acute Aortic Dissection. Long-term survival in patients presenting with type B acute aortic dissection: insights from the International Registry of Acute Aortic Dissection. Circulation. 2006;114(21):2226–2231

41. Lansman SL, Raissi S, Ergin MA, Griepp RB. Urgent operation for acute transverse aortic arch dissection. J Thorac Cardiovasc Surg. 1989; 97(3):334–341

42. Kazui T, Tamiya Y, Tanaka T, Komatsu S. Extended aortic replacement for acute type A dissection with the tear in the descending aorta. J Thorac Cardiovasc Surg. 1996;112(4):973–978

43. Tsai TT, Isselbacher EM, Trimarchi S, et al; International Registry of Acute Aortic Dissection. Acute type B aortic dissection: does aortic arch involvement affect management and outcomes? Insights from the International Registry of Acute Aortic Dissection (IRAD). Circulation. 2007;116(11, Suppl):I150–I156

44. Kaji S, Akasaka T, Katayama M, et al. Prognosis of retrograde dissection from the descending to the ascending aorta. Circulation. 2003; 108(Suppl 1):II300–II306

45. Park KH, Lim C, Choi JH, et al. Midterm change of descending aortic false lumen after repair of acute type I dissection. Ann Thorac Surg. 2009;87(1):103–108

46. Tsai TT, Evangelista A, Nienaber CA, et al; International Registry of Acute Aortic Dissection. Partial thrombosis of the false lumen in patients with acute type B aortic dissection. N Engl J Med. 2007; 357(4):349–359

47. De Bakey ME, Cooley DA, Creech O Jr. Surgical considerations of dissecting aneurysm of the aorta. Ann Surg. 1955;142(4):586–610, discussion 611–612

48. Crawford ES, Crawford JL, Stowe CL, Safi HJ. Total aortic replacement for chronic aortic dissection occurring in patients with and without Marfan's syndrome. Ann Surg. 1984;199(3):358–362

49. Böckler D, Schumacher H, Ganten M, et al. Complications after endovascular repair of acute symptomatic and chronic expanding Stanford type B aortic dissections. J Thorac Cardiovasc Surg. 2006; 132(2):361–368

50. Nienaber CA, Rousseau H, Eggebrecht H, et al; INSTEAD Trial. Randomized comparison of strategies for type B aortic dissection: the INvestigation of STEnt Grafts in Aortic Dissection (INSTEAD) trial. Circulation. 2009;120(25):2519–2528

51. Eggebrecht H, Plicht B, Kahlert P, Erbel R. Intramural hematoma and penetrating ulcers: indications to endovascular treatment. Eur J Vasc Endovasc Surg. 2009;38(6):659–665

52. deMonyé W, Murphy M, Hodgson R, Holemans J, Mcwilliams R. Acute aortic syndromes: Pathology and imaging. Imaging. 2004;16:230–239

53. Svensson LG, Labib SB, Eisenhauer AC, Butterly JR. Intimal tear without hematoma: an important variant of aortic dissection that can elude current imaging techniques. Circulation. 1999;99(10):1331–1336

54. Sakamoto I, Sueyoshi E, Uetani M. MR imaging of the aorta. Radiol Clin North Am. 2007;45(3):485–497, viii

55. Song JK. Diagnosis of aortic intramural haematoma. Heart. 2004; 90(4):368–371

56. Song JK, Kim HS, Kang DH, et al. Different clinical features of aortic intramural hematoma versus dissection involving the ascending aorta. J Am Coll Cardiol. 2001;37(6):1604–1610

57. Ohmi M, Tabayashi K, Moizumi Y, Komatsu T, Sekino Y, Goko C. Extremely rapid regression of aortic intramural hematoma. J Thorac Cardiovasc Surg. 1999;118(5):968–969

58. Kang DH, Song JK, Song MG, et al. Clinical and echocardiographic outcomes of aortic intramural hemorrhage compared with acute aortic dissection. Am J Cardiol. 1998;81(2):202–206

59. Kaji S, Nishigami K, Akasaka T, et al. Prediction of progression or regression of type A aortic intramural hematoma by computed tomography. Circulation. 1999;100(19, Suppl):II281–II286

60. Shimizu H, Yoshino H, Udagawa H, et al. Prognosis of aortic intramural hemorrhage compared with classic aortic dissection. Am J Cardiol. 2000;85(6):792–795, A10

61. Svensson LG, Kouchoukos NT, Miller DC, et al; Society of Thoracic Surgeons Endovascular Surgery Task Force. Expert consensus document on the treatment of descending thoracic aortic disease using endovascular stent-grafts. Ann Thorac Surg. 2008;85(1, Suppl):S1–S41

62. Sundt TM. Intramural hematoma and penetrating atherosclerotic ulcer of the aorta. Ann Thorac Surg. 2007;83(2):S835–S841, discussion S846–S850

63. Coady MA, Rizzo JA, Hammond GL, Pierce JG, Kopf GS, Elefteriades JA. Penetrating ulcer of the thoracic aorta: what is it? How do we recognize it? How do we manage it? J Vasc Surg. 1998;27(6):1006–1015, discussion 1015–1016

64. Hayashi H, Matsuoka Y, Sakamoto I, et al. Penetrating atherosclerotic ulcer of the aorta: imaging features and disease concept. Radiographics. 2000;20(4):995–1005

65. Stanson AW, Kazmier FJ, Hollier LH, et al. Penetrating atherosclerotic ulcers of the thoracic aorta: natural history and clinicopathologic correlations. Ann Vasc Surg. 1986;1(1):15–23

66. Cho KR, Stanson AW, Potter DD, Cherry KJ, Schaff HV, Sundt TM III. Penetrating atherosclerotic ulcer of the descending thoracic aorta and arch. J Thorac Cardiovasc Surg. 2004;127(5):1393–1399, discussion 1399–1401

67. Tittle SL, Lynch RJ, Cole PE, et al. Midterm follow-up of penetrating ulcer and intramural hematoma of the aorta. J Thorac Cardiovasc Surg. 2002;123(6):1051–1059

68. Kleisli T, Wheatley GH III. Closure of a penetrating ulcer of the descending aorta using an Amplatzer occluder. Ann Thorac Surg. 2009;88(3):e18–e19

69. Gaubert JY, Moulin G, Mesana T, et al. Type A dissection of the thoracic aorta: use of MR imaging for long-term follow-up. Radiology. 1995;196(2):363–369

70. Sundaram B, Quint LE, Patel HJ, Deeb GM. CT findings following thoracic aortic surgery. Radiographics. 2007;27(6):1583–1594

71. García A, Ferreirós J, Santamaría M, Bustos A, Abades JL, Santamaría N. MR angiographic evaluation of complications in surgically treated type A aortic dissection. Radiographics. 2006;26(4):981–992

72. Spielvogel D, Mathur MN, Lansman SL, Griepp RB. Aortic arch reconstruction using a trifurcated graft. Ann Thorac Surg. 2003;75(3):1034–1036

73. Orton DF, LeVeen RF, Saigh JA, et al. Aortic prosthetic graft infections: radiologic manifestations and implications for management. Radiographics. 2000;20(4):977–993

74. Graham EM, Bandisode VM, Atz AM, Kline CH, Taylor MH, Ikonomidis JS. Percutaneous occlusion of a pseudoaneurysm evolving after homograft aortic valve and root replacement with the Amplatzer muscular ventricular septal defect occluder. J Thorac Cardiovasc Surg. 2006; 131(4):914–916

75. Atik FA, Navia JL, Svensson LG, et al. Surgical treatment of pseudoaneurysm of the thoracic aorta. J Thorac Cardiovasc Surg. 2006;132(2):379–385

76. Flick WF, Hallermann FJ, Feldt RH, Danielson GK. Aneurysm of aortic cannulation site. Successful repair by means of peripheral cannulation, profound hypothermia, and circulatory arrest. J Thorac Cardiovasc Surg. 1971;61(3):419–423

77. Dumont E, Carrier M, Cartier R, et al. Repair of aortic false aneurysm using deep hypothermia and circulatory arrest. Ann Thorac Surg. 2004;78(1):117–120, discussion 120–121

78. Murayama H, Watanabe T, Kobayashi Y, Matsumura Y, Kobayashi A. Nonmycotic false aneurysm of aortic cannulation site presenting 26 years postoperatively. Ann Thorac Surg. 2009;87(3):936–939

79. Reyes KG, Pettersson GB, Mihaljevic T, Roselli EE. A strategy for safe sternal reentry in patients with pseudoaneurysms of the ascending aorta using the PORT-ACCESS EndoCPB system. Interact Cardiovasc Thorac Surg. 2009;9(5):893–895

80. Gilkeson RC, Markowitz AH, Ciancibello L. Multisection CT evaluation of the reoperative cardiac surgery patient. Radiographics. 2003;23(Spec No):S3–S17

81. Gornik HL, Creager MA. Aortitis. Circulation. 2008;117(23):3039–3051

82. Katz ES, Tunick PA, Rusinek H, Ribakove G, Spencer FC, Kronzon I. Protruding aortic atheromas predict stroke in elderly patients undergoing cardiopulmonary bypass: experience with intraoperative transesophageal echocardiography. J Am Coll Cardiol. 1992;20(1):70–77

83. Kronzon I, Tunick PA. Aortic atherosclerotic disease and stroke. Circulation. 2006;114(1):63–75

84. Amarenco P, Cohen A, Tzourio C, et al. Atherosclerotic disease of the aortic arch and the risk of ischemic stroke. N Engl J Med. 1994;331(22):1474–1479

85. Di Tullio MR, Russo C, Jin Z, Sacco RL, Mohr JP, Homma S; Patent Foramen Ovale in Cryptogenic Stroke Study investigators. Aortic arch plaques and risk of recurrent stroke and death. Circulation. 2009;119(17):2376–2382

86. Tunick PA, Krinsky GA, Lee VS, Kronzon I. Diagnostic imaging of thoracic aortic atherosclerosis. AJR Am J Roentgenol. 2000;174(4):1119–1125

87. Lancaster G, Lovoulos CJ, Moussouttas M, et al. Aortic arch replacement for recurrent cerebral embolization. Ann Thorac Surg. 2002;73(1):291–294

14

Congenital Heart Disease in the Adult

Robert A. Quaife, C. Douglas Borg, Nicolas Hilpipre, and David Wang

As a result of improvements in diagnosis, surgical techniques, and management of congenital heart disease (CHD), the number of children with CHD surviving into adulthood has increased significantly over the past 50 years. It is estimated that there are now 800,000 adults in the United States living with simple CHD and 600,000 with moderate and complex cardiac lesions.[1] Although initial detection, follow-up, and treatment of CHD is largely performed by transthoracic echocardiography or transesophageal echocardiography (TEE), limitations with regard to spatial resolution, ultrasound windows in adults (especially post-surgery) and associated extracardiac anomalies render these techniques less valuable in adults than in children. Similarly, magnetic resonance imaging (MRI), although an excellent imaging modality that spares radiation exposure, may be contraindicated in those who are claustrophobic or dependent on an MRI-incompatible implanted medical device, such as a pacemaker.[2]

Applications of electrocardiographic (ECG)-gated cardiac CT have expanded dramatically over the past decade from assessment of coronary calcium and coronary stenosis to evaluation of cardiac anatomy, function, and structural abnormalities. When echocardiography is limited or MRI is contraindicated, cardiac CT can provide a wealth of information about the location and size of congenital cardiac defects, as well as an estimate of the degree of shunting. The full field of view obtained with high-spatial-resolution tomographic images acquired within a single breath-hold is well suited to depict surgical reconstructions and the myriad vascular anastomoses present in adult patients with complex CHD. This is particularly important in the pre-operative or preprocedural planning of interventional percutaneous or surgical procedures.[3]

◆ Congestive Heart Disease Cardiac CT Methodology

Using CT technology available in the 1980s, several groups reported the detection of interatrial shunts.[4,5] Since then, faster gantry rotation speed, increased numbers of detectors, and dual-source CT scanners have allowed improved spatial and temporal resolution in cardiac CT. The advent of multiphase contrast injectors and high-concentration contrast agents (350–370 mg/mL of iodine) have dramatically improved the image quality for delineation of fine structures and shunts (ie, atrial baffles in d-transposition of the great vessels).

Typical acquisition protocols for CHD require at least a 64-row multidetector CT scanner with high temporal resolution. Elimination of cardiac motion artifacts is accomplished by ECG gating. Oral or intravenous β-blockers that reduce heart rate can improve image quality but should be used with caution in patients with pulmonary hypertension, reduced ventricular function, or cardiac conduction abnormalities (ie, heart block with ventral septal defect [VSD] or tetralogy of Fallot [TOF]). Although prospective ECG gating with limited imaging during mid-late diastole may reduce radiation exposure, the dynamic nature of atrial septal defect (ASD) or VSD size may need to be assessed throughout the cardiac cycle. As with all applications of cardiac CT, it is important to tailor the examination to deliver the minimum radiation dose that will answer the clinical question. This is especially important in young individuals who, because of their disease, have often been subjected to multiple procedures using ionizing radiation.

A good two-phase power injector that allows two independent rates of contrast delivery is important for evaluation of CHD. Rapid delivery of an adequately dense-contrast bolus is needed to opacify the cardiac chambers. Dense-contrast material must be flushed out of the superior vena cava to avoid beam hardening artifact. When evaluating for a left-to-right shunt, it is important to flush contrast out of the right heart with a saline chaser to achieve an adequate contrast gradient between the two sides of the heart. In a typical cardiac examination using a 64-slice scanner, about 75 mL of iodinated contrast is injected in the right antecubital fossa at 5 mL per second, followed by a 30 to 50 mL saline chaser at 3 to 4 mL per second. In the presence of anomalous venous connections, the site of contrast injection (**Fig. 14.1**) may be key to the identification of different cardiac or surgical shunts.

Information regarding the direction of shunting in CHD is often determined from a dynamic contrast-enhanced

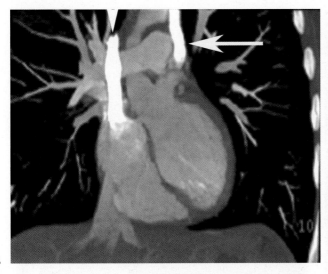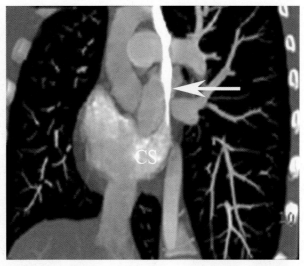

A

B

Fig. 14.1 Tailored contrast injection to demonstrate bilateral superior vena cavas (SVCs). Dual-contrast injection with right-arm power injection and hand injection in the left arm. **(A)** Oblique coronal view demonstrates opacification of the right-sided SVC (*arrowhead*) with a second opacified structure coursing around the pulmonary artery (*arrow*). **(B)** Oblique sagittal view demonstrates that this second opacified structure empties into the coronary sinus (CS), identifying it as a persistent left SVC (*arrow*). Prior knowledge of anatomic variations may be necessary to tailor the injection technique properly for cardiac CT.

cardiac CT. Shunt directionality may be demonstrated by comparing the density of right- and left-sided chambers at 5 and 30 seconds after contrast injection.[6] A triple-phase contrast protocol using 60 mL of full-strength contrast followed by 40 mL of dilute contrast (50:50 with saline) and a 50 mL of saline flush may be useful for demonstrating shunt directionality.[7] Furthermore, the orientation of a contrast jet on dynamic cardiac CT can be helpful in the differentiation of a secundum ASD from a patent foramen[8] and in the evaluation of other complex CHD.

◆ Atrial Septal Defects

ASD is the most common congenital heart anomaly in adults, after bicuspid aortic valve and mitral valve prolapse, comprising 30% of all congenital heart anomalies in adults older than 40 years.[2] This figure may underestimate the actual number of ASDs in adults because many are hemodynamically insignificant and found incidentally or on autopsy. Four main types of ASD have been described in the literature: ostium secundum, ostium primum, sinus venosus, and coronary sinus. Although ostium primum, sinus venosus, and coronary sinus ASDs have no gender predilection, ostium secundum defects, the most common form of ASD, are two to three times more common in women.[1]

Ostium secundum and ostium primum ASDs result from the variable growth and arrest of the septum primum and septum secundum during embryologic development. Sinus venosus and coronary sinus ASDs result from abnormal formation of the atriocaval junctions and coronary sinus, respectively. Patent foramen ovale (PFO) is frequently included in the discussion of ASD as a cause for interatrial

shunt, despite the lack of a structural abnormality in the interatrial septum.[7,8] ASDs may be associated with other anomalies, such as anomalous pulmonary venous connection or persistent left superior vena cava.

Undetected ASD can persist into adulthood and may manifest based on symptoms or an incidental finding at echocardiography. Symptomatic ASDs are usually characterized by exercise intolerance and exertional dyspnea. Additionally, longstanding ASD can result in atrial dilatation with subsequent atrial arrhythmia resulting in chest pain and shortness of breath. Less commonly, patients can present with cyanosis or paradoxical embolus. As a result of such symptoms, patients may be evaluated in the emergent setting by CT with the unexpected finding of an ASD.

◆ Atrial Septal Defect Types

Ostium Secundum

The secundum subtype accounts for 70% of ASDs.[9] Less than 10% of secundum ASDs are associated with an anomalous pulmonary venous connection.[10] The typical location for secundum ASD is in the region of the foramen ovale in the mid to cephalic portion of the interatrial septum (**Fig. 14.2**). Characterization of the quantity of tissue around the rim of the ASD is critical for the assessment of percutaneous therapeutic options (see following and Chapter 12).

Secundum ASDs arise from disproportionate resorption of the septum primum or incomplete development of septum secundum such that the foramen ovale is incompletely covered. Excessive perforation of the septum primum may also contribute to an enlarged ostium secundum and

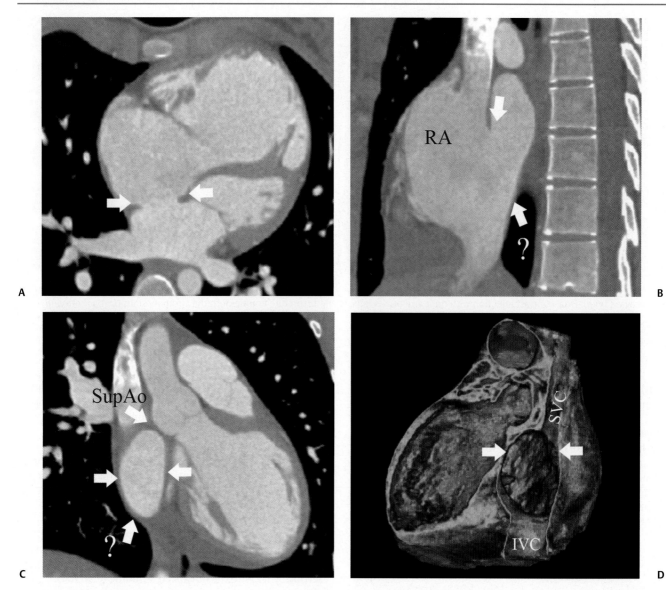

Fig. 14.2 Large secundum atrial septum defect (ASD). **(A)** ASD is depicted by arrows in this axial view. **(B)** Sagittal view demonstrates a small superior rim (*arrow*) with an absent inferior rim (*arrow?*). **(C)** Short axis through the ASD (*arrows*) with imaging of the aortic outflow demonstrates the close relationship of the superior ASD lip to the aortic root (SupAo). **(D)** Three-dimensional volume-rendered image cut to visualize the ASD looking from the left atrium into the right atrium (RA) at the mitral valve level. IVC, inferior vena cava; SVC, superior vena cava.

foramen ovale. In development of the atrial septum, small fenestrations develop in the septum secundum that coalesce to form foramen secundum. Occasionally, the fenestrations do not coalesce and the septum secundum is structurally weakened, resulting in a septal aneurysm (**Fig. 14.3**). This form of fenestrated ASD may be challenging to define, but the septal aneurysm is often large and markedly distorts the septal architecture.

Secundum ASDs are rarely symptomatic during infancy and early childhood; secundum ASDs are detected during childhood because of a murmur. When secundum ASDs persist into adulthood, left-to-right shunting can progress to right ventricular failure. Whether or not an ASD produces symptoms depends largely on the size of the defect. ASD defects smaller than 5 mm in diameter generally result in a negligible shunt, whereas larger ASDs (i.e., >20 mm) often result in hemodynamically significant shunting.[1] Over time, enlargement of the atria, right ventricle (RV), and pulmonary arteries results from increased flow volume (see **Figs. 9.18, 9.19,** and **9.20**). Longstanding secundum ASDs can produce chronic atrial dilatation, leading to atrial dysrhythmia and symptoms of easy fatigability and dyspnea, with ultimate progression to pulmonary arterial hypertension. Patients with hemodynamically significant shunts who develop right ventricular failure

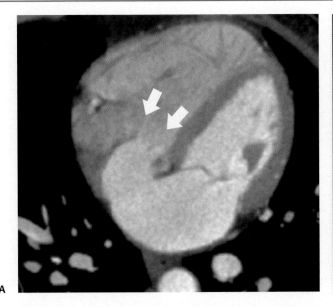

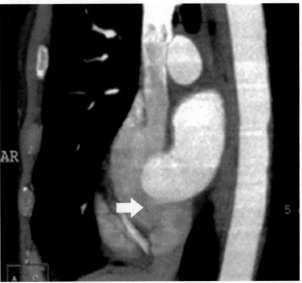

A   B

Fig. 14.3 Large atrial septal aneurysm with multiple fenestrations. **(A)** Axial image demonstrates a large interatrial septal aneurysm with bowing of the septum into the right atrium. Several small fenestrations are identified based on contrast extension into the right atrium (*arrows*). **(B)** Sagittal image again demonstrates contrast extension into the right atrium from the inferior aspect of the interatrial septal aneurysm (*arrow*).

and cardiac arrhythmias develop marked symptoms with death occurring in the fourth to sixth decades of life.[1]

Ostium Primum

Primum ASDs account for 20% of ASDs and arise from incomplete fusion of the free edge of the septum primum with the endocardial cushions. Primum defects are found at the caudal aspect of atrial septum near the atrioventricular (AV) septum and AV valve planes. When endocardial cushion abnormalities are present, there is abnormal development of the mitral valve; cleft mitral valve is commonly associated with primum ASDs.[11] Absence of the atrial septum at the level of the valve plane may result in prolapse of a mitral leaflet into the RV (**Fig. 14.4**).

Sinus Venosus

Sinus venosus ASDs account for 10% of all ASDs. Superior sinus venosus ASDs arise from abnormal development of the superior atriocaval junction such that the posterior and superior margins of the right atrial free wall are absent, resulting in a superior vena cava that may override both atria (see **Fig. 9.23**). Sinus venosus ASDs involving the inferior atriocaval junction are possible (see **Fig. 9.24**), although the superior type is far more common. Nearly all cases of superior sinus venosus ASDs are associated with anomalous drainage of the right upper pulmonary vein (**Fig. 14.5**).[12] Sinus venosus ASD is found in about 42% of patients with partial anomalous venous return from the right upper lobe.[13]

Coronary Sinus

Coronary sinus anomalies have been classified into four main types: enlarged coronary sinus with or without left-to-right coronary sinus shunt, absent coronary sinus (with an ASD in the expected region of the coronary sinus), atresia of the right coronary sinus ostium, and hypoplastic coronary sinus.[14] The rare coronary sinus ASD results from abnormal regression of the paired vitelline, umbilical, and cardinal veins, resulting in a partial or complete absence of the roof of the coronary sinus, which communicates directly with the left atrium (**Fig. 14.6**). The coronary sinus ASD is often associated with a persistent left superior vena cava (PLSVC). A morphologic classification of unroofed coronary sinus describes four subtypes: completely unroofed coronary sinus with PLSVC, completely unroofed coronary sinus without PLSVC, partially unroofed midportion of the coronary sinus, and partially unroofed terminal portion of the coronary sinus.[15]

Patent Foramen Ovale

In about 10 to 25% of the general population, the foramen ovale fails to close normally.[16] PFO represents failure of the valve of the foramen ovale to fuse with the interatrial septum. Because there is no abnormality of the interatrial septum, PFO is not considered an ASD. A small study of 20 patients, including six patients with PFO, demonstrated the presence of a left atrial flap in the expected region of the septum primum in all six patients with PFO confirmed by TEE. Adding two additional CT criteria, the presence of a continuous column of contrast connecting the flap to the right atrium and a contrast jet into the right atrium, resulted

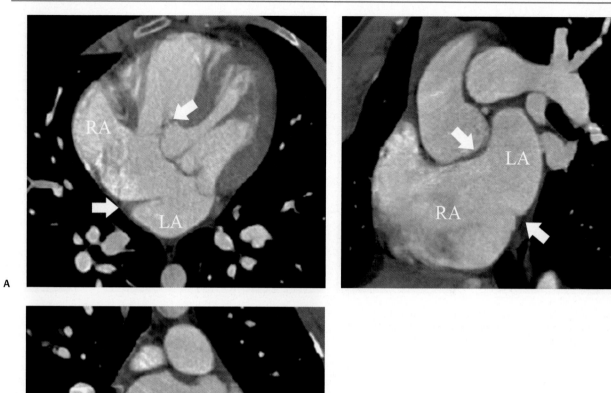

A

B

C

Fig. 14.4 Large primum atrial septal defect. **(A)** Axial image demonstrates a large defect (*between the arrows*) where the primum atrial septum should be present. Note the partial prolapse of the anterior mitral valve leaflet into the right ventricle. **(B)** Sagittal image again demonstrates absence of the atrial septum in its expected location (*arrows*) between the right atrium and left atrium **(C)** Coronal image again demonstrates the lack of an interatrial septum (*arrows*).

in greater specificity for the CT diagnosis but reduced the sensitivity for PFO detection to 66%.[17]

Pre-Procedural Planning

With the advent of closure devices,[18–21] most ASDs are now closed percutaneously.[22–26] Successful percutaneous closure of an ASD requires a clear understanding of the defect anatomy,[11] including the definition of specific rims (infero-posterior, near the inferior vena cava and anterosuperior, around the aorta) on which the closure device is secured. Inadequate rim tissue is a predictor of poor procedural success. In a study of large ASDs (>25-mm diameter), a small posterior rim was the most important limiting factor for successful device implantation.[27] In addition, proximity of the ASD to structures such as the aortic root, pulmonary

veins, or coronary sinus may significantly limit placement of occluder devices because of potential vascular obstruction or occlusion.[24,28]

Cardiac CT is well suited for pre-operative planning in the placement of an ASD occluder device as well as for post-procedure assessment (**Fig. 14.7**). In the pre-operative assessment, CT demonstrates the location and size of the ASD as well as its relationship to adjacent structures. The presence of multiple ASD fenestrations may also be detected (see **Fig. 9.17**). In the post-procedure assessment, CT provides a unique method to evaluate device placement along with the surrounding anatomic structures as an adjunct to echocardiography in symptomatic patients.[29] CT may demonstrate residual shunts or other complications such as obstruction of vascular structures, erosion through the atrial wall, or erosion into the aortic root.

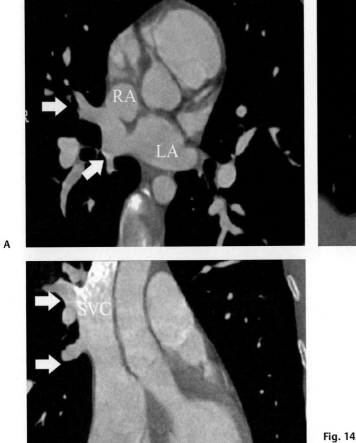

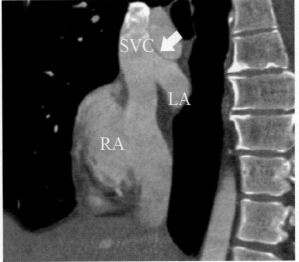

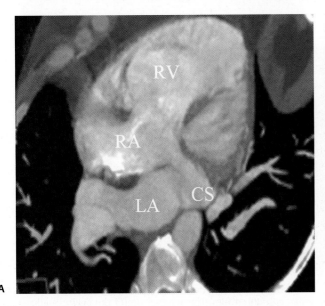

Fig. 14.5 Sinus venosus atrial septal defect. **(A)** Axial image demonstrates a communication between the right atrium (RA) and left atrium (LA) with anomalous pulmonary veins (*arrows*) emptying into the superior vena cava (SVC) at the level of the defect. **(B)** Sagittal view demonstrates that the SVC overrides both the RA and LA (*arrow*). **(C)** Coronary image demonstrates two pulmonary veins (*arrows*) emptying into the SVC. IVC, inferior vena cava.

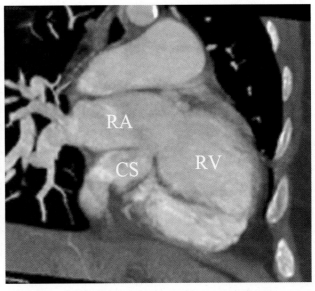

Fig. 14.6 Unroofed coronary sinus atrial septal defect. **(A)** Oblique image through the crux of the heart demonstrates a dilated coronary sinus (CS) leading into the right atrium (RA) but not clearly defined from the left atrium (LA). **(B)** Coronal view again demonstrates a dilated CS leading into the right atrium (RA). (*Continued on page 356*)

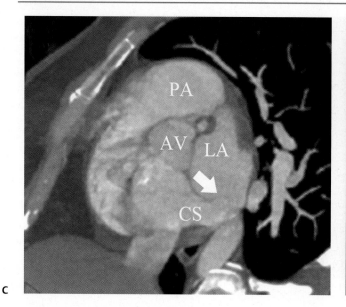

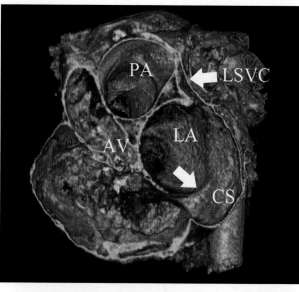

C   D

Fig. 14.6 (*Continued*) Unroofed coronary sinus atrial spiral defect. **(C)** Oblique view demonstrates a communication (*arrow*) between the CS and the LA. **(D)** Volumetric rendering demonstrates a persistent left superior vena cava (LSVC) draining into the LA (*upper arrow*) as well as the CS draining into the left atrium (*lower arrow*). Both of these connections shunt deoxygenated blood into the LA.

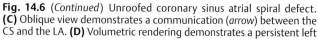

◆ Ventricular Septal Defects

VSDs are classified into four main types: (1) AV canal type, (2) muscular, (3) conoventricular, and (4) conal septal. AV canal type defects occur in the posterior ventricular septum at the inlet of the ventricle. Muscular ventricular septal defects occur in the muscular septum between the ventricular trabeculations, may present with multiple defects, and may have many different locations (**Fig. 14.8**). Conoventricular defects, often classified as perimembranous VSDs (see **Fig. 9.26**), lie between the ventricular septum and the conal septum (infracristal, or below the crista supraventricularis). They may be primarily membranous or associated with malalignment of the conal septum, wherein they involve more than just membranous septum. Conal septal (or supracristal) defects are the least common and are located in the septum between the aortic and pulmonary valves. A high perimembranous VSD may be difficult to distinguish from a supracristal defect by CT (see **Fig. 9.27** and **Fig. 14.9**). Complex defects may span different portions of the ventricular septum and may also involve the atrial septum.[30,31]

The severity of shunting through a VSD, the degree of LV enlargement, and patient symptoms determine whether the

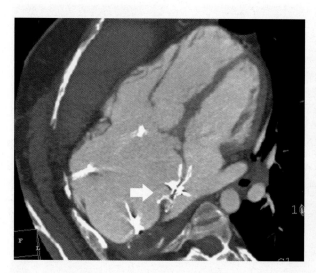

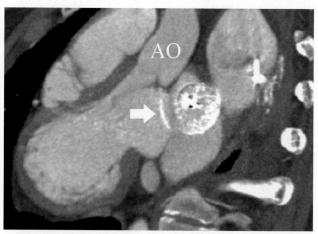

A   B

Fig. 14.7 Amplatzer atrial septal defect (ASD) closure device. **(A)** Axial image demonstrates a closure device (*arrow*) between the left atrium and the enlarged right atrium. **(B)** Modified three-chamber view again demonstrates a closure device (*arrow*) between the left atrium and the enlarged right atrium. The superior rim of the device is adjacent to the aortic root (AO).

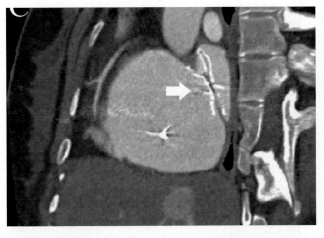

C

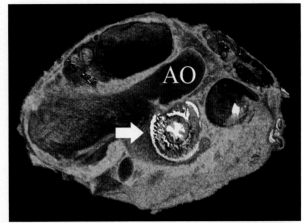

D

Fig. 14.7 (*Continued*) **(C)** Oblique view demonstrates the splay of the device around the aortic root at the superior rim of the ASD. **(D)** Volumetric rendering shows the device orientation adjacent to the mitral valve annulus and just inferior to the aorta.

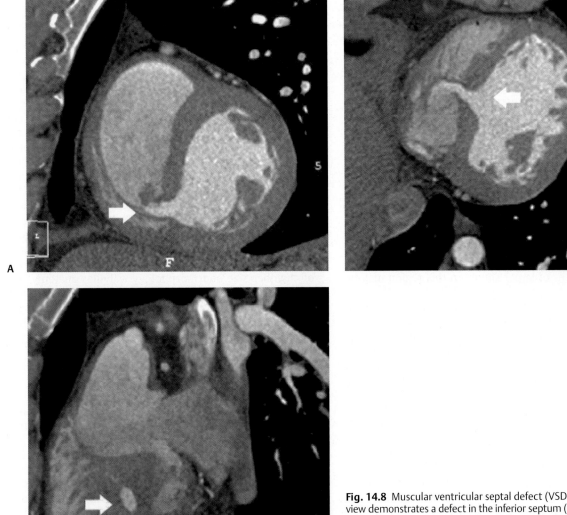

A

B

C

Fig. 14.8 Muscular ventricular septal defect (VSD). **(A)** Short-axis view demonstrates a defect in the inferior septum (*arrow*). **(B)** Axial image again demonstrates the inferoseptal VSD (*arrow*) with a windsock of tissue extending into the right ventricle. **(C)** Cross-section of the VSD in short axis (*arrow*) allows measurement of the VSD diameter.

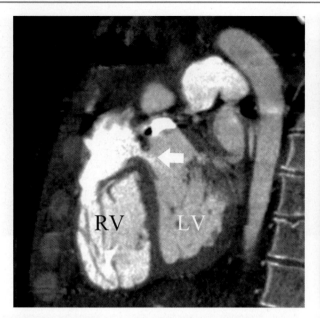

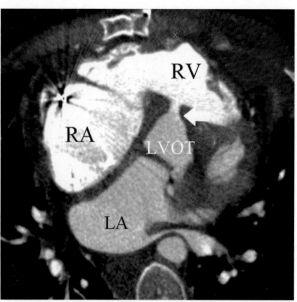

A   B

Fig. 14.9 High conoventricular (perimembranous) ventral septal defect (VSD). **(A)** Long-axis view of the left ventricle (LV) and right ventricle (RV) demonstrates the VSD (*arrow*) into the right ventricular outflow tract. **(B)** Short-axis view again demonstrates the VSD between the left ventricular outflow tract (LVOT) and upper RV. LA, left atrium; RA, right atrium.

defect should be closed using surgical or percutaneous techniques. Infracristal and muscular defects may naturally become smaller or spontaneously close over time. Large VSDs and supracristal defects are unlikely to become smaller over time. VSDs are most often surgically patched through the tricuspid valve with either fabric or pericardium or, less commonly, may be directly oversewn. Transcatheter occlusion of VSD is an evolving technology[32] mostly defined in muscular defects. High membranous defects often are in close proximity to the aortic valve and the septal leaflet of the tricuspid valve (see **Figs. 12.11** and **12.12**). Placement of a percutaneous closure device in a high membranous defect may result in impaired valve function such that surgical management of larger shunts in this region may be preferable.

Echocardiography demonstrates most VSDs but is limited in visualization of supracristal defects.[31] Cardiac MRI can clearly demonstrate VSDs and provide quantitation of any shunt. For optimal evaluation of a VSD by CT, the left ventricle should be well opacified with relatively little opacification of the RV to permit visualization of intracardiac shunting (**Fig. 14.8**).

Multiplanar reformatting is key to defining accurately the VSD anatomy, particularly for smaller defects or high perimembranous septal defects (**Fig. 14.9**). AV canal type defects may result in a common AV canal with an associated ASD or valve leaflet abnormalities. Clefts may be present in the septal leaflet of the tricuspid valve or the anterior leaflet of the mitral valve. Any abnormal attachment of the AV valves should be noted. Ventricular volumes and ejection fractions should be assessed. Initially left ventricular dilatation may occur with larger left-to-right shunts, but with time right ventricular dilatation results from the volume

overload and right ventricular hypertrophy develops secondary to pulmonary hypertension and elevated right-sided pressures (see discussion of right-sided volume and pressure overload and figures in Chapter 9). Large VSDs can result in pulmonary arterial hypertension which, if untreated, may progress to Eisenmenger syndrome with reversal of the interventricular shunt (right → left). Conoventricular and conal septal defects may be associated with prolapse of the right or noncoronary cusp of the aortic valve into the defect, leading to aortic insufficiency.[32] VSDs can also be associated with right or left ventricular outlet narrowing. Based on these associations with VSDs, CT assessment should include evaluation of the VSD location and size along with a review of chamber size and morphology, valvular anatomy, and careful assessment of the outflow tracts below the semilunar valves. Post-operative evaluation of VSD repair, although not routine, should focus on any leak around the patch or through the defect if primary closure was performed.

◆ Tetralogy of Fallot

TOF is the most common form of cyanotic CHD and is traditionally characterized by four abnormalities: (1) pulmonary stenosis, (2) overriding aorta, (3) VSD, and (4) right ventricular hypertrophy (**Fig. 14.10**), which is not an initial manifestation of TOF but usually develops after several weeks of life. It is thought that the tetralogy is actually caused by a single developmental abnormality (ie, underdevelopment of the subpulmonary infundibulum).[33] As patients grow, infundibular stenosis becomes progressively more obstructive. The most severe variant involves complete atresia of the pulmonary valve. The pulmonic valve is

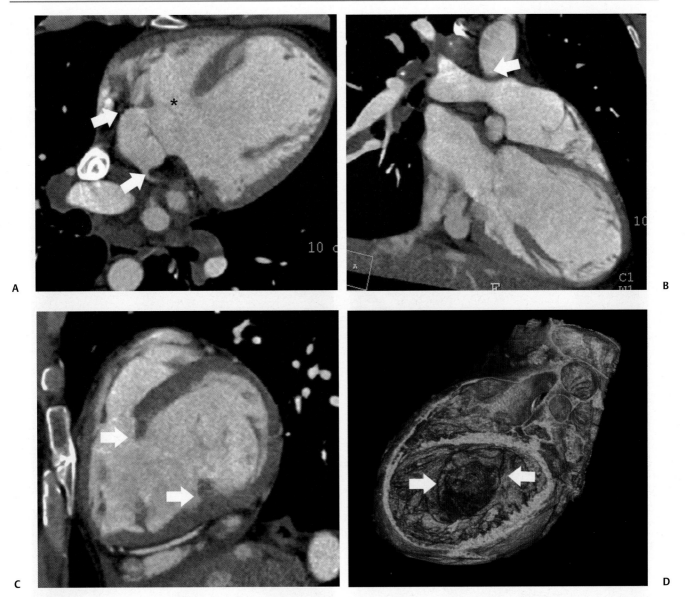

Fig. 14.10 Tetralogy of Fallot with large ventricular septal defect (VSD). **(A)** Axial image demonstrates a large VSD (*) with overriding aorta (*arrows*). **(B)** Coronal image demonstrates mild narrowing of the pulmonary outflow tract (*arrow*). **(C)** Short-axis image again demon-strates the large VSD (*arrows*). **(D)** Volumetric reconstruction views the VSD from the left ventricle side looking through the defect into the right ventricle, showing the massive size.

commonly bicuspid or unicuspid. Also, the central pulmonary arteries may be hypoplastic, diffusely or focally stenotic, discontinuous, or even absent. Pulmonary blood flow may be reliant on a patent ductus arteriosus, bronchial arteries, or aortopulmonary collateral vessels.[33]

The VSD of TOF is usually large and of the conoventricular type. The conal septum is misaligned with the muscular septum. In some patients, the right coronary cusp of the aortic valve may be fused to the VSD, resulting in aortic insufficiency. The overriding aorta is variable in severity but is generally rotated to the right and anteriorly, placing it more over the RV ("overriding"). This overriding must be differentiated from double-outlet RV (DORV) in that the aorta maintains fibrous continuity with the mitral valve in

TOF, whereas DORV has both a subaortic and subpulmonary conus. Thus the anterior portion of the aortic valve tilts superiorly in TOF, whereas it is horizontal in DORV.[34]

In 5 to 6% of patients, coronary artery anomalies are present with TOF, the most important being the left anterior descending artery arising from the right sinus of Valsalva, crossing the infundibulum (see **Fig. 4.19**).[33] Surgeons must be aware of this coronary anomaly before infundibulotomy to avoid injury to the left anterior descending artery. Other abnormalities that may be present with TOF include left superior vena cava, ASD, PFO, and right aortic arch.

In addition to assessment of cardiac morphology and coronary anatomy, cardiac CT may be most useful in visualizing pulmonary blood flow; transthoracic echocardiography is limited in evaluating extracardiac vessels and pulmonary vascular abnormalities, which may be quite complex in TOF. Low-level pulmonary arterial opacification may be achieved without substantial streak artifact by decreasing the rate of infusion for the saline chaser or by infusing dilute contrast in place of a saline chaser after the initial full-strength contrast injection. Because progressive right ventricular dysfunction is common in TOF, right and left ventricular volumes and function should be assessed both before and after surgery.[6]

Surgical repair of TOF usually involves patch repair of the VSD, infundibulotomy, and patch enlargement of the right ventricular outflow tract (RVOT) (**Fig. 14.11**). In the case of significant pulmonary valve stenosis, the valve annulus will be incised and the patch extended across the valve plane. The resulting chronic pulmonary regurgitation often necessitates valve replacement (**Figs. 14.11** and **14.12**). Surgical complications include VSD or RVOT patch leaks, aneurysm of the patch graft, pseudoaneurysm at the margins of the

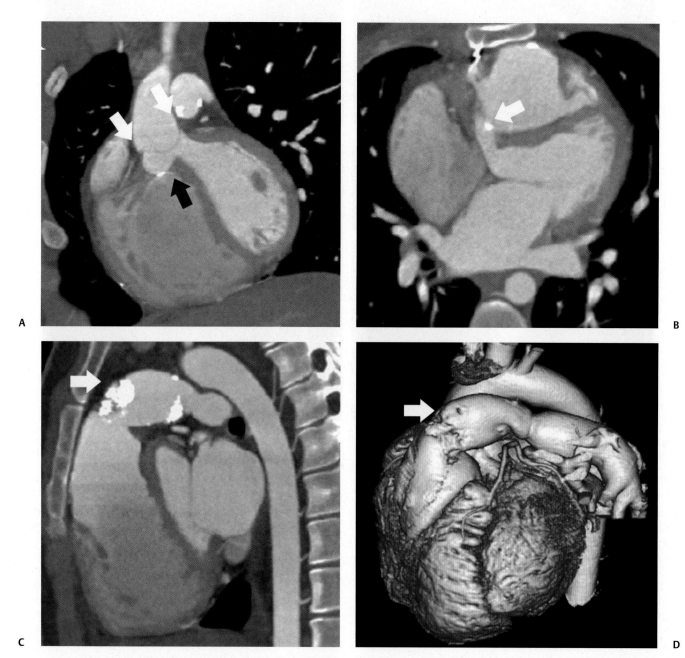

Fig. 14.11 Repaired tetralogy of Fallot. **(A)** Oblique view demonstrates overriding aorta (*white arrows*) with VSD patch (*black arrow*). **(B)** Axial view again demonstrates calcified VSD patch (*arrow*). **(C)** Sagittal view demonstrates the postoperative appearance of a pulmonary valve homograft with calcification in the valve and conduit (*arrow*). **(D)** Three-dimensional volumetric rendering of right ventricle outflow patch/homograft repair (*arrow*).

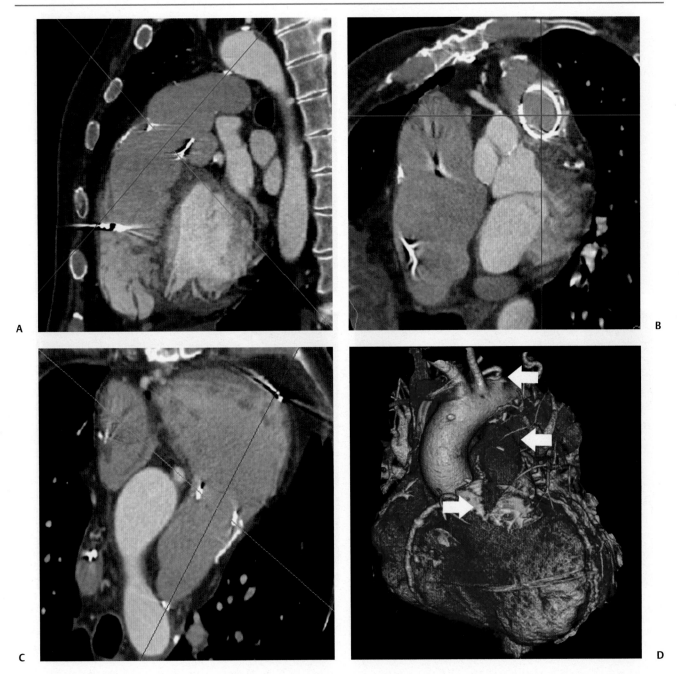

Fig. 14.12 Bioprosthetic pulmonary valve with right ventricular (RV) outflow patch. **(A)** Sagittal and **(B)** axial images demonstrate a bioprosthetic pulmonary valve at the level of the crosshair. The RV is dilated and hypertrophied. **(C)** Oblique view through the RV outflow tract again demonstrates the bioprosthetic valve ring at the crosshair with a dilated and hypertrophied RV. **(D)** Three-dimensional volume image shows the lack of left subclavian artery (*upper arrow*) and the site of surgical repair of the RV outflow (*lower arrows*).

patch, and akinesis of the adjacent RV. Downstream pulmonary artery (PA) aneurysms and pulmonary branch stenoses may also be seen.[33]

A valved conduit is often placed from the RV to the main PA to treat TOF with pulmonary atresia. Complications of conduit placement include leaks around the conduit and kinking or stenosis of the conduit. Other palliative shunts performed before full repair include the classic or modified

Blalock-Taussig (BT) shunt. The classic BT shunt involves ligation of the subclavian artery contralateral to the aortic arch, with an end-to-side anastomosis of the subclavian artery to the ipsilateral PA. The modified BT shunt involves leaving the subclavian artery intact and connecting a synthetic tube from the base of the inominate artery to the ipsilateral PA. Patency of the shunt should be assessed when imaging after surgery. These shunts are "taken down" at the

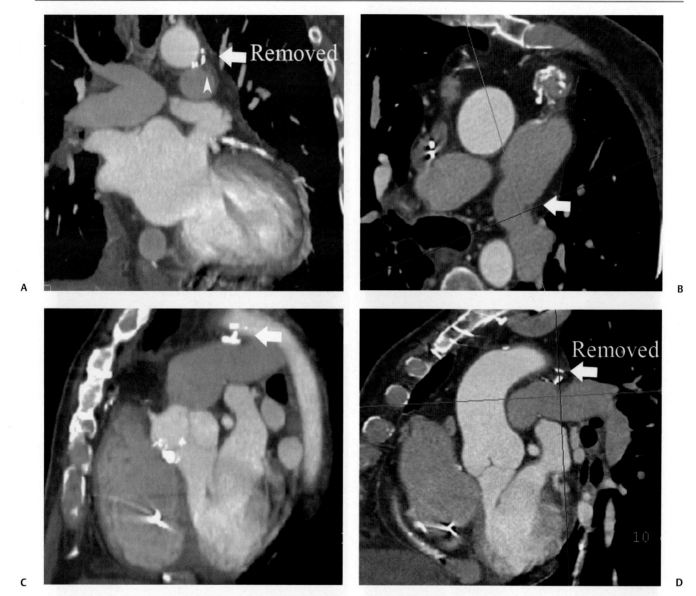

Fig. 14.13 Status post "take down" of Blalock-Taussig left subclavian artery to left pulmonary artery shunt for tetralogy of Fallot. **(A)** Coronal view demonstrates clips at the site of the previous Blalock-Taussig shunt, with mild irregularity in the pulmonary artery (*arrowhead*). The subclavian artery is no longer present. **(B)** Axial view, **(C)** sagittal view, and **(D)** oblique sagittal view again demonstrate post-operative narrowing at the origin of the left pulmonary artery (*arrow*). No significant enhancement is identified in the left pulmonary artery in this phase.

time of full repair, resulting in absence of the left or right subclavian artery (**Fig. 14.13**).

◆ Transposition of the Great Arteries

Transposition of the great arteries (TGA), the second most common cyanotic CHD, is defined by ventriculoarterial discordance, with or without AV discordance. When the AV arrangement is normal (ie, right atrium to RV and left atrium to left ventricle), the transposition is termed d-TGA or "complete transposition" because the morphologic RV is on the right side of the body and anterior to the morphologic left ventricle (see **Fig. 14.14**). Malpositioning of the great arteries in d-TGA results in isolated systemic and pulmonary blood circuits and must therefore be accompanied by a blood mixing shunt (ie, patent ductus arteriosus, ASD, or VSD). The incidence of VSD in d-TGA is about 45%; associated anomalies in d-TGA include coarctation or interrupted aortic arch in 12%, pulmonary stenosis in 5%, right ventricular hypoplasia in 4%, and juxtaposition of the atrial appendages in 2% (**Fig. 14.15**).[35] Pre-operative evaluation of TGA should specifically assess for these associated anomalies as well as coronary artery anomalies and fistulas that are common with TGA (see **Fig. 4.21**).

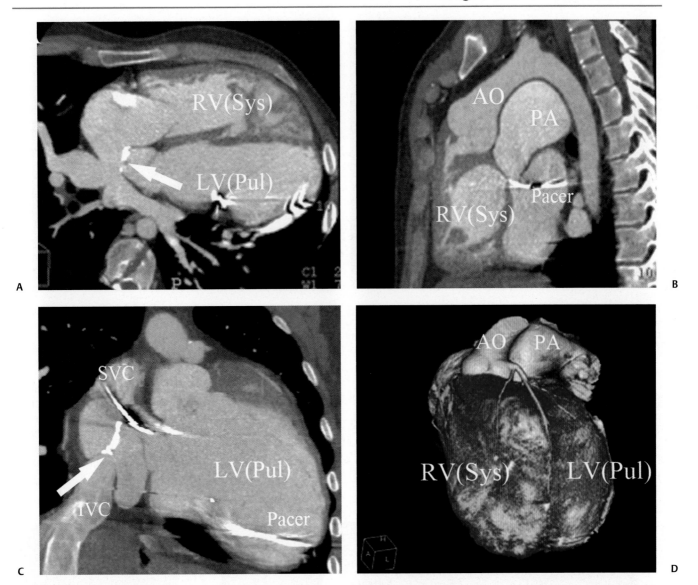

Fig. 14.14 Complete transposition of the great vessels (d-TGA) post atrial switch (Mustard/Senning). **(A)** Axial image demonstrates an anterior trabeculated chamber with a moderator band corresponding to the morphologic right ventricle (RV). The atrial baffle (*arrow*) redirects the inflow between the atria and the ventricles. **(B)** Sagittal image demonstrates the anterior aorta (Ao) connected to the morphologic RV with the pulmonary artery (PA) originating from the posterior chamber, defining arterial transposition. **(C)** The baffle (*arrow*) directs superior vena cava (SVC)–inferior vena cava (IVC) flow anteriorly and to the front into the morphologic left ventricle (LV). The pulmonary venosus flow is baffled to direct flow posteriorly in the atrium into the morphologic RV shown in (A). **(D)** Volumetric rendering of the anterior aorta connected to the anterior systemic ventricle (morphologic RV) is shown.

The first long-term palliative surgery developed for d-TGA was by Senning in 1958. The Senning procedure used native atrial tissue to create an interatrial baffle to direct systemic venous blood flow from the vena cava through the left ventricle to the pulmonary arteries and to direct pulmonary venous blood flow to the RV and aorta.[35] A similar operation was later developed by Mustard, involving excision of the atrial septum and creation of the atrial baffle using pericardium or synthetic material (see **Fig. 14.14**). The main complications of these so-called atrial switch procedures include late right ventricular dysfunction, tricuspid regurgitation, sinus node dysfunction, arrhythmias, obstruction of systemic or pulmonary venous flow, and baffle leaks.[35]

To avoid the late morbidity associated with the atrial switch procedures, Jatene et al described an alternative "arterial switch" operation in 1976.[36] The Jatene procedure, which has become the standard of care, involves transection of the great arteries above the sinuses and detachment of the coronary arteries with buttons of aortic tissue. The arterial positions are switched and the coronary arteries are reimplanted into the neoaortic root (pulmonary stump). A modification of this procedure

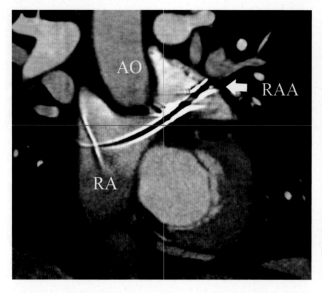

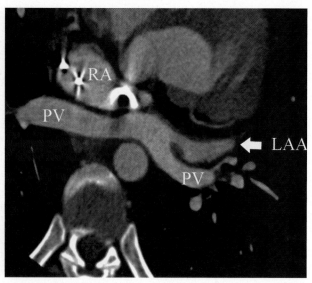

A

B

Fig. 14.15 Juxtaposed right atrial appendage (RAA) on the opposite side of the aorta (Ao) in a transposition of the great arteries (TGA) patient. **(A)** Coronal and **(B)** axial views demonstrate that the atrial lead of a pacemaker crosses the center of the atrium into this displaced appendage. RA, right atrium.

(Lecompte maneuver) straddles the right and left pulmonary arteries around the aorta (**Fig. 14.16**). Advantages of the Jatene operation include re-establishment of the left ventricle as the systemic ventricle and avoidance of extensive atrial suture lines. Complications of arterial switching include coronary artery stenosis, dilatation of the neoaortic root with aortic regurgitation, and PA stenosis.[35,37]

Post-operative CT should evaluate for any of the aforementioned anatomic complications, as well as for ventricular or valvular dysfunction, residual VSD, and aortic coarctation (if initially present). CT is particularly well suited to evaluate the coronary arteries for stenosis related to stretching or displacement of the vessels following a switch procedure (**Fig. 14.17**).[37]

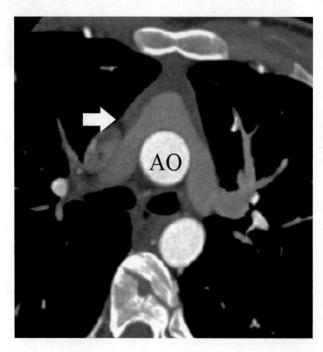

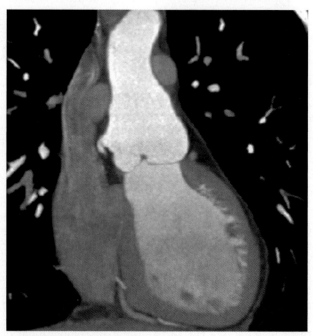

A

B

Fig. 14.16 Transposition of the great arteries after arterial switch procedure (Jatene). **(A)** Axial image demonstrates the pulmonary arteries (*arrow*) stretching around the aorta (AO). **(B)** Oblique coronal image demonstrates the aorta above the left ventricle.

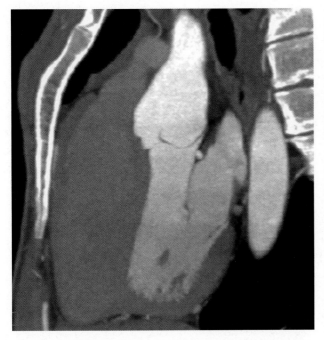

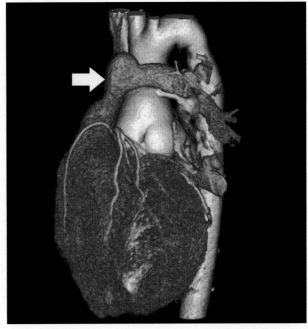

C

D

Fig. 14.16 (*Continued*) **(C)** Sagittal image again demonstrates the aorta above the left ventricle. The aorta is detached and moved posteriorly to the left ventricle and behind the crossing left pulmonary artery. **(D)** Three-dimensional volume rendering of the pulmonary arteries (*arrow*) indenting the aorta as they pass anteriorly.

TGA that occurs with AV discordance is termed l-TGA, ventricular inversion, or "congenitally corrected" TGA. Systemic venous blood returns to the heart through the right atrium, flows into the morphologic left ventricle, and then flows out through the PA. Pulmonary venous blood enters the left atrium, flows through the morphologic RV, and then flows out the aorta (**Fig. 14.18**). Although the morphologic RV is subjected to systemic arterial pressures, normal physiologic blood flow is maintained and patients may live into adulthood with unrecognized l-TGA if there are no other

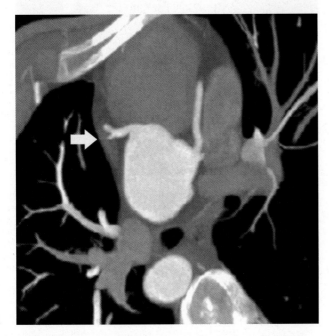

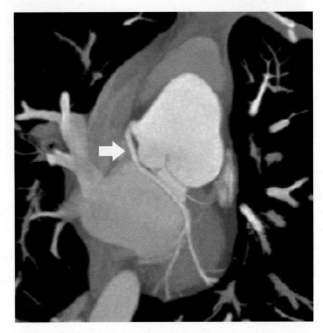

A

B

Fig. 14.17 Transposition of the great arteries after arterial switch with circumflex coronary artery anomaly. **(A)** Axial image demonstrates the right coronary artery origin from the right coronary sinus (*arrow*) as well as the left anterior descending artery origin from the left coronary sinus. **(B)** Oblique maximum intensity projection demonstrates the left circumflex artery (*arrow*) originating from the right coronary artery. The circumflex artery courses inferiorly and posterior to the aortic valve to supply the lateral wall of the left ventricle.

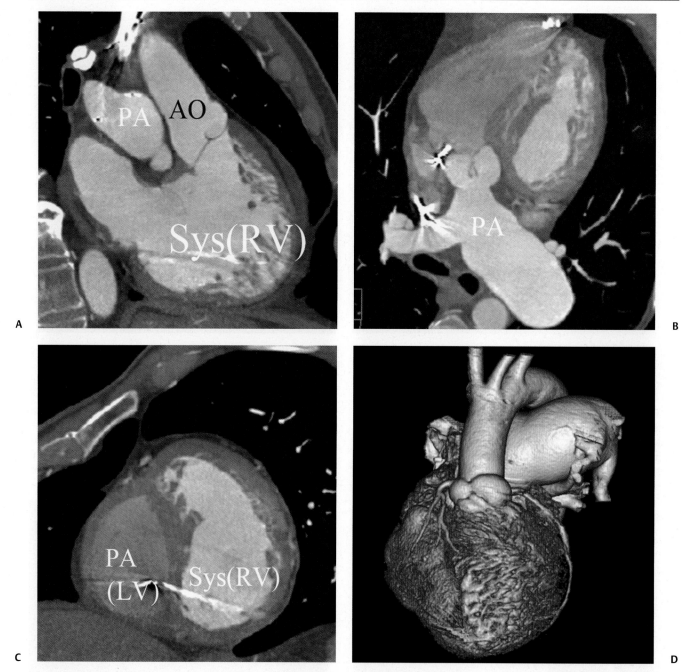

Fig. 14.18 Congenitally corrected transposition of the great vessels (CCTGV, l-TGA). **(A)** Sagittal image demonstrates the anteriorly positioned aorta (AO) arising from a dilated, trabeculated chamber, which represents the morphologic right ventricle (RV). An infundibulum divides the aortic valve from the tricuspid valve. The pulmonary artery (PA) arises more posteriorly. **(B)** Axial image demonstrates the PA arising from the anterior morphologic left ventricle (LV) with an aneurysm of the left PA. **(C)** Short-axis image through the ventricles demonstrates a trabeculated posterior ventricle with a moderator band, consistent with morphologic RV, which is opacified during the systemic phase of contrast distribution. A smooth anterior ventricle, consistent with the morphologic LV is not opacified because the contrast has been displaced from the right-sided circulation by the saline flush in the second phase of the injection. CCTGV is often called ventricular inversion. **(D)** Three-dimensional volume rendering of anterior aorta and posterior PA with left PA aneurysm.

major associated anomalies. In the third and fourth decades of life, the systemic RV function begins to fail, often resulting in the unexpected diagnosis of CHD.

Associated anomalies and complications of congenitally corrected TGA include systemic (tricuspid) AV valve dysfunction in 90%, VSD in 70% (usually conoventricular), pulmonary stenosis in 40% (usually subvalvular), and complete AV block.[35] Many patients may have their systemic AV valve displaced inferiorly toward the cardiac apex, mimicking Ebstein anomaly. The tricuspid valve is relatively delicate and prone to regurgitation when faced with systemic blood pressure and more so if an Ebstein anomaly is present. CT evaluation of a patient with l-TGA should evaluate for ventricular function, associated anomalies, complications of repair of any anomaly (eg, VSD patch leak), and coronary artery anatomy. Limited data suggest that these individuals may benefit from biventricular pacemakers to improve systemic ventricular function. Cardiac CT can identify the coronary sinus anatomy and define appropriate veins on the correct ventricular side for biventricular pacing (see the following).

◆ Complex Congenital Heart Disease

The heterotaxy and univentricular syndromes are a complex set of congenital defects, including abnormalities of the heart as well as the visceral organs (**Fig. 14.19**). These syndromes have classically been divided into the broad classifications of *asplenia* and *polysplenia*. However, there is such variability of both the intracardiac and extracardiac findings that these terms are rarely used to describe the phenotypes encountered. A hallmark of the heterotaxy

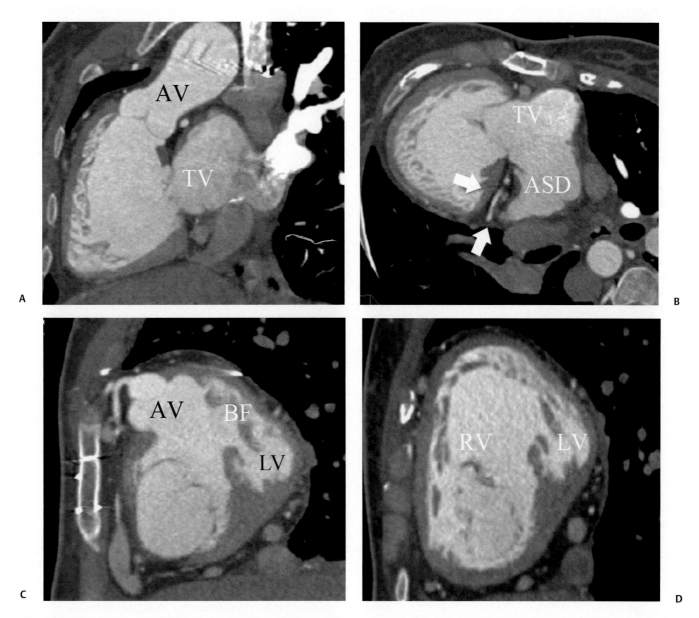

Fig. 14.19 Heterotaxy patient. **(A)** Coronal view demonstrates a right-sided liver with the cardiac apex on the right and the superior vena cava on the left. The aorta and aortic valve (AV) arise from the single trabeculated morphologic right ventricular (RV) chamber. **(B)** Axial image demonstrates mitral valve atresia (*arrows*) with a large atrial septal defect (ASD) between the atria. The mitral atresia results in marked hypoplasia of the left ventricle (LV). A single atrioventricular valve, the tricuspid valve (TV), is present. **(C)** Oblique sagittal view demonstrates a large bulboforaminal (BF) defect or VSD with a small left ventricle (LV), which is functionally part of the univentricle. The aortic root and AV are visualized rising from the ventricle. **(D)** Short-axis view demonstrates the single RV with hypoplastic LV.

syndromes is right-sided or left-sided atrial isomerism. In right-sided isomerism or bilateral "right-sidedness," typical broad-based right atrial appendages are present with pectinate muscles that extend around the vestibule of the AV junction. The position of the cardiac apex is variable, and levocardia, dextrocardia, or mesocardia may be encountered. Frequently encountered intracardiac abnormalities include an AV septal defect, mitral or tricuspid atresia with a concomitant VSD, varying degrees of right or left ventricular dominance, DORV, TGA, and an anterior aorta, often with subpulmonary stenosis or atresia. Additional alterations in vascular anatomy may include connection of the inferior vena cava to the right atrium while the superior vena cava drains to the opposing atrium, interrupted inferior vena cava with the hepatic veins draining directly to the atrium, and a dilated azygous or hemiazygous vein draining all venous blood from below the diaphragm. The abdominal aorta and inferior vena cava are frequently ipsilateral in relation to the spine. The pulmonary veins may be anomalous, draining to either atrium, and are frequently indirect or obstructed.[38]

Univentricular Congenital Heart Disease

The univentricular heart is a rare condition in which a single functional ventricle is present. A small remnant of the nondominant ventricle is usually present and variably located in relation to the dominant ventricle. Congenital cardiac syndromes that fit into this specific nomenclature include double-inlet AV connections (double-inlet left or RV), absence of or severe hypoplasia, one AV connection (mitral or tricuspid atresia), common AV valve and only one well-developed ventricle (unbalanced common AV canal defect), and only one well-developed ventricle with heterotaxy syndrome (single-ventricle heterotaxy syndrome). Despite the heterogeneity of the conditions associated with univentricular heart syndrome, surgical palliation is directed to establish separate pulmonary and systemic circulations. This process is often referred to as the *Fontan repair* and currently is performed in two or three stages, depending on the initial anatomy and physiology. Stages I and II are discussed here, and stage III is discussed more fully under the separate section "The Fontan Patient."[39,40]

Stage I palliation typically occurs in the first weeks of life with the palliative goals of creating unobstructed systemic outflow, unobstructed systemic and pulmonary venous return, and controlled pulmonary blood flow. Pulmonary banding may be performed if an excess of pulmonary flow is present but may later lead to late pulmonary subvalvular stenosis. If there is inadequate pulmonary blood flow, this first stage of repair consists of a classic BT shunt or a modified BT shunt, along with augmentation of the aortic arch as needed (usually in the case of left-sided obstructive lesions).

Stage II palliation, ideally after 4 months of life, converts this unstable circulation to a more stable circulation with a bidirectional Glenn shunt (with end-to-side anastomosis of the divided superior vena cava to the undivided PA) or hemi-Fontan procedure (incorporation of the roof of the

atrium into the PA anastomosis). BT shunt take down is also performed at this time. This procedure removes the superior vena cava circulation from the cardiac circuit but leaves the inferior vena cava connected to the atrial mass. Removing most of the systemic venous return from the cardiac circuit provides a significant reduction in workload for the single ventricle. Stage III of the repair, often termed *Fontan completion*, involves separating the inferior venous return from the cardiac circuit and connecting it directly to the pulmonary arterial circulation as well (**Fig. 14.20**). Evidence of these palliative procedures is visualized during CT examination in the adult patient with univentricular cardiac physiology. Signs of a ligated patent ductus arteriosus and creation of a common atrium will often be present as well.[38-40]

Cardiac CT evaluation of patients in whom a hemi-Fontan has been performed (but before Fontan completion) should evaluate the cardiac chambers and related vascular anatomy carefully because obstruction or dilatation of any segment may be present (**Fig. 14.21**). Specific details to be evaluated include identification of ventricular morphology, AV connections, and ventriculoarterial connections. It is important to define the characteristics of the RV (including trabeculation, presence of the moderator band, and an infundibulum separating the AV valve annulus from the semilunar pulmonic valve), the narrow neck of the left atrial appendage from the wide-based neck of the right atrial appendage, and the arterial connections.[39]

In patients with a double-inlet left ventricle (DILV; 75% of patients have a dominant left ventricle, 20% a dominant RV, and 5% have truly one ventricle), the ventricles are separated by a VSD; the size and location of this VSD should be visualized. In DILV the ventriculoarterial connections are most commonly discordant, with the aorta originating from the RV, which receives blood via a VSD. Subaortic stenosis, aortic hypoplasia, and arch anomalies are frequently present. In contrast to DILV, double-inlet RVs frequently have concordant ventriculoarterial connections with systemic outflow tract obstruction, and AV valvular abnormalities are common. The standard cardiac CT examination should assess ventricular volume, systolic function, and myocardial mass. However, the single versus independent chamber volumes are sometimes difficult to isolate with large "bulboforminal defects" or VSDs.[38,41]

The Fontan Patient

The Fontan procedure was initially performed to palliate and manage tricuspid atresia, but now it has been adapted to palliate patients with single-ventricle physiology when biventricular repair is not possible (**Fig. 14.21**). The principal goal of the Fontan procedure is to separate the pulmonary and systemic circulations by directing systemic venous return directly to the pulmonary circulation without the support of a subpulmonary ventricle.[38] The procedure is often performed in two stages. The first stage, at approximately 4 to 6 months of life, creates a bidirectional Glenn shunt (see preceding section on Univentricular Heart). In

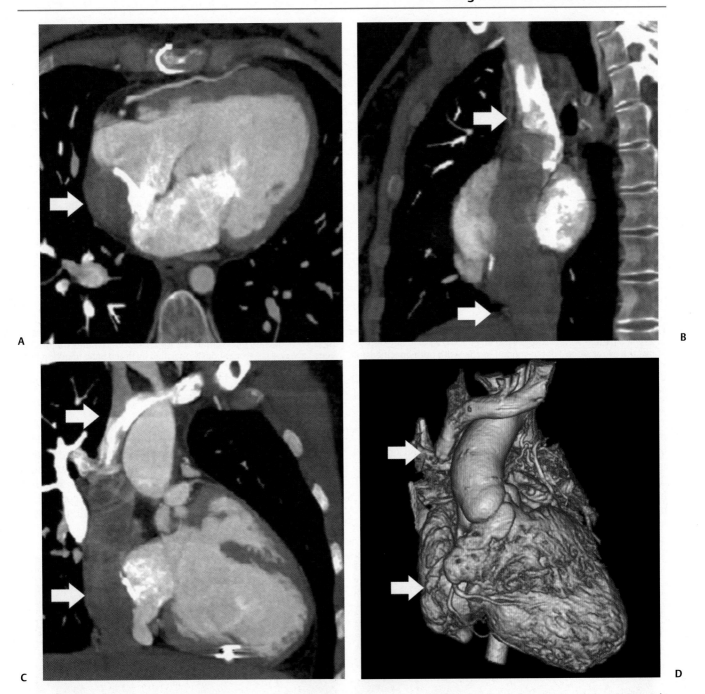

Fig. 14.20 Double-inlet left ventricle (LV) with a lateral tunnel Fontan surgical caval correction. **(A)** Axial view demonstrates a low-intensity structure behind the right atrium (*arrow*), corresponding to the bicaval Fontan connection. **(B)** Sagittal and **(C)** coronal views demonstrate the bicaval Fontan connection (*arrows*) traversing the posterior right atrium. Contrast is shown in the superior vena cava as well as within a right pulmonary artery branch. **(D)** Volumetric rendering again demonstrates the bicaval Fontan connection (*arrows*).

children this first stage removes most systemic venous return from the cardiac circuit so that the patient is able to grow appropriately but will remain cyanotic.

The final stage of the Fontan procedure, often termed *Fontan completion*, is performed between ages 3 and 15 years. The original procedure involved a right atrial to PA anastomosis, but modifications of this procedure include creation of an intracardiac total cavopulmonary connection (lateral tunnel)

or creation of an extracardiac total cavopulmonary connection. After the Fontan completion, the single ventricle pumps exclusively to the systemic circulation. Later modifications of the procedure exclude the right atrium from the pulmonary circuit and demonstrate improved hemodynamic properties. In many centers, a fenestration is created from the Fontan to the common atrium, providing right-to-left shunting and decompression of Fontan pulmonary pressure.

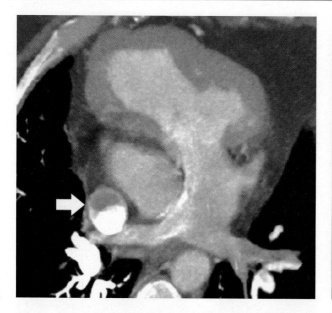

A

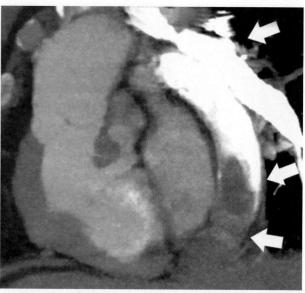

B

Fig. 14.21 Extracardiac Fontan conduit connected to the right pulmonary artery in a patient with tricuspid valve atresia. **(A)** Axial image demonstrates the extracardiac Fontan conduit (*arrow*) with both opacified and unopacified blood. **(B)** Coronal image shows the caval to pulmonary arterial connection with mild stenosis at the superior vena cava (SVC) anastomosis site (*just above the upper arrow*). The SVC was well opacified by power-contrast injection in the upper extremity, and the inferior vena cava was heterogeneously opacified by timed hand injection from the leg.

Assessment of flow by cardiac CT is challenging because most first-pass venous flow from the upper extremities bypasses the heart. Cardiac opacification is based on pulmonary venous return after the bolus of contrast has been dispersed during relatively slow flow through the lungs. It is important to note that the Fontan shunt may not be opacified because inflow from the inferior vena cava or the liver is unopacified (**Fig. 14.22**). The CT examination of patients who have undergone Fontan completion should be evaluated for segmental obstruction, intravascular or intracardiac thrombus, evidence of pulmonary or systemic embolism, and indirect evidence of increased pulmonary pressure.[41] Systemic venous pressure is elevated by virtue of a direct connection to the pulmonary circulation, and even slight alterations in

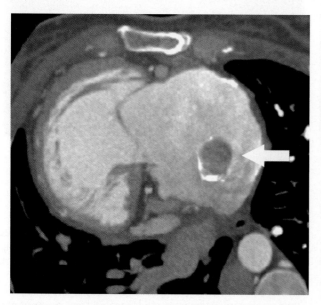

A

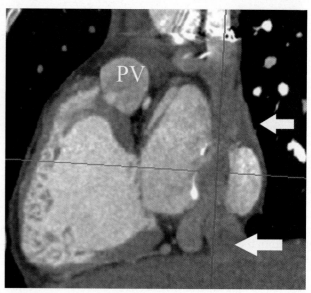

B

Fig. 14.22 Intracardiac Fontan caval anastomosis in a heterotaxy patient. **(A)** Axial image demonstrates the unopacified conduit (*arrow*) passing within the common atrium. **(B)** Oblique coronal image demonstrates the unopacified conduit arising from the left hepatic vein (*lower arrow*) and coursing superiorly (*upper arrow*).

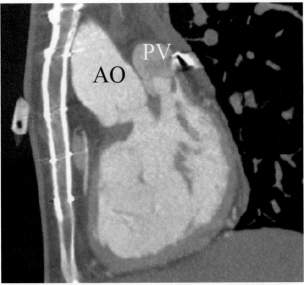
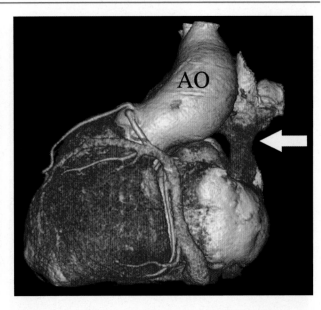

C

D

Fig. 14.22 (Continued) **(C)** Oblique sagittal view demonstrates stenosis at the level of the pulmonic valve (PV) with poor opacification of the pulmonary artery above the valve. **(D)** Volumetric rendering demonstrates the hepatic vein to left pulmonary artery Fontan conduit (arrow).

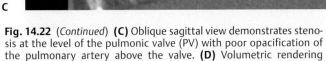

pulmonary pressure can cause significant symptoms. Mild Fontan stenosis or obstruction should be carefully sought because it can present as symptoms related to right-sided heart failure and exercise intolerance. The morphology of the systemic ventricle should be evaluated. Ventricular dysfunction and valvular regurgitation are common, more often in patients with a morphologic systemic RV. In some patients, a classic Glenn shunt (connection of the superior vena cava end to end with the right PA) may remain as part of the Fontan circulation and should be identified. With increasing time after placement of a Glenn shunt, the likelihood that pulmonary AV malformations are present increases and may represent the cause of late clinical deterioration. The aorta should be evaluated for both development of stenosis or aneurysm, both of which are sometimes seen post-operatively. Other possible findings include evidence of ASD closure, BT shunt ligation, and correction of a classic Glenn shunt.

Damus-Kaye-Stansel and Rastelli Repair

The Damus-Kaye-Stansel (DKS) repair involves end-to-side anastomosis between the divided PA and the ascending aorta to increase systemic blood flow (**Fig. 14.23**). This repair is performed in d-TGA for patients with a large VSD and significant subpulmonic (left ventricular outflow tract [LVOT]) obstruction or a hypoplastic ascending aorta. More commonly, the DKS repair is used for single RVs with a hypoplastic ascending and transverse aorta. Although the original procedure included an extracardiac conduit from the RV to the distal PA, this aspect has been replaced by a modified BT shunt, a bidirectional Glenn shunt, or an extracardiac Fontan, depending on age and other physiologic factors.[42–45]

CT offers a complementary imaging study to echocardiography for morphologic and functional information and the detection of extracardiac abnormalities following DKS repair. Whereas echocardiography is superior for definition of

semilunar valve dysfunction, CT can better delineate the geometrically distorted post-surgical anatomy. CT assessment should include evaluation of the pulmonary arterial-to-aortic anastomotic site for narrowing; the PA for residual stenosis from PA banding during early infancy; PA enlargement, which may be marked, depending on the degree of hypoplasia of the systemic outflow chamber; stenosis or occlusion of the branch pulmonary arteries, which can occur post-operatively; and ventricular systolic function, volume, and mass.[42–48] Shunts to the pulmonary circulation—a BT or bidirectional Glenn shunt, likely combined with an extracardiac Fontan—must also be evaluated.

The Rastelli operation was initially used for repair of d-transposition of the great vessels with a large VSD and pulmonary (LVOT) stenosis resulting in a reduction in pulmonary blood flow.[35,49,50] It has also been applied to other cardiac lesions characterized by two ventricles and an overriding aorta with pulmonary outflow tract obstruction, such as pulmonary atresia with a VSD or double-outlet RV with pulmonary stenosis or atresia. Initially an intracardiac baffle is placed to direct left ventricular blood flow through the VSD and out the aorta. The RVOT is sewn shut. The PA trunk is resected and connected to the RV via an external valved conduit, creating a small RV outflow pouch. Advantages of the Rastelli procedure include preservation of the left ventricle as the systemic pumping chamber and bypass of significant LVOT obstruction.[49,50]

Late complications of the Rastelli repair include RV to PA conduit degeneration and stenosis and LVOT obstruction. Subsequent ventricular dysfunction and sudden cardiac death have been associated with late mortality.[52] Ventricular dysfunction can be affected by an abnormal interventricular septum with a large prosthetic component (the VSD baffle) and the presence of RV hypertension, which impairs left ventricular filling and forces leftward septal displacement.[50,51] Pressure gradients are evaluated with echocardiography, but

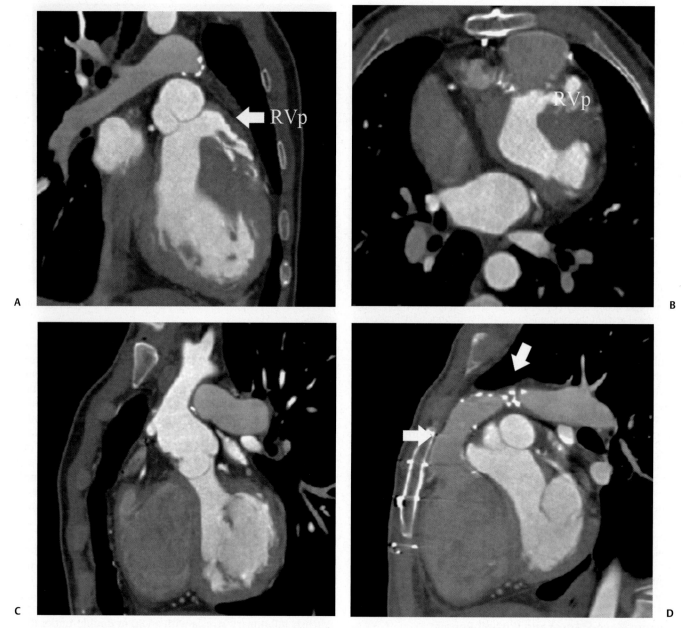

Fig. 14.23 Damus-Kaye-Stansel arterial switch in a patient with transposition of the great vessels and a large ventral septal defect (VSD). **(A)** Coronal image shows the small right ventricle pouch (RVp) with the large VSD. **(B)** Axial image demonstrates closure of the RV outflow tract, creating a small RVp. **(C)** Oblique sagittal view demonstrates reorientation of the aorta posteriorly, adjacent to the conduit to the pulmonary artery (PA). **(D)** Sagittal image demonstrates the Rastelli RV to the PA conduit (*arrows*) with mild narrowing at the anastomosis to the PA (*upper arrow*). The opacified aorta is present under the conduit.

CT better defines the anatomic relationships of the chambers and outflow channels and identifies patients who may be eligible for percutaneous intervention versus those who require surgical repair.

◆ **Pulmonary Vascular Disease**

The normal main PA is slightly smaller than the adjacent ascending aorta. The main PA is normally less than 28 mm in diameter, and the right and left main PA branches should be less than 16 mm in diameter.[52] When pressures in the pulmonary circuit are elevated, dilatation of all or some of the pulmonary segments may occur in association with dilatation of the right-sided cardiac chambers.

Congenital anomalies of the PAs may occur in isolation or in combination with other congenital cardiovascular anomalies. Unilateral proximal interruption of the proximal left or right PA is rare. Interruption of the left PA is associated with a right-sided aortic arch and often with TOF after ductal closure, which essentially causes coarctation of the proximal left PA. Another congenital anomaly is idiopathic dilatation of the pulmonary trunk, which is typically benign and nonprogressive. In this scenario, absence of pulmonary valve stenosis or other cardiac anomalies and the presence of normal PA pressure should be evaluated.[52]

PA aneurysms or pseudoaneurysms may be congenital or acquired and are typically related to a structural weakening of the vessel wall. PA aneurysms may be associated with CHD, such as patent ductus arteriosus, ASD or VSD, TOF, absent pulmonary valve syndrome, TGA, or pulmonary valve structural abnormalities leading to stenosis or regurgitation.[53] Acquired causes include traumatic aneurysms of the PAs, which may be related to injury during interventional procedures to correct stenosis. CT is the preferred examination to follow PA size over time or to assess for PA damage and hemorrhage.

PA branch stenosis may occur as an isolated finding (40%) or in association with CHD (60%), such as valvular pulmonary stenosis and left-to-right shunts, including ASD, VSD, and patent ductus arteriosus. Patients with TOF have a 20% incidence of branch pulmonary stenosis (**Fig. 14.24**).[54] Branch PA stenosis is often present in conjunction with supravalvuar aortic stenosis with genetic syndromes such as Williams

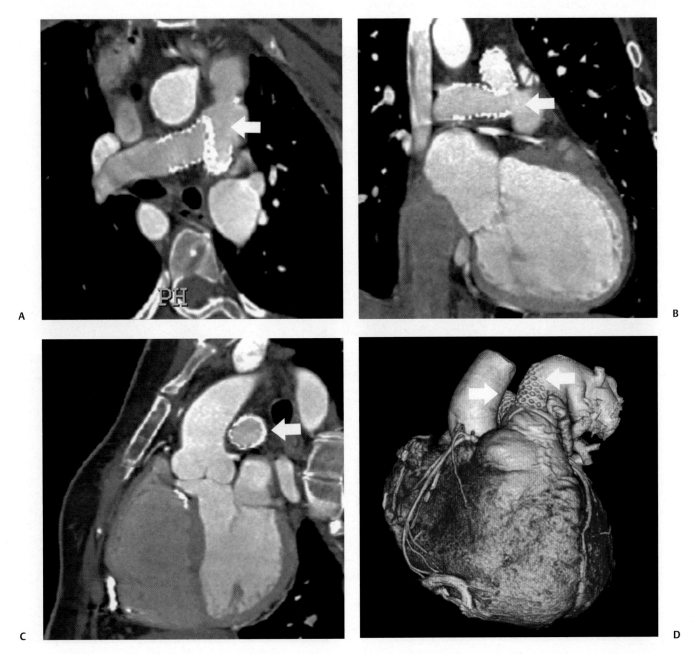

Fig. 14.24 Tetralogy of Fallot patient with stents in the pulmonary arteries (PAs) placed to treat bilateral branch stenosis of the PA. **(A)** Axial image demonstrates a stent in the proximal right PA (*arrow*). **(B)** Oblique sagittal image demonstrates a "kissing" stent in the proximal left PA (*arrow*), immediately adjacent to the right PA stent. Both stents are patent. **(C)** Sagittal image demonstrates the stented left PA (*arrow*) immediately behind the overriding aorta. Post-surgical changes just below the aorta mark the site of a ventral septal defect patch. **(D)** Volumetric rendering again demonstrates the stents in the proximal PAs (*arrows*).

syndrome.[57] Patients with CHD who have undergone surgical correction are also at high risk to develop PA or branch stenosis. The consequences of significant branch stenosis include placing the contralateral pulmonary circulation at risk for complications of increased pulmonary blood flow and pulmonary hypertension. Also, significant systemic to pulmonary collaterals may develop. Occasionally surgical correction of complex congenital defect involves bypass conduits to compensate for hypoplastic pulmonary vessels or valves (**Fig. 14.25**).

Although echocardiography may provide useful information regarding pressure gradients at the site of stenosis, it may incompletely evaluate the degree of stenosis and relationships to surrounding structures. Cardiac CT or MRI provides useful pre-operative information to clinicians regarding serial change and local anatomic relationships in preparation for surgical or percutaneous intervention.

◆ **Cardiac Vein Mapping in Congenital Heart Disease**

Patients with complex CHD have a propensity to develop systolic or even diastolic dysfunction as well as conduction abnormalities, especially if the morphologic RV is the sole supply of systemic circulation. Furthermore, patients with complex CHD have often endured multiple palliative surgical

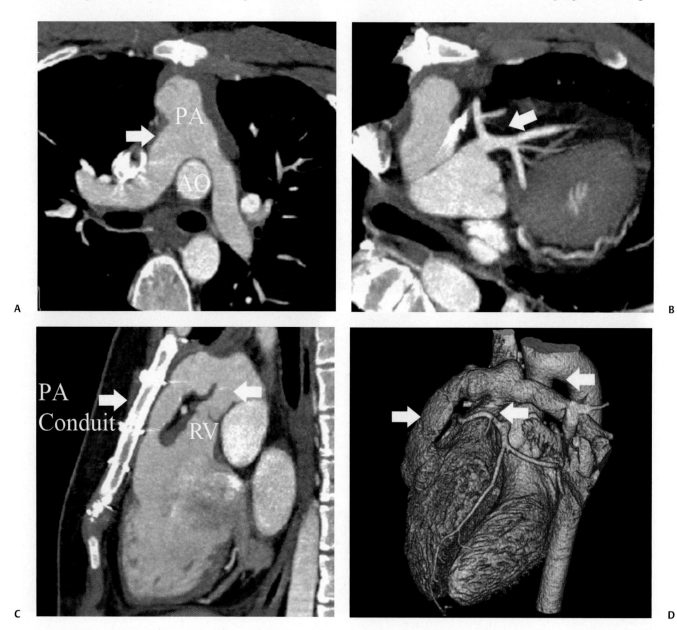

Fig. 14.25 Transposition of the great vessels with pulmonary artery (PA) and valve hypoplasia, status post Jetene procedure. **(A)** Axial image shows the classic arterial (Jatene) switch correction with the PA moved anteriorly and its branches wrapping around the aorta (*arrow*). **(B)** A single coronary artery was present supplying both the right and left coronary territories (*arrow*). **(C)** Sagittal image demonstrates an right ventricle (RV) to PA conduit creating dual RV outflow tracts as a corrective surgical variation. **(D)** Volumetric reconstruction again demonstrates the RV to PA conduit (*arrow on left*) and the single coronary artery (*middle arrow*). The PAs wrapping around the aorta (*arrow on right*).

procedures and are prone to disruption of normal atrial, AV, and interventricular conduction. These abnormalities may benefit from chronic dual-chamber pacing to improve ventricular dysfunction.[56]

In patients with moderate to severe systolic dysfunction and significant electrical and functional heterogeneity of contraction, a biventricular pacemaker may be attempted.[57] Given the variability in size and location of the coronary veins in this population, CT may be extremely helpful in identifying the presence and location of a lateral cardiac vein before attempting to place a biventricular pacemaker (**Fig. 14.26**).

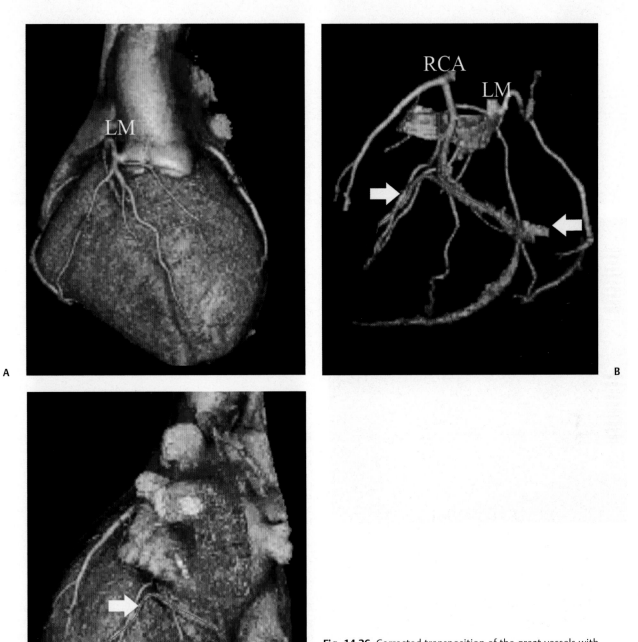

Fig. 14.26 Corrected transposition of the great vessels with venous mapping in a patient with a biventricular pacer. **(A)** Volumetric rendering viewed from an anterior approach demonstrates transposed great vessels with the left main coronary artery (LM) arising from the anterior aorta. **(B)** Segmented coronary arteries and cardiac veins are demonstrated (*arrows*) **(C)** Volumetric rendering demonstrates appropriate location of a pacer wire in a lateral coronary vein of the systemic ventricle (*arrow*). RCA, right coronary artery.

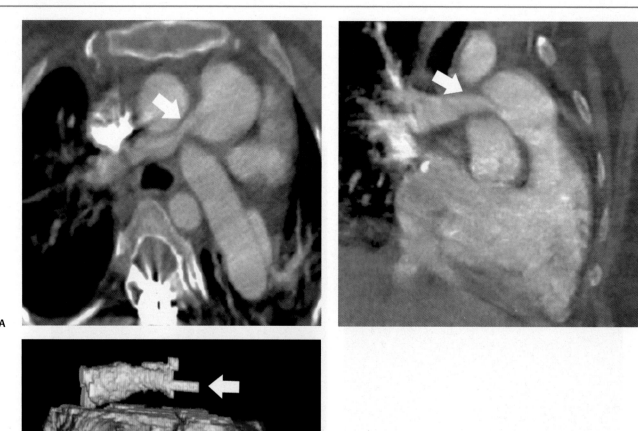

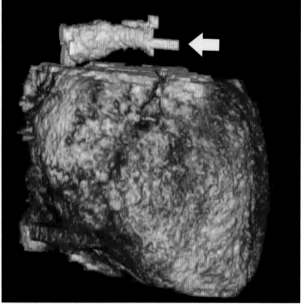

Fig. 14.27 Tetralogy of Fallot patient with stenosis at the origin of the right pulmonary artery (PA). **(A)** Axial image demonstrates stenosis at the origin of the right PA (*arrow*). **(B)** Oblique sagittal image again demonstrates stenosis at the origin of the right PA (*arrow*). **(C)** Using segmentation algorithms, volume rendering of the angulation and position of the stenosis (*arrow*) are characterized in preparation for importing the CT data into the interventional suite.

◆ Cardiac CT Planning and Guidance of Interventional Procedures

Cardiac CT is well suited to the diagnosis of many forms as CHD, as described in this chapter. The localization, sizing, and definition of approach for many cardiac procedures may be best performed with CT.[3,58] Three-dimensional evaluation of cardiac structures in relationship to venous and arterial connections allows for catheters or device selection before the actual interventional procedures.

As an example, in a TOF patient with pulmonary branch stenosis, pre-procedural cardiac CT defines the severity of stenosis as well as the potential path of a planned intervention for treatment of the stenosis (**Fig. 14.27**). Advanced planning is performed using software that integrates cardiac position in the CT data set with fluoroscopic imaging (**Fig. 14.28**). Accurate pre-procedure planning and intraprocedure guidance with CT may reduce procedural time and total radiation exposure while improving patient outcomes.[59]

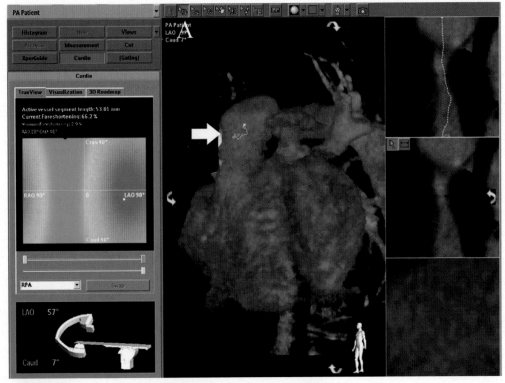

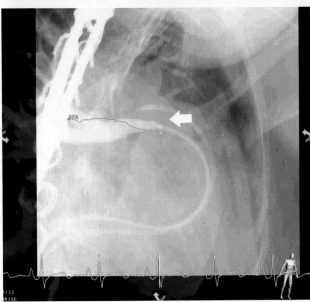

Fig. 14.28 Importation of cardiac CT data into the catheterization laboratory for treatment of right pulmonary artery (PA) stenosis (straight *arrows* in parts A and B). **(A)** TrueView display moves the CT data in relationship to the fluoroscopic imaging arm angulations. The centerline of the PA stenosis is shown in the small images along the right side of the display. **(B)** Selective pulmonary angiogram performed with appropriate angulation based on the CT image to visualize the PA stenosis without foreshortening.

◆ Conclusion

Cardiac CT can rapidly acquire important three-dimensional morphologic and functional cardiac images that are often complementary to echocardiography. When the cardiac CT examination is properly tailored to a clinical question, key data acquired by CT can be used to direct the appropriate management of CHD. These benefits of CT imaging in CHD often outweigh the potential risks of iodinated contrast and radiation exposure. Finally, pre-procedural planning and procedural guidance with cardiac CT are possible today and will probably revolutionize the diagnosis and procedural management of patients with complex CHD in the near future.

References

1. Pillutla P, Shetty KD, Foster E. Mortality associated with adult congenital heart disease: trends in the US population from 1979 to 2005. Am Heart J. 2009;158(5):874–879

2. Steiner RM, Reddy GP, Flicker S. Congenital cardiovascular disease in the adult patient: imaging update. J Thorac Imaging. 2002;17(1):1–17

3. Hudson PA, Eng MH, Kim MS, Quaife RA, Salcedo EE, Carroll JD. A comparison of echocardiographic modalities to guide structural heart disease interventions. J Interv Cardiol. 2008;21(6):535–546

4. Lipton MJ, Higgins CB, Farmer D, Boyd DP. Cardiac imaging with a high-speed cine-CT scanner: preliminary results. Radiology. 1984;152(3):579–582

5. Skotnicki R, MacMillan RM, Rees MR, et al. Detection of atrial septal defect by contrast-enhanced ultrafast computed tomography. Cathet Cardiovasc Diagn. 1986;12(2):103–106

6. Funabashi N, Asano M, Sekine T, Nakayama T, Komuro I. Direction, location, and size of shunt flow in congenital heart disease evaluated by ECG-gated multislice computed tomography. Int J Cardiol. 2006;112(3):399–404

7. Gade CL, Bergman G, Naidu S, Weinsaft JW, Callister TQ, Min JK. Comprehensive evaluation of atrial septal defects in individuals undergoing percutaneous repair by 64-detector row computed tomography. Int J Cardiovasc Imaging. 2007;23(3):397–404

8. Kim YJ, Hur J, Choe KO, et al. Interatrial shunt detected in coronary computed tomography angiography: differential features of a patent foramen ovale and an atrial septal defect. J Comput Assist Tomogr. 2008;32(5):663–667

9. Vick GW, Bezold LI. (2008, October 1) Classification and clinical features of isolated atrial septal defects in children. In: Basow DS, ed. UpToDate. Waltham, Mass: UpToDate; 2008

10. Webb GD, Smallhorn JF, Therrien J, Redington AN. Left to right shunts. In: Libby P, Bonow RO, Mann DL, Zipes DP, eds. Braunwald's Heart Disease: A Textbook of Cardiovascular Medicine. 8th ed. St. Louis: WB Saunders, 2007; 1577

11. Webb G, Gatzoulis MA. Atrial septal defects in the adult: recent progress and overview. Circulation. 2006;114(15):1645–1653

12. Green CE, Gottdiener JS, Goldstein HA. Atrial septal defect. Semin Roentgenol. 1985;20(3):214–225

13. Ho ML, Bhalla S, Bierhals A, Gutierrez F. MDCT of partial anomalous pulmonary venous return (PAPVR) in adults. J Thorac Imaging. 2009;24(2):89–95

14. Mantini E, Grontin CM, Lillehei CW, Edwards JE. Congenital anomalies involving the coronary sinus. Circulation. 1966;33:317–327

15. Thangaroopan M, Truong QA, Kalra MK, Yared K, Abbara S. Images in cardiovascular medicine. Rare case of an unroofed coronary sinus: diagnosis by multidetector computed tomography. Circulation. 2009; 119(16):e518–e520

16. Hagen PT, Scholz DG, Edwards WD. Incidence and size of patent foramen ovale during the first 10 decades of life: an autopsy study of 965 normal hearts. Mayo Clin Proc. 1984;59(1):17–20

17. Williamson EE, Kirsch J, Araoz PA, et al. ECG-gated cardiac CT angiography using 64-MDCT for detection of patent foramen ovale. AJR Am J Roentgenol. 2008;190(4):929–933

18. McMahon CJ, Feltes TF, Fraley JK, et al. Natural history of growth of secundum atrial septal defects and implications for transcatheter closure. Heart. 2002;87(3):256–259

19. Rickers C, Hamm C, Stern H, et al. Percutaneous closure of secundum atrial septal defect with a new self centering device ("angel wings"). Heart. 1998;80(5):517–521

20. Gupta A, Kapoor G, Dalvi B. Transcatheter closure of atrial septal defects. Expert Rev Cardiovasc Ther. 2004;2(5):713–719

21. Harper RW, Mottram PM, McGaw DJ. Closure of secundum atrial septal defects with the Amplatzer septal occluder device: techniques and problems. Catheter Cardiovasc Interv. 2002;57(4):508–524

22. Hein R, Büscheck F, Fischer E, et al. Atrial and ventricular septal defects can safely be closed by percutaneous intervention. J Interv Cardiol. 2005;18(6):515–522

23. Murphy JG, Gersh BJ, McGoon MD, et al. Long-term outcome after surgical repair of isolated atrial septal defect. Follow-up at 27 to 32 years. N Engl J Med. 1990;323(24):1645–1650

24. King TD, Thompson SL, Steiner C, Mills NL. Secundum atrial septal defect. Nonoperative closure during cardiac catheterization. JAMA. 1976;235(23):2506–2509

25. Moake L, Ramaciotti C. Atrial septal defect treatment options. AACN Clin Issues. 2005;16(2):252–266

26. Visconti KJ, Bichell DP, Jonas RA, Newburger JW, Bellinger DC. Developmental outcome after surgical versus interventional closure of secundum atrial septal defect in children. Circulation. 1999; 100(19, Suppl):II145–II150

27. Berger F, Ewert P, Abdul-Khaliq H, Nürnberg JH, Lange PE. Percutaneous closure of large atrial septal defects with the Amplatzer Septal Occluder: technical overkill or recommendable alternative treatment? J Interv Cardiol. 2001;14(1):63–67

28. Knirsch W, Dodge-Khatami A, Valsangiacomo-Buechel E, Weiss M, Berger F. Challenges encountered during closure of atrial septal defects. Pediatr Cardiol. 2005;26(2):147–153

29. Zaidi AN, Cheatham JP, Raman SV, Cook SC. Multislice computed tomographic findings in symptomatic patients after amplatzer septal occluder device implantation. J Interv Cardiol. 2009;22(1):92–97

30. Van Praagh R, Geva T, Kreutzer J. Ventricular septal defects: how shall we describe, name and classify them? J Am Coll Cardiol. 1989;14(5):1298–1299

31. Bremerich J, Reddy GP, Higgins CB. MRI of supracristal ventricular septal defects. J Comput Assist Tomogr. 1999;23(1):13–15

32. Wald RM, Powell AJ. Simple congenital heart lesions. J Cardiovasc Magn Reson. 2006;8(4):619–631

33. Van Praagh R, Van Praagh S, Nebesar RA, Muster AJ, Sinha SN, Paul MH. Tetralogy of Fallot: underdevelopment of the pulmonary infundibulum and its sequelae. Am J Cardiol. 1970;26(1):25–33

34. Dorfman AL, Geva T. Magnetic resonance imaging evaluation of congenital heart disease: conotruncal anomalies. J Cardiovasc Magn Reson. 2006;8(4):645–659

35. Warnes CA. Transposition of the great arteries. Circulation. 2006; 114(24):2699–2709

36. Jatene AD, Fontes VF, Paulista PP, et al. Anatomic correction of transposition of the great vessels. J Thorac Cardiovasc Surg. 1976;72(3):364–370

37. Ou P, Mousseaux E, Azarine A, et al. Detection of coronary complications after the arterial switch operation for transposition of the great arteries: first experience with multislice computed tomography in children. J Thorac Cardiovasc Surg. 2006;131(3): 639–643

38. Khairy P, Poirier N, Mercier LA. Univentricular heart. Circulation. 2007;115(6):800–812

39. Gaca AM, Jaggers JJ, Dudley LT, Bisset GS III. Repair of congenital heart disease: a primer-part 1. Radiology. 2008;247(3):617–631

40. Libby P, Bonow RO, Zipes DP, et al. Braunwald's Heart Disease, 8th ed. Philadelphia: Saunders and Elsevier; 2008

41. Spevak PJ, Johnson PT, Fishman EK. Surgically corrected congenital heart disease: utility of 64-MDCT. AJR Am J Roentgenol. 2008;191(3): 854–861

42. Kaye MP. Anatomic correction of transposition of great arteries. Mayo Clin Proc. 1975;50(11):638–640

43. Subramanian VA. Surgery for transposition of great arteries (letter). Ann Thorac Surg. 1975;20:722–724

44. Stansel HC Jr. A new operation for d-loop transposition of the great vessels. Ann Thorac Surg. 1975;19(5):565–567

45. Laks H, Gates RN, Elami A, Pearl JM. Damus-Stansel-Kaye procedure: technical modifications. Ann Thorac Surg. 1992;54(1):169–172

46. McElhinney DB, Reddy VM, Silverman NH, Hanley FL. Modified Damus-Kaye-Stansel procedure for single ventricle, subaortic stenosis, and arch obstruction in neonates and infants: midterm results and techniques for avoiding circulatory arrest. J Thorac Cardiovasc Surg. 1997;114(5):718–725, discussion 725–726

47. Brawn WJ, Sethia B, Jagtap R, et al. Univentricular heart with systemic outflow obstruction: palliation by primary Damus procedure. Ann Thorac Surg. 1995;59(6):1441–1447

48. Fraser CD Jr. Management of systemic outlet obstruction in patients undergoing single ventricle palliation. Semin Thorac Cardiovasc Surg Pediatr Card Surg Annu. 2009;12:70–75

49. Rastelli GC, McGoon DC, Wallace RB. Anatomic correction of transposition of the great arteries with ventricular septal defect and subpulmonary stenosis. J Thorac Cardiovasc Surg. 1969;58(4):545–552

50. Kreutzer C, De Vive J, Oppido G, et al. Twenty-five-year experience with rastelli repair for transposition of the great arteries. J Thorac Cardiovasc Surg. 2000;120(2):211–223

51. Palik I, Graham TP Jr, Burger J. Ventricular pump performance in patients with obstructed right ventricular-pulmonary artery conduits. Am Heart J. 1986;112(6):1271–1278

52. Castañer E, Gallardo X, Rimola J, et al. Congenital and acquired pulmonary artery anomalies in the adult: radiologic overview. Radiographics. 2006;26(2):349–371 Review

53. Makaryus AN, Catanzaro J, Boxt L. Pulmonary artery aneurysm evaluated by 64-detector CT 254 in a patient with repaired tetralogy of Fallot. Tex Heart Inst J. 2007;34(2):254–255

54. Bacha EA, Kreutzer J. Comprehensive management of branch pulmonary artery stenosis. J Interv Cardiol. 2001;14(3):367–375

55. Beuren AJ, Schulze C, Eberle P, Harmjanz D, Apitz J. The syndrome of supravalvular aortic stenosis, peripheral pulmonary artery stenosis, mental retardation, and similar facial appearance. Am J Cardiol. 1964;13:471–483

56. Hsieh MJ, Yeh KH, Satish OS, Wang CC. Permanent pacing using a coronary sinus lead in a patient with univentricular physiology: an extended application of biventricular pacing technology. Europace. 2006;8(2):147–150

57. Dubin AM, Janousek J, Rhee E, et al. Resynchronization therapy in pediatric and congenital heart disease patients: an international multicenter study. J Am Coll Cardiol. 2005;46(12):2277–2283

58. Kim MS, Hansgen AR, Wink O, Quaife RA, Carroll JD. Rapid prototyping: a new tool in understanding and treating structural heart disease. Circulation. 2008;117(18):2388–2394

59. Chen SJ, Hansgen AR, Carroll JD. The future cardiac catheterization laboratory. Cardiol Clin. 2009;27(3):541–548

15

Triple Rule-Out CT Angiography for Evaluation of Acute Chest Pain and Suspected Acute Coronary Syndrome

Ethan J. Halpern*

◆ Essentials

1 The primary goal of "triple rule-out" (TRO) CT in the emergency department (ED) is to facilitate the safe, rapid discharge of patients judged to be at low to intermediate risk of acute coronary syndrome (ACS).

2 The detection of noncoronary lesions that explain the presenting complaint is a major advantage of the TRO-CT over nuclear stress testing.

3 TRO studies are most appropriate and cost-effective when there is a suspicion for ACS along with other diagnoses, such as pulmonary embolism, acute aortic syndrome, or nonvascular pathology in the thorax.

4 An optimized TRO protocol provides excellent image quality for aortic, coronary, and pulmonary arterial evaluation while minimizing contrast dose and radiation exposure.

5 Attention to the details of patient preparation, contrast administration, and timing of the scan is the key to high-quality TRO studies.

TRO-CT angiography (CTA) can provide cost-effective evaluation of the coronary arteries, aorta, pulmonary arteries, and adjacent intrathoracic structures for the patient with acute chest pain. It is most appropriate for the patient who is judged to be at low to intermediate risk for ACS and whose symptoms may also be attributed to acute pathology of the aorta or pulmonary arteries. Although a regular cardiac rhythm remains an important factor in coronary CT image quality, newer CT scanners with 64 or more detector rows afford rapid electrocardiographic (ECG)-gated imaging to provide high-quality TRO-CT in patients with heart rates up to 80 beats per minute. Injection of iodinated contrast material (≤100 mL) is tailored to provide simultaneous high levels of arterial enhancement in the coronary arteries and aorta (>300 Hounsfield units [HU]) as well as the pulmonary

arteries (>200 HU). To limit radiation exposure, the TRO-CT does not include the entire chest but is constrained to incorporate the aortic arch down through the heart. Scan parameters, including prospective ECG tube current modulation and prospective ECG gating with the "step and shoot" technique, are tailored to reduce radiation exposure (optimally 5–9 mSv). When performed with appropriate attention to timing and technique, TRO-CT provides coronary image quality equal to that of a dedicated coronary CTA and pulmonary arterial evaluation that is free of motion artifact related to cardiac pulsation. In an appropriately selected ED patient population, TRO-CT can safely eliminate the need for further diagnostic testing in more than 75% of patients.

Evaluation of chest pain in the ED is a public health issue of great consequence. Based on the most recent available health statistics report from the Centers for Disease Control and Prevention, evaluation of acute chest pain and related symptoms was the second most common reason for a visit to the ED by adult women and the most common reason for a visit to the ED by adult men in the United States in 2006.[1] Chest pain accounted for 6,392,000 ED visits and 1,976,000 hospital admissions. Overall, suspected heart disease and chest pain were the most common reason for direct admission from the ED and accounted for 2,492,000 hospital admissions in 2006.

The differential diagnosis of chest pain is a complex problem for the ED physician. The diagnosis of ACS includes unstable angina, non–ST-elevation myocardial infarction, and ST-elevation myocardial infarction. Among patients presenting to the ED with symptoms of ACS, only 25% ultimately have a confirmed diagnosis of ACS on discharge.[2] The failure rate for diagnosis of ACS among patients presenting to the ED is in the range of 2 to 5%[3,4] but may be as high as 29% in low-volume centers.[5] Patients in whom the diagnosis of ACS is missed tend to be younger, with an atypical presentation and a nondiagnostic ECG.[6] The missed diagnosis of ACS is a common reason for litigation against ED physicians, accounting for up to 25% of the total malpractice liability of ED physicians.[7]

* Adapted with permission from Radiology. 2009 Aug;252(2):332–45

On the other hand, uncertainty in the diagnosis of ACS results in the practice of defensive medicine and begets an increased number of diagnostic tests and hospital admissions.[8] The cost of negative inpatient cardiac evaluations is estimated at $6 billion in the United States each year.[9]

◆ Clinical Role of TRO-CT

Numerous studies have demonstrated good to excellent diagnostic accuracy of dedicated coronary CT (cCTA) for evaluation of coronary disease,[10] with excellent negative predictive value.[11,12] However, few reports have described the application of CT as part of the TRO examination with a dedicated TRO injection and scan protocol.[13] TRO-CT is a tailored ECG-gated examination designed to evaluate the aorta, coronary circulation, pulmonary arteries, and the mid to lower portion of the chest with a single scan. Application of the TRO for evaluation of suspected ACS in the ED is possible because of advances in CT technology that provide greater z-axis coverage with improved temporal resolution and decreased radiation dose. A recent survey of radiology practices found that 33% used CT in the ED for the workup of chest pain and that 18% were using the TRO study.[14]

All patients with ACS require hospital admission, and many will benefit from rapid triage to cardiac catheterization and intervention. On the other hand, when the patient's presentation clearly suggests a noncardiac diagnosis, coronary evaluation is not required and is not cost-effective. The remaining patients with suspected ACS must be cleared of this diagnosis before discharge. Given the potentially life-threatening consequences of missing the diagnosis of ACS, a high negative predictive value is critical for discharging patients with suspected ACS. The negative predictive value of cCTA for ACS will depend on the prevalence of coronary disease in the study population. A recent multicenter trial demonstrated a 99% negative predictive value of cCTA for coronary disease at both the patient and vessel level in a population with a disease prevalence of less than 25%, establishing cCTA as an effective noninvasive examination to rule out obstructive coronary artery stenosis.[15] Although another recent multicenter trial demonstrated a negative predictive value of only 83% for cCTA, this study evaluated a population with a high (56%) prevalence of obstructive coronary disease.[16] Based on these studies of dedicated cCTA, it is likely that TRO-CT will be most effective in a population with a low prevalence (<25%) of obstructive coronary disease.

For patients with low risk of ACS who are evaluated with conventional nuclear stress testing, only one third of patients with a positive or indeterminate stress test are found to have significant coronary disease on catheterization.[17] For the evaluation of patients presenting to the ED who are judged to be at low risk of ACS, coronary CTA is at least as accurate as nuclear imaging,[18] and it allows the safe, rapid discharge of low to intermediate risk ACS patients.[19–21] A recent study suggests that in low to moderate risk patients a CT triage model is less costly and more effective than strategies based on either stress echocardiography or stress ECG testing.[22] Another recent study concludes that "compared to the other strategies, immediate CTA is safe, identified as many patients with coronary disease, had the lowest cost, had the shortest length of stay, and allowed discharge for the majority of patients."[23] TRO-CT precludes the need for additional diagnostic testing in over 75% of patients with low to intermediate risk of ACS, and provides the additional advantage of finding noncoronary diagnoses that explain the presenting complaint in 11% of ED patients.[24] TRO-CT avoids the need for separate dedicated studies for coronary disease, aortic dissection, pulmonary embolism, and other acute chest pathology. In a properly selected population, coronary CT can provide cost-effective evaluation[25] with reduced diagnostic time, lower costs, and fewer repeat evaluations for recurrent chest pain compared with standard diagnostic evaluation.[26]

Among patients who present to the ED with a low to moderate risk of ACS and who are evaluated with TRO-CT, a minority (<10%) are subsequently evaluated with conventional cardiac catheterization. Among those ED patients who are studied with both TRO-CT and cardiac catheterization, few normal cardiac catheterization studies would be expected.[24] Because it would not be ethical to subject most patients with a low to moderate risk of ACS to cardiac catheterization, there are no studies that confirm the negative predictive value of TRO-CT relative to conventional arteriography in the ED population. Nonetheless, if the quality of coronary imaging obtained with TRO-CT is equivalent to that of dedicated cCTA, one would expect the same high diagnostic accuracy and negative predictive value that has been documented with dedicated cCTA.

Injection and scanning techniques for TRO-CT studies vary considerably from one institution to another, resulting in inconsistent image quality. Some radiologists are reluctant to perform TRO studies because of an impression that the TRO is too technically challenging or that the quality of the coronary artery study is compromised in the TRO examination. The goal of this "how I do it" chapter is to discuss various approaches to patient preparation, bolus timing, contrast administration, and ECG gating and to describe a straightforward, optimized technique for performance of TRO-CT studies. An "optimized" TRO protocol should minimize contrast dose and radiation exposure to the patient while providing coronary arterial image quality equivalent to that of a dedicated cCTA, pulmonary arterial image quality equivalent to that of a dedicated CT pulmonary arteriogram, and high-quality imaging of the thoracic aorta without pulsation artifact.

◆ Patient Selection

Appropriate patient selection is crucial to the cost-effective application of TRO-CT (**Table 15.1**). Patients who are at high risk for ACS with elevated cardiac biomarkers or acute ECG changes should be admitted to the hospital and are likely to benefit from direct triage to cardiac catheterization for diagnostic purposes and timely intervention. In the remaining patients with suspected ACS, the goal of TRO-CT is to exclude the diagnosis of coronary disease or to define an

Table 15.1 Patient Selection Criteria for Triple Rule-Out CT

- Clinical presentation: low to moderate risk of acute coronary syndrome (ACS)

- Clinical presentation: non-ACS diagnosis considered

- Negative biomarkers (myoglobin and troponin-I)

- Normal electrocardiographic (ECG) or nonspecific changes

- No history to suggest extensive coronary calcium

- Not recommended for patients with bypass or stents

- Patient able to tolerate CT and hold breath

- Cardiac rhythm acceptable for ECG-gated scan

- Adequate renal function

alternative diagnosis that might explain the presenting symptoms. Patients who are likely to have a high burden of calcified coronary plaque based on known coronary disease (previous myocardial infarction, chronic angina, stented patients, and post-bypass patients) are less likely to benefit from the coronary imaging performed with TRO-CT, although the TRO study may still be useful with respect to the aorta, pulmonary arteries, and other intrathoracic pathology. The degree of coronary disease is often overestimated in these patients as a result of blooming of calcified plaque such that it is impossible to exclude significant coronary disease. Older patients with multiple cardiac risk factors are more likely to have extensive coronary calcification.[27] An indeterminate coronary CT evaluation is much more likely in patients with an elevated calcium score (above 400–1000).[28] In such patients, a calcium scoring study may be useful before performing TRO-CT to determine whether the patient is a candidate for TRO-CT.

An acceptable clinical history for TRO-CT includes a symptom complex that raises the suspicion of ACS, including symptoms such as chest pain; shortness of breath; syncope or near syncope; or neck, shoulder, back, or arm pain not appearing to be musculoskeletal in nature. Patients should have negative initial cardiac biomarkers (myoglobin and troponin-I) and should not have new ECG changes suggestive of myocardial ischemia. Ideally, these patients should have signs, symptoms, and laboratory data that might be interpreted as consistent with ACS or other causes of chest pain, including pulmonary embolism and acute aortic syndrome. In selected patients with low levels of positive biomarkers, TRO-CT may be appropriate when the clinical impression favors pulmonary embolism or acute aortic syndrome; there is a need to exclude ACS, but there is no immediate intention of sending the patient for invasive cardiac catheterization. When clinical suspicion is truly limited to ACS, a dedicated coronary CTA is preferred because it will use less contrast material and expose the patient to a lower radiation dose. Age, gender, and clinical presentation are well-validated parameters that can be used to define a

population with suspected ACS that would be appropriate for TRO-CT.[29] Although traditional cardiac risk factors such as a family history of coronary disease, hypercholesterolemia, or hypertension are important long-term prognostic markers, such risk factors are of limited clinical value in diagnosing ACS in the ED setting and in triaging these patients.[30]

The presence of a cardiac arrhythmia presents a challenge for ECG-gated coronary imaging, but it is no longer an absolute contraindication. Sinus bradycardia is the preferred heart rhythm for TRO-CT. In the absence of a clinical contraindication, a β-blocker should be administered before performing TRO-CT. Both heart rate and ectopy are reduced after treatment with an intravenous β-blocker.[31,32] New scanner technology provides improved temporal resolution with the capability of scanning the entire heart in one or two heartbeats (compared with four to five beats for most 64-slice scanners). This new technology has reduced the required phase window for diagnostic imaging of the coronary arteries along with the impact of variability in heart rhythm on coronary image quality.[33] The decision as to whether a patient should be excluded from the TRO-CT on the basis of a cardiac arrhythmia must be based on an assessment of the magnitude of the arrhythmia and the specific capabilities of the scanner that will be used for the study. Regular heart rates up to 80 beats per minute are no longer a contraindication for many new scanners, including dual-source scanners and single-source scanners with gantry rotation times less than 300 msec. Irregular tachyarrhythmias pose a more difficult problem, but the degree of contraindication depends on the frequency of ectopic beats.

Allergies to contrast material and renal insufficiency are relative contraindications to administration of iodinated contrast for TRO studies. The presence of asthma, acute heart failure, severe cardiomyopathy, and hypotension may limit the use β-blockers to control heart rate and thus may reduce the quality of the TRO examination. A history of recent cocaine use or a positive drug screen for cocaine is also a relative contraindication to the use of β-blockers for the scan,[34] although this contraindication remains controversial.[35] Recent use of a phosphodiesterase inhibitor is a relative contraindication to the administration of nitroglycerin for coronary vasodilatation during CT, but this does not represent a contraindication to TRO-CT.

◆ CT Hardware and Radiation Issues

TRO-CT studies require a longer scan length than dedicated coronary CTA. A mean scan length of 20 cm is required to image the chest from above the aortic arch through the caudal aspect of the heart. To perform this scan during a single breath-hold, the scanner should be capable of imaging the required volume with ECG-gated technique in no more than 15 seconds. This requirement limits TRO-CT studies to scanners with at least 64 detector rows.

TRO studies are associated with a higher radiation dose compared with dedicated coronary CTA examinations

Table 15.2 Patient Preparation for Triple Rule-Out CT

- Withhold caffeine and other cardiac stimulants before the study
- Good intravenous (IV) access (preferable 18-gauge)
- Proper positioning of the arm with the IV line, directly in front of the patient and resting on the gantry, to avoid subclavian vein compression
- Saline injection at rapid rate to test IV
- Electrocardiographic lead placement for clear R-waves
- β-blockers (2.5–30 mg IV) to achieve sinus bradycardia
- Sublingual nitroglycerin 2–3 min before CT angiography
- Practice a small breath-hold for 15 s

Table 15.3 Scan Location, Timing, and Parameters

- Heart is positioned at the center of the gantry to maximize resolution
- Acquisition begins 1–2 cm above the aortic arch
- Caudal extent is programmed to extend through the base of the heart, but real-time monitoring is used to terminate the scan as soon as the base of the heart is imaged
- CT angiography begins 5 s after contrast enters the left atrium
- Cranial-to-caudal direction of acquisition is preferred
- Standard scan parameters: mean effective mA of 600 at 120 kVp

because of the longer scan length. Our typical scan parameters include a tube voltage of 120 kVp and a mean effective tube current of 600 mA per slice (where effective mA = tube mA × gantry rotation time/pitch). Heavier patients weighing over 200 pounds are scanned with higher tube current of 800 to 1000 mA based on a subjective estimate of patient body habitus by the attending radiologist. In our experience, mean effective TRO radiation dose for patients evaluated in helical scan mode without tube current modulation averages 18 mSv and is decreased to 8.75 mSv among patients evaluated with tube current modulation.[36] Mean effective tube current or tube voltage can be decreased in smaller patients to reduce radiation dose.

Until recently all cCTA studies were performed with a helical scan acquisition (with or without tube current modulation). In patients with stable heart rates, newer scanners can acquire TRO-CT with prospective ECG gating using the "step and shoot" axial mode to further reduce radiation dose to 5–6 mSv. Prospective ECG gating should be reserved for patients with a stable heart rate because any change in cardiac rhythm will either prolong the scan time (as the scanner waits for the next "normal" heartbeat) or result in degraded image quality from cardiac motion. Images obtained with prospective ECG gating are more sensitive to minor variations in heart rate and cannot provide information about cardiac function and regional wall motion. Nonetheless, in appropriately selected patients evaluated with proper attention to technique, prospective ECG gating

of coronary CTA can be used to reduce radiation dose while maintaining image quality.[37,38]

CT imaging, and coronary CT in particular, have been criticized as an important source of radiation exposure to the population.[39,40] Recent advances in CT technology, however, allow a dramatic decrease in radiation dose with coronary CT. The effective radiation dose for a TRO-CT with a state-of-the-art scanner compares favorably with the dose of a nuclear stress test, which has been reported to range from 10 to 17 mSv.[41] When one considers that the conventional workup of a chest pain patient presenting to the ED is likely to include a negative nuclear stress test as well as another diagnostic radiologic examination such as a chest CT or VQ study, application of TRO-CT studies to an appropriate patient population may actually reduce the per patient radiation exposure for diagnostic studies during the ED evaluation.

◆ TRO Technique and Image Quality

High-quality coronary imaging is essential to distinguish patients with coronary disease from those in whom ACS may be excluded. Careful attention to patient preparation (**Table 15.2**), scan technique (**Table 15.3**), and injection technique (**Table 15.4**) will result in optimal, homogeneous aortic, coronary, and pulmonary arterial opacification and in coronary image quality that is equal to that obtained by dedicated coronary CTA.[42] ECG gating of TRO studies

Table 15.4 Contrast Injection Protocol for Triple Rule-Out (TRO) CT

Protocol	First phase	Second phase	Injection rate
Dedicated coronary CT angiography	70 mL I-350 mg/mL	40 mL saline	5.5 mL/s
TRO-CT	70 mL I-350 mg/mL	50 mL dilute contrast (25 mL I-350 + 25 mL saline)	5.0 mL/s
Extended TRO-CT18–20 s (see Fig. 15.8)	80 mL I-350 mg/mL	70 mL dilute contrast (35 mL I-350 + 35 mL saline)	5.0 mL/s

eliminates motion artifact related to cardiac pulsation and therefore provides superior definition of the pulmonary arterial tree compared with dedicated pulmonary CTA without ECG gating. The discussion that follows is directed primarily toward performance of the TRO study with a 64-slice scanner.

◆ Patient Preparation and Monitoring

To minimize ectopy in the cardiac rhythm during coronary CTA studies, patients should refrain from stimulants such as caffeine on the day of the scans. However, unlike typical outpatients scheduled for coronary CTA, TRO-CT patients typically present directly from the ED and cannot be instructed to modify their dietary intake before the study. Nonetheless, the use of intravenous β-blockers allows rapid control of heart rate and reduction of ectopy in ED patients sent for TRO-CT.

Adequate intravenous access is necessary to deliver a rapid contrast bolus for coronary CTA. An 18- to 20-gauge intravenous line is placed into a large vein in the antecubital fossa. The intravenous line should be tested with a rapid saline flush to ascertain that there is no extravasation and that the patient does not experience pain with injection. A painful intravenous line can result in a sudden change of heart rate during contrast injection, with degradation of image quality. To reduce inadvertent compression of the subclavian vein during contrast injection, the arm with the intravenous line should not be extended above the patient's head. With the patient lying in a supine position, I prefer to extend the arm with the intravenous line directly in front of the patient. To keep the patient comfortable and keep the arm out of the gantry, the extended hand is rested on the gantry during the scan.

ECG leads are positioned above and below the level of the scan to avoid streak artifact. The ECG tracing should be evaluated immediately prior to the scan with the patient's arms raised into the position that will be used for the scan. It is important to be certain that the ECG leads will not be pulled off of the patient when the table moves for the scan. A clearly defined R-wave is necessary to insure adequate ECG-gating. If necessary, leads should be repositioned to obtain a clearly defined R-wave.

Baseline heart rate and blood pressure are obtained before administration of β-blockers, during administration of β-blockers, and following the procedure. A stable blood pressure should be documented before the patient is returned to the ED.

The ideal heart rate for ECG-gated studies is a slow regular rhythm, usually a sinus bradycardia at 50 to 60 beats per minute.[43] Although precise control of heart rate may be less critical with dual-tube scanners or with newer scanners that have a faster gantry rotation and improved temporal resolution, image quality is optimized and radiation dose is minimized with a regular cardiac rhythm. Oral β-blockers may be given in the ED at least 1 hour before the scan for control of heart rate. However, heart rate often increases with the level of anxiety when the patient is placed on the

CT table. I prefer to administer metoprolol intravenously when the patient is on the CT table. Intravenous metoprolol has an onset of action within 1 to 3 minutes (compared with 1 to 2 hours for an orally administered dose) and allows better titration of heart rate before contrast injection. β-blockers may alter vascular tone, cardiac rhythm, and myocardial contractility and can promote bronchospasm. Metoprolol should be used with caution and may be contraindicated in patients with heart block, uncompensated heart failure, or asthma.

In the interest of improving patient throughput, administration of metoprolol is performed during acquisition of the scout topogram and setting up of the bolus tracking images before performing coronary CTA. Patients who arrive with a heart rate in the range of 60 to 65 beats per minute are given an initial intravenous dose of 2.5 mg of metoprolol. Patients who arrive with a heart rate greater than 65 beats per minute are given an initial intravenous dose of 5 mg. After allowing several minutes to observe the effect of the first dose, additional doses of 5 mg are administered every 3 to 5 minutes until the target heart rate is achieved. A minority of patients with acute chest pain or shortness of breath will present with a tachycardia that does not respond to β-blockade. It is unusual to administer more than 20 mg of metoprolol because patients who do not respond with a lower heart rate after the first 10 to 20 mg are unlikely to respond to a higher dose. For patients who continue to respond slowly to administration of an intravenous β-blocker, my maximum intravenous dose is 30 mg. The patient's heart rate and blood pressure are monitored after every dose, and no further β-blocker is given if systolic pressure falls below 100 mm Hg.

To achieve maximum coronary vasodilatation for the study, sublingual nitroglycerin is administered 2 to 3 minutes before initiating the TRO-CT.[44] A recent study suggests that pre-treatment with sublingual nitroglycerin may improve the diagnostic accuracy of coronary CT.[45] As with metoprolol, nitroglycerin is not administered if the systolic blood pressure falls below 100 mm Hg. Although nitroglycerin and β-blockers can combine to cause hypotension, this is not generally a problem on the CT table with the patient in supine position. Nitroglycerin does result in a reflex tachycardia, but this is not generally a problem when patients have received a β-blocker before the study. Relative contraindications to nitroglycerin include clinical scenarios such as hypovolemia and idiopathic hypertrophic subaortic stenosis or patients who have recently taken a phosphodiesterase inhibitor, in whom nitroglycerin may induce profound hypotension.

After administration of nitroglycerin, I generally practice the breath-hold with the patient. The patient is instructed to take a slow, small breath and to hold it for 15 seconds. A large inspiratory effort draws more unopacified blood from the inferior vena cava and may reduce the level of intravascular opacification during the scan.[46] If the patient takes a large practice breath, I ask the patient to repeat the practice exercise and take a smaller breath. Although the breath-hold may seem like a trivial detail, it is important to practice the breath-hold so that the patient is prepared for the length of the breath-hold that will be required for the scan.

Setting up the Scan

The TRO-CT must include the entire thoracic aorta as well as the heart. Based on the scout topogram, TRO scans are programmed to start 1cm above the aortic arch, usually at the inferior margins of the clavicular heads (**Fig. 15.1**). Because the radiation dose to the patient is directly proportional to the length of the scan, the lung apices above the level of the aortic arch are not included. Although 5% of patients with pulmonary embolism have an isolated upper lobe embolus,[47] an isolated subsegmental pulmonary embolus above the level of the aortic arch is extremely uncommon and is unlikely to be detected by CTA. In the early days of spiral CT, before the introduction of multislice CT scanners, dedicated pulmonary CTA was generally limited to a distance of 10 to 12 cm from the aortic arch down through the inferior pulmonary veins.[48] Excluding the apices from TRO-CT reduces the scan length by about 4 to 5 cm, which we estimate is associated with a reduction in effective radiation dose by 15 to 20%.

Many centers traditionally scan CT pulmonary arteriography studies in the caudal-to-cranial direction to reduce the impact of respiratory motion in the lower lobes.[49,50] Others have suggested advantages to scanning in the cranial to caudal direction for CT pulmonary arteriography.[51] As discussed later, the cranial-to-caudal scan direction is favored for TRO studies because of additional considerations related to timing of the contrast injection and patient heart rate. Although the scan is programmed to continue through the base of the heart, the TRO-CTA acquisition is monitored in real time and is manually stopped as soon as the base of the heart is imaged. Manually stopping the scan at the heart base can reduce scan length by 1.5 to 2 cm. The radiation dose estimates of 8.75 to 18 mSv cited previously were obtained before we routinely began terminating the scan in real time once the base of the heart was imaged. We estimate that the use of real-time monitoring to reduce acquisition length can reduce the radiation dose by another 7 to 10%.

Contrast Injection and Timing of Image Acquisition

The goal of contrast administration for dedicated coronary CTA is to maintain a high level of enhancement in the coronary arteries.[52] Coronary opacification demonstrates a strong correlation with the rate of injection as well as the concentration of iodine within the contrast material.[53,54] For TRO-CT studies, a reasonable enhancement goal is a density level above 300 HU in the coronary arteries and above 200 HU in the pulmonary arteries. Standard injection techniques used for dedicated coronary CTA result in suboptimal opacification of the pulmonary arterial circulation.[55] Opacification of the pulmonary arteries requires an extended contrast injection to maintain contrast on the right side of the heart during the scan. However, it is important not to have full-strength contrast in the superior vena cava at the time of the scan because this can cause streak artifact that can limit image quality.

Studies of aortic CTA have demonstrated an advantage to the biphasic injection of contrast material.[56] High-rate, uniphasic injection of contrast material results in a peak of contrast enhancement during a short interval, with attenuation minima at the beginning or end of the acquisition. A biphasic injection protocol can be tailored to provide a more homogeneous enhancement profile over time. To optimize both coronary and pulmonary arterial enhancement for TRO-CT, I prefer a biphasic contrast injection protocol to provide an intense, homogeneous level of contrast enhancement in the left-sided circulation (aorta and coronary arteries), with a slightly lower, homogeneous level of enhancement in the right-sided circulation. A rapid flow rate is maintained throughout the injection to minimize the effect of venous return from the inferior vena cava. Although pre-heating of contrast material is not required to obtain a rapid flow rate, pre-heating up to a temperature of 37° C before injection reduces viscosity of the contrast material and facilitates a rapid flow rate at lower injection pressures.[57]

The biphasic injection is timed so that the first phase of the injection opacifies the left side of the heart while the second phase opacifies the right side during TRO-CT. More specifically, for a 64-detector scanner the biphasic injection consists of 70 mL of undiluted contrast material (350 mg of iodine per milliliter) followed by 25 mL of contrast diluted with 25 mL of saline, all injected at 5.0 mL per second (**Table 15.4**). To make efficient use of the contrast bolus, imaging is triggered based on opacification of the left atrium, which begins 2 to 3 seconds before opacification of the descending aorta. The scan begins 5 seconds after the contrast enters the left atrium (**Fig. 15.1**) so that the aorta and coronary arteries are in the plateau phase of peak enhancement during CTA acquisition. The injection volume and rate are optimized for a scan time of about 14 to 15 seconds. In the event of a significantly longer scan time, as may occur if there is an arrhythmia when using prospective ECG gating or when the CTA is extended in length, the injection would need to be prolonged to ensure adequate pulmonary opacification (**Table 15.4**). When the TRO study is properly timed, the first phase of the injection opacifies the coronary arteries during image acquisition (**Figs. 15.2** and **15.3**); the second phase of the injection provides simultaneous homogeneous enhancement of the pulmonary arteries (**Figs. 15.4** and **15.5**). The thoracic aorta is also homogeneously enhanced and optimally evaluated (**Figs. 15.6** and **15.7**). A review of our TRO studies demonstrates that this technique provides a mean enhancement level of 300 to 350 HU in the aorta, pulmonary arteries, and coronary arteries.

Several variations of this biphasic injection protocol have been proposed. In one variation, a biphasic injection is used with undiluted contrast material (320 mg of iodine per milliliter), but the flow rate starts at 5 mL per second and is then reduced to 3 mL per second to avoid overloading the right side of the heart and superior vena cava (SVC) with dense contrast.[58,59] The reduced flow rate in the second phase of the injection provides a longer injection time and reduces streak artifact from the SVC. A 50-mL saline flush is applied as a third phase to flush the contrast that remains in the arm veins into the right-sided heart. An alternative

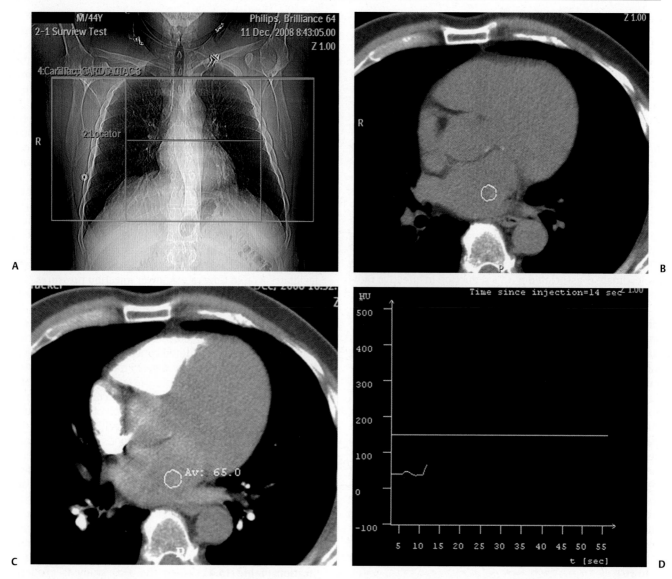

Fig. 15.1 Scan setup and bolus tracking images. **(A)** Scout topogram. Scan levels are planned within the green rectangle. The starting level for the scan is at the inferior margin of the clavicular heads, just above the aortic arch. The inferior margin of the scan is set below the base of the heart. To limit radiation to the patient, CT angiography (CTA) acquisition is monitored in real time and manually stopped as soon as the base of the heart is imaged. Note that the setup specifies two different reconstruction fields of view. The smaller 25-cm field of view is used for evaluation of the aorta and coronary anatomy. The larger field of view is used to evaluate the pulmonary arteries, lungs, and chest wall. **(B)** Pre-contrast image for bolus tracking. Table height and patient position are adjusted so that the heart is centered within the scan. CT resolution is maximized in the center of the gantry. A region of interest is defined within the left atrium (*circle*). **(C)** Low-dose bolus tracking images are obtained every 2 seconds, beginning 5 seconds after the start of the contrast injection. This bolus tracking image demonstrates early opacification of the left atrium. The CTA acquisition was manually started at this time. **(D)** The scan is programmed to begin 5 seconds after initial opacification of the left atrium reaches a level 100 HU above baseline (horizontal line at 150 HU in this plot). However, to maximize use of the contrast dose, the scan is manually started by the technologist as soon as contrast enters the left atrium. This manual start time is about 2 seconds earlier than the density would have triggered an automatic start to the scan. The programmed start line serves as a backup in the event the technologist fails to start the scan earlier.

triphasic technique uses a first phase with 50 mL of undiluted contrast material (350 mg of iodine per milliliter) followed by 50 mL of 60% contrast/saline and 30 mL of saline, each injected at 4.5 mL per second.[60] Contrast is diluted in the second phase of the injection to reduce streak artifact from the SVC. The use of dilute contrast material with a faster flow rate has a theoretical advantage over the use of full-strength contrast material at a slower rate. The faster injection rate results in greater filling of the venous system from the injection, more filling of the right atrium from the SVC, and less variation related to unopacified venous flow from the inferior vena cava.

Although I use a saline flush for dedicated cCTA, I do not use a saline flush for TRO studies. In my experience the

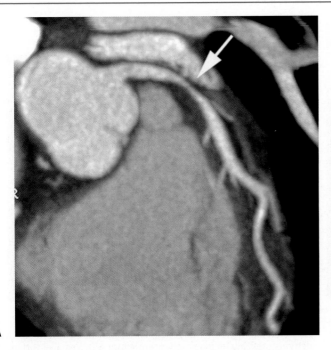

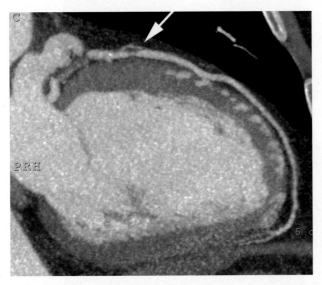

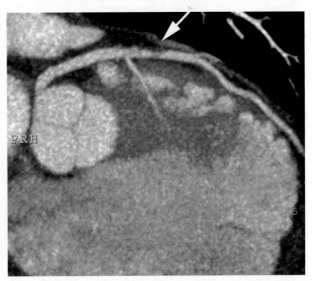

Fig. 15.2 Triple rule-out (TRO) CT angiogram of a 37-year-old woman with no significant prior cardiac history presenting with sudden onset of chest pain while at work. TRO demonstrates a smooth 75% stenosis of the left anterior descending artery (*arrows*). Patient was treated with angioplasty. **(A)** Slab maximum intensity projection (MIP) of the left anterior descending artery (LAD) in the long axis of the aortic root. **(B)** Slab MIP of the LAD in an orthogonal obliquity in the short axis of the aortic root.

saline flush can result in complete washout of contrast from the right side of the heart and can result in a nondiagnostic pulmonary arteriogram when the scan acquisition time is prolonged or when the start of image acquisition is delayed by a slow right-to-left contrast transit time. I prefer to leave some of the dilute contrast material from the second phase of injection in the patient's arm rather than risk using a saline flush that may wash the contrast out of the pulmonary circulation. When scan time must be increased for additional z-axis coverage, the injection may be prolonged

Fig. 15.3 Triple rule-out (TRO) CT angiogram of a 51-year-old athletic man with no prior significant cardiac history presenting with atypical chest pain while resting at home. TRO demonstrates an irregular narrowing of the left anterior descending artery (LAD) (*arrows*). Patient was treated with angioplasty. (The bright spots projecting just below the LAD correspond to contrast material within the interstices of the right ventricle between trabeculations adjacent to the interventricular septum. These are imaged along with the septum because of the thickness of the slab MIP projection.) **(A)** Slab MIP of the LAD along the long axis of the left ventricle. **(B)** Slab MIP of the LAD in an orthogonal obliquity in the short axis of the aortic root.

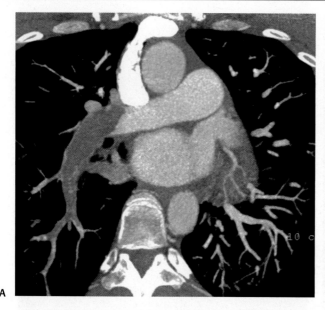

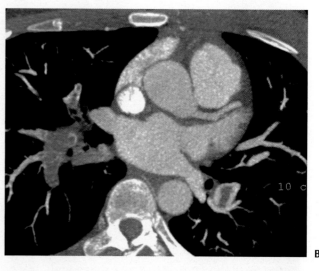

Fig. 15.4 Triple rule-out (TRO) CT angiogram of a 31-year-old woman with chest pain that was atypical for angina but with no significant shortness of breath. TRO demonstrates bilateral pulmonary embolism with a normal aorta and coronary arteries. **(A)** Oblique coronal slab maximum intensity projection (MIP) demonstrates a large thrombus in the right pulmonary artery and the interlobar pulmonary artery with extension into right lower-lobe segmental branches. **(B)** Axial slab MIP demonstrates bilateral pulmonary embolism with a smaller thrombus also present in the left pulmonary artery.

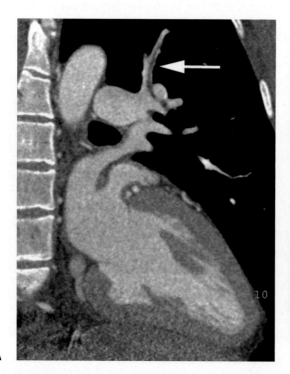

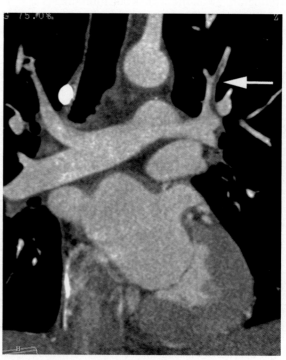

Fig. 15.5 Triple rule-out (TRO) CT angiogram of a 40-year-old man with chest pain and tachycardia. TRO demonstrates left upper-lobe pulmonary embolus extending into an apical segmental branch of the left pulmonary artery (*arrows*). Coronary arteries and aorta were normal. **(A)** Sagittal slab maximum intensity projection (MIP). **(B)** Coronal slab MIP.

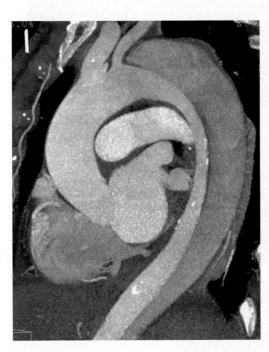

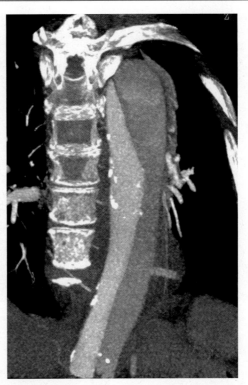

A

B

Fig. 15.6 Triple rule-out (TRO) CT angiogram of a 79-year-old woman with recent onset of vague chest discomfort. TRO demonstrates a type B aortic dissection extending from the distal aortic arch into the descending aorta. **(A)** Oblique slab maximum intensity projection (MIP) demonstrates the entire aortic arch with a dissection flap extending into the abdomen. **(B)** Coronal slab MIP again demonstrates the dissection with asymmetric enhancement of the true and false lumens.

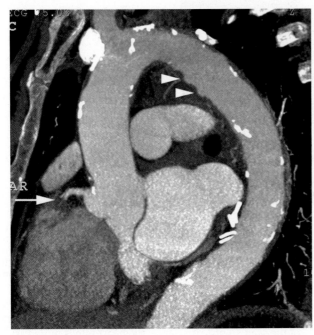

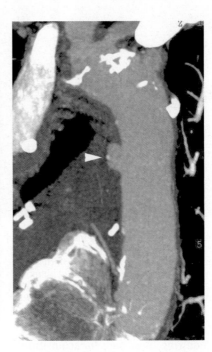

A

B

Fig. 15.7 Triple rule-out (TRO) CT angiogram of a 74-year-old man with a history of coronary disease and prior pulmonary embolism who presents with progressive chest pain over 6 months, which became acutely worse on the day of presentation. The diagnosis of pulmonary embolism, a primary clinical consideration, was excluded by CT. **(A)** Oblique slab maximum intensity projection (MIP) demonstrates an ectatic aortic arch with atherosclerotic calcification and a suggestion of two areas of aortic ulcertation (*arrowheads*). The proximal right coronary artery is visualized (*arrow*). **(B)** A different obliquity on the slab MIP demonstrates one of these ulcers that measured 10 mm wide and extended 8 mm beyond the expected contour of the aorta (*arrowhead*). Comparison with prior studies demonstrated no significant change in the appearance of the aortic ulcers. (*Continued on page 390*)

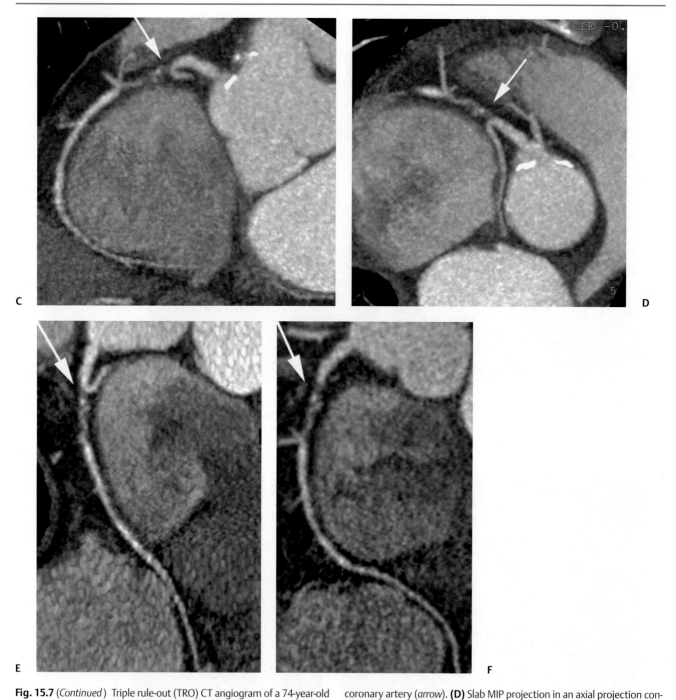

Fig. 15.7 (*Continued*) Triple rule-out (TRO) CT angiogram of a 74-year-old man with a history of coronary disease and prior pulmonary embolism who presents with progressive chest pain over 6 months, which became acutely worse on the day of presentation. The diagnosis of pulmonary embolism, a primary clinical consideration, was excluded by CT. **(C)** Slab MIP projection in a left anterior oblique projection demonstrates a high-grade stenosis or possible proximal occlusion in the proximal right coronary artery (*arrow*). **(D)** Slab MIP projection in an axial projection confirms the high-grade stenosis or possible proximal occlusion in the proximal right coronary artery (*arrow*). **(E,F)** Curved MIP images of the right coronary artery confirm the lesion in the proximal right coronary artery (*arrows*). The presence of ischemia in the inferior wall and inferoseptum was confirmed by stress testing.

with additional contrast material (**Fig. 15.8** demonstrates a carotid + TRO study requiring 20 seconds for acquisition).

Different centers use different approaches to the directionality used for scanning of TRO studies. If the patient is unable to told his or her breath for the full scan, it is best to scan from caudal to cranial so that the heart is imaged before the patient begins to breath. The cranial-to-caudal scan direction used in my protocol introduces an additional

5 seconds between the breath-hold and the cardiac portion of the scan. In my experience, the heart rate is more variable when the patient first takes a breath and tends to plateau at a rate slightly below the baseline level 5 to 15 seconds after the patient takes a breath. For most patients who have no trouble holding their breath, scanning in a cranial-to-caudal direction affords better coronary image quality by imaging the heart during this respiratory-induced plateau of the

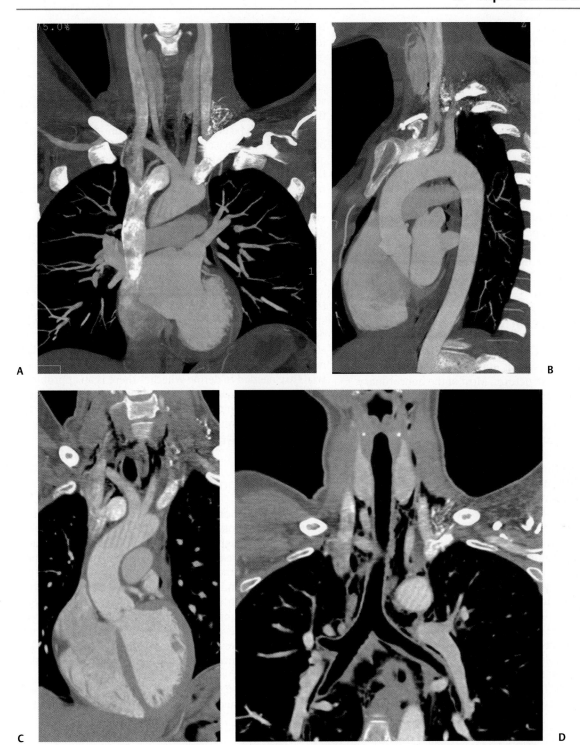

Fig. 15.8 Triple rule-out (TRO) CT angiogram of the neck and chest in a 24-year-old woman with a history of Marfan syndrome who presented with acute onset of chest pain radiating into the neck. Clinical suspicion was high for aortic dissection with possible extension into coronary arteries or into the great arteries in the neck. This scan was obtained with prospective electrocardiographic gating using 120 mL of iodinated contrast. The first phase of the injection was increased to 80 mL of contrast; the second phase of the injection was increased to 40 mL of contrast mixed with 40 mL of saline to compensate for the increased scan time to include the carotid arteries. **(A)** Coronal slab maximum intensity projection (MIP) demonstrates enhancement of the aorta and pulmonary arteries as well as the great vessels extending from the arch with no dissection. **(B)** Oblique slab MIP demonstrates a normal aortic arch and descending thoracic aorta. **(C)** Oblique coronal slab MIP demonstrates a normal left ventricular outflow tract extending into the proximal aortic arch. However, there is air within the tissues of the neck surrounding the great vessels. **(D)** Coronal slab MIP through the trachea demonstrates extensive emphasematous changes in the mediastinum. On further questioning, the patient complained of an episode of intense coughing the previous night just before the symptoms began. The mediastinal air was believed to represent the cause of symptoms and likely related to a ruptured pulmonary bleb (never seen). The patient recovered without any further interventional therapy.

heart rate. Furthermore, because contrast material must pass through the pulmonary arterial tree before it enters the coronary arteries, optimal enhancement in the pulmonary circulation is achieved before optimal coronary arterial enhancement. A scan performed in the cranial-to-caudal direction can be started a few seconds earlier than a scan performed in the caudal-to-cranial direction and can take advantage of the earlier enhancement in the pulmonary circulation to reduce the overall contrast load.

Timing of contrast injection and image acquisition is a critical component of the study. When the scan is timed to begin 5 seconds after contrast first appears in the left atrium, image acquisition corresponds to the "peak plateau" of contrast enhancement in the coronary circulation. The entire TRO study can be performed with 100 mL of contrast material with current 64-slice scanners. Even faster scan times with shorter injections can be achieved with newer CT systems using 256- or 320-slice detectors.

◆ Image Interpretation

Interpretation of TRO-CT studies includes interpretation of the coronary arteries as well as interpretation of other vascular and nonvascular structures. Most of the noncoronary structures are interpreted with axial 3- to 5-mm-thick images. Thinner sections may be obtained when needed for further evaluation of abnormalities detected on the 3- to 5-mm sections. For patients without substantial coronary disease, I prefer to evaluate the coronary arteries with a combination of the thin-section 0.6- to 0.8-mm axial images and 5-mm slab maximum intensity projection (MIP) reconstructions (**Figs. 15.2** and **15.3**). Slab MIP images are reconstructed in real time during the interpretation session so that no additional technologist effort is required. It is important to be certain that each segment of each coronary artery is evaluated in multiple projections by rotating the slab MIP images on a workstation. The aorta and pulmonary arteries are evaluated with the same viewing tools used for the coronary circulation (**Figs. 15.4, 15.5,** and **15.6**). For more complicated cases that have vascular calcifications or complex plaque, vessel-tracking software is useful to create curved MIP views that facilitate visualization of the coronary arteries in multiple planes (**Fig. 15.7**).

For cases scanned with a conventional helical acquisition, multiphase reconstructions are obtained at 10% increments throughout the cardiac cycle. Cardiac wall motion is evaluated

on a workstation in standard echocardiographic projections, including a four-chamber view, a three-chamber view, a two-chamber view, and a short-axis view. Any abnormality of regional wall motion should be correlated with the corresponding vessel in the cCTA to search for or confirm a stenosis. Identification of a wall motion abnormality can confirm that a coronary artery lesion is functionally significant.

In a patient who does not have a high pre-test likelihood of obstructive coronary disease, a normal cCTA serves to obviate any further need for a diagnostic coronary workup.[61] In the practice at my institution, the diagnosis of ACS is effectively "ruled out" by a TRO-CT that demonstrates normal coronary arteries or no more than minimal coronary disease (<25% stenosis). When there is more than minimal disease, further cardiac workup may be appropriate. Although both calcified and noncalcified plaque may be associated with ACS, mixed calcifying and noncalcifying plaques with a predominantly noncalcifying component are better correlated with ACS.[62] One recent study suggests that positive vascular remodeling, low plaque density, and spotty calcification in coronary plaque are associated with ACS.[63] Unfortunately, the anatomic information provided by cCTA in the presence of substantial coronary disease might not be definitive for the functional diagnosis of ACS. Clinical trials are needed to define whether there is an appropriate appearance of coronary plaque or degree of coronary stenosis that can definitively include or exclude ACS. In the future, CT perfusion will be combined with cCTA to provide a more accurate diagnostic tool for evaluation of ACS.

◆ Conclusion

TRO-CT examination can be a powerful tool for evaluation and triage of patients presenting with low to moderate risk of ACS in whom diagnostic catheterization is not indicated. However, compared with most CT studies that can be performed by the technologist by simple protocol, TRO-CT studies require more individualized attention. Careful attention to patient selection, patient preparation, injection technique, and scanning technique will result in high-quality TRO-CT examinations to evaluate the aorta, coronary circulation, pulmonary arteries, and adjacent intrathoracic pathology. Compared with conventional management of acute chest pain in the ED, appropriate application of TRO-CT can reduce (1) time for patient triage, (2) the number of required diagnostic tests, (3) ED costs, and (4) radiation exposure to the patient.

References

1. Pitts SR, Niska RW, Xu J, Burt CW. National Hospital Ambulatory Medical Care Survey: 2006 emergency department summary. Natl Health Stat Report. 2008;(7):1–38

2. Pope JH, Selker HP. Acute coronary syndromes in the emergency department: diagnostic characteristics, tests, and challenges. Cardiol Clin. 2005;23(4):423–451, v–vi

3. Pope JH, Aufderheide TP, Ruthazer R, et al. Missed diagnoses of acute cardiac ischemia in the emergency department. N Engl J Med. 2000; 342(16):1163–1170

4. Christenson J, Innes G, McKnight D, et al. Safety and efficiency of emergency department assessment of chest discomfort. CMAJ. 2004;170(12):1803–1807

5. Schull MJ, Vermeulen MJ, Stukel TA. The risk of missed diagnosis of acute myocardial infarction associated with emergency department volume. Ann Emerg Med. 2006;48(6):647–655

6. Rusnak RA, Stair TO, Hansen K, Fastow JS. Litigation against the emergency physician: common features in cases of missed myocardial infarction. Ann Emerg Med. 1989;18(10):1029–1034

7. Karcz A, Korn R, Burke MC, et al. Malpractice claims against emergency physicians in Massachusetts: 1975-1993. Am J Emerg Med. 1996;14(4):341–345

8. Katz DA, Williams GC, Brown RL, et al. Emergency physicians' fear of malpractice in evaluating patients with possible acute cardiac ischemia. Ann Emerg Med. 2005;46(6):525–533

9. Storrow AB, Gibler WB. Chest pain centers: diagnosis of acute coronary syndromes. Ann Emerg Med. 2000;35(5):449–461

10. Meijer AB, O YL, Geleijns J, Kroft LJ. Meta-analysis of 40- and 64-MDCT angiography for assessing coronary artery stenosis. AJR Am J Roentgenol. 2008;191(6):1667–1675

11. Marano R, De Cobelli F, Floriani I, et al; NIMISCAD Study Group. Italian multicenter, prospective study to evaluate the negative predictive value of 16- and 64-slice MDCT imaging in patients scheduled for coronary angiography (NIMISCAD-Non Invasive Multicenter Italian Study for Coronary Artery Disease). Eur Radiol. 2009;19(5):1114–1123

12. Hamon M, Morello R, Riddell JW, Hamon M. Coronary arteries: diagnostic performance of 16- versus 64-section spiral CT compared with invasive coronary angiography—meta-analysis. Radiology. 2007;245(3):720–731

13. Gallagher MJ, Raff GL. Use of multislice CT for the evaluation of emergency room patients with chest pain: the so-called "triple rule-out". Catheter Cardiovasc Interv. 2008;71(1):92–99

14. Thomas J, Rideau AM, Paulson EK, Bisset GS III. Emergency department imaging: current practice. J Am Coll Radiol. 2008;5(7):811–816, e2

15. Budoff MJ, Dowe D, Jollis JG, et al. Diagnostic performance of 64-multidetector row coronary computed tomographic angiography for evaluation of coronary artery stenosis in individuals without known coronary artery disease: results from the prospective multicenter ACCURACY (Assessment by Coronary Computed Tomographic Angiography of Individuals Undergoing Invasive Coronary Angiography) trial. J Am Coll Cardiol. 2008;52(21):1724–1732

16. Miller JM, Rochitte CE, Dewey M, et al. Diagnostic performance of coronary angiography by 64-row CT. N Engl J Med. 2008;359(22):2324–2336

17. Khare RK, Powell ES, Venkatesh AK, Courtney DM. Diagnostic uncertainty and costs associated with current emergency department evaluation of low risk chest pain. Crit Pathw Cardiol. 2008;7(3):191–196

18. Gallagher MJ, Ross MA, Raff GL, Goldstein JA, O'Neill WW, O'Neil B. The diagnostic accuracy of 64-slice computed tomography coronary angiography compared with stress nuclear imaging in emergency department low-risk chest pain patients. Ann Emerg Med. 2007;49(2):125–136

19. Rubinshtein R, Halon DA, Gaspar T, et al. Usefulness of 64-slice cardiac computed tomographic angiography for diagnosing acute coronary syndromes and predicting clinical outcome in emergency department patients with chest pain of uncertain origin. Circulation. 2007;115(13):1762–1768

20. Hollander JE, Chang AM, Shofer FS, McCusker CM, Baxt WG, Litt HI. Coronary computed tomographic angiography for rapid discharge of low-risk patients with potential acute coronary syndromes. Ann Emerg Med. 2009;53(3):295–304

21. Chang SA, Choi SI, Choi EK, et al. Usefulness of 64-slice multidetector computed tomography as an initial diagnostic approach in patients with acute chest pain. Am Heart J. 2008;156(2):375–383

22. Khare RK, Courtney DM, Powell ES, Venkatesh AK, Lee TA. Sixty-four-slice computed tomography of the coronary arteries: cost-effectiveness analysis of patients presenting to the emergency department with low-risk chest pain. Acad Emerg Med. 2008;15(7):623–632

23. Chang AM, Shofer FS, Weiner MG, et al. Actual financial comparison of four strategies to evaluate patients with potential acute coronary syndromes. Acad Emerg Med. 2008;15(7):649–655

24. Takakuwa KM, Halpern EJ. Evaluation of a "triple rule-out" coronary CT angiography protocol: use of 64-Section CT in low-to-moderate risk emergency department patients suspected of having acute coronary syndrome. Radiology. 2008;248(2):438–446

25. Ladapo JA, Hoffmann U, Bamberg F, et al. Cost-effectiveness of coronary MDCT in the triage of patients with acute chest pain. AJR Am J Roentgenol. 2008;191(2):455–463

26. Goldstein JA, Gallagher MJ, O'Neill WW, Ross MA, O'Neil BJ, Raff GL. A randomized controlled trial of multi-slice coronary computed tomography for evaluation of acute chest pain. J Am Coll Cardiol. 2007;49(8):863–871

27. Wexler L, Brundage B, Crouse J, et al; Writing Group. Coronary artery calcification: pathophysiology, epidemiology, imaging methods, and clinical implications. A statement for health professionals from the American Heart Association. Circulation. 1996;94(5):1175–1192

28. Hecht HS, Bhatti T. How much calcium is too much calcium for coronary computerized tomographic angiography? J Cardiovasc Comput Tomogr. 2008;2(3):183–187

29. Fraker TD Jr, Fihn SD, Gibbons RJ, et al; 2002 Chronic Stable Angina Writing Committee; American College of Cardiology; American Heart Association. 2007 chronic angina focused update of the ACC/AHA 2002 guidelines for the management of patients with chronic stable angina: a report of the American College of Cardiology/American Heart Association Task Force on Practice Guidelines Writing Group to develop the focused update of the 2002 guidelines for the management of patients with chronic stable angina. J Am Coll Cardiol. 2007;50(23):2264–2274

30. Han JH, Lindsell CJ, Storrow AB, et al; EMCREG i*trACS Investigators. The role of cardiac risk factor burden in diagnosing acute coronary syndromes in the emergency department setting. Ann Emerg Med. 2007;49(2):145–152, e1

31. Fenster PE, Quan SF, Hanson CD, Coaker LA. Suppression of ventricular ectopy with intravenous metoprolol in patients with chronic obstructive pulmonary disease. Crit Care Med. 1984;12(1):29–32

32. Quan SF, Fenster PE, Hanson CD, Coaker LA, Basista MP. Suppression of atrial ectopy with intravenous metoprolol in chronic obstructive pulmonary disease patients. J Clin Pharmacol. 1983;23(8-9):341–347

33. Steigner ML, Otero HJ, Cai T, et al. Narrowing the phase window width in prospectively ECG-gated single heart beat 320-detector row coronary CT angiography. Int J Cardiovasc Imaging. 2009;25(1):85–90

34. Lange RA, Hillis LD. Cardiovascular complications of cocaine use. N Engl J Med. 2001;345(5):351–358

35. Dattilo PB, Hailpern SM, Fearon K, Sohal D, Nordin C. Beta-blockers are associated with reduced risk of myocardial infarction after cocaine use. Ann Emerg Med. 2008;51(2):117–125

36. Takakuwa KM, Halpern EJ, Gingold EL, Levin DC, Shofer FS. Radiation dose in a "triple rule-out" coronary CT angiography protocol of emergency department patients using 64-MDCT: the impact of ECG-based tube current modulation on age, sex, and body mass index. AJR Am J Roentgenol. 2009;192(4):866–872

37. Hirai N, Horiguchi J, Fujioka C, et al. Prospective versus retrospective ECG-gated 64-detector coronary CT angiography: assessment of image quality, stenosis, and radiation dose. Radiology. 2008;248(2):424–430

38. Shuman WP, Branch KR, May JM, et al. Prospective versus retrospective ECG gating for 64-detector CT of the coronary arteries: comparison of image quality and patient radiation dose. Radiology. 2008;248(2):431–437

39. Brenner DJ, Hall EJ. Computed tomography—an increasing source of radiation exposure. N Engl J Med. 2007;357(22):2277–2284

40. Einstein AJ, Henzlova MJ, Rajagopalan S. Estimating risk of cancer associated with radiation exposure from 64-slice computed tomography coronary angiography. JAMA. 2007;298(3):317–323

41. Thompson RC, Cullom SJ. Issues regarding radiation dosage of cardiac nuclear and radiography procedures. J Nucl Cardiol. 2006;13(1):19–23

42. Halpern EJ, Levin DC, Zhang S. Comparison of image quality and arterial enhancement with a dedicated coronary CTA protocol versus a triple rule-out coronary CTA protocol. Proceedings of the 94th Annual Meeting of the Radiological Society of North America. Chicago, November 2008

43. Ferencik M, Nomura CH, Maurovich-Horvat P, et al. Quantitative parameters of image quality in 64-slice computed tomography angiography of the coronary arteries. Eur J Radiol. 2006;57(3):373–379

44. Dewey M, Hoffmann H, Hamm B. Multislice CT coronary angiography: effect of sublingual nitroglycerine on the diameter of coronary arteries. Rofo. 2006;178(6):600–604

45. Chun EJ, Lee W, Choi YH, et al. Effects of nitroglycerin on the diagnostic accuracy of electrocardiogram-gated coronary computed tomography angiography. J Comput Assist Tomogr. 2008;32(1):86–92

46. Wittram C, Yoo AJ. Transient interruption of contrast on CT pulmonary angiography: proof of mechanism. J Thorac Imaging. 2007;22(2):125–129

47. Oser RF, Zuckerman DA, Gutierrez FR, Brink JA. Anatomic distribution of pulmonary emboli at pulmonary angiography: implications for cross-sectional imaging. Radiology. 1996;199(1):31–35

48. Remy-Jardin M, Remy J. Spiral CT angiography of the pulmonary circulation. Radiology. 1999;212(3):615–636

49. Washington L, Goodman LR, Gonyo MB. CT for thromboembolic disease. Radiol Clin North Am. 2002;40(4):751–771

50. Wittram C. How I do it: CT pulmonary angiography. AJR Am J Roentgenol. 2007;188(5):1255–1261

51. Hargaden GC, Kavanagh EC, Fitzpatrick P, Murray JG. Diagnosis of pulmonary emboli and image quality at CT pulmonary angiography: influence of imaging direction with multidetector CT. Clin Radiol. 2006;61(7):600–603

52. Cademartiri F, Mollet NR, Lemos PA, et al. Higher intracoronary attenuation improves diagnostic accuracy in MDCT coronary angiography. AJR Am J Roentgenol. 2006;187(4):W430-3

53. Rist C, Nikolaou K, Kirchin MA, et al. Contrast bolus optimization for cardiac 16-slice computed tomography: comparison of contrast medium formulations containing 300 and 400 milligrams of iodine per milliliter. Invest Radiol. 2006;41(5):460–467

54. Rist C, Becker CR, Kirchin MA, et al. Optimization of cardiac MSCT contrast injection protocols: dependency of the main bolus contrast density on test bolus parameters and patients' body weight. Acad Radiol. 2008;15(1):49–57

55. Dodd JD, Kalva S, Pena A, et al. Emergency cardiac CT for suspected acute coronary syndrome: qualitative and quantitative assessment of coronary, pulmonary, and aortic image quality. AJR Am J Roentgenol. 2008;191(3):870–877

56. Fleischmann D, Rubin GD, Bankier AA, Hittmair K. Improved uniformity of aortic enhancement with customized contrast medium injection protocols at CT angiography. Radiology. 2000;214(2):363–371

57. Cademartiri F, Mollet NR, van der Lugt A, et al. Intravenous contrast material administration at helical 16-detector row CT coronary angiography: effect of iodine concentration on vascular attenuation. Radiology. 2005;236(2):661–665

58. Vrachliotis TG, Bis KG, Haidary A, et al. Atypical chest pain: coronary, aortic, and pulmonary vasculature enhancement at biphasic single-injection 64-section CT angiography. Radiology. 2007;243(2):368–376

59. Haidary A, Bis K, Vrachliotis T, Vrachiolitis T, Kosuri R, Balasubramaniam M. Enhancement performance of a 64-slice triple rule-out protocol vs 16-slice and 10-slice multidetector CT-angiography protocols for evaluation of aortic and pulmonary vasculature. J Comput Assist Tomogr. 2007;31(6):917–923

60. Litmanovich D, Litmanovitch D, Zamboni GA, et al. ECG-gated chest CT angiography with 64-MDCT and tri-phasic IV contrast administration regimen in patients with acute non-specific chest pain. Eur Radiol. 2008;18(2):308–317

61. Achenbach S. Computed tomography coronary angiography. J Am Coll Cardiol. 2006;48(10):1919–1928

61. Feuchtner G, Postel T, Weidinger F, et al. Is there a relation between non-calcifying coronary plaques and acute coronary syndromes? A retrospective study using multislice computed tomography. Cardiology. 2008;110(4):241–248

63. Motoyama S, Kondo T, Sarai M, et al. Multislice computed tomographic characteristics of coronary lesions in acute coronary syndromes. J Am Coll Cardiol. 2007;50(4):319–326

16

Innovations in Cardiac CT: Slice Wars, Dual Energy, Myocardial Perfusion, and Targeted Contrast Agents

Jacob Sosna, Galit Aviram, and Ethan J. Halpern

The field of cardiac imaging has advanced rapidly over the past few decades. The latest innovations in technology provide better image quality with noninvasive techniques using lower doses of radiation compared with techniques used in the recent past. Innovations from the past two decades provide the basis for most of this text. New innovations in the coming years will expand further the clinical applications of cardiac CT to provide a comprehensive anatomic and functional examination of the heart. This chapter reviews several key innovations in CT technology as they are applied to cardiac imaging.

◆ More Slices, More Resolution, and Flat-Panel CT

To increase z-axis coverage, new scanners have been developed with larger detector panels that can image the entire heart at once. Extended z-axis of up to 16 cm of coverage has several potential advantages for cardiac imaging. Because the entire heart can be imaged at one time, coronary CT angiography (CTA) may be obtained in a single heartbeat, thus minimizing the impact of an arrhythmia on scan quality as well as reducing radiation. With sufficient temporal resolution, coronary CTA with extended z-axis coverage might be possible without electrocardiographic (ECG) gating. Because the entire scan can be acquired with a single axial scan using prospective ECG triggering, extended z-axis detectors should eliminate additional radiation exposure related to the overlap between the sequential axial acquisitions that would be required when using a scanner with a shorter z-axis coverage. Furthermore, simultaneous imaging of the entire heart during the same arterial phase of contrast arrival should facilitate more accurate perfusion CT imaging of the myocardium.

Scanners with 128 rows of detectors and a z-axis wobble that acquires 256 slices are commercially available. These scanners have a detector element that is 8 cm in the z-axis and can acquire a complete coronary CTA in two steps with prospective ECG gating (**Fig. 16.1**). Although the detector element is 8 cm long, the actual coverage in two steps is reduced by 2 to 3 cm (less than the 16-cm coverage that might be expected) because of the overlap required by the cone beam reconstruction algorithm. A recent study estimated an effective dose of 3.2 mSv for prospective ECG gating with a 256-slice scanner with 80-mm detector coverage.[1] A phantom model study suggests that scanners with 256 detector rows may provide cardiac imaging during a single heartbeat without ECG gating, thereby eliminating artifacts related to ectopy and variability of heart rate.[2] This nongated approach has yet to be validated in an in vivo clinical trial.

One vendor has introduced a 320-detector row scanner (16cm detector) capable of imaging the entire coronary circulation in a single axial acquisition (**Fig. 16.2**).[3] Coronary imaging with this scanner has been described as providing excellent diagnostic quality with axial scanning using both ECG-gated and nongated modes.[4] The ability to perform coronary CTA during a single cardiac cycle should result in more reliable imaging of the coronary circulation in patients with cardiac arrhythmias. Furthermore, the injected contrast volume can be minimized as long as the injection is optimized to ensure optimal opacification of the entire coronary tree during the single cardiac cycle used for imaging.

CT evaluation of small coronary arteries and stents is currently limited by scan resolution. Although conventional coronary angiography has a resolution of about 0.2 mm, the detector elements in multislice CT provide a z-axis slice thickness of no less than 0.5 to 0.75 mm. In-plane resolution for conventional scanners is limited by the scanner sampling rate (number of samples per rotation) and by pixel size, which is typically on the order of 0.5 mm (using a 250-mm field of view with a 500 × 500 pixel image). Coronary vessels are 3 to 4 mm wide, corresponding to six to eight pixels in current technology. Thus, a difference in stenosis of between 60 and 80% may correspond to a difference of only a single pixel.

Vendors have increased the in-plane resolution on commercial systems based on multislice detectors by increasing sampling rates per gantry rotation for newer systems. This sampling rate may be limited by the afterglow time of detector material or by the speed of the electronics that must transmit the data from the detector to the processing computer. Flat-panel detector technology currently under development has the potential to provide superior resolution in all planes compared with current multiple-row detector technology. In vivo implementation of this flat-plate technology, however, is limited by the extremely rapid sampling rates that are required for flat plate technology.

A prototype flat-panel unit that has been used to image explanted human heart specimens provides an isotropic

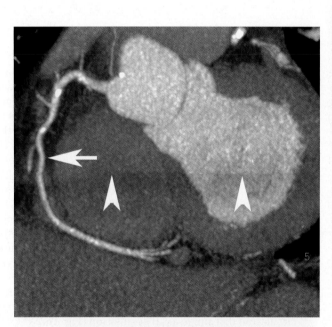

A

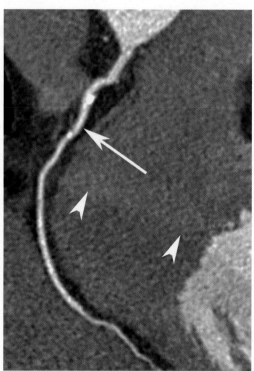

B

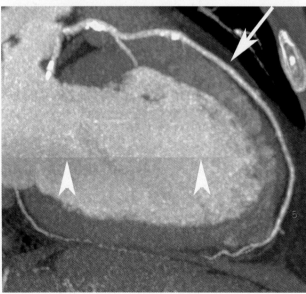

C

Fig. 16.1 Coronary CT angiography (CTA) acquisition in two steps with prospective electrocardiographic (ECG) gating. The step artifact is most visible on images that are rendered in a plane perpendicular to the z-axis. **(A)** Slab maximum intensity projection (MIP) left anterior oblique projection of the right coronary artery (RCA) (*arrow*). The demarcation between the two steps is visible (*arrowheads*) but does not interfere with interpretation as long as the vessel is well aligned in the two steps. **(B)** Curved multiplanar reformat (MPR) of the RCA (*arrow*) based on vessel tracking. The demarcation between the two steps is present but not as visible (*arrowheads*). **(C)** Slab MIP right anterior oblique projection of the left anterior descending artery (LAD) (*arrow*). The demarcation between the two steps is again visible (*arrowheads*), but this does not interfere with evaluation of the LAD.

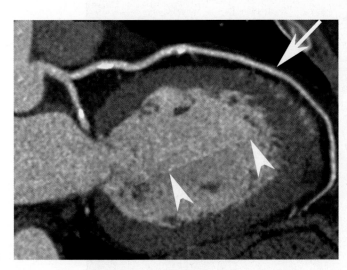

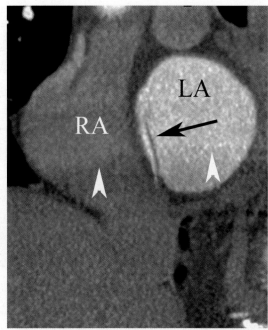

D

E

Fig. 16.1 (*Continued*) **(D)** Curved MPR of the LAD (*arrow*) based on vessel tracking. The demarcation between the two steps is only visible within the left ventricular cavity (*arrowheads*) and is less obvious than in part C. **(E)** Oblique sagittal view through the right atrium (RA) and left atrium (LA) in the same patient demonstrates that the septum primum (*arrow*) is not fused to the septum secundum, resulting in a patent foramen ovale. The step artifact (*arrowheads*) is present but less well defined in parts (B), (D), and (E) because the image is rendered in a plane that is oblique to the step artifact. A smoothing filter can be used to remove this "step artifact," but the edges of the coronary arteries may not be as sharply defined in the smoothed image.

voxel with 0.25-mm resolution.[5] Another study using flat-panel technology imaged an excised pig heart with visualization of coronary arteries down to fifth-degree branches.[6] The superior resolution of flat-panel technology can minimize blooming artifact associated with vascular calcifications and stents, thereby providing improved visualization of the vessel lumen.[7] A recent study demonstrated the application of flat-panel imaging to the coronary arteries in 25 isolated hearts removed during autopsy.[8] This study suggests that flat-panel volume CTA may have sufficient resolution to detect reliably the lipid pool within coronary plaque. Temporal resolution of these prototype systems, as well as image artifacts, currently limits their clinical application, but these are likely to improve in the near future.

◆ Dual-Energy and Spectral CT

Various tissues demonstrate differences in radiographic attenuation based on a range of Compton and photoelectric effects at different energies. Multienergy techniques exploit these differences to provide improved image quality or additional tissue characterization.[9] Although dual-energy CT applications were described more than 30 years ago,[10] advances in technology have only recently made these applications a reality for cardiac imaging. Dual-energy CT refers to the synchronous acquisition of CT data at two different ranges within the spectrum of roentgen tube energies (**Fig. 16.3**). Perhaps the most important application of dual-energy imaging is for the improved visualization of iodine. The radiographic attenuation of iodine is much greater at 80 kVp compared with 140 kVp, but the relative change in radiographic attenuation as a function of kVp is different for iodine compared with water or calcium. Based on these differences in relative attenuation at low and high kVp, dual-energy data may be mathematically processed with material decomposition algorithms that enhance or suppress iodine relative to water or tissue or iodine relative to bone (**Fig. 16.4**).[11-13] Material decomposition may be used to identify tissues that would be very difficult to distinguish on conventional single-energy scan (**Fig. 16.5**). As an extension of this process, dual-energy post-processing may be used to provide "iodine maps" and quantitative estimates of iodine concentration in tissue (**Fig. 16.6**). Further processing of dual-energy CT images may be performed to provide "monoenergetic" images that are created to simulate the image that would be obtained using a single keV radiographic source. Such monochromatic images may be useful to eliminate artifacts related to beam hardening.

Several options for acquiring dual-energy CT data for cardiac imaging have been implemented. The first commercially available dual-energy system was based on a dual-source CT scanner with two different roentgen tubes and two sets of detectors. Although the dual-source design was initially implemented to improve temporal resolution at a

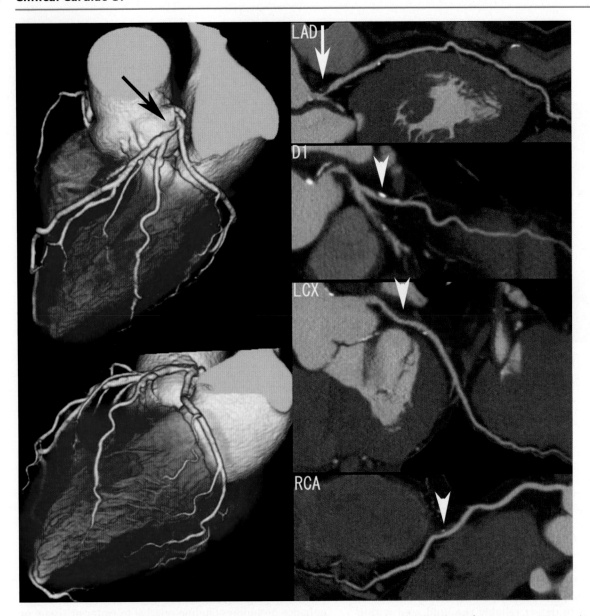

Fig. 16.2 Single heartbeat acquisition of the entire coronary circulation. The two panels on the left demonstrate volumetric renderings of the coronary circulation with the underlying cardiac chambers. A focal stenosis is present in the proximal left anterior descending artery (*black arrow*). The four right-sided panels demonstrate curved maximum intensity projection renderings of the left anterior descending artery (LAD), first diagonal branch (D1), left circumflex artery (LCX), and right coronary artery (RCA). Moderate to severe narrowing in the proximal LAD is clearly defined (*arrow*), as is the presence of calcified plaque in D1 (*arrowhead*) and noncalcified plaque in the LCX and RCA (*arrowheads*). Note that there is no "step artifact" in this one-step acquisition. Acquisition of the entire scan within a single cardiac cycle limits the negative impact of cardiac arrhythmia. (Figure supplied courtesy of Toshiba Medical Systems, Japan.)

single kVp, the two roentgen tubes may be operated at different kVp settings to obtain dual-energy information. An interesting advantage of this approach is the ability to process information selectively from either one or both radiographic sources to optimize temporal resolution versus energy-specific information (see below for application to myocardial perfusion imaging). A disadvantage of this approach is the slight difference in the time of acquisition for two co-registered data sets based on the additional quarter revolution of the gantry between the two sources.

The lack of precise co-registration limits this vendor's ability to combine dual-energy raw data in "projection space" during the reconstruction phase of CT processing. Dual-energy data may still be combined in "image space" by post-processing of the images obtained from the two radiographic sources to perform material decomposition and to provide monochromatic images.[14] Clinical studies are needed to determine the relative advantages of dual-energy reconstructions in raw data projection space versus image space.

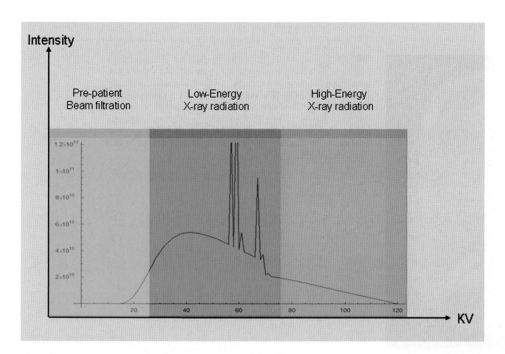

Fig. 16.3 Spectrum of radiographic energies received by a CT detector. Although a single kVp is applied across the roentgen tube to generate the roentgens for the scan, the polychromatic beam contains a spectrum of energies. Pre-patient beam filtration is used to remove low-energy photons that would contribute little information to a scan but increases patient's radiation exposure. Multienergy techniques measure the selective absorption of the radiographic beam in different portions of the spectrum. Dual-energy techniques divide the spectrum into high- and low-energy components.

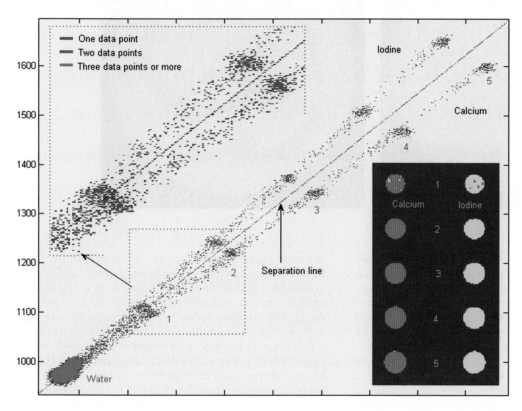

Fig. 16.4 Processing of dual-energy CT data obtained from a mixture of calcium and iodine. A graphical plot of the low-energy versus high-energy attenuation values within a region of interest on a dual-energy scan is displayed. Although the calcium and iodine may have similar CT numbers in an image that is created from the entire spectrum of the polychromatic X-ray, the CT numbers differ when the low-energy and high-energy components of the spectrum are processed independently. Because calcium and iodine differ in their absorption characteristics for photons of different energies, it is possible to distinguish pixels that contain calcium from those that contain iodine based upon a separation line in the graph.

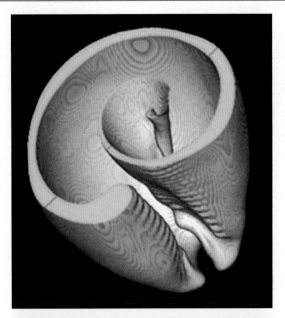

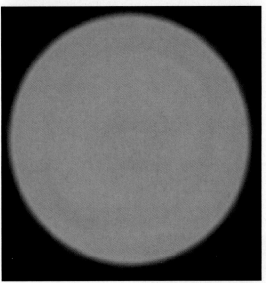

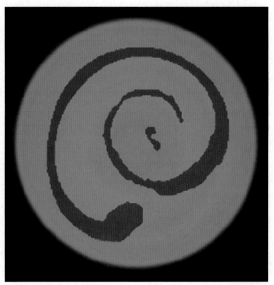

Fig. 16.5 Tissue decomposition used to distinguish a seashell from iodinated contrast material. **(A)** Volumetric rendering of a seashell imaged with a conventional single-energy technique. **(B)** Axial image from a conventional single-energy CT of the seashell submerged in iodinated contrast material. The density of the contrast solution was intentionally equalized to that of the seashell. **(C)** Spectral analysis with dual-energy CT can be used to identify the sea shell, which is defined by a color map.

A

B   C

Other methods for acquisition of dual-energy data may offer advantages in terms of improved temporal registration of the data. A second vendor recently introduced a commercial system capable of dual-energy imaging based on a single radiographic source with rapid kVp switching. A rapid sampling rate of 0.5 msec provides good co-registration of raw data acquisition at the two different energy levels. Thus, the dual-energy data from this system may be processed in either the raw data projection space or in image space.

Dual-energy scanning based on a dual-source scanner or a single-source scanner with kVp switching may require a tradeoff of temporal resolution or sampling frequency to operate in dual-energy mode. An interesting solution to this problem has been developed for the dual-source scanner that combines data from the two different energies to maintain temporal resolution for the coronary CTA. A prototype system from a third vendor provides simultaneous acquisition of dual-energy data based on a single radiographic source and a double-layered, 32-row detector panel. The "double-decker" detector acquires low- and high-energy radiographic photons simultaneously. A preponderance of low-energy photons are processed by the upper detector, which the photons encounter first. Higher-energy photons pass through to the deeper detector. This design allows simultaneous detection of both energies and should therefore provide the best co-registration for dual-energy processing.

In theory this ability to perform tissue decomposition within a CT image and to create monoenergetic images would be even better with a spectral CT scanner that would include independent measurements of roentgen absorption

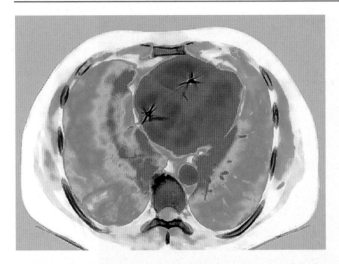

Fig. 16.6 Iodine map in tissue. Dual-energy CT can be used to define the concentration of iodine in tissues. This dual-energy section through the chest demonstrates a much higher iodine concentration within the chambers of the heart and the aorta compared with the lungs.

at multiple different energy levels (**Fig. 16.7**). This future technology may be achieved with photon-counting techniques that can separate the radiographic spectrum to various desired energy levels. In clinical practice, however, commercially available scanners use no more than two different energy levels.

Several studies have demonstrated that CT characterization of the coronary lumen,[15] calcified coronary plaque,[16] and the coronary stent lumen[17] may be improved with dual-energy imaging. Selective classification of calcification from adjacent iodinated contrast material in the coronary arteries has been performed using a dual-energy scanner (**Fig. 16.8**). A recent study by our group, however, failed to demonstrate improved visualization of the lumen inside a coronary stent with dual-energy imaging.[18]

◆ Myocardial Perfusion Imaging

A true comprehensive examination of the heart should include evaluation of myocardial perfusion in addition to coronary anatomy. Coronary CTA is highly sensitive for the presence of stenosis with greater than 50% diameter reduction, but the presence of stenosis does not necessarily imply myocardial ischemia. The extent of inducible ischemia associated with coronary disease is predictive of the risk of a coronary event as well as the expected benefit of revascularization compared with medical therapy.[19,20] In the ideal study, evaluation of myocardial perfusion obtained during coronary CTA could be used in place of a nuclear stress test to establish whether a stenosis is responsible for clinical symptoms. This ideal study would take advantage of the complementary nature of the anatomic and functional information, both of which are present in a coronary CTA study with the added benefit of reduced radiation.

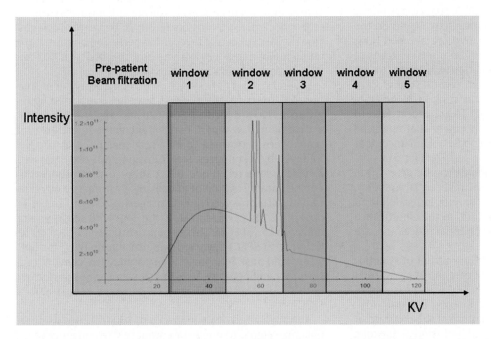

Fig. 16.7 Spectrum of radiographic energies received by a CT detector. Although a single kVp is applied across the roentgen tube to generate the roentgens for the scan, the polychromatic beam contains a spectrum of energies. Photon counting techniques classify the photons that are detected into multiple bins, corresponding to different energy levels. The ability to obtain independent measurements of tissue absorption at multiple different energies should allow for improved separation of tissues based on their different absorption characteristics and for more accurate tissue decomposition.

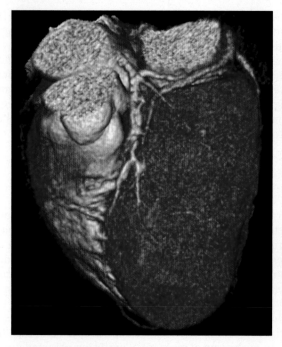
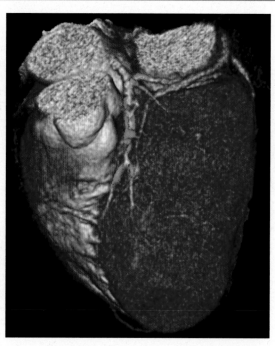

A   B

Fig. 16.8 Identification of coronary calcium with dual-energy CT. **(A)** Surface-rendered image in the left anterior oblique projection demonstrates the bifurcation of the left main coronary artery into the left anterior descending and circumflex arteries. Vascular calcification cannot be distinguished from contrast-enhanced lumen in the standard surface volumetric rendering technique. However, even when other rendering techniques are used, the CT attenuation of vascular calcification may be similar to that of the contrast-enhanced lumen, limiting the assessment of vascular stenosis. **(B)** Surface rendering of the same patient with color highlighting of vascular calcification based on a dual-energy CT acquisition. Calcified plaque may be distinguished from enhanced vessel lumen based on differential attenuation of different radiographic energies by calcium and radiographic contrast material.

Various methods have been proposed to perform myocardial perfusion imaging with CTA. In theory, a dynamic CT evaluation of myocardial enhancement would be the most accurate method to quantify myocardial blood flow, but dynamic acquisition would require multiple scans of the heart with a relatively high radiation exposure to measure changes in iodine concentration. Several studies have used a two-phase examination consisting of blood-pool imaging during the arterial phase of CTA and repeat delayed imaging to demonstrate late enhancement that might be associated with infarction.[21] The blood-pool enhancement during the arterial phase is used as a surrogate for true perfusion imaging, which would require a dynamic acquisition of several scans. For assessment of myocardial viability, low-dose CT late enhancement scanning is feasible and adds valuable diagnostic information on the significance of coronary stenoses before interventional procedures are performed.[22]

A Japanese group has promoted the concept of systolic–diastolic perfusion imaging for the detection of myocardial ischemia.[23] Subendocardial CT intensity was measured in both systolic and diastolic phase images. Ischemic myocardium was characterized by a pattern of subendocardial hypoperfusion at systole and normal perfusion at diastole. In a more recent study of 75 patients using a single-source 64-detector row scanner, the same group demonstrated a sensitivity of 90% and specificity of 83% for CT detection of myocardial ischemia as defined by nuclear perfusion imaging.[24] A recent study at Johns Hopkins University used a transmural perfusion ratio during adenosine stress CT (subendocardial attenuation density/subepicardial attenuation density) to detect myocardial perfusion abnormalities and demonstrated a sensitivity and specificity of 86% and 92%, respectively, in a per-patient analysis.[25]

Several studies of first-pass perfusion during adenosine-induced stress myocardial CTA have been reported by the group at Harvard Medical School using single-energy CT on a dual-source scanner. Two independent injections and scans were performed to obtain adenosine stress images followed by rest images. Stress imaging was obtained with a helical scan technique using tube-current modulation during administration of adenosine. Rest images were obtained with prospective ECG triggering. Overall radiation dose of 12.7 mSv was similar to the dose with single-photon emission CT (SPECT). These scans demonstrate good correlation with SPECT myocardial perfusion imaging for both stress and rest imaging.[26] Compared with conventional coronary angiography, stress perfusion studies performed with CT demonstrate diagnostic accuracy comparable to SPECT.[27]

Although a relatively high kVp of 100 to 120 is useful to optimize signal to noise for coronary CTA, imaging of the blood pool in the myocardium may benefit from the greater sensitivity to iodine that is obtained with lower kVp.[28] The group at Medical University of South Carolina has used a dual-source scanner with different kVp settings

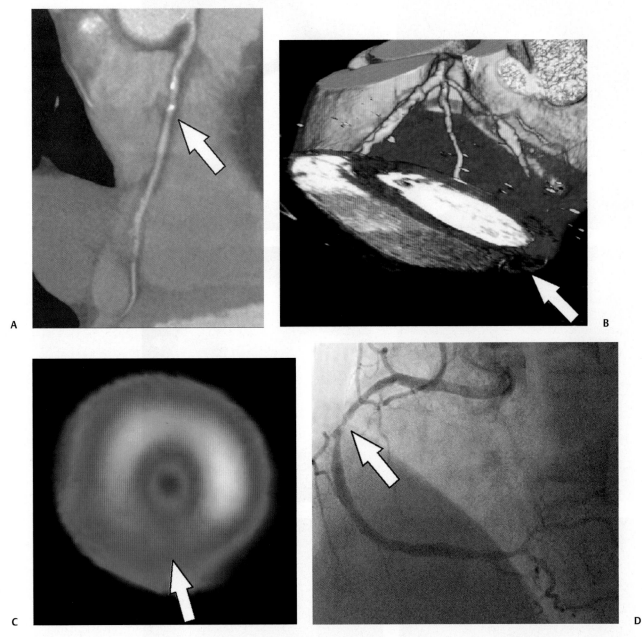

Fig. 16.9 Dual-energy CT angiography (CTA) with perfusion obtained during adenosine infusion in a patient with significant disease of the right coronary artery (RCA). The CTA and perfusion map are acquired during a single scan through the heart. **(A)** Curved maximum intensity projection image of the RCA generated from a combination of the high-energy and low-energy spectral components demonstrates calcified plaque (*arrow*) with findings suspicious for significant stenosis. **(B)** Iodine map based on the low-energy components of the dual-energy scan demonstrates inferior ischemia (*arrow*). **(C)** Conventional single-photon emission CT stress study confirms the presence of inferior ischemia. **(D)** Conventional arteriogram demonstrates a high-grade lesion in the RCA, corresponding to the findings on CTA. (Figure supplied courtesy of Balazs Ruzsics, MD, PhD, and U. Joseph Schoepf, MD, Medical University of South Carolina.)

on the two tubes of a dual-source system to improve the sensitivity of CT perfusion imaging (**Figs. 16.9** and **16.10**). A low-kVp image is obtained from one tube to improve sensitivity for myocardial perfusion defects; a combination of high (140) and low (80) kVp data from both tubes is used to achieve better signal to noise and higher temporal resolution of the coronary arteries. The low-energy "iodine perfusion map" is displayed as a color overlay on the high-resolution coronary CTA image for this "dual-energy" display. Dual-energy iodine maps of the myocardium compared favorably with SPECT perfusion scans for the identification of myocardial blood pool deficits (sensitivity 91%, specificity 92%).[29] In a more recent study by the same group, dual-energy blood pool maps demonstrated an

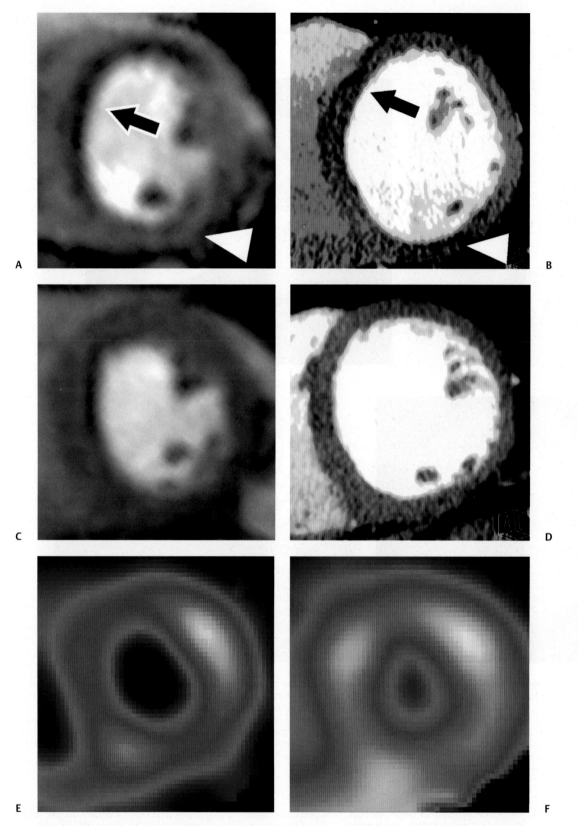

Fig. 16.10 Stress-rest dual-energy CT perfusion in a patient with anteroseptal and inferior ischemia. **(A)** Short-axis image of the left ventricle during infusion of adenosine demonstrates decreased perfusion in a large territory involving the anteroseptum and extending into the anterior wall (*arrow*). A subtle endocardial perfusion defect may be present in the inferior wall (*arrowhead*). **(B)** Iodine map of the stress image again demonstrates the anteroseptal perfusion defect (*arrow*) but more clearly identifies a perfusion deficit in the inferior wall (*arrowhead*).

(C) Short-axis image at rest demonstrates substantial normalization of the perfusion pattern. **(D)** Iodine map at rest confirms that there is no perfusion defect. **(E)** Stress single-photon emission CT (SPECT) confirms a large area of ischemia in the anteroseptal and anterior walls. **(F)** Rest SPECT images demonstrate perfusion to the ischemic areas, confirming the findings of CT perfusion. (Figure supplied courtesy of Balazs Ruzsics, MD, PhD, and U. Joseph Schoepf, MD, Medical University of South Carolina.)

overall sensitivity and specificity of 92% and 93%, respectively, for SPECT perfusion defects, with a sensitivity of 88% and specificity of 89% for reversible SPECT defects.[30] Of note, reversible SPECT perfusion defects were detected on dual-energy iodine maps without stress imaging. The authors suggest that CTA may be more sensitive to perfusion defects without stress imaging because of superior spatial resolution, a wider dynamic range for rates of myocardial perfusion, or the intrinsic vasodilatory effects of iodinated contrast.[31] Although the theoretical benefit of the dual-energy approach is obvious, a clinical trial with direct comparison of single-energy and dual-energy techniques is needed to demonstrate whether this dual-energy approach provides a true advantage over the single-energy technique used by the Harvard group.

The dual-energy technique reported above does use low kVp scanning to optimize visualization of myocardial enhancement, but it does not exploit the dual-energy acquisition to provide selective imaging of iodine or to reduce beam-hardening artifact. As described in the previous section, the information in a dual-energy acquisition may be processed with material decomposition algorithms to enhance the visualization of iodine relative to water and other soft tissues in an image. Selective iodine maps should provide optimized visualization of iodine and allow evaluation of even subtler changes in myocardial perfusion. Monoenergetic images obtained from a dual-energy data set should reduce beam-hardening artifact that can occur at the interface between the densely enhanced lumen of the left ventricle and the adjacent endocardium. Ultimately, dual-energy technology may be combined with low-dose dynamic imaging of the myocardium to quantify iodinated contrast material and blood flow in the myocardium. It is likely that the combination of stress CTA imaging with dynamic dual-energy perfusion analysis will result in further improvements in the diagnostic accuracy of CTA for detection of myocardial perfusion deficits.

◆ New Contrast Agents

Iodinated contrast agents have been used for many years in conventional CT to demonstrate the presence of blood or tissue perfusion. These agents provide excellent contrast to delineate the lumen of a patent vessel, but they are not selective for imaging the inflammatory process associated with atherosclerotic disease. Recently, macrophage-specific contrast agents have been shown to be of value in imaging metabolic processes within atherosclerotic plaque. Macrophage-enriched plaque can be selectively enhanced with iodine nanoparticles.[32] Furthermore, the intensity of CT enhancement with this macrophage-specific agent correlates with $_{18}$F-FDG uptake and with macrophage infiltration, suggesting that this type of selective enhancement may identify vulnerable plaque, which is likely to represent the culprit lesions in acute coronary syndrome.[33] Our group recently showed that the addition of dual-energy CT can improve the visualization of macrophage-specific contrast agents in a rabbit model of atherosclerosis (**Fig. 16.11**). Other potential steps in the evolution of the vulnerable plaque can be a target for specific contrast agents to be developed in the future. These include intraplaque bleeding as well as high-density lipoprotein. It is envisioned that future imaging of vulnerable plaques will be used in clinical practice to predict patients at risk and to monitor therapy and intervention.

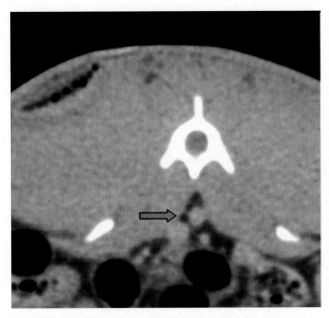
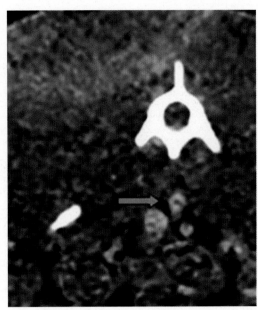

A

B

Fig. 16.11 Model of atherosclerosis imaging in the aorta of a rabbit. **(A)** Conventional CT scan of the rabbit demonstrates the aorta in cross-section (*arrow*). **(B)** Macrophage-enriched plaque is selectively enhanced with iodine nanoparticles along the wall of the aorta.

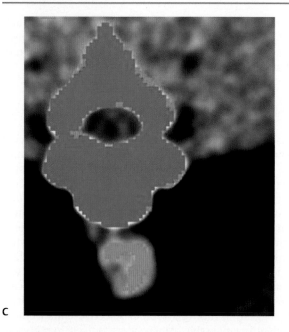

C

Fig. 16.11 (*Continued*) Model of atherosclerosis imaging in the aorta of a rabbit. **(C)** Tissue decomposition based on a dual-energy scan provides a color map of the iodine nanoparticles along the wall of the aorta, improving discrimination of the location of enhancement.

◆ Conclusion

Technical innovations in CT scanners and contrast agents have advanced rapidly over the past few decades. Image quality has improved with faster scans and lower doses of radiation. Myocardial perfusion CTA combines two complementary examinations—coronary anatomy and perfusion—to provide a more comprehensive evaluation of cardiac health, more accurate diagnosis of coronary artery disease, and improved patient risk stratification. Dual-energy techniques have the potential to characterize tissues better and to enhance the conspicuity of contrast agents used during myocardial perfusion imaging. Finally, targeted contrast agents may be useful in high-risk patients to allow more appropriate targeting of invasive therapy.

References

1. Efstathopoulos EP, Kelekis NL, Pantos I, et al. Reduction of the estimated radiation dose and associated patient risk with prospective ECG-gated 256-slice CT coronary angiography. Phys Med Biol. 2009;54(17):5209–5222

2. Mizuno N, Funabashi N, Imada M, Tsunoo T, Endo M, Komuro I. Utility of 256-slice cone beam tomography for real four-dimensional volumetric analysis without electrocardiogram gated acquisition. Int J Cardiol. 2007;120(2):262–267

3. Rybicki FJ, Otero HJ, Steigner ML, et al. Initial evaluation of coronary images from 320-detector row computed tomography. Int J Cardiovasc Imaging. 2008;24(5):535–546

4. Hein PA, Romano VC, Lembcke A, May J, Rogalla P. Initial experience with a chest pain protocol using 320-slice volume MDCT. Eur Radiol. 2009;19(5):1148–1155

5. Nikolaou K, Flohr T, Stierstorfer K, Becker CR, Reiser MF. Flat panel computed tomography of human ex vivo heart and bone specimens: initial experience. Eur Radiol. 2005;15(2):329–333

6. Knollmann F, Pfoh A. Image in cardiovascular medicine. Coronary artery imaging with flat-panel computed tomography. Circulation. 2003;107(8):1209

7. Mahnken AH, Seyfarth T, Flohr T, et al. Flat-panel detector computed tomography for the assessment of coronary artery stents: phantom study in comparison with 16-slice spiral computed tomography. Invest Radiol. 2005;40(1):8–13

8. Knollmann FD, Wieltsch A, Peters S, Mahlke A, Niederberger S, Kertesz T. Flat panel volume computed tomography of the coronary arteries. Acad Radiol. 2009;16(10):1251–1262

9. Yeh BM, Shepherd JA, Wang ZJ, Teh HS, Hartman RP, Prevrhal S. Dual-energy and low-kVp CT in the abdomen. AJR Am J Roentgenol. 2009;193(1):47–54

10. Chiro GD, Brooks RA, Kessler RM, et al. Tissue signatures with dual-energy computed tomography. Radiology. 1979;131(2):521–523

11. Johnson TR, Krauss B, Sedlmair M, et al. Material differentiation by dual energy CT: initial experience. Eur Radiol. 2007;17(6):1510–1517

12. Tran DN, Straka M, Roos JE, Napel S, Fleischmann D. Dual-energy CT discrimination of iodine and calcium: experimental results and implications for lower extremity CT angiography. Acad Radiol. 2009; 16(2): 160–171

13. Lell MM, Hinkmann F, Nkenke E, et al. Dual energy CTA of the supraaortic arteries: technical improvements with a novel dual source CT system. Eur J Radiol. 2009;October 8 (Epub ahead of print)

14. Maass C, Baer M, Kachelriess M. Image-based dual energy CT using optimized precorrection functions: a practical new approach of material decomposition in image domain. Med Phys. 2009;36(8):3818–3829

15. Boll DT, Hoffmann MH, Huber N, Bossert AS, Aschoff AJ, Fleiter TR. Spectral coronary multidetector computed tomography angiography: dual benefit by facilitating plaque characterization and enhancing lumen depiction. J Comput Assist Tomogr. 2006;30(5):804–811

16. Boll DT, Merkle EM, Paulson EK, Mirza RA, Fleiter TR. Calcified vascular plaque specimens: assessment with cardiac dual-energy multidetector CT in anthropomorphically moving heart phantom. Radiology. 2008;249(1):119–126

17. Boll DT, Merkle EM, Paulson EK, Fleiter TR. Coronary stent patency: dual-energy multidetector CT assessment in a pilot study with anthropomorphic phantom. Radiology. 2008;247(3):687–695

18. Halpern EJ, Halpern DJ, Yanof JH, et al. Is coronary stent assessment improved with spectral analysis of dual energy CT? Acad Radiol. 2009;16(10):1241–1250

19. Hachamovitch R, Hayes SW, Friedman JD, Cohen I, Berman DS. Comparison of the short-term survival benefit associated with revascularization compared with medical therapy in patients with no prior coronary artery disease undergoing stress myocardial perfusion single photon emission computed tomography. Circulation. 2003;107(23): 2900–2907

20. Hachamovitch R, Kang X, Amanullah AM, et al. Prognostic implications of myocardial perfusion single-photon emission computed tomography in the elderly. Circulation. 2009;120(22):2197–2206

21. Ko SM, Seo JB, Hong MK, et al. Myocardial enhancement pattern in patients with acute myocardial infarction on two-phase contrast-enhanced ECG-gated multidetector-row computed tomography. Clin Radiol. 2006;61(5):417–422

22. Kopp AF, Heuschmid M, Reimann A, et al. Evaluation of cardiac function and myocardial viability with 16- and 64-slice multidetector computed tomography. Eur Radiol. 2005;15(Suppl 4):D15–D20

23. Nagao M, Matsuoka H, Kawakami H, et al. Quantification of myocardial perfusion by contrast-enhanced 64-MDCT: characterization of ischemic myocardium. AJR Am J Roentgenol. 2008;191(1):19–25

24. Nagao M, Matsuoka H, Kawakami H, et al. Detection of myocardial ischemia using 64-slice MDCT. Circ J. 2009;73(5):905–911

25. George RT, Arbab-Zadeh A, Miller JM, et al. Adenosine stress 64- and 256-row detector computed tomography angiography and perfusion imaging: a pilot study evaluating the transmural extent of perfusion abnormalities to predict atherosclerosis causing myocardial ischemia. Circ Cardiovasc Imaging. 2009;2(3):174–182

26. Okada DR, Ghoshhajra BB, Blankstein R, et al. Direct comparison of rest and adenosine stress myocardial perfusion CT with rest and stress SPECT. J Nucl Cardiol. 2010;17(1):27–37

27. Blankstein R, Shturman LD, Rogers IS, et al. Adenosine-induced stress myocardial perfusion imaging using dual-source cardiac computed tomography. J Am Coll Cardiol. 2009;54(12):1072–1084

28. Gorgos A, Remy-Jardin M, Duhamel A, et al. Evaluation of peripheral pulmonary arteries at 80 kV and at 140 kV: dual-energy computed tomography assessment in 51 patients. J Comput Assist Tomogr. 2009;33(6):981–986

29. Ruzsics B, Lee H, Zwerner PL, Gebregziabher M, Costello P, Schoepf UJ. Dual-energy CT of the heart for diagnosing coronary artery stenosis and myocardial ischemia-initial experience. Eur Radiol. 2008;18(11):2414–2424

30. Ruzsics B, Schwarz F, Schoepf UJ, et al. Comparison of dual-energy computed tomography of the heart with single photon emission computed tomography for assessment of coronary artery stenosis and of the myocardial blood supply. Am J Cardiol. 2009;104(3):318–326

31. Baile EM, Paré PD, D'yachkova Y, Carere RG. Effect of contrast media on coronary vascular resistance: contrast-induced coronary vasodilation. Chest. 1999;116(4):1039–1045

32. Hyafil F, Cornily JC, Feig JE, et al. Noninvasive detection of macrophages using a nanoparticulate contrast agent for computed tomography. Nat Med. 2007;13(5):636–641

33. Hyafil F, Cornily JC, Rudd JH, Machac J, Feldman LJ, Fayad ZA. Quantification of inflammation within rabbit atherosclerotic plaques using the macrophage-specific CT contrast agent N1177: a comparison with 18F-FDG PET/CT and histology. J Nucl Med. 2009;50(6):959–965

Index

Note: Page numbers followed by *f* and *t* indicate figures and tables, respectively. Narratives for cineangiography are indicated by page numbers followed by *ca.*

Brief DVD Contents